HEALTH CARE
ECONOMICS

WILEY SERIES IN HEALTH SERVICES

Stephen J. Williams, Sc.D., Series Editor

HEALTH CARE ECONOMICS

SECOND EDITION

Paul J. Feldstein, Ph.D.

Professor
School of Public Health and Department of Economics
The University of Michigan
Ann Arbor, Michigan

A WILEY MEDICAL PUBLICATION
JOHN WILEY & SONS
New York · Chichester · Brisbane · Toronto · Singapore

Cover design: Wanda Lubelska
Production Supervisor: Audrey Pavey

Preparation of the first edition was assisted by a grant from the Robert Wood Johnson Foundation, Princeton, New Jersey. The opinions, conclusions, and proposals in the text are those of the author and do not necessarily represent the views of the Robert Wood Johnson Foundation.

Library of Congress Cataloging in Publication Data:

Feldstein, Paul J.
  Health care economics.

  (Wiley series in health services) (A Wiley medical
publication)
  Includes index.
  1. Medical economics. 2. Medical economics—United
States. I. Title. II. Series. III. Series: Wiley
medical publication. [DNLM: 1. Economics, Medical—
United States. W 74 F312h]

RA410.F44 1983   338.4′736210973 83-6842
ISBN 0-471-87279-2

Printed in the United States of America

10 9 8 7 6 5 4 3 2 1

To Anna

Preface
to the Second Edition

Among the several reasons for revising the first edition, perhaps the most compelling is to keep up with the changes occurring in the health care sector. Health policy is currently changing. Politically, national health insurance (NHI) is no longer an issue whose time has come; when NHI is discussed, it is more in reference to constraining expenditures than as a means of increasing access. Competition is now the new area of policy focus. Whereas a few years ago it appeared that health care regulation was going to become more pervasive, there is now greater interest in the use of market forces for restructuring the delivery system. The concern over a shortage of physicians has changed to a concern with an impending surplus of physicians. From being reimbursed on a cost-plus basis, hospitals are now facing prospective reimbursement; from a system of many free-standing community hospitals, the trend is now toward greater consolidation. Multi-institutional systems are becoming more common. These are some of the changing forces in the health care system that have been incorporated into this revision.

just since '79

A chapter on the pharmaceutical industry has also been added. This chapter examines both the performance of the industry as well as federal regulation of drug safety. In addition, the other chapters have all been updated with more recent data and references to current articles.

In writing this book and in teaching my course, I have benefited from the work of other health economists. Some measure of that debt is indicated by the numerous references to others' work found throughout the book. In preparing this new edition, I wish to thank all those who gave me comments on the first edition. I particularly want to thank Jeremiah J. German for his extensive suggestions. Darrell Graham, my research assistant, provided invaluable service in working with me on this revision. Leslie Hamilton cheerfully gave of her time in typing the various revisions.

Paul J. Feldstein

Preface
to the First Edition

This book grew out of a course on the economics of health services that I have taught at The University of Michigan for many years. During this period the health economics literature has grown rapidly, eventually resulting in a course reading list sufficiently large to cause my students concern. As the literature increased, so did its technical content, often assuming a background students lacked. In addition, the literature developed unevenly, leaving gaps which this book is designed to fill. This introductory text attempts to provide an analytical approach to the study of medical care and, through the use of numerous applications, to illustrate the usefulness of economics to the understanding of public policy issues in medical care.

The material in this book presumes familiarity with some of the economic concepts presented in a microeconomics course at the undergraduate level. I have, therefore, tried to refresh students' memory of these concepts when discussing the applicability of economics to health care. Since institutional knowledge of medical care issues is generally not uniform among students, particularly undergraduates, I have defined concepts and described legislation that would be more familiar to students in a School of Public Health.

This book is meant to be used for a one-semester course in health economics. Realizing that professors' preferences for topics to include in such a course may differ, I have included more of them than would normally be covered in one semester. For the interested student, several topics have been treated in greater depth.

While writing this book I have tried to clarify those subjects found by my students to be most difficult and most inadequately explained in the classroom. If the reader has difficulty understanding certain sections, he or she will have developed a better appreciation for my students' experience. For example, as a result of student comments I became aware of the need to make explicit the relationship between economic analysis and the value judgments underlying different public policies. For this reason, I have tried to stress these issues in the various subjects discussed.

The emphasis in this book is on the financing and delivery of personal medical services, rather than on the broader issues of health and health services. This narrower focus reflects the almost exclusive emphasis of federal and state legislation and of the current policy issues, such as increasing health care costs and national health insurance, on personal medical services rather than health and health services, which might well be more appropriate. The relationship of personal medical services to health is discussed in an early chapter; thereafter, the material emphasizes the definition, measurement, and selection of public policies to achieve economic efficiency and equity in the financing and delivery of personal medical services.

Paul J. Feldstein

Contents

Tables

Figures

HEALTH CARE
ECONOMICS

CHAPTER 1

An Introduction to the Economics of Medical Care

TRENDS IN MEDICAL EXPENDITURES

Expenditures on personal medical services have risen more rapidly than expenditures on most other goods and services in the economy. Annual expenditures on personal medical services have increased from $10.8 billion in 1950 to $255 billion in 1981. A large part of this dramatic increase has occurred in the last 10 years. In 1967, $44 billion or 5.6 percent of the gross national product (up from 4.1 percent in 1950) was being spent on personal medical services. (See Table 1-1.) By 1981, 8.7 percent of the GNP was being allocated to personal medical services. If the current rate of increase in medical care expenditures continues at approximately 15 percent per year, personal medical services will consume an increasing portion of all goods and services produced in the United States.

Part of the increase in total medical care expenditures is the result of increases in the population receiving such services. When we adjust for such population increases by examining expenditures on a per capita basis, we find that the annual percentage increase in per capita medical expenditures over the past 10 years is still very close to the annual percentage increase in total medical expenditures. Per capita medical expenditures have risen from $70.37 in 1950 to $1089.93 in 1981.

Not all of the increase in medical expenditures represents an increase in the quantity of services per capita. A substantial part of the expenditure increase has been due to an increase in prices for the same services, as well as a change in the type of services provided. The price of medical care, as measured by the Consumer Price Index, has been increasing quite rapidly. Starting in 1966, the price of medical care began to increase more rapidly than it had in the past; this acceleration in medical prices continued until the early 1970s, when federal price controls were imposed on the economy. The Economic Stabilization Program lasted longer for the medical sector than for the rest of the economy, from

1

[handwritten marginal note: "This table is too complex and too many years — students audience doesn't need this much."]

TABLE 1-1. Trends in Personal Medical Care Expenditures[a]

(1) Calendar Year	(2) Total (Billions)	(3) Annual % Increase Total	(4) % of GNP	(5) Per Capita Total	(6) Annual % Inc. Per Capita Total	(7) Annual % Inc. in CPI Medical Care	(8) Private Expend. (Billions)	(9) Annual % Increase Private	(10) % of Total Private	(11) Per Capita Private	(12) Annual % Inc. Per Capita Private	(13) Public Expend.	(14) Annual % Inc. Public	(15) % of Total Public	(16) Per Capita Public	(17) Annual % Inc. Per Capita Public	(18) Federal Expend. (Billions)	(19) Annual % Inc. Per Capita Federal	(20) State and Local Expend. (Billions)	(21) Annual % Inc. State
1950	$ 10.9		3.8	$70.37			$ 8.5		77.6	$54.59		$ 2.4		22.4	$15.78		$ 1.1		$ 1.3	
1955	15.7	7.6	3.9	93.29	5.8	3.8	12.1	7.3	77.0	71.86	5.7	3.6	8.5	23.0	21.43	6.3	1.6	5.9	2.0	9.0
1960	23.7	8.6	4.7	128.81	6.7	4.1	18.5	8.9	78.2	100.76	7.0	5.2	7.6	21.8	28.05	5.5	2.2	4.1	3.0	8.5
1965	35.8	8.6	5.2	180.73	7.0	2.5	28.1	8.7	78.4	141.75	7.1	7.7	8.2	21.6	38.98	6.8	3.6	8.9	4.1	6.5
1966	39.6	10.6	5.2	197.61	9.3	4.4	29.5	5.0	74.3	146.92	3.7	10.1	31.2	25.7	50.69	30.0	5.3	43.3	4.9	19.5
1967	44.4	12.1	5.6	219.29	11.0	7.1	29.3	-0.7	66.0	144.71	-1.5	15.1	49.5	34.0	74.58	47.1	9.5	78.6	5.6	14.3
1968	50.2	13.1	5.7	245.50	12.0	6.1	32.5	10.9	64.6	158.66	9.6	17.7	17.2	35.4	86.84	16.4	11.4	18.7	6.4	14.3
1969	56.9	13.4	6.0	275.64	12.3	6.9	36.8	13.2	64.6	178.05	12.2	20.1	13.6	35.4	97.59	12.4	13.2	14.6	7.0	9.4
1970	65.1	14.4	6.6	312.29	13.3	6.4	42.6	15.8	65.5	204.57	14.9	22.5	11.9	34.5	107.72	10.4	14.5	9.2	7.9	12.9
1971	72.0	10.6	6.7	340.64	9.1	6.5	46.4	8.9	64.4	219.50	7.3	25.6	13.8	35.6	121.14	12.5	16.8	13.9	8.8	11.4
1972	80.2	11.4	6.7	375.53	10.2	3.2	51.4	10.8	64.0	240.47	9.6	28.8	12.5	36.0	135.06	11.5	18.9	11.7	9.9	12.5
1973	88.7	10.6	6.7	411.20	9.5	3.9	56.7	10.3	63.9	262.62	9.2	32.0	11.1	36.1	148.58	10.0	21.1	10.2	11.0	11.1
1974	101.0	13.9	7.0	463.84	12.8	9.3	62.4	10.1	61.8	286.69	9.2	38.6	20.6	38.2	177.15	19.2	25.8	12.1	12.8	16.4
1975	116.8	15.6	7.5	530.97	14.5	12.0	70.7	13.3	60.5	321.20	12.0	46.1	19.4	39.5	209.77	18.4	31.4	20.8	14.7	14.8
1976	131.8	12.8	7.7	593.67	11.8	9.6	80.3	13.6	60.9	361.60	12.6	51.5	11.7	39.1	232.07	10.6	36.1	13.9	15.4	4.8
1977	148.7	12.8	7.8	663.16	11.7	9.6	90.8	13.1	61.1	404.96	12.0	57.9	12.4	38.9	258.20	11.3	41.0	12.2	16.9	9.7
1978	166.7	12.1	7.7	735.57	10.9	8.4	101.5	11.8	60.9	447.86	10.6	65.2	12.6	39.1	287.71	11.4	46.4	12.1	18.8	11.2
1979	189.1	13.4	7.8	825.68	12.3	9.3	114.7	13.0	60.7	500.95	11.9	74.4	14.1	39.3	324.73	12.9	53.1	13.2	21.3	13.3
1980	217.9	15.2	8.3	940.62	13.9	10.9	131.5	14.7	60.4	567.66	13.3	86.4	16.1	39.6	372.96	14.9	62.5	16.5	23.9	12.2
1981	255.0	17.0	8.7	1089.93	15.9	10.7	152.1	15.7	59.6	649.68	14.5	102.9	19.1	40.4	439.82	17.9	74.6	18.1	28.3	18.4

Sources: Robert M. Gibson and Daniel R. Waldo, "National Health Expenditures, 1980," *Health Care Financing Review* 3 (September 1981): 36–38, Table 4; U.S. Department of Health and Human Services, *HHS News* (newsletter released July 26, 1982); U.S. Bureau of the Census, *Statistical Abstract of the U.S.*, 1981, 102 ed. (Washington, D.C.: U.S. Government Printing Office, 1981), p. 467, Table 779.

[a]Personal Medical Care Expenditure is equal to Total Health Care Expenditures less expenditures for Prepayment and Administration, Government Public Health Activities, and Research and Constructions of Medical Facilities.

1971 until 1974. Since the removal of those price controls, the annual percentage increase in medical prices has been approximately two-thirds of the annual percentage increase in total medical expenditures.

In 1966, the passage of Medicare and Medicaid introduced an important change to the medical sector. Medicare is a federal program for financing the medical services of the aged; Medicaid is a federal-state financing program for the medically indigent. The extent of the changes effected by Medicare and Medicaid is indicated by the changing share of the financing of medical services. In 1965, 80 percent of medical expenditures were privately financed. By 1981, although the private sector had increased its total expenditures (from $28 billion in 1965 to $152 billion in 1981), this total represented a declining share of total medical expenditures, 60 percent. The federal rather than state government is paying an increasing share of total medical expenditures.

These increases in government expenditures, particularly the federal government's, are far larger than increases in the private sector. In 1965, the federal government spent $3.6 billion on personal medical services, while the states spent $4.1 billion. By 1981, the federal government was spending $74.6 billion a year and the states were spending $28.3 billion.

The rapid and continuing increase in the amount of our nation's resources being devoted to personal medical services and the increasing role of government in financing personal medical services (over 40 percent of total medical care expenditures) raise several important policy questions.* For example, are the large annual percentage increases in medical prices, which contribute to the increase in expenditures, justified? Could a greater amount of medical services be provided, for the same amount of expenditures, if those resources were allocated differently? To analyze these issues we must examine the efficiency with which the medical sector produces its output.

We may further ask, should the government be spending an increasing share of its limited resources on personal medical services when there are competing needs, such as those for education and welfare reform? To answer this question, it is necessary to first determine the amount of medical services redistribution that should occur and the population groups to be served. Once these value judgments have been stated explicitly, economics can determine the most efficient way to achieve a given equity goal.

Economics offers two basic tools and a set of criteria with which to analyze issues of efficiency and distribution. The first tool is techniques of optimization. Optimization techniques specify the appropriate criteria to be used when allocating scarce resources so as to minimize the cost of achieving a given objective. We can use techniques of optimization to evaluate the efficiency of the

---

*Public expenditures on health and medical care services as a percentage of all federal and of all governmental (including state and local) expenditures have been increasing rapidly since 1966. Prior to 1966, government medical expenditures, as a percentage of all governmental expenditures, remained steady at approximately 3.7 percent. Federal medical expenditures, as a percentage of all federal expenditures, remained steady at approximately 3.0 percent. By 1980 the percentages were 0.9 percent and 11.9 percent, respectively. U.S. Bureau of the Census, *Statistical Abstract of the United States, 1981,* 102 ed. (Washington, D.C.: U.S. Government Printing Office, 1981), p. 275, Table 467; Robert M. Gibson and Daniel R. Waldo, "National Health Expenditures, 1980," *Health Care Financing Review* 3 (September 1981): 36, Table 4.

current system of medical services delivery. Similarly, optimization techniques can be used by governments and other organizations to determine the most efficient allocation of medical and nonmedical resources to achieve a given objective, such as an increase in the health status of the population.

The second economic tool is the determination of equilibrium situations, by which, for example, economists can predict the final result of a change in demand for a service. Predicting new equilibrium situations involves the use of the familiar tools of supply and demand analysis. The use of supply and demand analysis should point to the causes for the rapid increases in medical care prices and expenditures and should enable us to predict prices and expenditures in the years ahead. Supply and demand analysis is also used for estimating the consequences, in price, quantity of service, and total expenditure, of policies governing the redistribution of medical services in the population, such as through national health insurance.

Implicit in the use of the above analytical tools is a set of criteria for evaluating economic welfare. These welfare criteria are used to determine whether someone is made better or worse off as a result of a particular action or policy and to evaluate the performance of an industry. Welfare criteria and the explicit statement of the assumptions that underlie their use contribute to the study of medical care. Much public policy is based on the values held by individuals and their perception of the most efficient method for achieving the given set of values. A specific set of welfare criteria provides the means by which differences in values and differences in methods for achieving a set of values can be separately evaluated.

BASIC CHOICES THAT MUST BE MADE WITH REGARD TO MEDICAL SERVICES

Problems of scarcity are the basis for the development and use of the economist's tools and criteria. The economist's skill in using optimization techniques, forecasting, and criteria for evaluating economic performance is useful and necessary regardless of how medical care is organized and provided in a country. The decisions that must be made in any medical system are the same whether they are made by consumers or by government.

Three basic choices determine the organization of health and medical services (and other sectors of the economy). The first choice is determination of both the amount to be spent on health and medical services and the composition of those services. The second choice is a selection of the best method for producing medical services; two such methods are prepaid group practice and fee-for-service. Even within a given delivery system, choices must be made regarding the amounts of capital and equipment to use relative to the amounts and types of labor in providing a service. The third choice is a selection of the method for distributing health services among the population. The first two choices are concerned with issues of economic efficiency, the third with equity in use of health services.

Every country must decide on how much it wants to spend on medical services and the best methods for producing and distributing them. A crucial assumption underlying the application of economics to this decision making process is that alternatives exist for each of the three basic decisions to be made. If there were no alternatives, then economics would not be of use to decision-making in a situation of resource scarcity. It is important to determine whether or not there are choices in medical care for making the above decisions. A discussion of choices in medical care should also clarify whether differences in selecting the choices to be made result from differences in values or a disagreement over the method of achieving an agreed-on set of values. In the following discussion of these three sets of medical care decisions, the economic tools discussed above will be used to illustrate the usefulness of economics both in clarifying and in making those choices.

DETERMINING THE OUTPUT OF MEDICAL SERVICES

The first set of medical care decisions to be made is referred to as the determination of output: how much should be allocated to and what should be the composition of medical services. In a medical system using a price system for resource allocation, consumer and physician decisions determine the quantity and quality of medical services. Theoretically, the consumer will select those services which, given his or her income and the prices of different services, maximize satisfaction. It is assumed that consumers make such choices rationally, and that they have information on both the benefits derived from different services and the prices of those services. If these assumptions are correct, then consumers will allocate their scarce resources (both time and income) to those services and activities that provide them with the greatest amount of benefits. The accuracy of these assumptions with respect to medical services will be discussed below.

In order to understand the allocation process used by consumers when selecting among various commodities, including both goods and services, and also to be able to predict changes in consumer allocation, it is necessary to understand marginal analysis, which is the basis of the optimization technique. Consumers' purchases provide them with benefits, or utility; additional purchases of those same services provide additional benefits, but these additional benefits decline as more units are purchased. The benefits derived from consuming the first unit of a commodity are high; subsequent units of that same commodity provide smaller benefits. Although total benefits increase with additional units of the same commodity, the marginal benefit of additional units declines. This relationship between marginal benefits and additional units of a service is shown in Figure 1-1A. The marginal benefit from consuming OA units of the particular commodity represented in Figure 1-1A is MB_1. If additional units are consumed, the marginal benefit received from those additional units declines, from MB_1 to MB_2.

The consumer receives benefits from many different commodities. To maximize the total benefits from all commodities purchased, the consumer will allocate his or her limited resources to ensure that the marginal benefits received from all commodities purchased are equal.* This optimization rule for equating

---

*For the sake of simplicity, it is here assumed that the prices of the different commodities are equal.

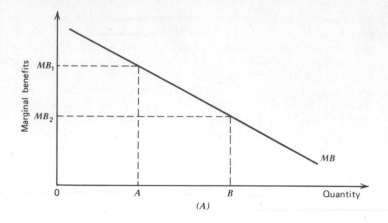

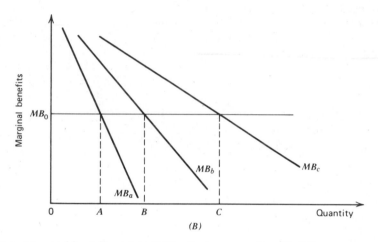

Figure 1-1. Marginal benefit curves of (A) a single commodity, (B) different commodities.

the marginal benefits of the last units of different commodities does not mean that the same number of units of each commodity will be consumed. It is more likely that when the marginal benefits of different commodities are equal, the buyer will be consuming differing quantities of the commodities purchased. The reason is that the marginal benefits decline at different rates for different commodities. The consumer is likely to purchase more units of those commodities with a gradual decline in marginal benefits than of those with a very sharp decline. As shown in Figure 1-1B, the marginal benefits are equal at MB_0 for different commodities when the consumer is purchasing OA units, OB units, and OC units of three different commodities. Any other allocation process would result in a lower total level of benefits. The consumer therefore maximizes the amount of benefits for a given income by allocating it across commodities to ensure that the marginal benefits from the last units are equal.

To allow for differences in commodity prices, the consumer must compare not only the marginal benefits of different commodities but also the ratio of the marginal benefit to the price of each commodity (*MB/P*). When this is done, the marginal benefit per dollar spent will be equal for all commodities. (It should be noted that the marginal benefits received from the purchase of a commodity vary among consumers. These differences may be illustrated with reference to Figure 1-1*B*. The marginal benefit curves of Figure 1-1*B* in this case represent the marginal benefits received from the same commodity by different consumers.)

The consumer evaluates the marginal benefits of a purchase in relation to its price, or stated differently, the consumer compares the ratio of marginal benefit to marginal cost for each purchase with the ratio of every other purchase. The marginal cost to the consumer is the price he or she must pay for that commodity. When the consumer has equated the marginal benefits and the marginal costs of each purchase, then his or her scarce resources have been allocated to maximize total benefits. In an equilibrium situation, when the quantity demanded equals the quantity supplied, the equilibrium price reflects the value placed on the last units purchased by all consumers, since all consumers face the same price in a given market. In a competitive market, prices represent the costs of production. The costs of production in turn reflect the value of other goods and services that might have been produced with the same resources. When an efficient price system is used for allocating resources, the marginal benefits to consumers of purchasing the last unit equal the marginal costs of the resources used to produce it.

Any of the following changes in factors affecting consumers' allocation decisions would cause a change in their purchasing behavior: a change in the price of one commodity relative to that of other commodities, a change in income, or a change in perception of the benefits to be derived from consuming additional units. Economic tools, which provide criteria that enable a consumer to allocate resources so as to maximize benefits, also provide the basis for understanding changes in consumer demand. It is in this way that the two tools of economics—optimization techniques and the determination of equilibrium situations—are related.*

The above description of the consumer choice process in a market system illustrates the importance of price in making choices. A nonmarket approach toward determining the amount of resources to be allocated to medical care requires a substitute mechanism that will perform the price function—that is, that will provide an incentive to consumers to limit their use of services to the point at which the cost of those services equals their value. Such a mechanism must also ration that available quantity of services among consumers and provide information to providers of changes in their demand. Although the functions that prices perform must still be performed under a nonmarket system, alternative mechanisms to perform these functions have generally been found to be unsatisfactory.

---

*This discussion of marginal analysis is not meant to imply that *every* consumer continuously undertakes an exact system of calculation for purchasing all commodities. Consumers, on the average, do consider such factors as marginal benefits, relative prices, and their level of income when making their purchase decisions. Psychological and sociological variables are also included in economic models as predictors of consumer behavior. However, to the extent that consumers have information and act to maximize their total benefits, predictions based on changes in relative prices and income will result in more accurate predictions of consumer demand than will other (e.g., psychological or sociological) models of consumer behavior that exclude such economic variables.

HOW BEST TO PRODUCE MEDICAL SERVICES

The second set of decisions that must be made in any health system is selection of the best method for producing the amount of medical services to be provided. Medical services can be provided in different organizational settings, including prepaid group practice or solo practitioners practicing under a fee-for-service arrangement. Even within a particular delivery system, the combinations of health personnel and equipment can vary. If the providers of medical services have the incentive to minimize their costs, then they will use the various inputs—health personnel and capital—according to their relative costs and productivity. The method of optimization used by the provider will be similar to that used by the consumer of medical services. In place of marginal benefits and relative prices on the consumer side, marginal productivity of inputs and their relative costs will be used by providers to determine the least costly method of providing a service. The decision rule will also be the same. When the ratio of the marginal productivity of an input to its wage is equal to that of other inputs, then the firm is minimizing its costs of providing medical services.

When the provider's costs are minimized, the combination of services (hospital and physician care) and the inputs (types of health personnel and capital) used to provide medical care will be both technically and economically efficient. Technical efficiency means that the medical services will be produced using the minimum number of inputs of any given proportion. However, several different combinations of inputs may be technically efficient. To minimize the cost of providing medical services, it is necessary to be not only technically but also economically efficient. The decisionmaker must choose among the several combinations of inputs, each of which is technically efficient, to determine which combination is also economically efficient—that is, least costly. To do so, the decisionmaker must consider the relative costs of the different inputs as well as their productivities.

When the economist applies the tools for optimization to the set of choices governing the production of medical services, several problems of medical services delivery are brought into sharper focus. Some medical care professionals have proposed the use of certain standards in the delivery of medical services: four hospital beds per thousand population is one such standard; specified lengths of stay, by diagnosis, for hospitalized patients is another example; and ratios of the number of registered nurses per hospitalized patient is a third. Standards such as these imply that medical services can or should be produced by only one method. If the provision of medical services were actually subject to such fixed proportions, then no choice of production methods would exist, and the effectiveness of the economist's tools for minimizing medical care costs would be very limited. It is, however, unlikely that the choices for producing medical care are so limited. Depending upon the illness being treated, ambulatory care and nursing home services can be substituted for hospital care, with no decrease in the quality of treatment. Lengths of stay can be varied depending upon the availability of other facilities in the community and someone to care for the patient at home. Other kinds of nursing personnel can substitute for registered nurses in the care of the hospitalized patient. Presently, wide variations exist across communities in lengths of stay by diagnosis, in use of registered nurses, and in number of hospital beds per thousand population. Substituting medical services and personnel without decreasing their quality is more possible than some would have us believe.

If greater substitution in the production and delivery of medical services is possible, then using the standards described above will hinder economic efficiency in providing medical care. Using inputs without regard to their relative costs is unlikely to result in the least-cost combination. The cost of hospital care relative to the cost of ambulatory and nursing home services has been increasing very rapidly. If four hospital beds per thousand population was the least costly input ratio 30 years ago, then changes in the relative costs of hospital care and other services would seem to require that inputs be combined differently to achieve the least costly method today. A similar analysis could determine the optimum number of registered nurses per patient relative to other types of nursing personnel. As the relative costs (and productivities) of inputs change over time, it is to be expected that the combination of inputs that is least costly for providing medical services will change also. The economist's tools of optimization can determine which combination of services and inputs is most efficient for providing medical care. Similarly, the concepts embodied in these tools provide a decisionmaker with vital information about the costs of different choices, which can be used to decide how best to deliver medical services.

The second of the economist's tools, the prediction of new equilibrium levels of prices and quantities, can be used to anticipate changes required in the production of medical services. A change in the price of an input will, as discussed above, result in a change in the combination of inputs that is least costly to use in producing medical care. It is also possible to analyze the new equilibrium situation that will result from the change. An increase in the price of an input will cause a reduction in the quantity demanded of it and an increase in demand for those inputs whose prices have not changed. If the higher-priced inputs are mainly used in the provision of one type of service, such as hospital care, we would then expect to observe a reduction in the quantity demanded of that service because its inputs have become more costly. As the cost of medical services increases, the supply curve of medical care will shift upward. Assuming no change in the demand for medical services, the price of medical care will increase and the quantity demanded will decrease. The extent of the actual change in prices and quantities of medical care will depend upon the elasticities of supply and demand.

The tools of demand and supply can be used to trace the consequences of a change in input prices throughout the medical system. They can also be used to anticipate the effects of changes in medical technology on productivity, medical prices, and quantities of services. Such equilibrium analyses are particularly helpful in anticipating future expenditures for medical care to be borne either by patients or by the government, such as those that would occur under a system of national health insurance.

THE DISTRIBUTION OF MEDICAL SERVICES

The third set of decisions that must be made in any medical system govern the distribution of the system's output. We must select from a number of alternatives when making this decision. We can provide medical care free of charge to all persons; we can distribute medical care in accordance with consumers' willingness to spend their incomes for it. We can also increase the medical care use of those consumers with incomes that are insufficient to purchase the amount of medical care society deems appropriate and necessary.

Economics can clarify the issues involved in the distribution of medical services by providing a set of criteria for determining whether or not a person's welfare is improved by a particular policy. If the purpose of that policy is to improve the person's welfare, economic criteria will suggest the most efficient means for accomplishing that goal. Two value judgments govern the distribution of medical services. The first is whether or not consumers should determine the amount they wish to spend on medical services. The second concerns the method and size of subsidy to be extended to those low-income consumers whose use of medical services is below what society believes it should be. The economist cannot decide which values are preferable; however, economics can help make the process of choosing more rational by providing information on the costs and the implications of different sets of values, and also by providing criteria for determining the most efficient method for achieving a given set of values.

Chapter 20, "National Health Insurance," contains a more complete discussion of the different values underlying the subsidies designed to redistribute medical services in the population. It also contains an analysis of the economic efficiency of existing methods of financing medical services as well as of those proposed under alternative approaches to national health insurance.

THE APPLICABILITY OF ECONOMICS TO THE STUDY OF MEDICAL CARE

Critics have questioned the applicability of economics to the study of medical services on two levels: first, they have questioned the accuracy of the assumptions underlying economic behavior of consumers and medical providers, and second, they have challenged the implicit values, such as consumer sovereignty, that influence the goal to be achieved, i.e., consumer satisfaction. For example, critics have claimed that it is inaccurate to assume that the consumer of health services is rational, and that he or she has sufficient information when deciding on use of services. Such critics also claim that the purchaser of medical services is not the consumer, as in nonmedical markets, but the physician, who also has a financial interest in the services to be purchased. With regard to economists' traditional assumptions about providers of medical services, critics claim that these providers are organized as nonprofit organizations and therefore do not have the same motivations as for-profit firms in other industries. Further, since consumers may be irreparably harmed by incompetent providers, more stringent controls must be exercised over the provision of medical services than over nonmedical goods and services. Lastly, such critics claim that access to medical services is considered a right by society and its distribution cannot be left solely to the marketplace.

It is important to distinguish between criticism directed at the validity of economic assumptions and criticism of the use of economic criteria for evaluating medical system performance. If economic analyses are undertaken, they will be based upon a given set of assumptions, which will lead us to predict a certain outcome. If the observed behavior is different from what was expected, the assumptions are reexamined to determine whether a different assumption could explain the divergence between the expected and observed behavior. For example, one factor affecting the performance of an industry is whether entry is permitted into that industry. An economic analysis would initially assume that entry into a market, such as the physician market, is free. Based on this assumption, we expect to observe certain measures of performance in that market; high physician incomes relative to other occupations would lead to increased enrollment in medical schools. If what we observe is different from what we have predicted, we then examine whether the free-entry assumption is accurate. Thus, economic analysis isolates those assumptions to be reexamined when a divergence occurs between expected and observed behavior.

If the observed performance of an industry is different from what we would expect in a competitive market, then public policy may be required to change that industry's performance. Some public policy prescriptions attempt to make structural changes that will bring an industry's actual performance into greater conformity with its expected performance. If, for example, an industry is observed to provide its services inefficiently, we examine whether efficiency incentives exist in that industry. If such incentives are lacking, then one appropriate policy prescription would be to improve the incentives for efficient operation.

For each of the aspects of medical care to be analyzed, the expected performance of consumers and providers will be contrasted with the observed performance. When a divergence is discovered between the two, the underlying assumptions will be reexamined to account for the observed behavior. The specific assumptions regarding consumer information, incentives for efficiency, and barriers to entry can thus be examined to determine what effect these factors have on the economic performance of the medical care sector when they differ from their theoretical assumptions.

The medical care market is also acknowledged to be different from other markets because it includes a greater demand for consumer protection. However, different approaches to providing consumer protection are available. These alternative approaches, together with other, possibly unique aspects of medical care, will be analyzed with respect to their impact on the performance of the medical care sector.

Criticisms of the values underlying the use of economic criteria for evaluating medical system performance are more difficult to resolve. Given a scarcity in the availability of resources for providing medical services, what criteria should society use for making the three basic medical care decisions? A medical system which values economic efficiency in consumption and production will base its choice of the amount to spend on medical services on the criteria of satisfying consumer preferences; it will base its method of providing services on the criteria of least cost; and it will base its choice of the amount and method of medical services redistribution on the criteria of consumer preference. Under this value system, medical services benefits are defined by consumer preference rather than by government or health agency perception of consumer preference.

If decisionmakers reject the foregoing criteria, new criteria must be specified. The criterion of efficiency in production is more likely to be acceptable than is the criterion of satisfying consumer preferences. In this latter case, the alternative that proponents are likely to substitute is a needs approach to the allocation of medical services. Under a needs approach, the value placed on medical services and the resources necessary to satisfy those needs are centrally determined. Because resources are insufficient to satisfy all medical needs, an additional decision rule must be developed that will enable the decisionmakers to choose which needs and population groups will be given highest priority.

The replacement of one set of values by another does not influence the usefulness of economics in the decisionmaking process; its value lies in its ability to make that process more rational by showing what the costs of different choices are. To the extent that economic analysis can clarify the cost of alternatives and make the values underlying those alternatives explicit, it is a useful approach to the study of medical care.

THE TRADE-OFF BETWEEN QUANTITY AND QUALITY IN THE PROVISION OF MEDICAL SERVICES

The following example of the trade-off between quantity and quality illustrates the kinds of choices that must be made with regard to medical services. One of the choices that any medical system must make in determining the use of its limited resources is the combination of quantity and quality of medical services it wishes to provide. If the length of training of health professionals is long, and if the equipment and facilities used are the most technically advanced, then fewer services will be available to the entire population. This trade-off between quantity and quality (which actually refers to the level of training of health professionals—a process measure, not an outcome measure, of quality) is shown in Figure 1-2. Point A represents a combination where quality is relatively high and is received by a small percentage of the population. Point B represents a different combination: a large percentage of the population receives some medical services, while the quality of those services is relatively low. The quantity-quality trade-off curve in Figure 1-2 is referred to as a production possibilities curve.*

What criterion should determine the combination of quality and quantity of medical services that a society should choose? If the criterion were the maximizing of consumer preferences, then, assuming adequate information and proper safeguards, consumers would be the appropriate group to select the quantity-quality combination that should prevail.† Alternatively, health professionals can

---

*The curve is shaped as it is (concave to the origin) because the resources used in producing quantity and quality (which are equivalent to two different outputs) are not completely substitutable for one another. As more of one combination of services is produced (as represented by points A or B), the resources are switched from producing one type of services to the other. The released resources are more specialized, hence more efficient, in producing their previous output. Moving those same resources into the production of a different good or service will cause them to be less efficient in the production of that new service. Thus, the costs of producing more of the new output are increased.

†The resultant quantity-quality combination would maximize consumer satisfaction because the marginal benefits of those services (to the consumer) would equal the marginal cost of resources used in their production.

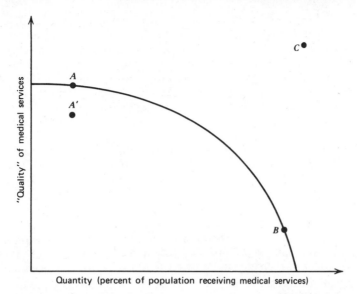

Figure 1-2. The quantity–quality tradeoff in medical care.

select the quantity-quality trade-off, as they now often do in the United States. For example, health professionals establish the educational requirements and determine the number of educational institutions through their accreditation policies. There are fewer health professionals than there would be if educational requirements were more flexible and if fewer restrictions were placed on entry into the health professions and on the tasks that professionals are permitted to perform.

The discussion of the quantity-quality trade-off can also be used to illustrate the second set of choices that must be made in any medical care system— namely, how best to produce medical services. Any quantity-quality combination on the production possibilities curve is assumed to have been produced in the least costly manner. The amount of resources devoted to medical services is represented by the area under the curve. If, owing to the placement of restrictions on the least costly manner of production or the use of a method of provider reimbursement that removes efficiency incentives, the providers of medical services are not as efficient as they might be, then fewer medical services will be produced for the same amount of resources. This situation is shown in Figure 1-2, where A' represents the same amount of resources as used at point A but the output is less than that achieved at point A. A' is obviously inefficient in that resources are being wasted; either more medical services or medical services of higher quality could be produced with the same quantity of resources. It is important to determine whether the current medical care system is at point A or A' and the reasons why it is.

The third set of choices concerning medical services distribution might be illustrated by a quantity-quality analysis of the statement, "All Americans should receive the highest quality of medical care." The highest quality of medical care to all would be represented by point C in Figure 1-2, which is equivalent to 100 percent of the population (furthest to the right on the horizontal axis), and by the highest point on the quality axis. To achieve such a goal, additional resources equivalent to the distance between point C and the current production possibilities curve would be required. These additional resources would be financed either by an increase in taxes or by decreased expenditures on other programs. These choices provide differing marginal benefits. Who is to decide their relative benefits? Health professionals attach greater benefits to medical as opposed to other services; however, they do not bear the costs of their decisions. Consumers, who will bear the costs, may not share their estimate of the relative benefits.

Each medical system must make choices in three areas: how much to spend on medical services, how best to produce those services, and how to distribute them. People differ in their values as to how those choices should be made. To evaluate how the medical system performs with respect to each of those choices, it is necessary to establish criteria for what is considered good performance. The performance criteria used by economists are based upon a set of values incorporated into their definition of economic efficiency—namely, maximizing consumer satisfaction and using the least costly method of production. If decision-makers disagree over these values, then it is necessary to state explicitly an alternative set of values. People can then decide whether they prefer one set of values over another. For any alternative set of values, it is also necessary to state the criteria to be used for evaluating the performance of the medical system. The debate over appropriate public policy in medical care is often confused because a clear distinction is not made between differences in values and differences in the best way to achieve a particular set of values. Clarification of these differences should sharpen the debate over the most appropriate public policies for medical care.

CHAPTER 2

The Production of Health: The Impact of Medical Services on Health

MEDICAL CARE AS AN OUTPUT OF THE MEDICAL SERVICES INDUSTRY AND AS AN INPUT TO HEALTH

The first of two alternative ways of looking at medical care is to regard it as the final output of the medical care industry. When viewing medical care as an output, it is important to determine how efficiently it is produced. Industry analyses of the factors affecting the supply of and demand for physician services, hospital care, and the various manpower markets enables us to infer the performance of the medical care industry; that is, we can compare the price and output of the industry as it now exists with the price and quantity (as well as quality) that might exist if the medical care industry underwent a structural change. A structural change would be said to have occurred if physicians, who were predominantly in solo practice and were reimbursed under a fee-for-service arrangement, organized into larger groups, such as prepaid group practices, that included other providers, such as hospitals. Many lesser structural changes can also occur, such as changing the state practice acts, which determine the tasks that different health professionals can perform, or changing the requirements for entering a health profession. All of these proposals affect the structure, hence the performance, of the medical services industry. When medical care is viewed as the output of the medical services industry, our understanding of the structure of that industry (and of its component industries) enables us to evaluate its performance.

15

The second way of looking at medical care is to view it, not as a final output, but rather as one input among many, all of which contribute to an output referred to as "good health." Improvements in health status may be achieved by providing medical services, undertaking medical research, instituting environmental health programs, such as those which control air pollution, and by conducting health education programs aimed at changing the lifestyle of consumers.

other inputs to health.

When determining the amount of resources to be allocated to the medical services sector if the objective is to ensure an increase in health, it is best to view medical care as one of many factors that can improve health status. This approach helps us to determine those program inputs to which resources should be allocated in order to improve health. This allocation question is different from that contained in the first view, which is concerned with the appropriate structure of the medical services industry and the allocation of resources for producing medical care itself. These two different ways of viewing medical care should be recognized explicitly, as each one is useful for different public policies. To determine whether medical care is being produced efficiently, one must examine it as a final output; to determine the most efficient way to allocate resources to increase health, one must view medical services as one of several inputs for achieving that goal.

The second, or input, view will be adopted in the remainder of this chapter, which will first present a theoretical approach for determining how many resources should be allocated to medical care; second, review empirical estimates of medical care's marginal contribution to increased health; and third, discuss applications and implications of those findings.

DETERMINING THE ALLOCATION OF RESOURCES TO MEDICAL CARE USING A HEALTH PRODUCTION FUNCTION

To determine among which inputs the allocation of resources would be least costly for achieving an increase in health levels, it is necessary to understand the concept of a "health production function." A production function describes the relationship between combinations of inputs and the resulting output; it is to be distinguished from a production possibility curve which describes the trade-off between different outputs from a given set of resources. Health can be produced using different combinations of inputs. (It is assumed in empirical studies of health production functions that the estimated relationships are technically efficient; i.e., the inputs produce the maximum possible output.) The economist (and the policymaker) is interested in determining which combination of inputs is economically efficient—that is, least costly, for producing the output, health. Before we can determine the least costly combination of inputs for producing a given level of health, we must determine the production function for health. Once it has been determined, and estimates have been developed for the marginal effects of each of the inputs on health, comparisons can then be made between increasing expenditures on different inputs. The process of allocating resources to increase health can be improved once information becomes available on both the relative costs of different programs and their effects on health status. Often the real intent of a program's expenditures may be inferred by determining the effect of its resources.

Several studies have attempted to estimate a health production function. However, before reviewing the results and limitations of these studies, it would be useful to discuss the concept itself. A health production function is an analytical method for determining how to allocate resources among alternative programs to achieve an increase in health. The analytical method involves two steps: specifying, first, what information is required, and second, how that information is to be used for allocating resources. Once the empirical studies of health production functions have been reviewed, those results will be used to determine whether increased expenditures on medical services offer a greater or lesser return for achieving an increase in health levels than would expenditures on alternative programs.

The first step in using a health production function for making allocation decisions is to state a specific function—that is, to define the output (or objective) to be achieved and the alternative approaches for achieving it. In order to arrive at alternative approaches, the desired output must be explicitly defined. For example, if the objective is increased health of the population, then the alternatives will also be fairly general: a better environment, improved nutrition, greater emphasis on preventive care, improved access to medical services, and better personal health habits. For policymakers, however, these alternative policies are not sufficiently specific to indicate which environmental, preventive, or medical care programs to undertake in order to have an impact on the health levels of specified population groups. Unless the health objective is defined by age and sex groupings (and probably location), it will not be possible to determine which project—a cancer screening program or a maternal and child health project—will have the greatest effect on health status.

Health professionals and others knowledgeable about health programs are best able to specify which health programs are alternatives for increasing the health status of a particular age-sex population group. By using optimization tools, the economist can determine how to allocate limited health funds among alternative programs to achieve the largest possible increase in health status.

The discussion that follows illustrates the approach that should be used to allocate expenditures among alternative programs to achieve the maximum possible increase in the policy objective. Assuming the policy objective is to decrease the infant mortality rate, on which type of programs should additional funds be spent? For illustrative purposes, let it be assumed that only two programs exist for reducing infant mortality rates: one is to establish additional intensive care units in selected hospitals for infants of high risk; the other is to increase funding for maternal and child health programs (to expectant mothers and children up to five years of age) in health shortage areas. The following approach demonstrates the type of information and analysis required to determine how best to allocate limited funds between these two programs (1).

The relationship between spending additional funds on each program and their impact on infant mortality rates is shown in Figure 2-1. When a program is relatively small, additional inputs devoted to that program are likely to result in relatively large increases in the program's output (decreased infant mortality rates). As additional resources are allocated to that program, the output will continue to increase, but at a more gradual rate. Finally, increases in output will

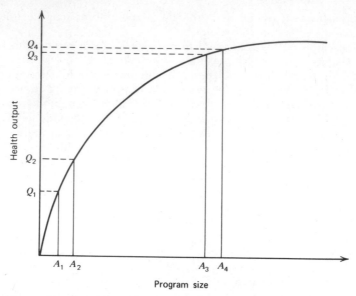

Figure 2-1. The relationship between total output and program size.

become negligible even though the program's inputs continue to increase. The relationship between program inputs and program output has a curvilinear shape because eventually it becomes more difficult to find high-risk infants, as is illustrated by the establishing of additional intensive care units (ICU). Placing a third intensive care unit for infants in an area may result in a decrease in use of all three units, even when formerly two units had been fully utilized. Thus, with a third unit, the output per ICU unit falls. Or, if use does not decrease, it will expand to include infants of lower risk than those admitted when there were fewer such units. With maternal and child health programs, initial programs are likely to provide care for those patients most likely to benefit from them. As additional resources are devoted to maternal and child health, it either becomes more costly to find recipients who will benefit most from these programs, or recipients whose need is not as great begin to use the program. In either case, the output of the program per unit of input begins to decline as the size of the program is increased. It is thus inappropriate to assume that there is a constant (i.e., linear) relationship between a program's inputs and its output. Additional resources spent on health programs are unlikely to produce the same increase in output as did previous increases in the program's expenditures.

Since the relationship between total program output and program input is curvilinear, as shown in Figure 2-1, it must be determined at which point on that total output curve a particular program is operating. If the size of the program is relatively large, as shown by point A_3, then adding resources equivalent to A_3–A_4 will result in an increase in total output of the magnitude Q_3–Q_4. If the program is smaller—for example, at size A_1—then the same increase in program resources will result in a larger increase in total program output, from Q_1 to Q_2.

Still using the simplified example, if it costs the same to increase the inputs

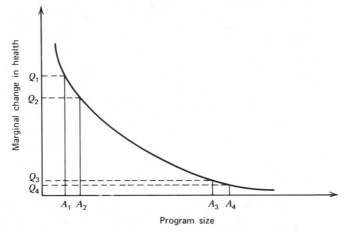

Figure 2-2. Marginal effects on health with a change in program size.

in two health programs, but one program (e.g., the intensive care unit program) is at size A_3, while the other (i.e., the maternal and child health program) is at size A_1, to which of the two programs should additional resources be allocated? Given the output and input relationship for both, as shown in Figure 2-1, the allocation of a given amount of resources to the program at point A_1 would result in the largest change in health output. Thus, the decision rule for allocating resources between the two programs (when the cost of changing either program is the same) is to select that program whose change in total output would be greatest.

It has sometimes been suggested that additional resources should be allocated to those programs whose total output is the largest. Such a decision rule, however, would not necessarily result in the largest increase in output for a given expenditure. Allocating additional resources among programs does not mean that those which receive little or no increase in their resources have to close down, thereby losing their entire output. Allocation decisions are based not on the total output of competing programs, but rather on changes in total output of competing programs. The total output achievable from all programs will be at its maximum only when additional resources are allocated to programs whose increase in total output is greatest.

Another way of illustrating how the above allocation technique results in the largest increase in total output is to examine the marginal relationships between inputs and outputs of the various programs. The marginal changes between total inputs and total outputs of each program are shown in Figure 2-2. These marginal relationships, which reflect the change in total output resulting from a unit increase in a program's inputs, eventually decline with increased program size for the same reason that the total output curve shown in Figure 2-1 increases at a decreasing rate. The marginal relationship shown in Figure 2-2 is the slope of the curve shown in Figure 2-1.

Once it is understood that marginal analysis is the tool for maximizing total output, the implications of allocation decisions based upon a need criterion

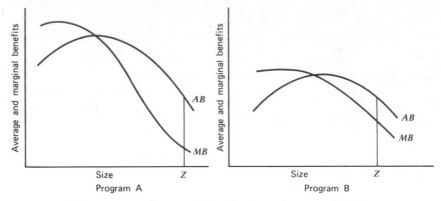

Figure 2-3. Average and marginal benefits from alternative health programs.

become clear. If additional resources were devoted to intensive care units, an increase in infant health levels from Q_3 to Q_4 would result. As long as further increases in total output beyond Q_4 could be achieved, its advocates, using the need criterion, would recommend additional resources for such programs. Scarce resources, however, have a "cost." The additional resources required to increase the ICU program beyond size A_4 could be spent on programs whose change in total output would have been greater. The real cost of the resources devoted to increasing the size of the ICU program is the benefit (output) that could have been achieved if those resources had been spent on alternative programs.

Resources will be allocated in an optimal manner when the additional output produced by resources in one program equals the foregone benefits of using those same resources on alternative programs. This approach toward allocating resources differs from that of health professionals, who generally see only the unmet needs that could be eliminated by devoting still more resources to their own programs.

Since empirical studies on the relationship between total program output and program inputs are not always available, it is difficult to develop estimates of the marginal effect of increased program resources. Data are more likely to be available on the program's total output and total expenditures. Analysts are therefore able to calculate the *average* benefits of the program (total output/total inputs). Because of the greater availability of average measures, they are often used as the basis for comparing the benefits of and allocating resources to competing programs. The use of such average measures, however, can result in an incorrect allocation of resources among health programs.

The average and marginal benefits of two programs are shown in Figure 2-3. At point Z (equivalent to a certain program size) the two programs could appear to be identical because their average benefits are equal. However, at point Z, the marginal benefits of program B are greater than those of program A. Since resource allocations made on the basis of marginal benefits result in the greatest increases in total output, using average benefits (perhaps as a proxy for marginal benefits) can result in error, as this example illustrates.

In Figure 2-1 it was assumed for the sake of simplicity that the cost of increasing the size of the two programs was the same. This is generally not the case. When the costs of increasing a program's size are not equal, the comparison cannot simply be made between the changes in the output of the two programs. The relevant criterion for allocating resources to programs having different benefits and costs is to select those programs whose marginal benefit per dollar spent is greatest. For example, assume that an increase in program A would result in a decrease in infant mortality of 30 infants. The marginal cost of achieving that increased benefit is $300,000. An increase in program B yields, as a marginal benefit, a decrease in infant mortality of 20 infants at a marginal cost of $100,000. The marginal benefits per dollar spent are larger for program B; a decrease in infant mortality of two per $10,000 as compared with one per $10,000 under program A.*

Based upon the foregoing discussion, we can summarize the type of information needed to allocate scarce resources among alternative health programs. First, the particular population group whose health is to be affected must be specified. The disease category for that given population group must also be specified so as to be able to form a health production function. Third, the marginal effect on health of each of the health programs should be empirically estimated. Unfortunately, very little information exists among health professionals or economists about the marginal impacts of alternative health programs. Thus, allocation decisions are currently being made with little or no information about their marginal effects. Determining the marginal impact on health of increased expenditures on medical services and on alternative health programs is an important area for research. Some general information is available on the overall marginal effect of medical services on health. For decisionmaking, however, information is required on the marginal effect that specific medical and other health programs have on disease-specific illness rates for particular population groups.†

---

*For the sake of simplicity, this discussion has assumed that the input-output relationship for each program is independent of changes in scale in the other programs. In actuality, this is not so. For example, if one health program emphasizes prevention, then an increase in resources for this program is likely to affect the productivity of others, such as acute care services. These interrelationships between health programs may cause the input-output curve of particular programs to shift either to the left or to the right; that is, the marginal benefits of the affected program may be increased or decreased without changing expenditures for that program.

In some cases acute care programs may become more productive, as for example after an increase in knowledge or technology (perhaps resulting from increased expenditures on research programs). An increase in knowledge or technology may enable a provider to see more patients or to have a more favorable effect on the outcome of the treatment provided. Alternatively, an increase in preventive programs may decrease the need for acute treatment in the population, thereby lowering the number of patients treated in existing acute care programs. The productivity of existing programs would therefore be lessened.

†Given the very limited data on the marginal effects of alternative health programs, only the grossest comparisons can be made. Ideally, with more appropriate data, additional refinements can be incorporated into the comparisons. For example, differences over time in both the stream of benefits and costs of alternative programs should be discounted. Unfortunately, the analyst may place too great an emphasis on such refinements when the basic data used in the analysis are subject to strong limitations. This results in attributing an unwarranted degree of credibility to the analytical results. The large variability in estimates of a program's effects may outweigh the consequences of those refinements.

If decisionmakers are to allocate scarce resources to produce the maximum possible increase in health levels, they must understand the economic concepts underlying their allocation and they must also generate the information needed to enable appropriate analyses to be undertaken (2). Program managers often avoid generating useful information because they do not want their program to be compared with competing health programs. They believe that the uncertainty of their program's effects will enhance their bargaining position.

The foregoing description of the information requirements of a health production function and the application of that information for allocating resources among alternative health programs provides a background for evaluating the empirical studies to be discussed.

EMPIRICAL STUDIES OF A HEALTH PRODUCTION FUNCTION

The justification often given for government intervention designed to provide more medical services to the population in general and to underserved population groups in particular is the desire to improve health status. If the objective of government expenditures is to increase health levels, then it is important to derive empirical estimates of the net impact that medical care has on health.

Empirical studies attempting to estimate the marginal contribution of medical services to increased health have been conducted at two levels of aggregation. The more aggregate studies of health production have used counties, states, and even countries as the basis of analysis (3). In these studies, the empirical analysis attempted to estimate the independent effect that each of the various factors, including medical services, has had on health levels. Each of the factors affecting health, including measures of health itself, were based on averages of the level of aggregation (i.e., state or county) used as the unit of observation. The less aggregate studies of health production, "microanalyses," used individuals as the unit of measurement (4).

The important distinction between the macro and micro studies of health production lies in the variables used to measure health status. No single measure of health can adequately represent the concept of health status; instead, it is described by certain of its quantifiable aspects. It is always implicitly assumed that these quantifiable measures are closely related to other aspects of health. On an aggregate level, available health measures are those collected by government agencies as part of vital statistics. These measures, such as births and deaths, also tend to be more accurate than others. Morbidity and disability measures of health are generally unavailable on an aggregate level, and they are not likely to be as reliable as mortality data. When mortality rates are used as the measure of health, the simplest such index is the crude death rate, which is the number of deaths per 1,000 population. More useful health indices are those that are age-sex specific. Such population-specific death rates, unlike the crude death rate, would not be affected by changes in the overall composition of the population (5). When studies of health production use individuals as the unit of observation, mortality rates cannot be meaningfully used. Instead, the measures of health used are generally time-loss indicators, such as the number of work-loss days, the individual's own evaluation of health status, and the number of chronic conditions.* The unavailability of data needed to measure health status adequately has led to the practice of measuring health by the use of negative health indices. These measures are obviously incomplete in their assessment of what is believed to constitute good health.

In addition to medical services, other factors affecting age-sex specific mortality rates in studies of health production include: lifestyle variables, such as income, occupation, cigarette smoking and alcohol consumption; environmental variables, such as the quality of housing and urbanization (which, in addition to capturing the effect of pollution, might also represent such offsetting factors as increased access to medical care); and an efficiency factor, measured by the number of years of formal education, which assumes that persons who are more efficient at producing health can do so at a lower cost. The better-educated person may not only be able to recognize symptoms and seek treatment earlier than others, but may also be more likely to use preventive services.

Health production studies generally measure the contribution of medical services to health in several ways: by quantities of the individual components of medical services, such as the number of physicians and hospital beds per thousand population; by the utilization of medical services, such as the number of physician visits or hospital patient days; or by aggregate expenditures on medical services, which include changes in prices, utilization of services, and differences in quality of services. Unfortunately, because of the unavailability of data, such studies have been unable to analyze the effect on health of specific medical services, such as prenatal care.

Auster, Leveson, and Sarachek analyzed interstate differences in age-sex adjusted mortality rates for 1960 (6). Their principal purpose was to estimate the elasticity of health with respect to medical services, which is the percentage change in mortality rates that would occur as a result of a 1 percent change in medical services. The authors used multivariate analysis and included measures of medical services, as well as a number of environmental factors, believed to affect health.† The medical services input was measured in two ways: as expenditures on medical services and as a separate production function for medical

---

*In his study on work-loss rates, M. Silver found that work-loss was positively correlated with income but negatively correlated with the earnings rate (a weekly wage measure). Although Silver acknowledges that this finding may be caused by a combination of incentives and causations—higher earnings make work-loss more expensive, while higher income may carry with it some health risks—he claims that recovery at home is a "superior" good. Therefore, the positive association of income with work-loss represents normal economic behavior rather than a health risk. Silver therefore concludes that work-loss may be an unreliable measure of true health status because it is too greatly affected by economic behavior.

†An important assumption in such cross-sectional studies, of which the authors are well aware, is that the mortality rate is related only to the quantity of medical services used in the particular year for which the study was undertaken. In reality, it is likely that the amount of medical services and influence of environmental factors over the lifetime of the population, rather than just the current period, will affect the population's health status in a given year.

services (which included as inputs into that production function the number of physicians per capita, the number of paramedical persons per capita, and so on).

The statistical results of the Auster, Leveson, and Sarachek study, which accounted for more than 50 percent of the interstate differences in mortality rates, indicated that environmental and personal factors had a greater effect than medical services on mortality rates. The specific findings for some of the more important factors affecting interstate differences in mortality rates were: 1) expenditures on medical care had an elasticity of approximately −.1, meaning that a 1 percent increase in medical expenditures would lead to a .1 percent decrease in age-sex adjusted mortality rates; 2) the elasticity of mortality rates with respect to education was almost twice as large as for medical services, −.2; 3) cigarette consumption per capita resulted in a positive increase in mortality rates (i.e., the elasticity estimate was +.1, meaning that a 1 percent increase in cigarette consumption per capita results in a .1 percent increase in mortality rates); and 4) family income also had a positive effect on mortality rates (i.e., the income elasticity was +.2). The authors explain the positive effect of income on mortality rates by associating high income with a lifestyle that includes adverse diets and fast cars. Occupations with higher incomes might also be associated with more stress and less exercise. The effect of income on health status probably differs according to level of income. At low levels, a rise in income would have a positive effect on health status; persons could afford more nutritious diets, improved housing, and better sanitation facilities. After a certain level of income has been reached, the effect of income on health probably becomes negative. Adverse diet, lack of exercise, and increased stress decrease health status. In the Auster, Leveson, and Sarachek study, the total effect of environmental and personal factors (e.g., income, education, and cigarette consumption) outweighed the marginal contribution of medical services to health status.*

Using individuals as the unit of measurement, Michael Grossman estimated the individual's demand for healthy time. Good health, or healthy time, in Grossman's model is demanded both because it enters the individual's utility function directly for its consumption value and because, as an investment, it increases the time available for other activities. Grossman found that education increases efficiency in producing health and that the elasticity of health with respect to medical services varies between .1 and .3. Grossman also found, as did Auster, Leveson, and Sarachek, that the income elasticity of health is negative, in spite of a positive income elasticity with respect to medical services.

Grossman has conducted several other studies on the determinants of health. In a study of child and adolescent health, Grossman and others found that

the home environment in general and mother's schooling in particular played an extremely important role. . . ." Holding other factors constant, "Children and teenagers of more-educated mothers have better oral health, are less likely to be

---

*Since smoking generally begins early in life, Grossman, Lewit, and Coate have estimated the price elasticity of demand for teenage smoking. With respect to teenage smoking participation, the price elasticity is −1.2, and is −1.4 with respect to the quantity of cigarettes smoked. Thus increasing cigarette taxes can have an important effect on reducing smoking by teenagers. This study is summarized, along with others, in Michael Grossman, "Government and Health Outcomes," *American Economic Review* (May 1980): 194.

obese, and less likely to have anemia than children of less-educated mothers. Father's schooling plays a much less important role. (7)

In another study, Grossman and Jacobowitz examined the effects of five programs and policies on the rapid decline in the neonatal mortality rate (deaths in the first 27 days of life per 1,000 live births) after 1963 (8). The programs and policies examined were Medicaid, subsized family planning services for low-income women, maternal and infant care programs, abortion reform, and physicians per capita. Using county data for 1971, they conducted a cross-sectional analysis to determine the effects of each of the above on neonatal mortality rates. The results of their empirical study can be expressed as follows: 1) the increase in the legalization of abortion among states has been the primary factor in the decline in the neonatal mortality rate; 2) subsidized family planning services have had a significant negative effect on mortality; and 3) increased medical care services, in the form of Medicaid and maternal and infant care programs, have had only small effects on neonatal mortality rates.

A problem with cross-sectional studies that attempt to measure the effect of medical services on health status is that, at any point in time, greater use of medical services may represent increased use by those whose health is poor. Further, increased use of medical services may have an effect on health status over a period longer than that in which they are used. To correct for these problems in interpreting the effect of increased use of medical services on health status, Lee Benham and Alexandra Benham studied the change in health status of groups of individuals during the period 1963 to 1970 (9). Using data from two different surveys, the authors classified individuals into 28 education-age categories (consisting of four education and seven age groupings) and attempted to determine the impact that increased use of medical services had on the health status of each education-age category between 1963 and 1970. (Education was considered as a proxy measure for permanent income.)

During the period studied, 1963 to 1970, two large government programs were started (Medicare and Medicaid) to finance increased use of medical services for the poor and elderly. The measures of health status used were: health status reported, the number of symptoms reported, and disability days reported during the previous year. The contribution of medical services was measured by the number of nonobstetric physician visits and nonobstetric hospital utilization.

The authors' statistical analysis related the (average) health status of each education-age group in 1970 to the (average) health status of that same group in 1963 and to changes in that group's utilization of medical services between 1963 and 1970. The authors assumed that increased utilization of medical services between 1963 and 1970 was primarily the result of an increase in government financing of medical services to the poor and elderly rather than a response to changes in that group's health status. The results of the Benham and Benham study were consistent with the findings from the previously mentioned studies. Increased use of medical services did not result in an improvement in health status during the period studied.

Perhaps more persuasive than these statistical attempts to determine the contribution of medical services to increased health is Victor Fuchs's excellent discussion of the causes of death by age (10). Fuchs examines the contribution of living standards, lifestyle, and medical services to the decline in infant mortality rates since 1900 and to causes of adult deaths. The large decline in infant mortality rates from 1900 to the present* has been due largely to rising living standards, the spread of literacy and education, a large decline in the birth rate, possibly chlorination of the water supply and pasteurization of milk, and the introduction of antimicrobial drugs in the 1930s. "It is important to realize that medical care played almost no role in this decline" (11). It was not until fairly recently (late 1960s) that maternal and infant services were extended to underserved families and intensive care units were provided for premature infants who are at high risk. Fuchs also points out that in other developed countries with fewer medical services than the United States and a large proportion of home births delivered by a midwife, infant mortality rates are lower than in the United States. Specific medical service programs targeted to high-risk pregnancies are likely to make a larger contribution to decreases in infant mortality rates than merely making more medical services generally available to the entire population. For example, in countries where medical services are provided free, as in Great Britain, the infant mortality rate is still not as low as that achieved in other developed countries. The lowest infant mortality rates in 1977 (between 8.0 and 8.9 per 1,000 live births) were those of Sweden, Switzerland, Denmark, and Japan.

When Fuchs examined mortality rates by cause of death for different age groups—adolescents and young adults (15–24 years of age), middle-aged persons (35 to 44), and late-middle-aged persons (55–64)—he again concluded that increased use of medical services has a smaller impact on health than the way in which people live. In the younger age groups, accidents (particularly from use of automobiles), suicides, and homicides are the major causes of death. In middle age, heart disease is the leading cause of death; accidents, suicides, cirrhosis of the liver (caused by alcoholism), and lung cancer are the other major contributors. Among nonwhites, homicides are the second leading cause of death. Again, the major causes of death may be attributed to behavioral factors. For persons in their late middle age, heart disease is again the leading cause of death; neoplasms are second.

Fuchs compares causes of death by age group in the United States and Sweden with interesting results (12). The major factors explaining the lower Swedish mortality rates in each of the various age groups are again determined to be behavioral (Swedes are less violent and have fewer accidents) and attributed to lifestyle (diet, exercise, smoking, and stress). "At present . . . the greatest potential for reducing coronary disease, cancer, and the other major killers still lies in altering personal behavior." Fuchs further notes, "Given our present state of knowledge, even the most lavish use of medical care would not bring the U.S. rate more than a small step closer to the Swedish rate" (13).

The studies employing statistical techniques to estimate a health production function and the discussion by Fuchs on the leading causes of death both suggest that health status is more importantly related to lifestyle factors than to increments of medical services. While the total benefit of medical services may be large, allocation decisions are rarely all-or-nothing decisions; instead, they are

---

*For example, the infant mortality rate in New York City declined from 140 per 1,000 live births in 1900 to 21.9 per 1,000 in 1968. By 1981 the mortality rate had declined to 15.7 per 1,000 live births.

incremental. If policymakers have an increase in health status as their objective, an increased provision of medical services is likely to have a relatively smaller impact on health than will alternative policies. Further, these additional expenditures on medical services are not without a cost; greater increases in health status could be achieved if these same funds were spent on other programs.

APPLICATIONS OF A HEALTH PRODUCTION FUNCTION (14)

One type of analysis that can be undertaken using information developed from a health production function is to determine from among which alternative health programs to allocate additional resources. The empirical studies discussed earlier estimated the elasticity of health with respect to medical services at approximately .1; with respect to education it was estimated at .2. The 1980 economic cost of mortality in the population was estimated at $152.6 billion; the economic cost of morbidity was estimated at $90.7 billion (15). If a 1 percent increase in medical expenditures resulted in a decrease of .1 percent in mortality, and presumably also in morbidity, then such an expenditure would save $243.3 million ($152.6 million from a decrease in mortality and $90.7 million from a decrease in morbidity). The cost of a 1 percent increase in medical expenditures that totaled $235.6 billion in 1980 would be $2.356 billion.

To determine whether to allocate funds to medical services or to alternative health programs, it is necessary to compare the costs of increasing other health programs to achieve the same economic benefits. Since the elasticity of health with respect to education is twice as large as it is for medical services (.2 as compared with .1), education expenditures would have to be increased by only .5 percent to achieve the same economic benefits as medical services.

In 1980, expenditures on education totaled $166.2 billion. One-half percent of that amount would be $831 million. To achieve an increase in health output equal to $243.3 million would have required a $2.356 billion medical expenditure and only a $831 million educational expenditure. Allocating additional funds to education would, at the margin, appear to be preferable to spending those funds on medical services.

The foregoing discussion illustrates the type of analysis to perform when determining how to allocate additional funds. This cost-benefit analysis assumes that no additional economic effects result from an increase in health and that no other reasons exist for undertaking the investment expenditure. It also assumes that the economic value of an increase in health is conceptually correct and accurately measured. All of these caveats are meant to indicate the limitations of such gross cost-benefit analyses. Before one actually allocated funds among education and medical services programs, it would be necessary to have more precise information as to which educational programs have an impact on health levels; the same would be true for medical services programs. Such broad categorizations as education or medical services are not useful for making allocation decisions.

Another application of a health production function explains the recent decline in age-adjusted mortality rates. As shown in Table 2-1, age-adjusted mortal-

TABLE 2-1. Contribution of Selected Medical Services and Environmental Factors to Changes in the Age-Adjusted Death Rate, 1965–1980

	Percentage Change in Variable	Percentage Change in Mortality Per Percentage Change in Variable	Percentage Change in Mortality
Actual change in U.S. death rate[a]			− 19.6%
Health care expenditures per capita, deflated by CPI for medical care[b]	+ 70.3%	− .1%	− 7.0%
Median family income, deflated by CPI for all items[c]	+ 15.7%	.2%	+ 3.1%
Education (median number of school years completed 25 and over)[d]	+ 5.9%	− .2%	− 1.2%
Cigarette consumption per capita[d]	− 9.3%	.1%	− .9%

Sources:

[a]National Center for Health Statistics, *Health—United States, 1981* (Hyattsville, Md.: U.S. Department of Health and Human Services, 1981), p. 117, Table 14; "Annual Summary of Births, Deaths, Marriage, and Divorces: United States, 1980," *Monthly Vital Statistics Report* 29 (September 17, 1981): 3.

[b]Robert M. Gibson and Daniel R. Waldo, "National Health Expenditures, 1980," *Health Care Financing Review* 3 (September 1981): 18, 19, Table 1.

[c]U.S. Bureau of the Census, *Statistical Abstract of the United States, 1981*, 102 ed. (Washington, D.C.: U.S. Government Printing Office, 1981), p. 436, Table 736.

[d]U.S. Bureau of the Census, *Statistical Abstract of the United States, 1981*, p. 141, Table 229; *Statistical Abstract of the United States, 1966* (Washington, D.C.: U.S. Government Printing Office, 1966), p. 113, Table 155.

ity rates declined 19.6 percent between 1965 and 1980. Using the empirical estimates developed in the Auster, Leveson, and Sarachek article, the decline in mortality over this period can be accounted for by the following factors. Expenditures per capita for medical services (adjusted for price increases) increased 70.3 percent during the 1965–1980 period. Based on an elasticity estimate of − .1, the effect of such increased expenditures is an estimated reduction in mortality of 7 percent during this period. The increase in real family income of 15.7 percent, based on an elasticity estimate of .2, is expected to have resulted in an increase in the mortality rate of 3.1 percent. An increase in education in the population of 5.9 percent, based on an elasticity of − .2, was expected to result in a decline in mortality of 1.2 percent. Per capita cigarette consumption declined by 9.3 percent, leading to a .9 percent decline in mortality rates, based on an elasticity estimate of .1 percent.

The percentage decline in mortality rates during this period not accounted for by the above factors is relatively large: 13.6 percent, or approximately 1 percent per year. During the period for which Auster, Leveson, and Sarachek calculated their results, 1955–1965, the unexplained percentage decline in the mortality rate was 5.0 percent. Auster et al. attributed the unexplained portion of the decreased mortality rate to technological change. The 19.6 percent decline in mortality rates during the 1965–1980 period was much greater than for the previous 10-year period, when it was only 3.9 percent. An important factor contributing to the overall decline in mortality rates in the more recent period was the decrease in infant mortality rates, which declined from 26.4 per 1,000 live births in 1955, to 24.7 in 1965, to 16.1 in 1975 to 12.5 in 1980 (16). It has been suggested that this more rapid decline in infant mortality rates is in part the result of improved contraception and liberalized abortion laws (17). The sharp decline in overall mortality rates in the more recent period cannot be explained by declines in infant mortality rates alone. The largest decline in mortality rates has been due to reductions in heart disease. According to two studies, changes in lifestyle factors, such as reduced smoking, lower serum cholesterol levels, control of hypertension, and improvements in the number and quality of coronary care units are the main contributing factors to the decline in heart disease (18).

These applications illustrate the types of analyses that could be undertaken based on knowledge of a health production function. To be useful for policymakers, more specific information on health production functions, by disease categories and for different population groups, is required. Before more precise estimates of health production functions can be derived, however, it is necessary for policy analysts to understand the types of data that need to be collected and how they will be useful for decision making.

The remainder of this book will examine the efficiency with which medical care is produced by the medical care industry. Even though the marginal impact of medical services on health may be relatively small, the increase in private and governmental financing of medical services has been large. The contribution to health of such expenditures will be even further reduced if increased prices of medical services absorb most of the increase in expenditures. The need to examine the efficiency of medical services and the equity of their distribution is addressed in the remaining chapters.

REFERENCES

1. For a more complete discussion of how economic analysis has been used by the government for the allocation of resources between health programs, see Robert N. Grosse, "Cost Benefit Analysis of Health Services," *Annals of the American Academy of Political and Social Science* 399 (January 1972): 89–99. For a more complete discussion of the principles and applications of cost-benefit analysis, see: Kenneth E. Warner and Bryan R. Luce, *Cost-Benefit and Cost-Effectiveness Analysis in Health Care* (Ann Arbor, Mi.: Health Administration Press, 1982).

2. Joseph Lipscomb has developed a resource allocation model that can be used for determining the optimal allocations of resources among various medical care programs so as to maximize a society's health status. He uses linear and integer programming methods to solve the model. For a detailed explanation of the model, see: Joseph Lipscomb, "Health Resource Allocations and Quality of Care Measurement in a Social Policy Framework," *Policy Sciences* 9 (1978): 19–43; and Joseph Lipscomb, et al., "Health Status Maximization and Manpower Allocations," in Richard Scheffler, Ed., *Research in Health Economics*, Vol. 1 (JAI Press, 1979), pp. 301–401.

3. Examples of health production functions using macro data are given by Mary Lou Larmore, "An Inquiry into an Econometric Production Function for Health in the United States" (unpublished doctoral dissertation, Northwestern University, 1967); Richard Auster, Irving Leveson, and Deborah Sarachek, "The Production of Health, an Exploratory Study," *The Journal of Human Resources* IV (Fall 1969): 411–436; and Charles T. Stewart, Jr., "The Allocation of Resources to Health," *The Journal of Human Resources* VI (Winter 1971). See also a critique of the Stewart article by Edward Meeker, "Allocation of Resources to Health Revisited," *The Journal of Human Resources* VIII (Spring 1973): 257–259.

4. Joseph P. Newhouse, "Determinants of Days Lost from Work Due to Sickness," in Herbert E. Klarman, Ed., *Empirical Studies in Health Economics, Proceedings of the Second Conference on the Economics of Health* (Baltimore: The Johns Hopkins Press, 1970), pp. 59–70; Morris Silver, "An Economic Analysis of Variations in Medical Expenses and Work-Loss Rates," in Klarman, Ed., *ibid.*, pp. 121–140; Michael Grossman, "On the Concept of Health Capital and the Demand for Health," *Journal of Political Economy,* March–April 1972; Lee Benham and Alexandra Benham, "The Impact of Incremental Medical Services on Health Status, 1963–1970," in R. Andersen, J. Kravitz, and O. Anderson, Eds., *Equity in Health Services: Empirical Analysis of Social Policy* (Cambridge, Mass.: Ballinger Publishing Co., 1975).

5. For a more complete review of health measures, their definitions and attendant difficulties, see Daniel F. Sullivan, *Conceptual Problems in Developing an Index of Health,* Public Health Service Publication No. 1000, Series 2, No. 17 (Washington, D.C.: Government Printing Office, May 1966). Also see Milton M. Chenn and James W. Bush, "Health Status Measures, Policy, and Biomedical Research," in Selma J. Mushkin and David W. Dunlap, Eds., *Health: What Is It Worth? Measures of Health Benefits* (New York: Pergamon Press, 1979), pp. 15–41.

6. Auster, Leveson, and Sarachek, "The Production of Health."

7. Michael Grossman, "Government and Health Outcomes," *American Economic Review* (May 1982): 192.

8. *Ibid. p.* 193.

9. Lee Benham and Alexandra Benham, "The Impact of Incremental Medical Services."

10. Victor R. Fuchs, *Who Shall Live?* (New York: Basic Books Inc., 1974), pp. 30–55. The data presented by Fuchs represent average relationships and do not indicate the relative marginal costs of achieving changes in health status. For policy purposes, it would be desirable to know the marginal effects of each of the variables on health status.

11. Fuchs, *Who Shall Live?*, p. 32.

12. *Ibid.*, p. 45.

13. *Ibid.*, p. 46.

14. The applications in this section are based on the article by Auster, Leveson, and Sarachek. The data, however, have been updated.

15. The 1980 estimates of economic cost of mortality and morbidity (which represents the discounted value of future earnings) were calculated by assuming a ten percent annual rate of increase in the 1972 estimates published by Barbara S. Cooper and Dorothy P. Rice, "The Economic Cost of Illness Revisited," *Social Security Bulletin* (February 1976): 21–36. When an annual rate of increase of 14 percent is assumed, the 1980 economic costs of mortality and morbidity are $203.1 billion and $120.6 billion, respectively.

16. U.S. Department of Health and Human Services, "Annual Summary of Births, Deaths, Marriages, and Divorces: United States, 1980," *Monthly Vital Statistics Report* 29 (September 17, 1981): 6. For a more detailed discussion of the reasons for the decline in infant mortality rates, see Jeffrey E. Harris, "Prenatal Medical Care and Infant

Mortality," and Mark R. Rosenzweig and T. Paul Schultz, "The Behavior of Mothers as Inputs to Child Health: The Determinants of Birth Weight, Gestation, and Rate of Fetal Growth," in Victor R. Fuchs, Ed., *Economic Aspects of Health* (Chicago: The University of Chicago Press, 1982).

17. Fuchs, *Who Shall Live?*, p. 33. Also see Michael Grossman and Steven Jacobowitz, "Variations in Infant Mortality Rates Among Counties of the United States: The Roles of Social Policies and Programs," National Bureau of Economic Research (NBER) Working Paper Series No. 615 (Cambridge, Mass.: National Bureau of Economic Research, 1981), p. 23.

18. Michael Stern, "The Recent Decline in Ischemic Heart Disease Mortality," *Annals of Internal Medicine* 91 (October 1979): 630–640; Joel Kleinman, Jacob Feldman, and Mary Monk, "The Effects of Changes in Smoking Habits On Coronary Heart Disease Mortality," *American Journal of Public Health* 69 (August 1979): 795–802.

CHAPTER 3

An Overview of the Medical Care Sector

DESCRIPTION OF THE MEDICAL CARE MARKETS

EXPENDITURES ON THE MAJOR COMPONENTS OF MEDICAL CARE

As an introduction to the medical care sector, let us examine the magnitude and changing composition of expenditures on the major components of medical care. As shown in Table 3-1, the two largest components of medical care, hospital and physician services, accounted for 40 and 20 percent of the $286 billion of total medical expenditures in calendar year 1981.* Current expenditures on hospital care, $118 billion, are twice as large as those for physician services, $54.8 billion. The relative proportions of expenditures on hospital, physician, and other medical services have not been constant over time. In 1965, before the large scale involvement of government in financing medical care for the indigent and elderly, total medical expenditures were $41.7 billion and expenditures for hospital care represented 33 percent of that amount; at that time hospital expenditures were only 64 percent greater than those for physician services. By 1981, the expenditures for hospital care had increased more rapidly (750 percent over 1965), than expenditures for all of the remaining components of medical services (506 percent over 1965).

Patients' and physicians' lessening concern with the price of hospital care contributed to the more rapid increase in hospital expenditures. Government expenditures on total medical services increased from $10.8 billion in 1965 to

---

*Personal health care expenditures were approximately $30 billion less than total health care expenditures. The difference between the two are in the "all other" category. Under personal health care expenditures the "all other" category excludes expenses for prepayment and administration, government public health activities, and research and medical facilities construction.

32

TABLE 3-1. Total Private and Public Expenditures for Medical Care by Type of Expenditure and Source of Funds, Calendar Years 1965 and 1981 (in Billions of Dollars)

	1965			1981		
	Total[a]	Private	Public	Total[a]	Private	Public
Hospital care	13.9	8.5	5.4	118.0	53.9	64.1
Physician services	8.5	7.9	.6	54.8	39.8	15.0
Dentist services	2.8	2.8		17.3	16.6	.7
Drug/drug sundries	5.2	5.0	.2	21.4	19.5	1.9
All other	11.3	6.7	4.6	75.1	34.3	40.8
Total	41.7	30.9	10.8	286.6	164.1	122.5

Sources: Robert Gibson and Daniel Waldo, "National Health Expenditures, 1980," *Health Care Financing Review* 3 (September 1981): 20–30, Table 2; U.S. Department of Health and Human Services, *HHS News* (newsletter dated July 26, 1982), Table II.

[a]The individual categories may not add up to their totals because of rounding.

33

$122.5 billion in 1981. Of the $122.5 billion, 52 percent went for hospital services—a $59 billion increase over 1965. The largest portion of this increase can be attributed to Medicare and Medicaid payments for personal health care. In 1965, before the introduction of Medicare and Medicaid, government expenditures for personal health care were only 22 percent of total personal health care expenditures, but in 1981, 15 years after the initiation of these two programs, the government share of personal health care expenditures climbed to 43 percent, nearly doubling its 1965 percentage. Private insurance payments also increased during this time period. By 1981, patient payments accounted for only 10.8 percent of the total hospital bill, the remainder of which was paid either by government (54.3 percent) or by private insurance (41.1 percent). As shown in Table 3-2, direct patient payments were smaller for hospital care than for any other medical service. On the average, patients are responsible for 38 percent of expenditures for physician services and 82 percent of expenditures for drugs. As the portion of the hospital bill paid for directly by the patient declines, so does the patient's or physician's incentive to question the prices charged by hospitals.

The patient's use of the hospital is generally believed to be less responsive to the price charged than is the use of most other medical services. The declining portion of the hospital bill for which the patient is responsible, together with the small effect that price has on hospital use, have removed patient and physician incentives to be concerned with how rapidly hospital prices are increasing or with the relative costs of hospitals. Under these circumstances, a more rapid increase in hospital expenditures would be expected. Conversely, a slower rate of increase in expenditures would be expected for medical services whose use is more affected by higher prices and for which patients pay a larger fraction of the bill. These factors are important for understanding the changing composition of medical expenditures.

Over time, as shown in Table 3-3, direct patient payments for all medical services have declined from 52 percent in 1955 to 45 percent in 1965 to 29 percent in 1981. As more of the bill for medical services is paid for by government and private insurance, the influence of price on the patients' use of the service and choice of a provider from whom to purchase that service diminishes. The removal of price incentives from patients and the increase in the ability of providers to pass on higher prices to third-party payors and government have important implications for the performance of the medical care market.

The government's financing of medical services is not uniform for each of the components of medical care; it is most concerned with cost containment in those areas to which it is financially committed. Higher prices for hospital services are of greater financial consequence and therefore of greater concern to the government than are similar price increases for dental services, whose financing is predominantly private.

The sharp increase and change in composition of medical care expenditures indicate a need for a set of economic tools to predict equilibrium situations. To understand why expenditures have increased so rapidly it is necessary to determine why prices and quantities of medical care have been changing. Understanding the reasons for such changes is essential for forecasting and for anticipating the effects of public policy on prices, quantities, and expenditures in each of the medical markets.

TABLE 3-2. Amount and Percentage of Personal[a] Health Care Expenditures Met by Third Parties, by Type of Expenditure, Calendar Year 1981 (in Billions of Dollars)

Type of Expenditure	Total[b]	Direct Payments	Third Party Payments							
			Total[b]	Private Health Insurance	Government Expenditures					
					Total[b]	Federal			State	Other[e]
						Medicare	Medicaid	Other[d]		
Total	255.0	81.7	173.2	66.8	102.9	43.5	16.4	14.7	28.3	3.5
Hospital care	118.0	12.8	105.2	39.4	64.1	31.4	5.9	11.3	15.4	1.7
Physicians' services	54.8	20.8	34.0	19.0	15.0	9.6	1.5	.5	3.3	
Dentists' services	17.3	12.3	5.0	4.3	.7		.3	.1	.3	
Drug/drug sundries	21.4	17.1	4.3	2.4	1.9		.9		.9	
All other services[c]	43.5	18.7	24.7	1.7	21.2	2.5	7.8	2.8	8.4	1.8
				Percentage Distribution						
Total	100.0	32.0	67.9	26.2	40.4	17.1	6.4	5.8	11.0	1.4
Hospital care	100.0	10.8	89.2	33.4	54.3	26.6	5.0	9.6	13.1	1.4
Physicians' services	100.0	38.0	62.0	34.7	24.4	17.5	2.7	.9	6.0	
Dentists' services	100.0	71.1	28.9	24.9	4.0		1.7	.6	1.7	
Drug/drug sundries	100.0	79.9	20.1	11.2	8.9		4.2		4.2	
All other services[c]	100.0	43.0	56.8	3.9	48.7	5.7	17.9	6.4	19.3	4.1

Source: U.S. Department of Health and Human Services, *HHS News* (newsletter dated July 26, 1982): Table III.

[a]Excludes expenses for prepayment and administration, government public health activities, and research and medical facilities construction.

[b]The various categories may not add up to their totals because of rounding.

[c]Includes other professional services, eyeglasses and appliances, nursing home care, and other health services.

[d]Includes expenditures for maternal and child health programs, vocational rehabilitation programs, temporary disability insurance, Public Health Service activities, Indian Health Service programs, workers compensation programs, Veterans Administration Services, and Alcohol, Drug Abuse and Mental Health Administration programs.

[e]Includes expenditure for industrial in-plant health services and contributions from private philanthropic organizations.

TABLE 3-3. Percentage Distribution by Source of Expenditures for Medical Care in the United States, 1955, 1960, 1965, 1970, 1975, and 1981

Source	1955[a]	1960[a]	1965	1970	1975	1981
Total						
Amount (billions of dollars)	17.3	25.9	41.7	74.7	132.7	286.6
Percent[b]	100.0	100.0	100.0	100.0	100.0	100.0
Private	74.5	75.3	74.1	62.8	57.6	57.3
Direct payments	51.9	48.6	44.4	34.8	29.4	28.5
Insurance benefits	13.6	18.2	24.0	22.9	24.4	25.5
All other	9.0	8.5	5.8	5.1	3.8	3.2
Public	25.5	24.7	25.9	37.2	42.4	42.7
Federal	11.2	11.3	13.2	23.7	28.0	29.3
State and local	14.3	13.4	12.5	13.5	14.4	13.5

Sources: Barbara S. Cooper, Nancy L. Worthington, and Mary F. McGee, *Compendium of National Health Expenditure Data*, DHEW Publication No. (SSA) 76-11927 (Washington: U.S. Government Printing Office, 1976); Robert Gibson and Daniel Waldo, "National Health Expenditure, 1980," *Health Care Financing Review* 3 (September 1981): 20–31, Table 2; and U.S. Department of Health and Human Services, *HHS News* (newsletter dated July 26, 1982), Table II.

[a]The values for 1955 and 1960 are for fiscal years beginning in July and ending in June. All other figures are for calendar years.

[b]The percentages may not add up to 100 percent because of rounding.

THE INTERRELATIONSHIP OF THE DIFFERENT MEDICAL CARE MARKETS

Medical care, which is the output of the overall medical care market, is, in fact, the outcome of several interrelated markets. These include the markets for registered nurses, hospital services, physician services, and even the market for health professional education. To be able to forecast the effects of a change in government policy on the medical care sector or to determine the effects of a natural change such as an increase in the aged population, it is necessary to have a model of the medical care sector that describes the relationship of various submarkets and components of medical care to each other. The model which follows describes the various submarkets that comprise the medical care sector, demonstrates the way in which these different sectors are interrelated, and illustrates the usefulness of such a framework for forecasting and policy analysis (1). This overview of the medical care sector will also indicate the various subject areas to be covered in this book.

Three types of markets are present in the medical care sector as shown in Figure 3-1. The patient's demand for a medical treatment (for a particular diagnostic category) is expressed by going to a physician whose determination of how to treat him is based on both economic and noneconomic characteristics. The physician's selection of one or more of several institutional settings—hospitals, outpatient facilities, nursing homes, the physician's office, or even home care— is based on the relative prices of each of those settings, the relative costs to the physician, and their efficacy in treatment. The demand for institutional care will depend on patient demand factors, physician considerations, and the relative price and efficacy of treatment in the different institutional settings. These in-

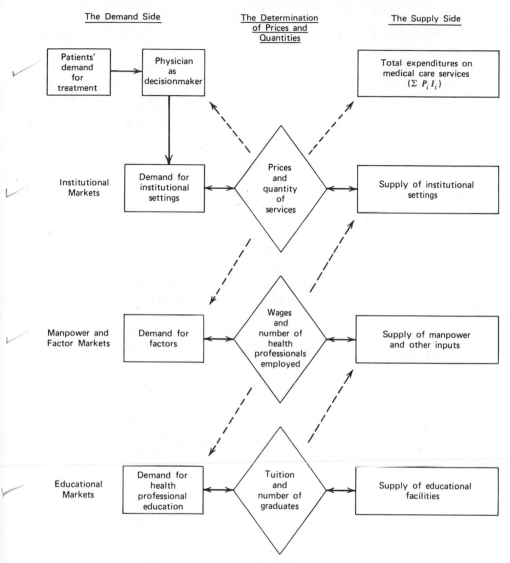

Figure 3-1. An overview of the medical care sector.

stitutional settings may thus be seen both as complements to and substitutes for one another.

A change in the demand for different institutional settings that is the result of, for example, a change in the age of the population, will be reflected in institutional demands for manpower and other factor inputs (e.g., capital and supplies). These comprise the second set of markets to be analyzed. Such institutional demands for manpower and other inputs represent the demand side of the health manpower (and inputs) markets. The demand for a particular health manpower category, for example, will depend upon factors relating to the patient's (and/or their physicians') demand for the institutional settings in which that manpower group is employed, the wages of the group, and the relationship of their wages to those of other health workers.

The demand for an education by prospective health professionals will depend upon the demand for health professionals in the market just described. The demand for a health professional education, which is the amount that a person is willing to pay in terms of tuition and foregone income, is determined by the expected income and wages that might be earned (as determined in the manpower market) and by noneconomic motivating factors.

The supply side of each of these markets works as follows. The supply of health professional educational institutions (in terms, for example, of institutional capacity and faculty) and the demands for such education determine the number of graduates and the tuition rate to be charged. The number of graduates (the time required to educate each category of health manpower will, of course, vary) plus the existing stock of health manpower (less deaths and retirements) comprise the supply of health manpower at any given time. The supply of each category of health manpower in conjunction with the demands for such manpower will determine incomes and wages as well as employment (the participation rate). The outcomes of the health manpower (and other input) markets will affect the supply of services offered in different institutional settings. The cost of providing care in a given institutional setting will rise as the wages for a given manpower group rise and as more members of that manpower category are used to provide care. In each institutional setting, the costs of providing care together with the demands for care will determine how much care is provided; this is the outcome of the institutional markets. Total expenditures for medical care consist, then, of the prices of each institutional setting multiplied by the quantity of care provided in each setting.

To summarize the demand side of each of these separate markets, the demand for institutional care is derived from the initial demands for medical treatments. The demand for health manpower is similarly derived from the demand for institutional care, and the demand for a health professional education is derived from the demand for each health manpower profession. Similarly, the supply of medical services is based upon the availability of the supplies in each of these other markets and upon their costs.

In order to forecast the consequences of change in the demand or supply side of any part of this model, it is necessary to understand how the markets in each of the sectors operate. For example, legal restrictions on the tasks health professionals are permitted to perform affect the demand for different health professionals, the wages they are paid, and, consequently, the price and availability of medical service. Similarly, past subsidies to medical schools that have enabled them to set low tuition levels and establish the number of educational spaces irrespective of the demand for those spaces has affected the availability of physicians, their incomes, and the fees they charge. The performance of each of the separate markets in the medical care sector—the different institutional markets, manpower markets, and educational markets—will influence each of the other markets and the final price and expenditures for medical care. A market in which price is higher and output is less than if it were functioning properly is subject to proposals for improving its performance.

APPLICATIONS OF A MODEL
OF THE MEDICAL CARE SECTOR

The effects of alternative public policies on the final market—that is, on the price and availability of medical services—can be predicted on the basis of an understanding of the different medical care markets and their interrelationships.

Our ability to forecast the likely consequences of changes in demand or supply conditions in medical care also requires an accurate overview of the medical care sector. Figure 3-2 describes the same markets discussed above by means of a different set of diagrams, showing each of the separate markets within the institutional, manpower, and educational markets in terms of a traditional supply and demand relationship.

A DEMAND POLICY

As a result of an increase in health insurance in the population, we would expect to observe an increase in the demand for medical care (as would be shown by a shift in demand in Figure 3-2A). How much the demand for medical care will increase will depend, in part, on the importance of price to increased utilization (i.e., the price elasticity of demand for medical care). As a result of an increase in demand, depending upon supply conditions in medical care, we would expect an increase in prices as well as an increase in medical care utilization. To forecast what will happen to prices and utilization for each component of medical care, we must examine how this increase in medical care demand is transmitted to each of the other markets. As a result of lower out-of-pocket prices to consumers for medical care, following greater insurance coverage, the demand for different institutional settings will increase; certain institutional settings will experience a larger increase in demand than others, depending, in part, upon which population groups will increase their demand, what types of medical treatments will be demanded, and how important price is to utilization in each market. As a result of the increased institutional demand, prices in these settings will increase, as will the quantity of services provided. The institutions affected will demand more inputs to supply that increased demand.

Various health professions will therefore experience an increase in demand for their services. Within each health manpower market, the employing institution's demand for a given health profession will be affected by the wages it would have to pay, the relative wages of other manpower groups that may be substituted for them, their relative productivity, the price of the output, and any legal restrictions which may prevent the use of certain personnel in performing specified tasks. With the increase in demand for health manpower and given the existing stock (i.e., currently trained professionals) of that manpower group, wages and the employment rate in each of the health manpower markets will increase. Exactly how much each will increase will depend upon the supply conditions (elasticity) and performance of each health manpower market. The resulting higher incomes will eventually increase the demand for an education leading to entrance into that profession. Thus, lowering an economic barrier to

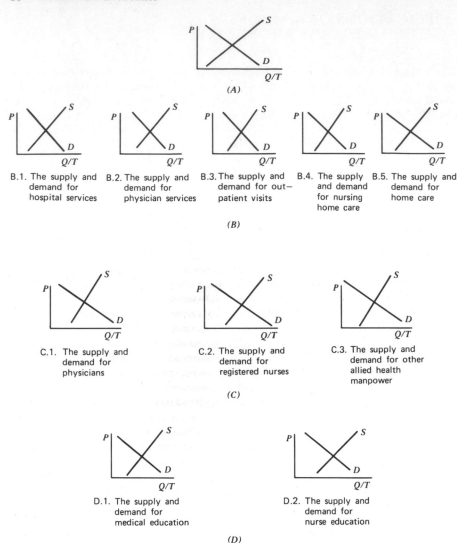

Figure 3-2. An economic model of the medical care sector: (A) the market for medical care services, (B) the markets for institutional services, (C) the markets for health manpower, (D) the markets for health professional education.

the use of medical care services by providing health insurance has increased demand for different institutional settings, manpower professions, and a health professional education.

The demand increases in each of the different markets will be followed by increases in prices as well as output. The size of the price and output increases in each market resulting from that initial increase in demand will depend upon the size of the demand increase and the responsiveness of supply (supply elasticity) within each market. The less elastic supply is, the greater the price increase and

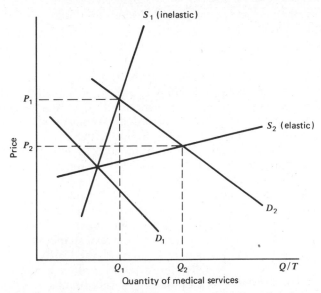

Figure 3-3. The effect on prices and medical services of an increase in demand when there are different supply elasticities.

the smaller the increase in output will be. It is precisely because of this effect on prices and output that an analysis of the efficiency of the supply side of each of the medical care markets becomes so important. If the supply side of the market is relatively inelastic—that is, if it takes a relatively large price increase to bring about an increase in output—then demand programs will result in large price increases and small output increases; consequently, it will cost a great deal of money to achieve an increase in output. For example, according to Figure 3-3, an increase in demand will affect prices and quantity of services differently, depending upon the elasticity of supply. If supply is relatively elastic (S_2), then an increase in demand, from D_1 to D_2, will be accompanied by a price increase, but it will be much less (P_2) than if supply were inelastic (S_1), in which case the new price would be (P_1). Similarly, a much greater increase in services provided will occur under conditions of elastic supply (Q_2 versus Q_1). If the increase in demand were to occur as a result of a government subsidy program, and if supply were inelastic (S_1), the increased government expenditures for that program would pay for higher prices (P_1) and less output (Q_1) than it would if supply were more elastic (S_2).

It is thus important to understand what the supply elasticity is for each of the medical care markets. If markets with relatively inelastic supply can be made more elastic, the potential benefits in terms of lower prices and increased output can be very great. Therefore we shall examine each of the medical care markets in terms of economic efficiency to determine how well each performs. We shall ask, how does each of these markets respond to changes in demand? Could their prices be lower and outputs greater if changes were made in their structure? By examining each of the medical care markets in terms of structure and performance, we can determine whether the efficiency of those markets can be improved and what mechanisms will be most useful for improving economic performance.

A SUPPLY POLICY

Such a model of the medical care sector is also useful in explaining how a supply subsidy might work. Typical governmental supply subsidies provide funds to educational institutions for increasing the number of health professionals. Such programs cause a shift to the right in the supply of the educational institutions and increase the schools' capacity for enrollments. The effect is to increase the number of graduates in the educational market. As the number of graduates (e.g., physicians or nurses) increases and the supply of those particular health professionals in the health manpower market shifts to the right, the wages or incomes of the subsidized health professionals become lower than they might otherwise have been. The larger number of health professionals (those that were subsidized) and their relatively lower wages will result in an increase in demand for them in the institutional market (a movement down the institutions' demand for such personnel); since they will be substituted for other health professionals whose wages and numbers were not affected by supply subsidies. The effect on the institutional sector will be a shift to the right in their supply curve, since they can presumably produce the same quantity of services at a lower price (or a greater quantity of services at the same price). This is because the price of one of their inputs has been reduced as a result of the subsidy. Institutions will be affected differently by such a subsidy, since some institutions use relatively more of the subsidized input (e.g., hospitals use relatively more registered nurses) than others. The subsidy program's overall effect on the final price and quantity of medical care will vary, depending upon how much of an increase in the input occurs as a result of that supply subsidy, how much of a decrease in the price of that input occurs, how much of that subsidized input is used in the production of medical care, and so on.

A completely specified model of the medical care sector should enable us to trace the effects of a supply subsidy program throughout each of the different medical care markets. We can then compare several supply subsidy programs on the basis of what it costs them to achieve a change in the final price and quantity of medical care services. Thus such a model of the medical care sector allows us to compare alternative government supply subsidies, each of which is designed to increase the availability of medical care. Such subsidy programs need not be directed solely at a manpower category; they may be directed at any number of inputs, such as lesser-trained personnel who increase the productivity of more highly trained professionals, or they may provide subsidies for hospital construction. An overall model of medical care thus allows any number of supply subsidy programs to be evaluated on the basis of the cost of the subsidy and its final effect on the price and availability of medical care.

CONCLUDING COMMENTS

The model of the medical care sector just described also serves to enumerate the different subject areas of this book. To understand the medical care sector it is

necessary to learn about the theory of demand for medical care and the consequent derived demands within each of the other markets. In the demand section,
as in all other sections, the theoretical discussion of demand will be followed by
a review of studies that have attempted to estimate the theoretical variables
discussed; the review will be followed by a summary of empirical estimates of
the factors that affect demand.

After explaining the demand side of the medical care sector we will examine
the supply side of the different markets. In this way we hope to be able to judge
the efficiency of each of the different medical care markets: hospital services,
physician services, the market for physicians, the market for registered nurses,
and the market for medical education. In addition to judging the efficiency of
each of these markets, we will evaluate the relevant government policies that
have an impact on these separate markets, such as the Hill-Burton program for
hospitals and health manpower legislation in the manpower markets. Lastly, we
will make public policy recommendations for improving efficiency within each
of these markets, based upon our analysis of their inadequate market performance.

This overview of medical care will also be used to discuss alternative approaches to its redistribution. Even though inefficiencies continue to exist in the
medical care market, society may decide to increase the consumption of medical
care to the population or to selected population groups. Such an overview suggests that it is possible to achieve an increase in consumption of medical care
services either by shifting the demands for care or by increasing the quantity of a
particular input on the supply side—i.e., shifting supply. Each of these policies
will result in an increase in the quantity of medical care services consumed, as
shown in Figure 3-4. For example, to increase the quantity of medical services
consumed from Q_0 to Q_1 (based upon a normative judgement that it is desirable
to do so), either the demand for medical care can be increased from D_1 to D_2, or
the supply can be increased from S_1 to S_2. Either of these policies will achieve

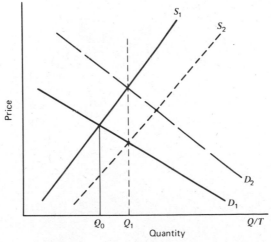

Figure 3-4. Alternative demand and supply policies to achieve a redistribution of medical
care.

the objective of increasing the use of medical care from Q_0 to Q_1. However, these different redistributive policies will differ in their costs and their effects on other population groups.

Public policies designed to redistribute care by means of supply subsidies will be analyzed in each of the sections devoted to particular markets. The last chapters in this book will analyze various demand subsidy programs, such as proposals for national health insurance.

The overview presented here illustrates why medical care is said to be the output of the medical care sector. The efficiency of the separate markets and their interrelationship affects the efficiency with which medical care is produced, the cost at which it is produced, and the growth of expenditures in this sector. The evaluation of the efficiency of each of these markets is, therefore, of prime concern for public policy.

The foregoing model of medical care also illustrates the alternative approaches that may be used to redistribute medical services and the means for evaluating them. These two concepts, efficiency and redistribution (equity), will be the basis upon which both the separate markets and government policies will be analyzed throughout this book.

REFERENCES

1. The description of the medical care sector in this section is based upon an article by Paul J. Feldstein and Sander Kelman, "An Econometric Model of the Medical Care Sector," in H. Klarman, Ed., *Empirical Studies in Health Economics* (Baltimore: Johns Hopkins University Press, 1970). Economists have developed other econometric models of the medical care sector. Perhaps the most ambitious of these is the one by D.E. Yett, L. Drabek, M.D. Intriligator, and L.J. Kimbell, *A Forecasting and Policy Simulation Model of the Health Care Sector* (Lexington, Mass.: Lexington Books, 1979).

CHAPTER 4

Measuring Changes in the Price of Medical Care

THE USES OF A DEFINITION OF THE PRODUCT OF THE MEDICAL CARE INDUSTRY

How has the price of medical care changed over time? Under what systems of reimbursement and what kinds of institutional arrangements is medical care produced most efficiently? What factors account for the differences in utilization of medical care among individuals and over time? These questions define major areas of research in the economics of medical care. They are of interest to policy-makers as well, given the current public concern with rising medical costs and inefficiencies and inequities in the production and distribution of medical care. In order to answer any of these questions, we must define the product of the medical care industry implicitly if not explicitly. Any discussion of medical care prices presupposes some choice of units. Similarly, any comparison of the productive efficiency of two medical care providers presupposes some standard for measuring their outputs.

The units in which medical care is traditionally measured, such as the different items that appear on a patient's bill after a stay in the hospital, are far from ideal indicators of health costs and efficiency. Some of them are not really homogeneous measures of anything. Exactly what a hospital patient purchases for the daily room charge, for instance, may vary with diagnosis, choice of hospital, and most certainly will vary over time. But more importantly, the traditional units used for payment purposes do not seem to be true units of output, if we define output as that which yields satisfaction or utility to consumers. The physician's visit, the hospital bed day, the diagnostic test, and the prescription drug are perhaps more properly viewed as inputs into the production of medical care than as final outputs themselves. After all, the typical consumer of medical care does not set out to purchase a specific bundle of services. From the patient's point of view, the demand for medical care is ordinarily the demand for a treatment for some perceived physical or mental disorder. After the patient consults a physician, a treatment is prescribed that often uses various inputs in combination.

If it were feasible, it would be more useful to measure the costs or prices of medical care in terms of final outputs rather than in terms of the inputs to the treatment process. Such an approach would reflect the effects on medical costs both of increases and decreases in input productivity and of technological advances. Similarly, efficiency studies and policies designed to promote efficiency ought to focus more on efficiently satisfying consumers' medical needs and wants than on the efficient production of particular medical inputs. When it is possible to substitute less costly inputs for more costly ones, without changing the treatment outcome—such as treating patients with relatively simple cases on an ambulatory rather than an inpatient basis, or using nursing home care or the services of a visiting nurse in place of the last few days of a hospital stay—such substitutions ought to be encouraged.

Viewing medical goods and services as inputs in the production of care is also useful in studying medical care utilization. For purposes such as manpower planning and investment in hospitals, it is important to forecast the utilization of particular components of medical care. Looking at these different segments of the industry as suppliers of inputs emphasizes their interrelationship. The availability and price of hospital services is likely to influence, and in turn be influenced by, the utilization of outpatient or ambulatory services and long-term care. Ideally, of course, equity in medical care should be defined by how well individuals' medical needs are met rather than by the number of physicians' visits or hospital days consumed by different segments of the population.

A measure of the output produced by the medical care industry could also be used to measure the price of medical care over time, to evaluate the efficiency of alternative methods of delivering medical care, and to explain variations in the use of specific medical services; however, medical economics has not yet satisfactorily devised such a measure. The word health is inevitably used to describe the output of the medical industry, but health, which is itself a difficult concept to measure, is not determined solely or even primarily by medical care consumption. The health of a population is not really a fair measure of the success of its medical care system.

Some have suggested that treatment ought to be considered the unit of output, since individuals ordinarily seek medical care in order to obtain treatment for actual or perceived, current or potential illnesses. Total output would then be a weighted sum of the number of cases of different types treated. In this way, we could make meaningful comparisons of the cost of medical care over time and could assess the relative efficiency of different medical care providers.

There are, however, several difficulties in measuring medical care output by the number of treatments. Because the quality of treatments of particular conditions may vary, institutions providing high-quality care at high unit costs might be automatically judged to be inefficient unless quality is included in the output measurements. Though not part of the treatment of existing illnesses, preventive care can affect the likelihood of future illnesses and the costs of treatment, and therefore should somehow also be included in an output measure. Although such problems have yet to be resolved, treatment is a better indicator of medical output than are the specific goods and services by which it is usually measured;

as it indicates both the interrelationships within medical care and how reimbursement policies for its improvement should be designed.

The rest of this chapter analyzes the measurement of prices, particularly in the field of medical care, beginning with a description of the functions and limitations of the Consumer Price Index (CPI). This is followed by a detailed discussion of the medical care component of the CPI, which is still the most widely used index of medical care prices. The final section describes and evaluates another approach to measuring the price of medical care—one which is based on the use of medical treatment as the most appropriate unit of medical care output.

THE CONSUMER PRICE INDEX

WHAT SHOULD THE CPI MEASURE?

The CPI is generally viewed as an index of the cost of living. The percentage change in the Index from one year to the next is taken as a measure of the rate of inflation—that is, of the rate at which a family's income would have had to increase just to keep up with rising prices. Many union contracts contain provisions for automatically increasing wages in line with increases in the CPI. Social security benefit levels are now keyed to it as well, as are the pensions of retired federal employees. In all, the incomes of about half of the U.S. population are directly affected by changes in the CPI. By 1980, a 1 percent change in the CPI was triggering an increase in payments under these various escalation provisions of at least $2 billion. Besides these direct effects on the economy, the CPI is viewed by makers of monetary and fiscal policy as an important indicator of the nation's inflation rate. It is also frequently used in social science research to deflate time series of money values, such as the average wage in a particular occupation over a period of years, and to express them in constant dollars.

These are some of the most prominent uses to which the CPI is put, but they don't exactly define what it is. The Bureau of Labor Statistics (BLS) calculates the Index in an attempt to measure changes in the price of that bundle of goods and services which was purchased on the average by members of a well-defined

---

*It can be expressed by the following formula:

$$I_t = \frac{\Sigma_i Q_{bi} P_{ti}}{\Sigma_i Q_{bi} P_{bi}}$$

where I_t = the value of the index in year t
Q_{bi} = the quantity of good i purchased in the base year
P_{bi} = the price of good i in the base year
P_{ti} = the price of good i in the year t

Such an index is often multiplied by some scaling factor so that it equals 100 in some particular year. Of course, if the index is multiplied by the same scaling factor in each year, percentage changes from year to year are not affected.

segment of the American population in a certain base year. A price index of this type, in which individual prices are weighted by base-year quantities, is called a Laspeyres index.* Thus, the CPI aims to measure how much the average household in its surveyed population will have to spend in order to buy the same market basket in the current year it bought in the base year. At first glance this might seem to be a logical measure of the change in the cost of living.

For several reasons, however, pricing a fixed market basket is not quite the same thing as measuring the cost of living. For one thing, the additional income required to purchase the base-year market basket in a later year will generally exceed the increase necessary to buy a market basket that is *equivalent in the eyes of the consumer* to that purchased in the base year. This is because consumers will substitute away from those items for which price is rising most rapidly and thus will lessen, to some extent, the impact of the general price increase.* If the price of beef rises particularly rapidly, for example, consumers will tend to buy less beef and more pork, chicken, or other meats.

More fundamentally, one may ask what a true cost-of-living index ought to measure. Economists often speak of a cost-of-living index as a measure of the cost of maintaining a given level of welfare or utility, of remaining on a certain indifference curve. If we take this point of view, the cost of living is influenced by much more than the prices of goods and services that consumers buy. Tax rates influence the amount of gross income needed to maintain a certain level of welfare. Taxes which directly influence the prices of products, such as sales taxes, are reflected in the index; income taxes are not. On the other hand, governmental provision of more free-of-charge services, such as better highways or better public schools, may increase the standard of living achievable at any level of income. One might argue that standards of living are also affected by changes in crime rates, environmental pollution, and other such factors essentially beyond the individual's control. It is not necessarily true that a household is better off when its gross income increases faster than the prices of the goods and services it buys (1).

Aware of the difficulty of measuring the cost of maintaining a level of welfare, the BLS attempts the more modest task of measuring the price of a fixed bundle of goods and services. Even this job, however, is not simple. The market basket purchased by the average household in the surveyed population is constantly changing, not only in response to price changes, but also in response to changes in incomes, tastes, and other factors as well. The quality of existing goods and services changes, and new products that had no counterparts in the past are introduced. It would be meaningless to go on pricing the same goods and services without making an allowance for these changes. In the succeeding section, we will discuss how the BLS resolves some of the major issues involved

---

*An index which used current-year quantities as weights would understate cost-of-living increases because it would put too much weight on items whose prices had increased relatively slowly. Such an index is called a Paasche index. Clearly, some sort of average of a Laspeyres and Paasche index will yield a better measure of cost-of-living changes than either one individually. The Laspeyres formula is used primarily because of the high cost of continually collecting information on weights. For a good discussion of index-number theory, see Kenneth Arrow, "The Measurement of Price Changes," in *The Relationship of Prices to Economic Stability and Growth,* Compendium of papers submitted by panelists appearing before the U.S. Congress Joint Economic Committee, March 31, 1958, pp. 77–87.

in constructing the CPI, and what the effects of these decisions on the performance of the index are likely to be.

ISSUES AND PROBLEMS IN CONSTRUCTING THE CPI

Population Coverage

The CPI has traditionally been designed with urban wage earners and clerical workers in mind, but the precise definition of the covered population has changed over time (2). Until 1964, only families were included. At that time, single persons were added and the stipulation that household income should be less than $10,000 was dropped. After the 1964 revision of the CPI, its coverage included about 45 percent of the total U.S. population.

In the latest revision, the results of which were incorporated in the published CPI in January 1978, the BLS has expanded the Index population to include all urban households in Standard Metropolitan Statistical Areas (SMSA) (3). This represents an addition of salaried and self-employed workers not previously included, the unemployed, and those not in the labor force (including retired people). Population coverage now includes about 80 percent of the total noninstitutional population. A separate index for wage earners and clerical workers has been continued. Because it claims that the more comprehensive index will rise more slowly than the traditional CPI, organized labor has supported the continued use of the traditional index in contract escalation provisions (4).

Sampling Problems

Although it currently makes greater use of them, the BLS has not always used probability sampling techniques in constructing the CPI. Several aspects of their sampling methodology may bias the Index (5). The BLS assigns weights to different items in the CPI based on data from periodic consumer expenditure surveys.* The major criticism of these surveys has been that, at 10-year intervals, they are not conducted frequently enough. The BLS's weighting system was, until very recently, still based on 1960–1961 information rather than on data from the 1972–1973 survey.

Table 4-1 indicates changes in the relative weights of major groups of items over the years. The years 1935–1939, 1952, 1963, and 1981 were chosen because they correspond to major revisions in the CPI growing out of new consumer expenditure surveys. The December 1981 weights are based on the 1972–1973 survey, and were first incorporated in the CPI in January 1978. It is interesting to note the similarity between the importance of the different components of the CPI for All Urban Consumers and the CPI for Urban Wage Earners and Clerical Workers. The similar weights indicate that the expenditure patterns of the two groups are relatively similar. This is expected since urban wage earners and clerical workers represent a large portion of urban consumers.

---

*The national CPI is built up from indexes calculated for a sample of cities. Separate city indexes are published. Differences between city indexes, however, do not measure price differences, but only differences in price *changes* between cities and over time for each city.

TABLE 4-1. Relative Importance of Major Components of the CPI, Selected Years (%)

Group	1935–1939	December 1952	December 1963	December 1981 CPI-U	December 1981 CPI-W
All items	100.0	100.0	100.0	100.0	100.0
Food and beverages	35.4	32.2	25.2	17.5	19.1
Housing	33.7	33.5	34.0	46.0	42.7
Apparel and upkeep	11.0	9.4	10.6	4.6	4.6
Transportation	8.1	11.3	14.0	19.3	21.8
Medical care	4.1	4.8	5.7	4.9	4.4
Entertainment[a]	2.8	4.0	3.9	3.6	3.4
Other goods and services[b]	4.9	4.8	5.7	4.0	4.0

Source: U.S. Department of Labor, Bureau of Labor Statistics, *Handbook of Labor Statistics*, 1980 (Washington, D.C.: U.S. Government Printing Office), p. 331; and *CPI Detailed Report*, 1982, pp. 10–11, Table 1, and pp. 31–32, Table 7.

[a]Called "Reading and Recreation" before December 1977.

[b]Includes "Personal Care," usually shown separately before December 1977.

The most striking trend in Table 4-1 is the decline in importance of food in consumer budgets. Its weight in total expenditures has fallen considerably despite the fact that, as Table 4-2 shows, its price has risen faster than the all-items index. The decline in the importance of food in consumer budgets probably reflects low income elasticity rather than high price elasticity. As per capita incomes have grown, a smaller fraction of them has been used to buy food. According to Table 4-1, the transportation component of expenditures has increased in relation to the food component as the latter has become less important. Food and housing remain, however, the most important elements in consumer budgets, together accounting for well over half of expenditures on the average.

Price data cannot be gathered on every purchased item represented in the consumer expenditure surveys. The CPI classifies goods and services into successively smaller subgroups, down to what is referred to as an expenditure class (EC), of which there are currently 68 (6). The EC is further subdivided into groups known as item strata. Finally, the item strata are divided into categories called entry level items. An example of an entry level item is a color television set. However, since there are many different models of color TV sets, the exact model to be priced is determined through a process which involves probability sampling, which was a change introduced in the latest CPI revision. The assumption is that the other items in the EC are changing in price, on the average, at the same rate as the item or items actually priced.

It is less expensive to collect price information from sellers rather than from consumers. But this introduces another sampling problem: from what outlets should price information be gathered? In this area, as well as for subcategories within an expenditure category, little attempt was made to apply probability sampling prior to the latest revision. A major difficulty was the absence of data on the outlets from which consumers purchased goods and services. Currently, a

Point-of-Purchase Survey is used to aid in choosing "price reporters" on a probability basis.

The Point-of-Purchase Survey and store-specific pricing, because they have introduced probability sampling to the CPI, have increased the likelihood that the prices used in determining the CPI represent the actual distribution of prices in the market. However, there is still the problem of outdated weights. Up until 1978 the weights for the CPI were based on the 15-year-old, 1962–1963 Consumer Expenditure Survey. Even the latest weights, which were first introduced in the 1978 CPI, were not current at their time of introduction. They were based on a survey that was already five years old. These outdated weights, because of the substitution effect, may lead to an upward bias, as has already been explained. To monitor and possibly correct any biases in the current weights, BLS has maintained continuing consumer expenditure and Point-of-Purchase Surveys, which are much smaller versions of the 1972–1973 surveys. These surveys may eventually lead to a more timely and inexpensive means of updating the CPI weights.

Quality Changes and New Products

As stated above, the BLS regards the CPI not as a true cost-of-living index, but as a price index for a bundle of goods and services. Even as an indicator of the rate of price increase in the economy, however, the contents of the bundle must be kept up to date with actual consumer purchases. For this purpose price changes that directly result from changes in product quality should be omitted from the index. For example, if a color television is substituted for a black-and-white one, the index should not reflect the full price difference between the two, since most of it will be due to product quality differences. Substitutions of new for old items are normally accomplished by linking. When the substitution is made, both the old and the new market baskets are priced. Percentage changes in the index prior to the link reflect percentage changes in the price of the old market basket; percentage changes after the link reflect percentage changes in the price of the new market basket. Thus, the price difference between the two market baskets at the time of the link is not reflected at all in the index.*

In many cases linking appears to be a good method of changing the CPI

---

*The following is a simple hypothetical example of linking. Suppose an EC has been represented by one item, black-and-white TV sets, and a decision has been made to price color sets instead. Let us say that the index for this EC was equal to 100 in year 1. The price of black-and-white sets rises from $150 to $165, from year 1 to year 2, which is an increase of 10 percent. The index, still based on black-and-white sets, rises to 110. At that point the link is made. Color sets go from $400 to $420, from year 2 to year 3, a 5 percent increase. The index, now based on the prices of color sets, increases 5 percent to 115.5 in year 3. The $235 difference between the prices of color and black-and-white sets in year 2 never shows up in the index at all.

An Example of Linking

Year	B & W TV Sets	Index	Color TV Sets
1	$150	100	—
2	$165	110	$400
3	—	115.5	$420

market basket. If the link is made at a time when one product is beginning to replace another in the market, but both are available and are purchased by some consumers, then the higher-priced one is worth the difference in price. The BLS has been criticized primarily for introducing new items too slowly (7); introductions occur at major revisions and when old items go off the market entirely. Based on the following description of events, it has been argued that the reluctance to introduce the new products imparts an upward bias on the CPI. Initially, a new item tends to have a relatively high price. This price falls as production expands, and an increase in the number of producers leads to greater price competition. Then, as newer products come to replace it in the market, its relative price may rise as the scale of production contracts. If consumers accept a new item while its price is relatively high, and if the item is absent from the index until after its price has fallen, then the index will fail to register that fall in price of an item already important in consumer budgets. This problem occurs, as will be discussed, with the introduction of new drugs.

A change in the quality of an existing product is similar in conception to the introduction of a new product. A problem arises, however, in the attempt to separate price change from quality change when an improved model of a commodity such as an automobile or refrigerator replaces the older model on the market. In practice, the BLS usually adopts one extreme measure or the other: in cases where price changes occur simultaneously with quality changes, it ignores the quality change or the price change entirely (8). In the latter case, the quality improved product is in effect treated as a new product and linked into the index in place of the old one.*

Table 4-2 presents values for the CPI and its major component groups during the 1935–1981 period. Since all the component indexes are scaled to equal 100 in 1967, those with the smallest values in 1935 increased the fastest over the 1935–1967 period. In 1982 BLS plans to change the base year to 1977, which means 1977 would then equal 100. The major component groups with the highest values in 1980 have increased the fastest since 1967. A one-point increase in an index is, of course, a smaller percentage increase today than it was in 1935. Table 4-2 shows that the indexes for the different major groups have had quite different patterns of increase over the years. Over the period as a whole, food and medical care have risen most rapidly, while each of the other indexes has increased more slowly than the all-items index.

---

*The issue of adjusting for quality changes in a price index has received a great deal of attention from economists and statisticians. One proposed method for making such adjustments is the so-called hedonic technique. It can be applied to products for which many types are available at any one time; automobiles are perhaps the best examples. Data are collected on the prices and characteristics of a number of different models at a point in time. Regression analysis is then used to estimate the contributions of different characteristics (in the case of the automobile, horsepower, fuel economy, interior room) to price. We can use this information to estimate what current models would have cost in the base year, based on their characteristics. The differences between these prices and the current-year prices would be estimates of the pure price changes. To date, this method has not been applied by the BLS. For a more complete discussion of this area see John Muellbauer, "Household Production Theory, Quality, and the Hedonic Technique," *American Economic Review* 64 (December 1974): 977–994, and Zvi Griliches, "Hedonic Price Indexes for Automobiles: An Econometric Analysis of Quality Change," in *The Price Statistics of the Federal Government*, Cambridge, Mass.: National Bureau of Economic Research, pp. 173–196.

TABLE 4-2. CPI and Major Groups, 1935–1981 (1967 = 100)[b]

Year	All Items	Food	Housing	Apparel and Upkeep	Transportation	Medical Care	Personal Care[d]	Entertainment[c]	Other[d]
1935	41.1	36.5	49.3	40.8	42.6	36.1	36.9	41.8	44.8
1945	53.9	50.7	59.1	61.7	47.8	42.1	55.1	62.4	56.9
1955	80.2	81.6	82.3	84.1	77.4	64.8	77.9	76.7	79.8
1965	94.5	94.4	94.9	93.7	95.9	89.5	95.2	95.9	94.2
1970	116.3	114.9	118.9	116.1	112.7	120.6	113.2	113.4	116.0
1972	125.3	123.5	129.2	122.3	119.9	132.5	119.8	122.8	125.5
1974	147.4	161.7	150.6	136.2	137.7	150.5	137.3	133.8	137.2
1976	170.5	180.8	177.2	147.6	165.5	184.7	160.5	151.2	153.5
1977	181.5	192.2	189.6	154.2	177.2	202.4	170.9	157.9	159.2
1978[a]	195.4	211.4	202.8	159.6	185.5	219.4	182.0	176.6	183.3
1979[a]	217.4	234.5	227.6	166.6	212.0	239.7	195.8	188.5	196.7
1980[a]	246.8	254.6	263.3	178.4	249.7	265.9	213.1	205.3	214.5
1981[a]	272.4	274.6	293.5	186.9	280.0	294.5	232.0	221.4	235.7

Sources: U.S. Department of Labor, Bureau of Labor Statistics, *Handbook of Labor Statistics, 1975–1980; CPI Detailed Report*, various issues. (Washington, D.C.: U.S. Government Printing Office.)

[a]CPI for All Urban Consumers.

[b]The 1978 revision brought about several definitional changes, which have made it impossible to directly link pre- and post-1978 indexes for "Entertainment" and "Other."

[c]"Entertainment includes most of what was called "Reading and Recreation." Entertainment excludes certain subcomponents found in "Reading and Recreation," such as TV and sound equipment, and TV repair and educational expenses.

[d]"Other" now includes educational and "Personal Care" expenses, which were previously found under other categories; it no longer includes alcoholic beverages.

53

THE MEDICAL CARE COMPONENT OF THE CPI (MCPI)

BACKGROUND ON THE MCPI

In 1981, medical care had a weight of 4.7 percent in the CPI, down from 6.4 percent in 1975. An increase of about 21.3 percent in the MCPI would, in and of itself, increase the CPI by 1 percent. Through its effect on the overall CPI, the MCPI influences not only wages and other payments to a large fraction of the population, but also public perceptions of the inflation rate in the economy. As the only major index of medical care prices, it is often cited as a measure of inflation in that sector.

The BLS views the MCPI, like the CPI, as an index of the price of a fixed bundle of goods and services. Periodic consumer expenditure surveys, the basic source of information for determining the CPI weights, provide information on the weights of particular items in the medical market basket of the relevant population; it is the movement in the price of this basket that the MCPI attempts to trace. Our discussion will center on how well this objective is carried out in practice, and on how well the MCPI approximates an index of the price of medical care.

Table 4-3 presents an overview of movements in the MCPI and its component items since 1940. A glance at the table reveals that the "Medical Services" category has increased much more rapidly than the "Medical Care Commodities" category. More specifically, while the "Professional Service" items have increased at roughly the same rate as the overall MCPI, "Hospital and other Medical Services," especially the "Hospital Room Rate," has increased much more rapidly.

Table 4-4 gives a breakdown of the relative weights of the items included in the MCPI as of December 1981. These weights are based on the 1972–1973 Consumer Expenditure Survey data on quantities of medical goods and services consumed, updated to 1981 prices. Notice once again that the weights for the All Urban Consumer Index and the Wage Earners and Clerical Workers Index are very similar. The significance of this similarity will become apparent in the next section.

CONSTRUCTING THE MCPI

Population Coverage

The population covered by the MCPI and the overall CPI is, of course, the same. Their traditional focus on urban wage earners and clerical workers has some important implications. Since at least one excluded group—the elderly—consumes large amounts of medical care relative to income, the weight assigned to medical care in the traditional CPI understates its importance in total consumption for the entire population. Within the MCPI itself, the relative weights of particular services are also different from the relative weights of those items in total U.S. medical care consumption. Hospital services, for example, are relatively more important for the elderly and unemployed than for urban wage earn-

TABLE 4-3. Trends in the MCPI, Selected Years, 1940–1981 (1967 = 100 unless noted)

Item	1940	1950	1960	1965	1970	1971	1972	1973	1974	1975	1976	1977	1978	1979	1980	1981
Medical care	36.8	53.7	79.1	89.5	120.6	128.4	132.5	137.7	150.5	168.6	184.7	202.4	219.4	239.7	265.9	294.5
Medical care commodities[a]	70.8	88.5	104.5	100.2	103.6	105.4	105.6	105.9	109.6	118.8	126.0	134.1	143.5	153.8	168.1	186.5
Prescription drugs	66.2	92.6	115.3	102.0	101.2	101.3	100.9	100.5	102.9	109.3	115.2	122.1	131.6	141.8	154.8	172.5
Nonprescription drugs and medical supplies (1977 = 100)[b]													103.6	110.5	120.9	133.6
Over-the-counter items[b]					106.2	110.2	111.3	112.4	117.5	130.1	138.9	148.5				
Medical care services	32.5	49.2	74.9	87.3	124.2	133.3	138.2	144.3	159.1	179.1	197.1	216.7	235.4	258.3	287.4	318.2
Professional services													208.8	226.8	252.0	277.9
Physicians' services	39.6	55.2	77.0	88.3	121.4	129.8	133.8	138.2	150.9	169.4	188.5	206.0	223.1	243.6	269.3	299.0
Dentists' services	42.0	63.9	82.1	92.2	119.4	127.0	132.3	136.4	146.8	161.9	172.2	185.1	198.1	214.8	240.2	263.3
Other professional services (1977 = 100)													104.0	111.1	123.6	135.2
Examination, prescription, and dispensing of eyeglasses[c]	58.1	73.5	85.1	92.8	113.5	120.3	124.9	129.5	138.6	149.6	158.9	168.2				
Other medical care services													267.6	296.4	330.1	366.9
Hospital and other medical services (1977 = 100)													106.2	117.6	133.5	152.5
Hospital service charge[d]							102.0	105.6	115.1	132.3	148.7	164.1				
Hospital room	13.7	30.3	57.3	75.9	145.4	163.1	173.9	182.1	201.5	236.1	268.6	299.5	332.4	370.3	418.9	481.1
Other hospital and medical care services (1977 = 100)													105.9	116.8	132.8	151.2

Sources: Department of Labor, Bureau of Labor Statistics, *Handbook of Labor Statistics*, 1975 and 1981 editions: *CPI Detailed Report*, various issues.

Note: The only indexes available prior to 1978 are for urban wage earners and clerical workers. However, the table uses the more comprehensive All Urban Consumer indexes, which were introduced in 1978, for the years 1978–1981.

a"Medical Care Commodities" was introduced as a new category in 1978. It took the place of the category "Drugs and Prescriptions." The index values for "Medical Care Commodities" from 1940 to 1977 are actually for the old "Drugs and Prescriptions" category.

b"Over-the-Counter Items" became part of the broader category "Nonprescription Drugs and Medical Supplies" in 1978.

c"Examination, Prescription, and Dispensing of Eyeglasses" was discontinued in 1978. The examination portion of this category was absorbed by the new category "Other Professional Services."

d"Hospital Service Charge" was replaced by the newly devised and more comprehensive "Hospital and Other Medical Services" category in 1978.

TABLE 4-4. Relative Weights of Items in the MCPI (as of December 1981)

	Weight as of December 1981	
Item	U (%)	W (%)
Medical care	100.0	100.0
Medical care commodities	16.4	16.6
Prescription drugs	7.6	7.0
Nonprescription drugs and medical supplies	8.8	9.6
Medical care services	83.0	83.2
Professional services	39.2	41.7
Physicians' services	19.6	21.7
Dental services	14.4	15.0
Other professional services	4.5	4.5
Other medical care services	43.8	41.5
Hospital and other medical care services	7.8	7.4
Hospital room	3.6	3.5
Other hospital and medical care services	4.1	3.9
Health insurance	36.0	34.0

U = All Urban Consumers Index; W = Wage Earners and Clerical Workers Index.

Source: U.S. Department of Labor, Bureau of Labor Statistics, *Relative Importance of Components in the Consumer Price Index,* 1977, Report 595. (Washington, D.C.: U.S. Government Printing Office.)

Note: The weights in the table are current to December 1981. They are based on the 1977 weights, found in the BLS Report 595, but they have been adjusted for differences in the rates of increase of prices of the MCPI Components with which they correspond.

ers and clerical workers. Dentists' fees are relatively less important. Thus, the MCPI cannot truly be considered a general price index for medical care consumed in the United States, although it is often used as though it were.

Nor will the weight of medical care and the relative weights within the medical care component in the expanded CPI more closely reflect the pattern of medical care consumption in total consumption. As a matter of policy, the BLS does not include changes in income taxes as changes in the cost of living, and it does not include governmental service provided free-of-charge as elements of consumer budgets. In expanding the population coverage of the CPI, the BLS has added groups for whom the government, through Medicare and Medicaid, pays a large portion of their medical care service. In keeping with its general policy, the BLS does not attempt to reflect these governmental expenditures in the CPI weights. The MCPI is not designed as an index of the price of the bundle of medical care services *consumed* by its target population, but of those services *purchased* by it.

The importance of some of these points is illustrated in Tables 4-5 and 4-6. Table 4-5 compares the weights of particular services in the MCPI* with the

---

*The weight given to hospital services includes the portion of the health insurance component representing hospital services. The weight given to physician fees includes the nonhospital services part of the health insurance component.

TABLE 4-5. Relative Weights of Items in MCPI, in Consumer Expenditures on Health Services and Supplies, and in Total National Expenditures on Health Services and Supplies, 1964, 1975, and 1981 (Calendar Years)

	1964			1975			1981		
	MCPI (December 1963) (1)	Consumer Expenditures (2)	Total Expenditures (3)	MCPI (December 1975) (4)	Consumer Expenditures (5)	Total Expenditures (6)	MCPI[a] (December 1981) (7)	Consumer Expenditures (8)	Total Expenditures (9)
Hospital services[b]	17.9	29.4	37.4	28.5	31.7	42.0	27.6	33.6	43.1
Physicians' services	28.1	29.1	23.9	28.5	25.7	20.3	28.6	25.7	20.0
Dentists' services	15.1	10.1	7.8	14.0	10.9	6.7	14.4	10.7	6.3
Medical care commodities (drugs and prescriptions)[c]	20.0	20.8	16.4	12.0	19.3	12.3	16.4	15.8	9.9
Nursing and convalescent homes[b]	0.0	3.0	3.5	0.0	6.0	8.2	<1.0	6.8	8.8

Sources: Robert Gibson, "National Health Expenditures, 1980," *Health Care Financing Review* (September 1981): 20–31, Table 2; R. Hanft, "National Health Expenditures, 1950–65," *Social Security Bulletin* (February 1967): 5; Department of Health and Human Services, *HHS News* (newsletter dated July 26, 1982): 00, Table II; U.S. Department of Labor, Bureau of Labor Statistics, *The Consumer Price Index: History and Techniques*, Bulletin 1517, 1966, p. 47; U.S. Department of Labor, Bureau of Labor Statistics, *Relative Importance of Components in the Consumer Price Index December 1975*, and U.S. Department of Labor, Bureau of Labor Statistics, *Relative Importance of Components in the Consumer Price Index, 1977*, Report 595 (1980) p. 5.

[a]The index for all urban consumers is used.

[b]Because of definitional changes "Hospital Services" does not include the same services in the 1978 revision that it did in the 1964 revision of the MCPI. The 1978 revision made "Hospital Services" a more comprehensive category. Although the room charge is still the major subcomponent, it includes a much broader range of hospital services than the 1964 revision. In addition, it includes other medical care services. These other services comprise only a small fraction of this index. One of the "other services" is Nursing and Convalescent Home Care, which was not included in the MCPI before the 1978 revision.

[c]"Medical Care Commodities" was first reported in 1978. See the footnotes to Table 4-3 for a description of how it has changed from the 1964 to the 1978 revision.

weights of similar services in national expenditures on health services and supplies. The weights are compared for 1964, 1975, and 1981, and the MCPI is compared both with consumer expenditures and with total national expenditures on health services and supplies.

Differences in weights between the MCPI and the Health Care Financing Administrations (HCFA) measures are due, in part, to measurement errors and to differences in category definitions. However, the primary reason for the differences between the MCPI (column 1) and Consumer Expenditures (column 2) is probably the difference in population included. The larger weight for hospital services in Consumer Expenditures reflects the relatively high consumption of such services by the groups excluded from the CPI. Total expenditures (column 3) also includes government expenditures, which are deliberately excluded from the CPI. It is clear that government expenditures for medical care were weighted heavily toward hospital services, increasing the weight for this component in column 3 to exceed even that in column 2. Correspondingly, the weights of dentists' fees and drugs fall as we move across the three columns. Note that nursing home services had no weight in the MCPI prior to the 1978 revision, which is not surprising given that the CPI was limited to wage earners and clerical workers. An index based on the column 2 or 3 weights would have increased faster than the MCPI did in the past decade, since the latter columns give a heavier weight to the rapidly rising hospital component.

The relative importance of items in the MCPI has changed from 1964 to 1975. The weights were still based on 1961–1962 consumer expenditure survey data, but because the prices of different services had changed at different rates, the implied expenditure weights were different in 1975. For example, the weight of hospital services increased considerably, since the prices for these services rose very rapidly. The weight of drugs and prescriptions fell, since their prices rose more slowly than the overall MCPI. Since the 1975 MCPI weights are based on a 15-year-old survey, they may not accurately reflect the breakdown of medical care expenditures by the covered population. The relative quantities of medical goods and services purchased may have changed in the meantime (partly in response to changes in relative prices), causing the true expenditure weights to vary from the MCPI weights. The similarity between columns 4 and 5 is surprising, given the population differences and the fact that column 5 is based on 1975 purchases and column 4 is intended to reflect 1960–1961 purchases at 1975 prices. If the narrowing gap between the hospital services weights in columns 4 and 5 and 1 and 2 reflects substitution away from increasingly expensive hospital services, then the 1975 MCPI weights overstate the percentage of medical care expenditures going for hospital services in the covered population. It may also reflect the increasing government role in financing hospital care for the poor and elderly. As column 6 demonstrates, government involvement in financing medical care is still strongly weighted toward hospital services. The weight for column (7) is based on the 1978 revision. It appears that the pattern that emerged prior to the 1978 revision continued. MCPI weights are not similar to the weights based on HCFA data. "Hospital Services" represents a much higher percentage of consumer and total expenditures when the HCFA data are used.

Table 4-6 demonstrates that the CPI weight of medical care might be different if the index covered the entire population and total consumption rather than consumer purchases. For 1964, 1975, and 1981, the CPI weight of medical care is

TABLE 4-6. Weights of Medical Care in CPI, in Personal Consumption, Plus Government Purchases, 1964, 1975, and 1981 (Calendar Years)

	1964	1975	1981
Weight of medical care in CPI	5.7	6.4	4.9[a]
Weight of consumer expenditure on health services and supplies in personal consumption	6.5	7.2[b]	8.7[b]
Weight of total expenditures on health services and supplies in personal consumption plus government purchases	6.5	9.3[b]	11.2[b]

Sources: U.S. Bureau of the Census, *Statistical Abstract of the United States: 1982.* U.S. Department of Commerce, Bureau of Economic Analysis, *Survey of Current Business* 62 (June 1982). Robert Gibson, "National Health Expenditures, 1980," *Health Care Financing Review* (September 1981): 20–31, Table 2. U.S. Department of Health and Human Services, *HHS News* (newsletter dated July 26, 1982): 00, Table II. R. Hanft, "National Health Expenditures, 1950–65," *Social Security Bulletin* (February 1967): p. 5. U.S. Department of Labor, Bureau of Labor Statistics, *The Consumer Price Index: History and Techniques,* Bulletin 1517, 1966) p. 47; U. S. Department of Labor, Bureau of Labor Statistics, *Relative Importance of Components in the Consumer Price Index, December 1975,* Report 439, and U.S. Department of Labor, Bureau of Labor Statistics, *Relative Importance of Components in the Consumer Price Index, 1977,* Report 595 (April 1980) p. 5.

[a]The CPI weight is for all urban consumers.

[b]Health expenditures data are for fiscal years, while total consumption figures are for calendar years.

compared with the weight of *consumer* expenditures on health services and supplies in personal consumption and with the weight of *total* expenditures on personal health care *plus* government purchases. Notice that in 1964, both of the latter weights are larger than the weight of medical care in the CPI, indicating that groups excluded from the CPI consumed more medical care relative to their total consumption than did those covered by the index. For 1975 and 1981 the divergence between the different weights becomes much greater. This reflects the increasing role of government in financing medical care, particularly for those groups traditionally excluded from the CPI. It appears that the CPI weight of medical care will continue to understate the importance of medical care in total consumption, particularly if the role of government in this sector continues to expand and the CPI fails to include such expenditures in determining its weights.

Sampling and the MCPI

The particular sampling problems of the all-items CPI already discussed are, of course, troublesome for the MCPI as well. We will now discuss the systematic biases between the calculated MCPI and the true one that the BLS attempts to measure. Until the 1978 revision, only a small sample of the wide variety of medical goods and services purchased by consumers was actually priced in the MCPI.*

---

*From 1939 to 1947, prices were obtained for the following items: physician home and office visits; obstetrical cases; surgical fees for appendectomy and tonsillectomy; several dental services; hospital

The BLS did not choose the items priced by probability sampling; they were selected "with the assistance of appropriate professional associations" (9). It is clear that the relatively simple, inexpensive, and frequently purchased goods and services were chosen for pricing, and the less common and more expensive ones were not. The extent to which this sampling procedure may have biased the index is not known, nor is the direction of the bias obvious. It is clear that the omitted goods and services were, on the average, more expensive than those priced, but it is the *rate of change* in price that the index measures, and it is not clear how this differed for omitted and included items.

The 1964 CPI revision expanded the number of items priced. The number of physician services priced, for example, was expanded to seven. The drugs and prescriptions sample was expanded from three to 16 (10). Hospital ward rates were dropped, but some additional hospital services were priced for use in computing the health insurance component.

Still, probability sampling techniques were not applied systematically in choosing the items for pricing until the latest revision (11). In this revision, the BLS has specified a much larger sample of medical care items for pricing. At each particular outlet, or provider of medical care, the item(s) to be priced are chosen by probability sampling from this larger group. Thus, contrary to past practice, not all general practitioners sampled are asked for their fees for the same services, nor are all drug outlets asked for the prices of the same drugs. In the case of physicians' fees, 10 physician service categories or specialties have been identified, as have a number of services in each category. The items for which prices are obtained from any particular physician in the outlet sample are chosen from the list of services corresponding to his or her specialty. Similar procedures are used in sampling the prices of drugs, hospital services, and other components of the MCPI. By choosing items for pricing by probability sampling from a large group, the BLS increases the probability that the calculated index will approximate the true one.

A 1958 review conducted of sampled physicians revealed that older doctors were overrepresented and that the sample was not properly distributed by geographic location within cities and metropolitan areas (12). Again, the direction of bias is not obvious, but if for some reason the prices charged by older physicians were changing at rates different from those charged by other physicians, or if prices were moving differently in different sections of cities, the calculated MCPI would provide a biased estimate of the true one. Paralleling its efforts in the rest of the CPI, the BLS has attempted in its last two revisions to broaden its use of probability sampling in choosing price reporters for medical services.

---

ward; private room, and semiprivate room rates; private nurse rates; eye examinations and glasses; and several drugs and prescriptions. In 1947, a budget cut forced the BLS to discontinue pricing dental charges for cleaning teeth, replacement lenses for eyeglasses, women's pay ward rates, and private nurse rates. Group hospitalization insurance was added in 1952, as was surgical insurance in 1958.

Though this sample provides at least some representation for a variety of services, it cannot be considered comprehensive. For example, the only physician services priced were an office visit, a home visit, an obstetrical case, and two surgical procedures. The first three (including the obstetrical case until 1961) were priced for general practitioners only, despite the fact that one-third of all private practice physicians in 1950 and over half in 1960 were specialists. For a more complete discussion of sampling, see Elizabeth Langford, "Medical Prices in the Consumer Price Index," *Monthly Labor Review* 80 (September 1957): 1953–1958, and Jeremiah German, "Some Uses and Limitations of the Consumer Price Index," *Inquiry* 1 (July 1964): 149–150.

Another problem which has drawn considerable attention in the area of physicians' fees is how to record a single provider's charges for a single service that vary with the recipient's ability to pay (13). The BLS currently gathers data from physicians on their usual or customary charges for particular services, but the average fee received by the physician (net of government payments) is a more relevant price, since it is also the average price paid by the consumer. Customary charges may differ from average prices *received* because customary charges may differ from average charges, and because not all charges are collected. Several authors have argued that over a long period the public and private expansion of insurance has reduced the importance of price discrimination and bad debts and has narrowed the gap between customary charges and average prices received (14). They claim that the physicians' fees component of the MCPI, based as it is on customary charges, has substantially understated the true increase in physicians' fees.

Quality Changes and New Products

In the MCPI, as throughout the CPI, the BLS intends to trace movements in the price of a *constant-quality* market basket of goods and services. It is particularly difficult, however, to measure the quality of most of the medical services priced. For example, how can we separate quality changes from price changes when a physician's office visit fee, a hospital's semiprivate room charge, or the premium on a health insurance policy changes? It is difficult to know when or how to introduce product and quality changes into the MCPI. In response to index critics who cite its handling of quality changes and new products as its most serious weakness, let us examine the problems of adjusting for such changes as they relate to the different components of the MCPI.

Drugs and Prescriptions.   It is widely agreed that, relative to their rapid development and adoption, the BLS has been slow to introduce new drugs into the MCPI. Critics also agree that a more rapid introduction of new products into this component would make the MCPI more representative of the market basket actually being purchased (15). Until changes were made in 1960, the entire drugs and prescriptions component consisted of only six items: aspirin, milk of magnesia, and multivitamins among nonprescriptions, and penicillin, a narcotic, and a nonnarcotic among prescriptions (16).

Skeptics have noted the disparity between movements in this index and price changes in drugs and prescriptions. Once again, no systematic bias in a particular direction is clearly evident. Some have argued that since new drugs initially tend to have relatively high prices, the failure of the MCPI to include them results in an understatement of price increases. But this is incorrect. For example, when a hospital purchases drugs, the prices it pays probably increase faster than the drug component of the MCPI because of the continuous introduction of relatively highly priced new drugs. The fact that the new drugs are purchased while the old ones are still available would seem to indicate that the price increases are offset by quality improvements. If so, the BLS's practice of linking new drugs and prescriptions into the MCPI after a considerable lag may actually lead to a slight *overstatement* of drug price increases. New drugs frequently come down in price after their introduction, as production expands and competition among sellers increases. An index that only picks them up slowly may do so after they have come down in price, and thus the index will rise more rapidly (or fall more slowly) than one which links in new drugs shortly after they are introduced. Since 1960 the BLS has considerably expanded its sample of drugs. It remains to be seen whether new products will be introduced into this component more rapidly in the future than they have been in the past.

Hospital Services.   It is also difficult to separate price from quality changes in hospital services. Prior to 1972, hospital services were represented in the MCPI by daily room charges only.* The index of semiprivate room charges was frequently cited as an index of the price of hospital care. This use of the semiprivate room charge not only ignored problems of quality change but also presumed that the prices of other services not included in the basic room charge were changing at the same rate.† In 1972, an expanded hospital service charge index was introduced. It included the semiprivate room charge, the operating room charge, and the charges for eight specific ancillary services. The latest revision has specified a much larger number of services for pricing. There are now 12 items in addition to hospital rooms for which data are gathered. At each hospital in the outlet sample, one or more items are chosen from this larger group for pricing by probability sampling.

    Nonetheless, the most important component in the new hospital service charge index will remain the basic room charge, which is not a constant-quality item. Adjusting for changes in the quantity of services provided under the daily room charge would seem consistent with the BLS's philosophy of attempting to price a constant-quality market basket. A recent study by the American Hospital Association suggests an approach to adjusting for quality change in a price index for hospital care (17). Instead of looking at charges, the investigators used cost data from the budgets of a fairly large but nonrandom sample of hospitals. They determined how many times, on the average, 37 different services were performed per patient day. By weighting the unit costs of these services by the frequency with which they were performed in a base year, the investigators arrived at what they considered a cost index for a constant bundle of services. That is, they estimated how much it would have cost to produce the 1969 patient day in 1974, based on the 1974 unit costs of services. As might have been expected, their index rose much more slowly (36.9 percent) than the hospital semiprivate room charge component of the MCPI (56.4 percent) during the period under study (1969–1974). These findings suggest that failure to account for quality improvements in computing the index of semiprivate room charges *may* lead to an index of hospital prices that is biased upward.

    There are problems in interpreting the results of this AHA study. For example, should all increases in service intensity be interpreted as quality improvements and therefore not be reflected in a pure price index? Or, what is essentially the same question, are all increases in the number of nursing hours,

---

*In the 1964 revision, operating room and x-ray diagnostic series charges were priced and used in the computation of the health insurance component.

†The room charge index is also sensitive to changes in hospital pricing policies that may not affect the overall level of hospital charges. The extremely rapid increase in the semiprivate room charge index immediately after the introduction of Medicare was probably due to a movement away from the traditional policy of keeping room rates below actual costs and overcharging on ancillary services.

diagnostic tests, and other services provided routinely by hospitals worth their price to consumers? If the market for hospital services conformed closely to the competitive model, the answer would be yes, since if the increased service intensity were not worth its price, consumers would not pay for it. But imperfections in this market—including the limited ability of consumers to judge the quality of hospital care and the incentive distorting effects of hospital insurance—make this conclusion less obvious.

Health Insurance.   The treatment of health insurance in the MCPI provides another example of the conceptual problems involved in adjusting for quality changes. Health insurance premiums may change in response to any of four types of changes: 1) changes in the price of medical services covered by the policy, 2) changes in the ratio of premiums collected to benefits paid out (the difference between the two is overhead expense), 3) changes in the comprehensiveness of the policy, and 4) changes in the average utilization of services by policyholders (18). Types 1 and 2 are clearly price changes and should be reflected in an index of the price of health insurance. A change of type 3 represents a change in the nature or quality of the policy and thus ought not to be reflected in the index. It is less clear how to classify type 4. Changes in the average utilization of services by policyholders might occur in response to any number of things, such as changes in the incidence of illnesses, advances in medical knowledge or technology, and changes in the availability of hospitals or physicians. One might argue that premium changes of type 4 are pure price changes, since the policy itself is unchanged. For the uninsured, however, increases in medical expenses due to increased consumption of services would not be considered price increases.

On balance, it is reasonable to make some adjustment for premium changes resulting from changes in average utilization of services, but how to make it is unclear. If premium increases due to utilization increases are not reflected at all in an index of health insurance prices, we are assuming that such increases are always worth their full price to policyholders. Conversely, if we treat all premium increases due to utilization changes as mere price increases, we are assuming that increased utilization is worth nothing.

From 1950 to 1964, the BLS included health insurance in the MCPI by pricing the most widely held Blue Cross–Blue Shield family plan in each sample area (note that the premiums of health insurance plans not priced were assumed to change at the same rate as those that were priced). All premium changes in the priced plans were reflected in the index, except those judged to be the result of changes in the comprehensiveness of policies, type 3 above. No attempt was made to adjust for premium changes of type 4, those due to changes in average utilization.

In the 1964 revision, the BLS discontinued a direct pricing of health insurance policies. Instead BLS decided to price a bundle of services representing those covered by health insurance, and to make periodic adjustments for changes in the weight of the overhead component of health insurance premiums. These steps were designed to account for premium changes of types 1 and 2 and to eliminate the need to adjust for premium changes of types 3 and 4, since these are not reflected in the index in the first place. Of the two methods that have been used, the former will show a more rapid increase during times of increasing health services utilization; the latter will show a more rapid increase when utilization is decreasing. Neither method is more obviously correct. The same method used in the 1964 revision has been carried over to the 1978 revision with only slight modification. The BLS is currently experimenting with different and hopefully better ways of calculating the price of health insurance.

Professional Services. Doctors frequently complain that the MCPI overstates the rate at which their fees are increasing because it does not account for quality improvements. They argue that physicians today are generally better trained than they were in the past and that, with the aid of an expanded body of knowledge and improved technology, they are providing better quality services. From their point of view, an office visit today cannot be considered the same product as an office visit of 15 years ago.

Such physicians may have a valid point. The quality of their services is difficult to judge, and the BLS has generally ignored the possibility of quality change in pricing the services of medical professionals.* Regardless of whether or not BLS believes physician fees should be quality adjusted, no method exists to measure and adjust for such changes.

In summarizing our discussion of the MCPI, we might emphasize three points. First, the MCPI is not designed as a comprehensive price index for all medical care consumed in the United States. Not only has it traditionally been targeted to a population that is not representative of the entire U.S. in terms of medical care consumption, but also it neglects the increasingly important share of medical care purchased by government. Second, the sampling procedures used are becoming more sophisticated, so that the MCPI is likely to resemble more closely the index that would have been calculated if all the relevant data (rather than samples) had been used. Third, the difficulty in accounting for quality change and the introduction of new products raises questions about what the MCPI does and what it ought to measure. These questions lead us into the next section, which is a discussion of an alternative measure of the price of medical care.

AN ALTERNATIVE MEDICAL CARE PRICE INDEX: THE COSTS OF TREATMENT OF A REPRESENTATIVE GROUP OF ILLNESSES

THE CONCEPT

Many of us choose intuitively to measure the product of the medical care industry by the number of episodes of illness treated rather than by the number of specific goods and services provided. When some mental or physical disorder is

---

*Except, apparently, when an obvious method of adjustment is available. For example, in 1961 obstetricians' fees for obstetrical cases were substituted for general practitioners' fees for the same service. The obstetricians' fees were linked in—that is, the difference between their fees and those of general practitioners was attributed entirely to a quality difference.

perceived, a consumer is prompted to seek medical care. The specific goods and services—physician visits, hospital bed days, prescription drugs, and so forth—function as inputs that are combined to produce treatments for such conditions. It is therefore reasonable to measure the cost of medical care by looking at specific illnesses and seeing how the average treatment costs per episode change over time. Many economists have found this cost-of-treatment approach to measuring medical care costs conceptually appealing.

In 1962, Anne Scitovsky detailed a proposal for an index of this type that would combine separate indexes of the treatment costs for specific illnesses into a composite index, weighting each component by the percentage of total medical expenditures spent on that illness in a base year (19). This procedure is analogous to the method by which the various component indexes are aggregated into the all-items CPI.*

While conceding that a costs-of-treatment index might be more expensive to construct, Scitovsky contended that its concept would be far superior to the traditional MCPI, since, unlike the MCPI, it could reflect quality changes in medical care and the introduction of new medical products and techniques. Since new goods and services are introduced over time and influence the costs of treating illnesses, their influence would automatically be reflected in a cost-of-treatment index. Similarly, if the quality of services—hospital bed days or physician visits, for example—improved over time, reducing the time and/or medical industry inputs required to treat illnesses, this change in input(s) quality would automatically be adjusted to the extent that it influenced costs of treatments. To compare the costs-of-treatment and MCPI approaches, suppose that hospital room charges increased, but that the increase was accompanied by a quality change that shortened hospital stays without requiring increases in the use of other inputs. The MCPI would show an increase because of the increase in room charges. The costs-of-treatment index would increase less and perhaps even decline, depending on the net effect of the changes on costs of treatments. It would thus adjust for this sort of quality change, whereas the traditional MCPI would not.

As long as the quality of *treatments* remained constant over time, this cost-of-treatment approach would appear to be a simple and direct method of adjusting for the effects on medical care price of changes in the quality of *inputs*. But not all changes in the amount or kinds of inputs used in providing treatments merely change the cost of producing an equivalent product. Many, perhaps most, such changes in methods of treatment change the product as well. They might change the probability of recovery or the amount of pain experienced in the course of the treatment, thus effectively changing the quality of the treatment itself. Even changes that alter the length of treatment affect not only treatment costs but quality too, since patients prefer shorter treatments to longer ones.

Recognizing that her proposed index would not adjust automatically for such changes in the quality of treatments, Scitovsky suggested that for each illness

---

*Scitovsky suggested that in order to minimize the cost of compiling such an index, illnesses might be grouped by similarity of treatment, with one or several illnesses chosen for actual pricing from each group. Such a procedure would involve an assumption that within groups, the costs of treatment of different illnesses would change at about the same rate over time.

included in the calculation of the index, a single objective indicator of quality be chosen. The average number of disability days might be appropriate for some infectious diseases or conditions requiring surgery; the number of live births per 100 pregnancies might be the quality measure for maternity cases. Using these quality indicators to adjust the individual costs-of-treatment indexes would have "the great merit of making possible more complete and systematic correction for quality changes," Scitovsky argued (20). As we shall see later, however, the issue of how to deal with changes in the quality of treatments has remained a major point of contention in the debate over the merits of this approach to measuring the cost of medical care.

A modification of the original Scitovsky idea arose out of a comment by Yoram Barzel. Using the example of polio, he argued that although the costs of treating individual cases of polio may not have fallen or may even have increased, the introduction of polio vaccine has led to a drop in the total cost of polio because its incidence has been curtailed. Barzel contended that it is more appropriate to look at the *expected* treatment costs of an illness rather than at the treatment costs of cases that actually occur (21). His suggestion has considerable merit. The prevention of a case or illness clearly represents an output that is superior to the successful treatment of a similar case, but if we concentrate on the costs per case of treating specific illnesses when they occur, we ignore the influence of preventive medical care. An index that measures the costs of medical treatments should reflect the role of preventive care, otherwise it gives a misleading view of changes in the price of care and the productivity of the industry.

In replying to Barzel, Scitovsky essentially agreed with him on this point and proposed a slight modification of her original approach (22). Instead of looking only at average treatment costs of illnesses when they occur, she would attempt to average all medical costs associated with particular illnesses, including the costs of preventive care, over the number of cases treated *plus* the number prevented. In theory, this would seem a reasonable way of accounting for preventive care in a costs of treatment index.

THE SCITOVSKY-McCALL FINDINGS

An actual costs-of-treatment index has not yet been constructed. Scitovsky and Nelda McCall have been involved, however in a study of the treatment costs of a selected group of illnesses in 1951, 1964, and 1971, a study that makes no adjustments for changes in treatment quality (23). The study was limited to cases treated by physicians at the Palo Alto Medical Clinic (PAMC)—a multispecialty, largely fee-for-service group practice of about 140 physicians in Palo Alto, California. Data on treatment costs were obtained from the records of PAMC and Stanford University Hospital, where nearly all patients requiring hospitalization were treated. Data on costs of treatment rendered outside PAMC or Stanford Hospital were obtained from the patients directly. Before attempting to generally evaluate the costs-of-treatment approach to measuring the cost of medical care, let us examine the Scitovsky-McCall findings.

Table 4-7 presents a summary of their findings on the changes in treatment costs for the conditions they studied. Disregarding, for the moment, the price columns and concentrating on the total percentage increase columns, it is strik-

TABLE 4-7. Changes in the Costs of Treatment of Selected Illnesses, 1951–1971

	Percentage Increase			
	1951–1964		1964–1971	
	Total	"Price"	Total	"Price"
Otitis media (children)	69	106	37	32
Appendicitis				
Simple	73	67	80	76
Perforated	86	72	115	89
Maternity care[a]	73	74	56	70
Cancer of the breast[b]	103	75	57	66
Forearm fractures (children)				
Cast only	53	53	17	14
Closed reduction no general				
anesthetic	85	36	102	64
Closed reduction, general				
or regional anesthetic	355	109	43	57
Myocardial infarction	NA	NA	126	70
Pneumonia (nonhospitalized)	NA	NA	13	32
Duodenal ulcer (nonhospitalized)	NA	NA	17	33
MCPI	55		47	

Source: Anne A. Scitovsky and Nelda McCall, "Changes in the Costs of Treatment of Selected Illnesses, 1951–1964–1971," Health Policy Program Discussion Paper, University of California School of Medicine, San Francisco, September 1975, pp. 10, 17.

[a]Exclusive of costs of outpatient drugs and prescriptions.

[b]Exclusive of costs of surgery performed independently from mastectomy.

ing that in so many cases the measured percentage increases in treatment costs exceed the percentage increases in the MCPI. Although results are more mixed in the later period, the Scitovsky-McCall estimates of increases in treatment costs exceed the increase in the MCPI in all but one instance for the 1951–1964 period. These earlier period results are at least a little surprising. Unless it can be shown that the quality of treatments for these illnesses improved substantially over the period, these results seem to belie the frequent allegation that the MCPI overstates increases in the price of medical care by failing to account for productivity improvements.

In fact, however, a number of possible explanations can be made for the differences between the rates of increase in the estimates of treatment costs and the MCPI. For example, Scitovsky and McCall found that the prices of ancillary hospital services were rising particularly rapidly. These services were not even priced by the BLS at that time, and the MCPI may have been biased downward by their omission. It is also possible that Scitovsky and McCall chose a sample of illnesses for which treatment costs rose faster than the cost of medical care in general.* Further, medical care prices tend to be higher in larger cities, and

---

* Scitovsky–McCall estimates are also based on small samples (ranging in size in 1951 from only three cases of forearm fractures, closed reduction, no general anesthetic, to 99 cases of simple appendicitis), and thus may contain some random error.

since Palo Alto doubled in size and became part of the San Francisco metropolitan area during the 1951–1964 period, part of the higher costs for the treatment approach may be a result of more rapid medical price increases in Palo Alto. The MCPI for San Francisco also increased faster than the national MCPI during this period (24).

The greater increase shown in the costs-of-treatment approach can also be attributed to a closing of the gap between customary and average charges for physicians' services. Scitovsky and McCall used data on actual charges for services* rather than customary charges as the BLS does. If it is true that average actual charges were increasing faster than customary charges—that the practice of cutting fees for low-income patients were becoming less prevalent—this might account for part of the differences in results. Scitovsky and McCall found some evidence to this effect. They found for example, that for pediatricians in PAMC from 1951 to 1964, the average charge increased 54 percent more than the customary charge for an office visit, and 31 percent more for a home visit (25).

A final reason why the costs-of-treatment approach rose more rapidly than the BLS index for medical care is that the latter measures only the price of an input, while the cost-of-treatment approach also includes the quantities of inputs used.

The figures in the price columns in Table 4-7 indicate how much treatment costs would have changed if the quantities of inputs used in the treatments (number of physician visits, number of hospital days, and so forth) had remained constant over time. In essence this is what the BLS attempts to measure. A comparison of the price and total increase columns in Table 4-7 is revealing. Though again the results are more mixed in the later period, from 1951 to 1964 the so-called price increases are generally *lower* than the total increases in treatment costs. This implies that changes in methods of treatment and in the quantities and types of inputs used generally tended to increase costs rather than lower them. Though this evidence is far from conclusive, it appears that changes in treatment methods that increase costs (presumably for the sake of improvements in treatment quality) are at least as common as changes that save inputs and thereby lower costs.

Tables 4-8 and 4-9 present a more detailed breakdown of changes in the methods of treatment in the illnesses that Scitovsky and McCall studied. They disclosed the following general trends. From 1951 to 1964 the number of physician visits used in treating cases tended to increase. Lengths of hospital stay generally fell, but total use of ancillary services tended to increase in those cases that required hospitalization. From 1964 to 1971 the trend toward shorter hospital stays continued, as did increases in the use of ancillary services. For some illnesses, the average number of physician visits continued to increase. Clearly, important changes in methods of treatment have affected costs in each direction, and cost-increasing changes have been quite common. It is interesting to note that when Scitovsky and McCall use their data to estimate changes in the price of specific goods and services from 1964 to 1971, the results are not very different from those calculated by the BLS. These findings are contained in Table 4-10.

---

*They used actual charges billed, not collected. Scitovsky suggests that because collection ratios were improving, the gap between customary charges and average charges collected was narrowing even faster than that between customary charges and actual charges billed (see Scitovsky, "Costs," p. 189).

TABLE 4-8. Average Number of Physician Visits and Average of Length of Hospital Stay Per Case, 1951, 1964, and 1971

Type of Service and Illness	1951	1964	1971
Average number of physician visits			
Appendicitis otitis media	1.8	1.7	1.9
Simple	2.9	5.6	5.5
Perforated	6.8	9.1	11.8
Maternity care (obstetrician)	12.7	14.5	14.9
Cancer of the breast			
Surgeons	12.6	13.7	12.0
Other MDs	1.3	3.1	1.9
Forearm fractures			
Cast only	5.3	4.5	4.4
Closed reduction, no general			
anesthetic	6.7	6.1	7.0
Closed reduction, general			
or regional anesthetic	5.8	7.9	8.1
Myocardial infarction	NA	27.6	26.0
Pneumonia	NA	3.0	2.6
Duodenal ulcer	NA	4.7	3.8
Average length of hospital stay			
Appendicitis			
Simple	4.3	4.2	3.8
Perforated	10.8	10.7	10.1
Maternity care	4.6	3.8	2.8
Cancer of the breast	12.7	10.2	8.9
Forearm fractures			
Closed reduction, general or			
regional anesthetic (all cases)	0.4	1.2	0.6
Closed reduction, general or			
regional anesthetic			
(hospitalized cases)	1.0	1.2	1.4
Myocardial infarction	NA	19.7	18.8

Source: Reproduced from Scitovsky and McCall, "Changes in the Costs of Treatment of Selected Illnesses, 1951–1964–1971," Health Policy Discussion Paper, University of California School of Medicine, San Francisco, September 1975, p. 28.

EVALUATING THE COST-OF-TREATMENT APPROACH

The results of the Scitovsky-McCall study clearly show that in the absence of adjustments for changes in treatment quality, a costs-of-treatment index might well rise even faster than the MCPI. However, if such adjustments were made, the index might rise more slowly than the BLS index. In evaluating the merits of the costs-of-treatment approach to measuring the cost of medical care, it is important to consider whether or not a legitimate basis and a practical method exist for making adjustments for changes in treatment quality.

Some argue that any increase in treatment costs that result directly from changes in the amounts or types of inputs used in treatments ought to be regarded entirely as quality improvements, not as price increases. This point of

TABLE 4-9. Number of Diagnostic and Other Services Per Case, Selected Illnesses, 1951, 1964, and 1971

Type of Service and Illness	1951	1964	1971
Laboratory tests			
Appendicitis			
Simple	4.7	7.3	9.3
Perforated	5.3	14.5	31.0
Maternity care	4.8	11.5	13.5
Cancer of the breast	5.9	14.8	27.4
Myocardial infarction	NA	37.9	48.5
Pneumonia	NA	3.0	2.3
Duodenal ulcer	NA	5.4	5.4
X-Rays			
Cancer of the breast			
Diagnostic	0.7	2.0	2.3
Radiotherapy	1.7	11.0	10.6
Forearm fracture			
Cast only	2.3	2.3	2.2
Closed reduction, no			
general anesthetic	3.7	2.7	3.9
Closed reduction, general			
or regional anesthetic	2.0	5.4	6.4
Myocardial infarction	NA	1.3	6.3
Pneumonia	NA	2.0	1.8
Duodenal ulcer	NA	2.4	2.2
Intravenous solutions			
Appendicitis			
Simple	0.1	2.4	4.6
Perforated	6.7	12.7	14.2
Cancer of the breast	1.0	1.7	1.7
Myocardial infarction	NA	1.6	10.6
Electrocardiograms			
Myocardial infarction	NA	5.4	9.0
Inhalation therapy			
Myocardial infarction	NA	12.8	37.5

Source: Reproduced from Scitovsky and McCall, "Changes in the Costs of Treatment of Selected Illnesses, 1951–1964–1971," Health Policy Discussion Paper, University of California School of Medicine, San Francisco, September 1975, p. 27.

view assumes that if the old treatment method for an illness is still available, consumers will not purchase a more input-intensive method of treatment unless the increase in quality is at least worth the increase in cost. Citing the Scitovsky-McCall data on the treatment of forearm fractures, Barzel points out that even though the differential in fees between general practitioner treatment and orthopedic surgeon treatment widened between 1951 and 1964, the percentage of cases treated by orthopedic surgeons increased. He interprets this as a shift in demand, and argues that it indicates that consumers value the additional quality of treatment by an orthopedic surgeon at its additional cost at least.

TABLE 4-10. Percentage Increase in Prices of Selected Medical Care Services, CPI and Scitovsky–McCall Data, 1964 to 1971

Type of Service	CPI	S-Mc Data
Medical care services	47.4	
Hospital service charges:		
Semiprivate room	128.7	114–142
Operating room charges	99.2	50
X-ray diagnostic series, upper G.I.	40.2	24
Professional services:		
General physician, office visits	56.0	71–91
Herniorrhaphy (adult)	39.7	
Tonsillectomy and adenoidectomy	42.4	
Radical mastectomy		36
Appendectomy		46
Obstetrical cases	49.0	45
Pediatric care, office visits	60.4	39–52
Other professional services:		
Routine laboratory tests	25.5	0–38
Drugs and prescriptions:	4.9	
Prescriptions	−2.0	−1
Over-the-counter items	13.4	3

Source: Reproduced from Scitovsky and McCall, "Changes in the Costs of Treatment of Selected Illnesses, 1951–1964–1971," Health Policy Discussion Paper, University of California School of Medicine, San Francisco, September 1975, p. 38.

Others are skeptical of whether medical care markets respond to consumer preferences so perfectly. Scitovsky claims that changes in methods of treatment are generally forced on consumers. She suggests, for example, that "the primary reason for the increased use of specialists is physicians' reluctance, not to say unwillingness, to treat cases outside their special field" (26). She does not deny that changes in methods of treatment are generally quality improvements, but (and here she reverses the position taken in her earlier paper) argues that since quality is forced on the consumer and since he or she does not really have the option of choosing the old treatment methods, an index of the cost of medical care should not be adjusted for such improvements in quality.

These two points of view—complete adjustment for cost-increasing changes in methods of treatment or no adjustment whatever—are the extremes on this issue, and neither of them seems entirely correct. Forced or not, if a change in treatment method really improves the quality of care, then the new treatment is a different and better product than the old. Comparing its price with the price of the old treatment overstates the increase in the price of a constant amount of medical care.

On the other hand, is it correct to assume that changes in treatment methods are always worth their full costs? This would be a reasonable assumption if medical care markets conformed closely to the competitive model. However, given that substantial third-party coverage for medical expenses exists and that consumers have little knowledge of medicine, patients are likely to accept the judgments of physicians as to what treatment methods are appropriate. Physicians, for their part, are not trained (and have little incentive) to weigh the benefits and costs of prescribing new methods of treatment; they apparently believe that any treatment change with an expected positive incremental benefit is justified, regardless of its additional costs. If patients pay little or nothing for care at the time they receive it, why should they not choose the method of treatment their physician feels is best, whatever its true cost? If medical care markets work in the manner just described, then we would expect that innovations in methods of treatment will tend to be quality-improving and that the improvements in quality may not always justify their true costs.* Thus, to adjust entirely for such cost-increasing changes in treatment methods in a medical care price index may be seriously misleading. Some middle ground between the two extremes of ignoring changes in treatment quality completely and assuming that they are always worth their full costs is more desirable than adopting either one.

Scitovsky's original suggestion that indexes of the treatment costs of specific illnesses be adjusted by some objective indicator of outcome quality is correct. However, three very serious problems still hinder the implementation of this approach. One problem is that the quality of a medical treatment is truly multidimensional; Scitovsky's suggestion that a single quality indicator for each illness be adopted might be too simplistic. Would it be proper to judge the quality of an automobile on its miles-per-gallon rating, or on any other single statistic? The probability of recovery, the expected number of disability days, the probable extent of physical impairments once recovery is completed, the painfulness of the treatment, and the amenities provided along with it are only some of the relevant aspects of the quality of a treatment. Determining how different treatment methods affect these different aspects of quality might be very costly, although such information would obviously be useful for other purposes besides the construction of a medical care price index.

The second problem, which would still be troublesome even if complete information existed on the technical aspects of the outcomes of different treatment methods, arises when placing values on differences in treatment quality. What value, for example, should be placed on a slightly lower probability of death from a particular disease, or on a little less pain? The problem of determining such values is as much conceptual as technical; its solution is not clear. For example, consider the suggestion by Scitovsky that, in order to hold quality constant, the costs of maternity care might be measured by the costs of handling all the pregnancies necessary to produce a certain number of live births (27). A reduction in the frequency of miscarriages certainly represents an improvement in the quality of maternity care, but should the cost-quality relationship be the one Scitovsky postulates? On what grounds can we assume that an obstetrician who is 99.9 percent successful in delivering babies is exactly twice as good as one who delivers only one live birth for every two cases handled? A doubling of

---

*This does not imply that the consumer is irrational. Each policyholder's individual consumption of medical care has a negligible effect on insurance premiums, and thus regardless of what the others do, each maximizes utility of consuming medical care to the point where to him or her, marginal benefit equals marginal cost (which is zero—neglecting time costs—if the insurance policy is comprehensive). When everyone acts in this way, premiums rise, and the whole group may be worse off than before the introduction of new methods of treatment.

the success rate in delivering babies or in treating an illness might imply more than a twofold increase in quality. But exactly how much more? This is the kind of question that must be answered if a cost-of-treatment index is to be adjusted correctly for changes in quality of treatments.

Third, it was suggested that the *expected* treatment cost of an illness is a more relevant measure than the average cost of cases actually treated. Since the expected cost is the probability of contracting an illness times the average cost of treatment, it can be influenced by preventive medical care. In principle, an expected-costs-of-treatment index could be calculated in the manner described earlier. For each illness, the total costs of treatment would be averaged over the number of cases treated plus the number of cases prevented. However, it is not simple to distinguish the number of cases eliminated by preventive medical care alone. Incidence rates of illnesses are influenced by many factors, including nutrition, personal health habits, lifestyle, and environmental factors such as pollution levels. The simple method of comparing the incidence of an illness in a base year with that in a later year and taking the difference as a measure of the effects of preventive care is not satisfactory. Other factors may be responsible for the difference. If birth rates go down and less is spent on maternity care, for example, does this mean that the medical care industry is more productive? Is it less productive if the nation increases its consumption of cigarettes and the incidence of lung cancer goes up? Surely the answer is no in both cases. Ideally, then, the effects of preventive care on incidence rates should be computed separately from those of other factors when preparing an index of expected treatment costs. Multivariate statistical techniques might be used for this task, but it is questionable whether precise estimates could be obtained.

Despite its limitations, the cost-of-treatment approach retains a theoretical appeal; it would enable more meaningful comparisons to be made of the cost of medical care, both cross-sectionally and over time. The fixed-bundle-of-goods-and-services method of pricing medical care used by the BLS yields results that are difficult to interpret meaningfully. The treatment of an illness seems a more appropriate notion of medical care output than the physician's visit, the hospital patient day, or the other more conventional units used by the BLS. Still, enormous practical difficulties and perhaps considerable cost would be involved in actually constructing a costs-of-treatment index as a substitute for the MCPI. In addition, some conceptual problems involved in this approach have not been solved adequately, most notably the issues of how to deal with changes in the quality of medical treatments and how to take account of the preventive aspects of medical care. However, the BLS is unlikely to embrace the costs-of-treatment approach in the near future.

APPENDIX: HEALTH INSURANCE PREMIUMS AS A MEASURE OF THE PRICE OF MEDICAL CARE

Another alternative approach to assessing the price of medical care, suggested by some economists, is to measure it in terms of health insurance premiums. Melvin Reder reasons that "if medical care is that which can be purchased by means of medical insurance, then its 'price' varies proportionately with the price of such insurance."* The apparent advantages of this price-of-insurance approach are its simplicity and the fact that productivity changes that influence the cost of providing care would automatically be reflected in the index. For example, technical changes that lower the costs of providing treatments would lead to downward pressure on insurance premiums and thus hold down the index of the price of medical care. Improvements in preventive care, which we have seen would be difficult to assess in a costs-of-treatment index, would also show up automatically in a price-of-insurance index. Preventive measures, to the extent that they lowered the expected cost of medical care, would also lower the cost of providing health insurance and would thus be reflected in this kind of index.

However, users of this approach will encounter the familiar conceptual problems involving the issue of quality change. A health insurance policy need not remain a constant-quality good over time, even if the language of the policy remains unchanged. Changes in the incidence of illnesses may occur, for example, for reasons beyond the control of the medical care industry. Such changes may affect the utilization of medical services and thereby raise or lower health insurance premiums. Alternatively, physicians may develop more input-intensive treatment methods over time, improving the quality of care but also raising insurance premiums. In neither case would it be correct to price the insurance policy as though it were a constant-quality item. Consider a third example: suppose there were increases in hospital capacity and physicians in a previously underserved area. It is likely that the amount of illness left untreated would drop, that treatments would generally be more complete, and that travel time and waiting time would decrease. Health insurance premiums would have to increase, but surely such premium increases would not be pure price changes. The improvement in care may more than compensate the population for the increase in premiums.

It appears, then, that the price-of-insurance approach is subject to the same basic problem that plagues the other methods of pricing medical care that we have examined: how can we quantify that component of price change that represents the value consumers place on increased quality (or the loss they attach to lower quality)? Adjusting a price-of-insurance index for quality change would be at least as conceptually and practically difficult as adjusting a costs-of-treatment index.

---

*"Some Problems in the Measurement of Productivity in the Medical Care Industry," *Production and Productivity in the Service Industries,* V. Fuchs (ed). New York, Columbia University Press, 1969, p. 98. In "Productivity and the Price of Medical Services," *Journal of Political Economy* 77 (November–December 1969): 1014–1027, Barzel also makes a case for this kind of index. In this same paper Barzel calculates an index of Blue Shield policy premiums from 1945 to 1964 and attempts to test the hypothesis that the physicians' fees component of the CPI overstates price increases for physicians' services by failing to adjust for improvements in the quality of services. He does find that premiums for Blue Shield group medical and surgical insurance policies increased on the average by only 66.5 percent from 1945 to 1964 compared with 85.3 percent for the physicians' fees component of the CPI. The implications of this finding are not so clear, however. The entire difference in percentage increases between the two indexes is accounted for in the first three years (both increase about 60 percent between 1948 and 1964). Were Blue Shield plans capturing economies of scale in claims processing from 1945 to 1948 (their membership tripled during that time)? Did Blue Shield plans obtain preferential prices for their members, who were at that time mainly low-income families? It should be noted that an index of Blue Shield premiums cannot be considered a comprehensive price index for medical care, since Blue Shield covers physicians' services almost exclusively.

Another kind of difficulty would arise by focusing exclusively on health insurance premiums. Since most individuals do not have complete insurance coverage for medical care, changes in insurance premiums are not the only factors that affect their cost of care. Many policies, for example, contain ceilings on the amounts the insurer will pay for specific services. If the service costs exceed those ceilings and continue to increase, the medical care costs will increase for the insured, since they will be forced to make up out-of-pocket what the policy does not cover. In the meantime, the insurance premium may not change. To avoid this kind of difficulty, the index might be based entirely on the premiums of very comprehensive prepaid insurance plans, without deductibles, coinsurance provisions, or ceilings. Since only a small percentage of the population is covered by such insurance plans, however, it is not clear how meaningful the index would be. There is little justification for assuming that the costs of medical care for those with no insurance coverage, for those with coverage for only specific types of services, and for those with less-than-complete coverage would always change in the same manner as the costs for those with comprehensive prepaid coverage.

REFERENCES

1. For a further discussion of the appropriateness of the CPI as a cost of living index see Janet L. Norwood, "Indexing Federal Programs: the CPI and Other Indexes," *Monthly Labor Review* 104 (March 1981): 60–65.

2. See *The Consumer Price Index: History and Techniques,* Bulletin No. 1517 U.S. Department of Labor, 1966, esp. p. 84.

3. For a general discussion of the latest revision of the CPI see the following: U.S. Department of Labor, Bureau of Labor Statistics, *Concepts and Content Over the Years,* Report 517 (May 1978); *The CPI—How Will the 1977 Revision Affect It,* Report 449 (1975). Also see John Laying, "The Revisions of the CPI," *Statistical Reporter* (February 1978): 140–148.

4. Julius Shiskin, "Updating the Consumer Price Index—an Overview," *Monthly Labor Review* 97 (July 1974): 3–4.

5. Philip McCarthy, "Sampling Considerations in the Construction of Price Indexes with Particular Reference to the United States Consumer Price Index," in *The Price Statistics of the Federal Government* (Cambridge, Mass.: National Bureau of Economic Research, 1961), pp. 197–232.

6. John Laying, "The Revision of the CPI," *Statistical Reporter* (February 1978): 143.

7. *The Price Statistics of the Federal Government,* pp. 37–39. (This useful report, prepared by a Price Statistics Review Committee of the National Bureau of Economic Research, if often referred to as the Stigler Report, after the committee chairman, George Stigler.)

8. Shiskin, "Updating the Consumer Price Index," p. 18.

9. Langford, "Medical Prices," p. 1056.

10. J. German, "Some Uses and Limitations of the Consumer Price Index," *Inquiry* (July 1964).

11. Daniel Ginsburg, "Revisions in the Medical Care Component of the Consumer Price

Index," Remarks delivered to the Blue Cross Conference on "Health Care in the American Economy: Issues and Forecasts," Hilton Head Island, S.C., January 18, 1977.

12. William Berry and James Daugherty, "A Closer Look at Rising Medical Costs," *Monthly Labor Review* 91 (November 1968): 6.

13. See, for example, Anne Scitovsky, "Changes in the Costs of Treatment of Selected Illnesses," *American Economic Review* 57 (December 1967): 1188–1189.

14. See the above reference and also Martin Feldstein, "The Rising Price of Physicians' Services," *Review of Economics and Statistics* 52 (May 1970): 122–123, and Victor Fuchs and Marcia Kramer, *Determinants of Expenditures for Physicians' Services in the United States 1948–68* (Washington: U.S. # DHEW, December 1972), pp. 7–9.

15. *The Price Statistics of the Federal Government*, pp. 37–39.

16. German, "Consumer Price Index," pp. 149–150.

17. P. Joseph Phillip, James Jeffers, and Abdul Hai, "Indexes of Factor Input Price, Service Intensity, and Productivity of the Hospital Industry," in *The Nature of Hospital Costs: Three Studies* (Chicago: Hospital Research and Educational Trust, 1976), pp. 201–262.

18. Ginsburg, "Revisions." The description of the handling of health insurance in the MCPI which follows is also based on information from this source.

19. "An Index of the Cost of Medical Care—A Proposed New Approach," in Solomon J. Axelrod, ed., *The Economics of Health and Medical Care* (Ann Arbor: Bureau of Public Health Economics, the University of Michigan, 1964), pp. 128–147.

20. "An Index of the Cost of Medical Care," p. 139.

21. "Costs of Medical Treatment: Comment," *American Economic Review* 58 (September 1968): 937–938.

22. "Costs of Medical Treatment: Reply," *American Economic Review* 58 (September 1968): 939–940.

23. Anne Scitovsky, "Changes in the Costs of Treatment of Selected Illnesses, 1951–65," *American Economic Review* 57 (December 1967): 1182–1195; and Scitovsky and Nelda McCall, "Changes in the Costs of Treatment of Selected Illnesses, 1951–1971," Health Policy Discussion Paper, University of California School of Medicine, San Francisco, September 1975.

24. Scitovsky, "Costs of Treatment, 1951–65," p. 1190.

25. *Ibid.*, p. 1188.

26. "Costs of Medical Treatment: Reply," pp. 938–939.

27. "Costs of Medical Treatment: Reply," p. 939.

CHAPTER 5

The Demand
for Medical Care

THE PURPOSE OF DEMAND ANALYSIS

One of the purposes of an analysis of the demand for medical care is to determine those factors which, on the average, most affect a person's utilization of medical services. At any point in time many factors influence the consumer's choice to seek medical treatment of a given intensity. It would be virtually impossible to explain completely every individual's utilization of medical services, but certain factors are important for most persons. Demand analysis seeks to identify which factors are most influential in determining how much care people are willing to purchase. The better our understanding of those factors is, the better able we will be to explain variations in utilization among population groups and between areas.

   Such an understanding will also enable us to forecast future utilization more accurately; to do so, each of the factors affecting demand is separately forecasted. If, for reasons of social policy, it were desirable to change a certain population group's utilization of medical care, then by our understanding of which factors affect demand, such a change could be wrought. Thus, an understanding of which factors affect demand, and to what extent, will enable us to explain variations in use of medical services. That knowledge can be used to forecast demand more accurately and to bring about changes in utilization if we desire.

He is terribly redundant

DEMAND VERSUS NEED AS BASIS FOR POLICY AND PLANNING

At various times it has been proposed that the planning of health facilities and health manpower be based solely upon estimates of need for medical care in the population. Need has generally been defined as the amount of medical care that medical experts believe a person should have to remain or become as healthy as

77

possible, based on current medical knowledge.* The Lee and Jones research of the 1930s (I) was one of the classic studies using medical need as the basis for determining physician requirements in the country. The Hill-Burton formula for planning hospital facilities also used need as the criterion for the number of beds required in an area. Four and one-half beds per thousand population was the standard adopted for determining whether additional beds should be built in an area. The only adjustment to this ratio was the population density in an area. If the density was fewer than six persons per square mile, then the standard became 5.5 beds per thousand population.

The assumption underlying the use of need as a basis for medical care public policy is that need itself is, or should be, the main determinant of hospital and physician use. However, since need is only one factor affecting demand for care, basing resource allocation decisions solely on medical need is likely to result in misallocation. If the estimated amount of services required to meet medical need exceeds the amount that people will actually use, then an allocation of facilities and manpower on the basis of need alone will result in an underutilization of those resources that could have been used elsewhere or in another manner. If, on the other hand, people use more medical care than would be provided based solely on a need criterion, then there will be an excess demand and increased waiting times. Shortages of facilities and manpower are costly because they waste a patient's time—time which could have been spent in a more productive manner.

Thus, planning based solely on medical need is likely to result in the use of either too few or too many resources. These consequences are shown in Figure 5-1. Planning according to medical need is shown by a vertical line, since need is independent of price. (Need is also independent of the prices of other services, of income, and of insurance coverage. Changes in these other factors would not change need, as medically defined.) The number of medical facilities determined by need is shown along the horizontal axis; e.g., Q_0 equals four beds per thousand population. If utilization is less than need (Q_1) or greater than need (Q_2) at a given price (P_0), then either too many ($Q_0 - Q_1$) or too few ($Q_2 - Q_0$) resources will be allocated to medical facilities.

When need is viewed as one factor affecting demand, then greater or lesser needs for care would be represented by different demand curves; for example, D_2 may include a greater amount of need than D_1. Changes in medical need cause a shift in the demand for care. If preventive care reduces the future need for acute medical services, then this may be shown by a shift to the left in the demand for acute care, e.g., from D_2 to D_1.

Planning according to demand would at least ensure against the wasting of resources and patients' time. If utilization is less than medical need (e.g., utiliza-

---

*Jeffers, J. et al. state, "An accurate specification of a population's 'needs' for medical services requires perfect knowledge of the state of its members' health, the existence of a well-defined standard of what constitutes 'good health,' and perfect knowledge of what modern medicine can do to improve ill (or below standard) health. It must be acknowledged that existing diagnostic procedures are not capable of providing perfect knowledge of the state of any population's, or even an individual's health. It also must be acknowledged that a clear-cut consensus as to what constitutes 'good health' does not exist among health professionals." James R. Jeffers, Mario F. Bognanno, and John C. Bartlett, "On the Demand Versus Need for Medical Services and the Concept of 'Shortage'," *American Journal of Public Health* 61 (1) (January 1971): 47.

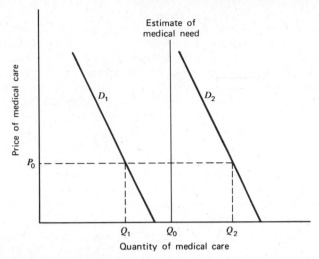

Figure 5-1. Need vs. demand as the basis for planning in medical care.

tion equals Q_1), then by understanding which factors affect demand and by knowing how much demand can be changed when one of these factors is changed, we can increase demand so that quantity demanded at the market price equals medical need. Conversely, if a decrease in utilization is desired where it exceeds need (e.g., utilization equals Q_2), then utilization can also be decreased by influencing one of the factors affecting demand. Using a demand analysis does not mean that medical need is disregarded in planning, only that other demand factors are incorporated in estimating what use will be. The emphasis, then, is accurately forecasting demand. Once demand has been forecast, we can decide, based on reasons of social policy, whether demand should be increased or decreased. Planning according to medical need alone is based on the assumption that medical need should be the only criterion for determining utilization, which is a value judgment that not everyone would share. Everyone may not place the same value on fulfilling all or even a certain percentage of their medical needs. Some may not be willing to pay the necessary price or to spend the necessary time to receive all the medical care that medical experts believe they should receive. Disregarding demand factors is likely to result in a waste of resources as well as a failure to ensure that those persons with the greatest need receive care.

If not need, should demand be the criterion for determining the quantity of medical services to be used? An assumption underlying all demand analysis is that people allocate their scarce resources among different goods and services in a way that maximizes their utility. Some persons might say, however, that medical care does not provide any utility, since the patient does not desire to purchase it. Many goods fall into this category: auto repair services, legal services, and home repairs. The desirability of the service is not relevant to the applicability of demand analysis. "Undesirable" services could simply be redefined as in the case of medical care to mean those services that provide benefits by alleviating or eliminating illness.

The marginal benefits derived from additional units of medical care differ. For example, the uncertainty of diagnosis lessens as more specialists' services and tests are used. In addition, the probability of recovery from particular illnesses will vary depending upon the quantity of medical care used. Some units of medical care provide large amounts of reassurance to patients; others provide the amenities. Some medical services are a substitute for services performed by the family in the home. Patients and their families differ in their perception of the value of these different aspects of medical care, which accounts for the differences in the amounts they are willing to pay for these perceived benefits. Similarly, if the price of medical care were reduced, then more people might be willing to buy more services of the abovementioned types.*

Since patients perceive the benefits to be derived from additional units of medical care differently, and since they are willing to pay different amounts for those additional services, who is to judge how much medical care should be used? If the patient makes this determination, then, as is the case in a market-oriented economy, he would use medical services to the extent that the marginal benefit of the last unit equals the price he must pay for those units. If, however, medical need is the criterion for rationing medical care use, then regardless of the patient's willingness to pay, he or she would not be allowed to receive more medical care than is needed.

In most markets in the United States, output quantity and quality are based upon the concept of consumer sovereignty. The assumption is that consumers are the best judges of how to use their resources to increase their own utility; how they choose to spend their money, together with the cost of producing those goods, will determine the variety and quality of the goods and services being produced.† The concept of consumer sovereignty in medical care is not uniformly accepted by health professionals, whose task it then becomes to develop an alternative set of criteria sufficiently specific to determine not only the quantity of resources to be spent on medical care but also the method by which these limited resources are to be allocated among different patients and institutional settings. These alternative criteria must substitute for all those allocative functions that would, in a system of consumer sovereignty, be performed by prices and differing consumer demands. In addition, an alternative system should make explicit the values underlying its distribution of medical care.

The determination of optimal output in a market, whether it is made with respect to medical care demand, the manpower markets, or the health education markets, is based upon the concept of marginal benefits and marginal costs. When the marginal benefits of a service are equal to the marginal costs of producing that service, then the amount of that service is considered to be optimal. If

---

*The great variability in the use of medical care due to the unpredictability of the individual incidence of illness should not lessen the usefulness of demand analysis. If we are interested in prediction, then the variability in medical care use and in the incidence of illness will average out over large groups of individuals. It will be possible to forecast the average demand for care, as opposed to the demand by any particular individual or family. The demand curve represents the average of many individuals' perceived benefits from additional units of medical care in relation to the price they are willing to pay for those additional benefits.

† Deciding whether incomes should be redistributed is independent of deciding who should determine the goods and services to be produced in society. If society determines that certain population groups do not have sufficient incomes, then their incomes can be supplemented.

the marginal benefits are either less than or greater than the marginal costs of producing a service, then consumption in that market is considered to be economically inefficient, i.e., resources are misallocated in that they are not placed in their highest valued uses. Efficiency in consumption, therefore, is one criterion by which the output of different medical care markets will be evaluated. The other criterion is efficiency in production: whether the output is produced at minimum cost. Economic efficiency in consumption and in production are criteria that economists use to evaluate the performance of different markets. In medical care, the criterion of efficiency in production is more widely accepted than is the criterion of efficiency in consumption, for which some persons would prefer to substitute a need criterion. Applying the criterion of efficiency in consumption to each medical care market, however, should sharpen the debate on the underlying values and criteria for defining optimal output in each market; should consumers' or health professionals' perception of marginal benefits prevail?

Whether or not people accept the criterion of efficiency in consumption, demand for medical services must still be analyzed if we are to be able to more accurately forecast use of services.

A MODEL OF THE DEMAND FOR MEDICAL CARE

THE DEMAND FOR MEDICAL CARE DERIVED FROM THE DEMAND FOR HEALTH

The traditional theory of consumer demand assumes that consumers purchase goods and services for the utility provided by those specific purchases. A more recent formulation of consumer demand, however, draws a distinction between goods and services purchased in the market and more fundamental objects of choice, referred to as commodities (2). If the commodity demanded by consumers is good health, then health can be produced by goods and services purchased in the market as well as by the time devoted to preventive measures. Within this framework, the demand for medical care is derived from the more basic demand for health.

According to Michael Grossman, (3), consumers have a demand for health for two reasons: 1) it is a consumption commodity; it makes the consumer feel better; 2) it is an investment commodity; a state of health will determine the amount of time available to the consumer. A decrease in the number of sick days will increase the time available for work and leisure activities; the return to an investment in health is the monetary value of the decrease in sick days.

A view of medical care demand as being derived from the demand for health implies the following. First, increases in age result in an increase in the rate at which a person's stock of health depreciates. Over the life cycle, people will attempt to offset part of the increased rate of depreciation in their stock of health by increasing their expenditures on, and use of, medical care. Second, the demand for medical care will increase with increases in a person's wage. The higher their wage, the greater the value of an increase in the number of healthy days. A consumer who is paid a high wage rate will also substitute purchases of medical care services for his or her own time when producing the commodity health. We would thus expect to observe a positive relationship between increased wages and greater expenditures on the demand for medical care. Third, it is hypothesized that education has a negative effect on the demand for medical care. More highly educated people are presumed to be more efficient in producing health. They are, therefore, likely to purchase fewer medical care services.

This is one that doesn't hold empirically

This view of medical care demand provides a rationale for including in the demand model certain factors believed to affect demand, traditionally known as taste variables, because they influence the individual's demand for health. The importance of the patient's time in relation to the demand for medical care will also be included in the demand model. Analyzing the demand for medical care as being derived from the individual's demand for health provides a better basis for determining which factors should be included in a model of demand for medical care, and for hypothesizing their effects.

DETERMINANTS OF THE DEMAND FOR MEDICAL CARE

A discussion of the demand for medical care requires an economic framework not only for surveying the literature on factors affecting demand, but also for evaluating empirical research on demand (4). If a demand study excludes relevant factors affecting demand, perhaps because they are not easily measured, or because the investigator is unaware of their importance, then its results are likely to be inaccurate.

Variations in the demand for medical care are determined by a set of patient and physician factors. The patient's demand for medical care is essentially the demand for a treatment, and variations in demand are a result of variations in the number, type, or quality of treatments demanded. This demand is typically initiated by the patient. The physician then combines various inputs to provide a treatment of a given quality. The patient's determinants of demand are his or her incidence of illness or need for care, a set of cultural-demographic factors, and economic factors. The role of the physician both as advisor to the patient and as a supplier of a service will be discussed separately below.

Empirical studies on the demand for medical care should thus describe, first, how different factors affect the patient's demand for medical care and, second, what determines how the physician will provide care for a given treatment. For purposes of clarity, the patient and physician phases will be described sequentially, although they occur simultaneously. The aim of empirical research, then, is to derive an estimate of the relationship between patient and physician factors and use of medical care.

The assumption of choice is implicit in studies of demand. Choices are made both of amounts of medical care purchased and of combinations of the components of care that produce a treatment. If choice in these areas were not possible, much less variation in medical care use would be observed when nonmedical factors, such as cultural and economic background, are analyzed. Less variation would also exist in the manner in which a treatment is provided. The patient's and physician's degree of choice depends on two factors: knowledge and the availability of substitutes. It is often assumed that no close substitutes within the field of medical care exist. Even if this were true, which it is not, families might still differ in their demand for medical services because they attach different values to the expected benefits of increased use or because their knowledge of these benefits varies. Within the field of medical care itself, the substitutability of components in providing a treatment appears to be increasing. Not only are ambulatory services and nursing home care partial substitutes for hospitalization, but also the increased use of outpatient surgery provides an additional substitute for hospital care. These, then, are the reasons underlying the assumption that the patient exercises choice in his or her demand for medical care and the physician exercises it in the treatment he or she provides.

Factors Affecting the Patient's Demand for Medical Care

As we have noted, the factors affecting a patient's demand for medical care are incidence of illness, cultural-demographic characteristics, and economic factors. The first two, stemming from the family's perception of a medical problem and their belief in the efficacy of medical treatment, shape the consumer's desire for medical care. When translating this desire into an expenditure, the family is limited by the extent of its available resources. Determining the amount to be spent for medical care becomes a part of the problem of allocating scarce resources among alternative desires. Each of these general factors affecting a patient's demand for care is discussed below.

Actual or perceived illness or desire for preventive medicine will determine whether or not an individual is in the market for medical care at any point in time. The onset of illness and the use of a hospital is for many people an unexpected occurrence. Thus, for individuals, illness may be considered a random event, but with respect to the age and sex of the population as a whole, illness has a fair degree of predictability. As individuals age, the incidence of illness increases and morbidity patterns change; chronic diseases become a more important determinant of the need for medical care. Although medical care expenditures are approximately the same for both sexes in the early years, there is a difference in the need for medical care among men and women, holding constant marital status and age. Later in life, expenditures incurred by women exceed those incurred by men primarily because of obstetrical charges, although the difference persists beyond the child-bearing ages. The relationship between age and use of medical services, however, is not simply linear nor is it the same for each type of medical service. For example, the relationship between age and use of hospital services is different from that which exists between age and the use of dental services. Even within the hospital component of care, differences in admissions and in length of stay exist for a given age group. Although these population characteristics may not affect each of the components of medical care in the same manner, they are important in explaining variations in the use of these services.

Marital status and the number of persons in the family also affect the demand for medical care. Single persons generally use more hospital care than married persons do. The availability of people at home to care for an individual may substitute for additional days in the hospital. Family size also affects demand; a larger family has less income per capita (although not necessarily proportionately less) than does a small family with the same income.

Education is also believed to affect the demand for medical services. A greater amount of education in the household may enable a family to recognize the early symptoms of illness, resulting in a greater willingness to seek early medical treatment. We might expect to observe such a family spending more for preventive services and less for more acute illnesses later on. Higher levels of education may also lead to increased efficiency in a family's purchase and use of medical services. Years of education in a household may be a proxy measure for a greater awareness of the need for medical care, for different attitudes toward seeking care, and for greater efficiency in its purchase and production. Differences in education among families are expected to result in differences in use and expenditures for medical care services.

Although it is important to our understanding to determine the effect that cultural-demographic factors have on the demand for medical services, such factors are not subject to sudden changes, nor are they generally the instrument of public policy. The age composition changes gradually, as attitudes do. The effect that economic factors have on the demand for medical services is of more immediate value for forecasting and policy purposes.

The economic factors contributing to medical services demand are income, prices, and the value of the patient's time. They affect not only whether a patient will seek medical care but also the extent of the care once treatment is undertaken. Economic factors may not have much of an effect on whether a maternity patient goes to a hospital (although they may influence the choice of hospital), but once she has been admitted, they may affect her length of stay. Each of these economic factors is briefly discussed below.

A number of studies have examined the relationship between family income and expenditures on medical care and also the effect of income on use of medical care. When these studies are based on survey data, it is often found that families with higher incomes have greater expenditures for medical care, although the percentage of income spent on medical care declines as income increases. In other words, the income elasticity of medical care expenditures is less than one; that is, the percentage increase in medical care expenditures is less than the percentage increase in income (5). The manner in which the family income is measured must be understood if the effect of income, as it is derived from medical care surveys, is to be interpreted correctly. A family's income in any given year may be abnormally low or high because of the temporary loss of employment, windfall gains, or other unexpected events. Empirical evidence suggests that total consumption is not raised or lowered to correspond with temporary changes in income. Rather, a family's level of consumption is determined primarily by its expected normal or permanent income (6). If transitory income has little or no effect on total expenditures, and families that are sick are likely to be below their normal incomes, then survey data that merely show the relationship between income and expenditures include both permanent and transitory income. Since transitory income is included in the income reported by the survey, although it presumably has little effect on expenditures, the reported survey relationship between income and expenditure is likely to be understated. If the effects of transitory income can be removed, the income elasticity of medical care expenditures will be increased. One important reason why estimates of the effect of income on medical care expenditures are low is that it is difficult to determine the relationship between permanent income and medical care expenditures from survey data.

Another reason why the estimate of income elasticity based on survey data is believed to be low is that employer contributions to health insurance premiums are not normally included in survey data. Such employer contributions do not constitute taxable income for the employee recipients. The higher the income tax bracket, the larger the potential tax saving to the employee and the greater the incentive to have payments for health insurance made by his or her employer. If, for persons with higher incomes, a greater proportion of medical expenditures is reimbursed by third-party payors, then survey data showing the relationship between family income and out-of-pocket expenditures will understate the true income elasticity.

not a big adjustment

Once the survey data are corrected for transitory income and employer paid health insurance premiums, it appears that the income elasticity of medical care expenditures is approximately "one," that is, a 10 percent increase in income will lead to a 10 percent increase in medical care spending.

It would be nice to see a citation to some real literature here — not just Paul's intuition

The price of a service and the use of that service are, according to economic theory, inversely related: as the price is reduced, purchase or use of the service will increase. Knowledge of price elasticity of demand for medical services is therefore of great importance for public policy. Many persons in medical care have generally assumed, however, that prices have very little effect on medical services use. If national health insurance is to result in greater use of medical services, then its proponents must assume that the use of medical services is responsive to changes in price; if not, national health insurance will not result in any changes in use but merely in a redistribution of income. Before discussing estimates of price elasticity of demand for medical services, it would be useful to discuss what the relevant price variable should represent.

price

The price or charges stated by a medical provider are often not what is paid by the patient. Part or all of the price (as in the case of Medicaid patients) is paid by a third-party payor or by the government on the patient's behalf. Any estimate of price elasticity of demand should be based upon the net or the out-of-pocket price paid by the patient. Health insurance is one of the most important factors reducing the patient's medical care prices. Insurance coverage represents a movement down the individual patient's demand curve, which increases the quantity of services demanded. For all individuals, the existence of insurance coverage represents a shift in the overall demand for medical care. The effect of insurance on the individual's demand for care and on the aggregate demand for care is explained graphically and more completely in the appendix to this chapter. Although, as will be discussed, estimates of price and insurance elasticities have generally been found to be inelastic with respect to demand for medical services, these estimates vary by type of medical service and by seriousness of illness.

Certain institutional settings can substitute for others in treatment of an illness. An analysis of the demand for any one component is incomplete if it omits the substitutability and demand for other components. Because a patient can be treated for an illness with different combinations of hospital care, outpatient services, and nursing home care, different lengths of stay in the hospital may reflect differences in the use of the other institutional settings. Therefore, a demand analysis of any one component of care should include the prices of its substitutes and complements. Again, the relevant price to the patient of these substitutes and complements is the net, not the stated, price.

One important reason why estimated price elasticities of demand for medical care are expected to be low is that time costs may represent a relatively large portion of the total price of medical care. In addition to prices and income, the consumer's time is a constraint that affects the type of goods and services the consumer purchases. Consumer time may be considered an input into the production of a good or service. Cooking a meal and consuming it at home, for example, requires more consumer time than eating in a restaurant. When people's time costs are high, they will substitute purchased services for their own time. Since time has an opportunity cost, it is also scarce and should be viewed as one of the resource constraints facing the consumer. The importance of including the time costs as well as the money costs of consuming a good or service is that it enables us to explain and predict consumer demand more accurately. If either the time or the money costs of a service decrease, it is to be expected that the quantity demanded would increase. People with higher earned incomes typically have a higher cost of time and will consequently have a higher demand for air travel than those with low time costs, such as students.

In medical care, time is used in traveling to a provider and waiting to be treated at the provider's setting. The following example illustrates how differences in time costs affect the price elasticity of demand for a service. Assume that the patient's out-of-pocket price for visiting a medical provider is $10 and that the time costs are equal to $20; the total price of the visit is therefore $30. If the elasticity of the medical service with respect to the total price were -1.0, meaning that a 10 percent change in the total price would result in a 10 percent change in use, and if the out-of-pocket price dropped 50 percent (from $10 to $5), the result would be only a 20 percent decrease in the total price of care (from $30 to $25). This 20 percent change in the total price would lead to a 20 percent change in use, because the price elasticity is -1.0. Thus, when an out-of-pocket price is reduced by 50 percent and use increases only 20 percent, the calculated price elasticity is $-.4$. The demand for that service is thereby estimated to be price inelastic. Thus, as time costs contribute a larger proportion of the total price, the calculated price elasticity of demand becomes smaller, while the time price elasticity increases (7).

As third-party coverage and government reimbursement cover more of the payment for medical service, time costs become a greater proportion of the total cost of using that medical service. The change in money and time costs has important implications for the consumption of medical services. Analyses of the impact on the demand for physician services of a change in insurance coverage, from no out-of-pocket price to the introduction of a 25 percent coinsurance provision, found that the use of such services substantially decreased, primarily among those enrollees with the lowest time costs (8). This increase in the money price of the service, to a 25 percent co-pay, represented a much larger increase in total price to persons with low time costs than it did for those with higher time costs. For example, home visits, which involve the lowest time costs, experienced twice as large a decline as other types of visits. Further, enrollees decreased "their demand for care of minor illnesses considerably more than their demand for medical care of other conditions" (9). Nonprofessionals (i.e., those with lower time costs) had a much greater reduction in the number of annual examinations as their out of pocket price increased. Female dependents, who have lower time costs than female subscribers, had a larger reduction in visits when the money price of a visit was increased.

This study, which was based on a natural experiment, was repeated four years later to determine whether the effect on physician visits of a 25 percent co-payment rate was temporary. The authors found that the 24 percent decline in per capita use of physician visits did not change four years later (10).

Three policy implications follow from the findings that time costs have an important effect on the demand for medical services. First, as the out-of-pocket prices to patients decrease, demand for medical care will become more responsive to the cost of time. If the quantity of medical care supplied does not increase sufficiently to meet increased demands, as is the case under a system similar to the British National Health Service, then the likely method of rationing is to allocate care to those who can afford to wait. Those with a low time cost are more likely to receive care than those with a high opportunity cost of time. Second, society has determined that certain population groups should increase their use of medical services. Although the money prices to these groups have been reduced, it may be desirable to increase further their use of services by reducing their time costs. Locating clinics closer to these population groups will lower their travel costs and increase utilization. Third, when medical care delivery systems are planned for, the patients' time cost should be considered, together with institutional costs, as the relevant costs for planners to minimize.* Consumers are willing to pay to decrease time costs. Unless these are included in the planning of medical care delivery systems, planners might attempt to lower the costs of hospital or other forms of care by building fewer though larger units, thereby increasing travel time costs to patients.

The Role of the Physician in the Demand for Medical Care

In nonmedical markets the consumer, with varying degrees of knowledge, selects the goods and services he or she desires. In medical care, however, the patient does not decide, for example, what hospital to enter or the form of treatment he or she is to receive; instead, the patient selects a physician who then makes these choices. In acting on the patient's behalf, the physician uses his or her awareness of the patient's financial resources and medical needs to act as the patient would if he or she had the knowledge and medical authority to make the decision.† When choosing the components of care to be used in treatment, the physician will be guided not only by their efficacy but also by their relative prices to the patient (11). For example, if a patient can be treated either as an outpatient or as an inpatient, but the patient's insurance coverage only covers inpatient hospitalization, then it would be less costly *to the patient* to be hos-

---

*A section on the planning of obstetric facilities in Chapter 11 explicitly incorporates the cost of time in determining the number and size of obstetric facilities in an area.

†The physician has been referred to in this role as a manager or agent for the patient. See *Report of the Commission on Cost of Medical Care* (Chicago: American Medical Association, 1964), Vol. I, pp. 9–21.

pitalized. This choice of treatment settings by the physician on the patient's behalf, however, would result in higher total health care costs.

Evidence that physicians make such choices on the patient's behalf is contained in the many studies that relate hospital utilization to the patient's insurance coverage. Although physicians' behavior will also be affected by other factors discussed below, we can use the fact that they often act in the patient's financial and medical interests to predict medical and hospital use according to the patient's financial, socio-demographic, and medical characteristics. The more likely a physician is to be aware of and to act in accordance with his or her patient's needs, desires, and financial interests, the stronger the empirical relationship should be between such patient characteristics and use of medical services.

With the growth of more comprehensive hospital insurance, financial constraints become less important, and physicians are able to prescribe the highest quality of medical care for their patients. This is rational behavior on the part of the physician and the patient, since the marginal benefit of care consisting of additional tests and other services, no matter how small, is still probably greater than the out-of-pocket price the patient must pay for it. The physician is able to practice what Victor Fuchs has referred to as the technologic imperative. In other words, medicine will prescribe the best care that is technically possible (12). It does not consider whether the marginal benefits of that additional care exceed the marginal costs of producing it.

However, other factors may prevent the physician from acting solely in the patient's interest. A physician may not have staff appointments at all of the hospitals in the community. If two hospitals provide similar care for their obstetrics patients, but one of them is more expensive than the other, then, unless the physician has a staff appointment at the less expensive hospital, his or her patient will be admitted to the more expensive hospital. Also, some hospitals may have utilization review committees that review the appropriateness of admissions and length of stay. In the face of an effective committee, a physician may find it difficult to prescribe hospital care and/or a length of stay that satisfies the patient's preferences. To the extent that such institutional arrangements and sanctions exist, the relationship between utilization and patient characteristics (both economic and noneconomic) will be less clear.

There is a more important reason why the physician may not act solely in the patient's interest. As one of the inputs into the patient's medical treatment, a physician has an economic interest in the manner in which a treatment is provided. In prescribing care to a patient, the physician is acting not only in the patient's interest as an advisor, but also in his or her own interest as a supplier of services. One of the more obvious examples of the effect of this dual role is the decrease in home visits. It is more convenient for a patient who is not seriously ill to be examined and treated by a physician at home. The physician, however, can achieve greater productivity, hence income, by staying in the office and seeing more patients instead of spending time in traveling. It is in the physician's economic interests to shift the travel costs to the patient. A physician may also shift certain costs to the patient and the patient's third party payor by prescribing a greater number of tests for the purpose of protecting himself against a possible malpractice suit.

Two controversial issues in the medical care literature, together with their policy implications, can be clarified when the dual role of the physician, as an advisor and as a supplier of a service, is used to explain them. The first relates to the idea that the supply of beds creates a demand for those beds, the second to the idea that physicians create demand. The ideas are related, but it is useful to separate them for purposes of analysis.

"A Built Bed Is a Filled Bed."   The hypothesis that the supply of beds creates a demand for those beds is associated with the work of Roemer and Shain (13). This belief has long been accepted by persons in the medical care field. Stated in its simplest fashion, it asserts that an increase in the supply of beds in an area will result in their being used. The empirical support for this hypothesis is the close statistical relationship between hospital beds and hospital utilization in an area.

According to this hypothesis, building beds eventually results in their being filled with patients whose hospitalization is not "medically" indicated. The resulting policy implication is that the number of beds in an area should be based upon a medical determination of the need for beds. Since medical need is believed to be similar in all areas, it suggests the establishment of hospital bed limits for each area in the form of bed to population ratios.

The supply-creates-demand hypothesis and its far ranging policy implications contains a number of conceptual and empirical problems. A simple correlation between beds and hospital use does not constitute empirical verification that they are causally related. The fact that the measures are correlated with one another might simply indicate that they are both affected by the same factors. Presumably, areas with a high demand for hospital care will generate an increase in supply to satisfy that demand; it would thus appear that areas with high demand will have a larger number of beds per capita than will areas with low demand.

It is more difficult to explain why increased demand appears to *follow* increases in the bed supply. There are three possible explanations for this observed phenomenon. First, the current demand for hospital care may exceed supply, in which case increasing the supply of beds satisfies existing demand. This situation is shown in Figure 5-2A. If the price of hospital care were set below the equilibrium level, at P_0, and the supply of beds were shown by S_0, hospital use would be Q_0. At a price of P_0, there would be an excess demand of $Q_3 - Q_0$. If the supply of beds were increased from S_0 to S_1, and subsequently to S_2 and S_3, hospital use would similarly increase from Q_0 and, eventually, to Q_3. Similar to the situation of continual excess demand is a situation in which supply expands in anticipation of increased demand. This situation is shown in Figure 5-2B. Initially, demand is represented by D_0 and supply by S_0; utilization is Q_0. If the supply of beds were increased to S_1 and then utilization increased to Q_1, it does not mean that supply created a new demand of D_1; rather, the supply of beds was built in anticipation of increased demand.

A second explanation of the apparent relationship between an increase in the bed supply and a subsequent increase in demand is that patients' travel costs have changed. If the additional beds are established in new, smaller hospitals that are closer to prospective patients, then travel costs to the hospital will decrease. Rather than creating a new demand (i.e., a shift of demand to the right), the increase in the supply of beds lowers the total price of hospital care to the

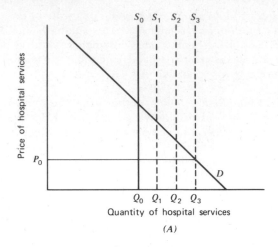

(A)

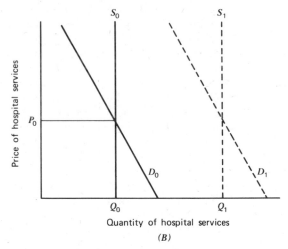

(B)

Figure 5-2. Change in the supply and demand for beds: (A) an example of excess demand for beds, (B) an increase in supply of beds in anticipation of an increase in demand.

patient by lowering the nonmonetary costs and is thus a movement down the patient's demand curve.

The third explanation focuses on the effect on the physician of an increase in beds. A physician can increase his or her productivity by hospitalizing patients instead of visiting them in their homes. Particularly in rural areas and in areas where physicians are few relative to the population, a physician is likely to admit more patients and keep them in the hospital longer because it is easier to monitor their illnesses while seeing more patients.

The hypothesis that an increase in the bed supply creates its own demand thus appears to be the recognition of a close relationship between beds and their use rather than the discovery of a causal relationship. To understand the reason for this close relationship and for the possibility that a bed increase may precede a use increase, it is necessary to examine what factors are affecting the patient's demand for care and what incentives are facing the patient's physician. Public policy that merely addresses the supply of beds without considering patient demand or physician incentive is likely to result in hospital use that is inequitable and inefficient. When hospital beds are purposely limited, the patients who receive care may not be those who are most in need of care. The value the patient places on hospital care should be related to the cost of providing that care. Arbitrary limits on hospital beds in an area are unlikely to be related either to demand factors or to the value a community has placed on its bed capacity.

Demand Creation. The second way in which the physician's role as the patient's advisor places the physician in conflict with his or her interests as a supplier of medical services has been referred to as *demand creation.* (This subject is also discussed in Chapter 9.) As a supplier of a service, the physician has a financial stake in those services used in treatment. It has been observed that with an increase in the supply of physicians in an area, both the price and quantity of physician services increase. Such a relationship would suggest a positively sloped demand curve. An alternative explanation of the relationship between the number of physicians and the price and quantity of their services suggests that consumers, lacking information on their diagnosis and treatment needs, are prescribed additional, unnecessary services (14). When faced with a relatively high demand for his or her services, a physician will have little incentive to prescribe additional treatments that may or may not be needed; however, when the supply of physicians increases in an area, then the demand facing each one of them decreases. Given the lack of patient information regarding treatment needs, the physician can exploit this ignorance by recommending additional services. This situation is shown graphically in Figure 5-3. The initial supply, demand, price, and quantity of physician services are indicated by $S_0, D_0, P_0,$ and Q_0, respectively. With an increase in the number of physicians, the supply shifts to S_1. Rather than face a decrease in the demand for his or her services (and a consequent fall in income), the physician, as the patient's advisor, recommends additional services. There is presumably a limit to how much additional demand the physicians can create. The new demand curve, D_1, shifts to the right. Thus, the price and quantity of services have increased with the increase in supply.

It may be rationalized that the additional demand created by the physician provides beneficial services; however, these additional services may be unnecessary and would not be provided were there sufficient demands of a more serious nature for the physician's services. One example of a physician-created demand is the recommendation that a patient return the week following an initial visit to enable the physician to determine that progress is satisfactory. A more serious example of demand creation is unnecessary surgery. Patients are least able to judge whether or not a surgical procedure is necessary. The patient may be able to determine whether additional home and office visits are providing any benefits, but in the case of surgery, the consequences of being mistaken may be more serious. The types of surgery that are likely to result from demand creation are tonsillectomies, appendectomies, and hysterectomies. The physician might rationalize that these surgical procedures are beneficial and do not affect the patient's ability to function. The patient would have no way of deter-

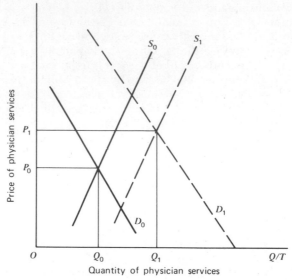

Figure 5-3. Demand creation with an increase in the number of physicians.

mining whether such surgery was useful, since his or her well-being would probably be unchanged after recovering from it.

A number of studies have shown that the rate of surgical procedures is higher when the physician is reimbursed on a fee-for-service basis. Between two population groups, with similar characteristics and similar physician and hospital coverage, the rate of surgical procedures varies according to the method of physician reimbursement: in one group, Health Insurance Plan of Greater New York (HIP), the physician is reimbursed on a capitation basis (the same rate of reimbursement regardless of the number of procedures performed); for the other group of patients, covered by Group Health Insurance in Washington, D.C. (GHI), the physician is reimbursed on a fee-for-service basis. The rate of hospitalized surgical procedures for HIP enrollees was 4.38 per hundred persons per year; for GHI it was 7.18. In another study of GHI and HIP populations, no significant difference was found in surgical procedures between adult males, but they were found between adult females—6.56 in GHI and 4.97 in HIP. In a third comparative study of physician reimbursement under a capitation system (Kaiser) and a fee-for-service method (Blue Cross–Blue Shield and commercial insurance), when patients had identical benefit coverage under all three plans, it was found that the hospitalized surgical procedure ratios per hundred persons per year were 3.3, 6.9, and 6.3, respectively. A fourth comparison was of two groups of federal employees with the same benefits, where one group belonged to a capitation plan while the other group belonged to a fee-for-service system. It was found that the rate of hospitalized surgical procedures was 3.9 in the capitation plan and 7.0 in the fee-for-service system. One-third of this difference in the rate of surgical procedures was a result of differences in the rate of surgical procedures for appendectomies (1.4 versus 2.6), tonsillectomies (4.0 versus 10.6), and "female surgery" (5.4 versus 8.2) (15). The above evidence appears to support the hypothesis that when patients lack knowledge and when the physician is both an advisor and a supplier of a service in which he or she has a financial interest, the physician can take advantage of the advisory role by creating additional demand.

This hypothesis has several implications for policymaking. First, increased patient knowledge would lessen the physician's ability to create additional demand. Pauly and Satterthwaite have found that the effect of increased physician supply in an area on patients' use of medical services declines with higher levels of patient education (16). As an alternative to education, the patient can obtain additional information by receiving a second opinion from another physician whenever surgery is recommended. When second opinions are used, it has been found that there is a lower surgical procedure rate (17). The second approach that has been suggested for reducing the amount of unnecessary surgery is to develop institutional arrangements such as tissue review committees. The problem with such review committees is that as long as other physicians in the hospital are financially unaffected by the medical practice of their colleagues, they have little incentive to become concerned with their colleagues' behavior. A third approach is to provide the physician with a financial incentive to avoid unnecessary surgery. One such financial incentive would be greater reliance on malpractice suits in cases of unnecessary surgery. Another approach would be to encourage other methods of physician reimbursement. Capitation-based reimbursement would be one such method, and is discussed more completely in Chapter 12 in the section on health maintenance organizations.

In summary, the physician's role as it affects the demand for medical care is potentially conflicting, as he or she is both an advisor to the patient and a supplier of a medical service.* To the extent that the physician acts in the advisory role, considering the patient's needs as well as resources, we would expect to find a strong relationship between the patient's characteristics and his or her demand for medical care. On the other hand, when the use of medical services differs from what we might initially expect, instead of abandoning the economic model of demand, we must examine the reasons for the unexpected use in terms of its effect on physician productivity and income. The important role of the physician in translating the patient's demand for care into use of medical services should not be forgotten in public-policy attempts to control medical costs and utilization. The fee-for-service physician determines the use of all medical resources, yet the physician does not bear fiscal responsibility for those decisions.

A Review of Selected Empirical Demand Studies

A number of studies have attempted to estimate price and income elasticities of demand for medical services (18). These studies have differed with regard to the theoretical variables included in the demand model, the measurement of the theoretical variables, data, statistical techniques, and methods used for analysis. Most of the demand studies have attempted to estimate the relationship between

---

*Many similar advisor-supplier relationships exist with purveyors of other goods and services that consumers purchase—for example, real estate agents and auto mechanics.

economic factors and either total medical care expenditures and separately for expenditures on hospital and physician services, while holding constant the effect of other, noneconomic factors. Very few studies have been able to measure the effect of economic factors by type of medical diagnosis or by seriousness of illness. Ideally, it would be desirable to know price elasticities at different deductible and coinsurance levels, holding constant such factors as health status, time prices, and noneconomic factors. It would then be possible to forecast more accurately changes in utilization if prices were increased or decreased, as under different national health insurance plans.

When expenditures, rather than visits or hospital utilization, are used as the dependent variable, estimated price and income elasticities are generally higher, presumably because expenditures include some measures of quality. Physician visits, hospital admissions, and patient days do not enable the investigator to differentiate between visits that include a greater intensity of services, use of specialists or changes in the length of the visit. Expenditure data reflect quality as well as quantity of services; therefore, price and income elasticity estimates based on expenditure data partly measure the demand for quality as well as the demand for quantity of services. When expenditure data are used, however, it is particularly important that prices be accurately measured. If, for example, a physician charges a higher price to higher-income persons, then part of the difference in expenditures between high- and low-income persons is a result of price differences and not of differences in quantity or quality.

The measurement of price has been troublesome for all demand studies. Ideally, the price should reflect the out-of-pocket price the patient pays, but estimates of out-of-pocket prices for each service used are generally unavailable. Instead, the stated price or an average price for all services is used, and whether or not the patient has any insurance coverage is separately included in the statistical analysis. For policy purposes it would be desirable to know the effect of deductibles and copayments (of different magnitudes) on utilization. The effect of a copayment will also vary depending upon the size of the patient's income. Recently, however, data have become available from the RAND Health Insurance Study that provide evidence of the effect of income-related copayments on medical services use and expenditures. The authors report that

> Interim results indicate that persons fully covered for medical services spend about 50 percent more than do similar persons with income-related catastrophic insurance. Full coverage leads to more services per user. Both ambulatory services and hospital admissions increase (19).

Data from the recently completed National Ambulatory Care Survey is also beginning to generate useful elasticity estimates.

The importance of time costs on demand has been included in statistical demand studies only recently. Only a few studies have estimated time price elasticities. As the importance of out-of-pocket price declines with the greater availability of health insurance, time costs will become an even more important determinant of utilization. Failure to include time explicitly as a factor affecting demand for services may also result in incorrectly attributing its effect to other factors.

Demand studies have also differed with respect to the inclusion of substitutes and complements in the demand model. The demand for hospital care will depend, in part, on the price of ambulatory services. The availability of data on substitutes and complements has generally been limited. Excluding such factors from the statistical estimation of demand may affect the price elasticities of demand for hospital services or for other services whose demand is being analyzed.

The measurement of income has also distorted the results of demand studies. Ideally, it is desirable to measure the effect of usual or permanent income, but when surveys collect income data, the incomes of those surveyed may be temporarily high or low. If, for example, a person is sick and their income is temporarily low, but their expenditures are related to their usual income, they will show up in the survey as having a low income but a high expenditure. Thus, if demands for medical services are related to usual and not temporary income, then the estimate of income elasticity will be too low when it is measured by using temporary incomes.

Data used in demand studies have also differed by level of aggregation. Some studies have been based on state averages, others have used individuals as the unit of observation. In those studies where the level of aggregation encompasses a state, certain factors known to affect demand, such as age, may turn out to be statistically insignificant because there is insufficient variation between states according to age. Use of individual data, however, has generally resulted in lower elasticity estimates. When individual data are used, many individuals in the sample may not have had any utilization during the period covered and it is often difficult to separate the effects of economic factors from all other variables that are included and that have an effect on demand.

The data bases from which elasticity estimates were derived have changed over time. Initially, researchers used state data which included only gross measures of prices and the degree of availability of insurance coverage. There were then a number of studies which used claims and premium data from specific insurance companies. Occasionally there were instances of a natural experiment, as when a copayment was introduced in the insurance plan for a particular group of people. Comparisons have also been made between individuals having different insurance policies. More recently, as in the RAND Health Insurance Study, a designed experiment was made possible. As the data have improved, it has become possible to develop better measures of prices, as well as to show the effect of income related copayments and health status.

The foregoing discussion of empirical demand studies provides some indication of the great variety of variables used, of how economic factors are measured, and of the source of data. Such studies have also used different methods of statistical estimation. Most studies have used a single-equation approach, although some have used simultaneous equations. Differences in statistical estimation methods could also result in different elasticity estimates. Given these differences in approach, data, and methods, it is not surprising that large variations exist in the statistical estimates of price and income elasticities.

A summary of some results of statistical demand studies is presented in Tables 5-1, 5-2, and 5-3. Generally, hospital and physician services are price inelastic. The price elasticity for patient days varies from $-.2$ to $-.7$; for admissions the variation in price elasticity is from $-.03$ to $-.5$; and for physician visits the price elasticity varies from $-.1$ to $-.2$. The estimate of income elasticity for medical care expenditures is approximately one ($+1.0$). The statistical effect of income appears to have declined over time as more of the patient's bill is paid for

TABLE 5-1. A Review of Some Empirical Results on Price Elasticities of Demand for Medical Care

Study	Hospital Admissions	Hospital Length of Stay	Hospital Patient Days	Hospital Expenditures	Physician Visits	Physician Expenditures	Physician and Hospital Expenditures	Nursing Home Services
B. Chiswick (1976)								−.23
K. Davis and L. Russell (1972)	−.50	−.24	−.32 to −.46					
M. Feldstein (1971)	−.43	−.23	−.67					
M.S. Feldstein (1977)	−.20	−.03	−.23					
P. Feldstein and R. Severson (1964)					−.13 to −.18			
F. Goldman and M. Grossman (1978)					−.03 to −.06 (pediatric visits)			
W.G. Manning et al. (1981)							−.20	
J. Newhouse and C. Phelps (1976)	−.17	−.02		−.24	−.16	−.42		
Newhouse, Phelps, and Marquis (1980)		−.06 to −.23			−.09 to −.13		−2.13 to −2.14	
C. Phelps (1975)		−.03			−.18	.19		

C. Phelps and
J. Newhouse (1974)
G. Rosenthal (1970)

−.14

−.00 to −.70
(depending on
diagnosis)

R. Rosett and
L. Huang (1973)

−.35
(at 20% co-ins)
−1.5
(at 80% co-ins)

Sources: B. Chiswick, "The Demand for Nursing Home Care: An Analysis of the Substitution Between Institutional and Noninstitutional Care," *Journal of Human Resources* (Summer 1976); Karen Davis and Louise Russell, "The Substitution of Hospital Outpatient Care for Inpatient Care," *Review of Economics and Statistics* 54 (1972); M. Feldstein, "Hospital Cost Inflation: A Study of Nonprofit Price Dynamics," *American Economic Review* (December 1971); M. Feldstein, "Quality Change and the Demand for Hospital Care," *Econometrica* (October 1977); P. Feldstein and R. Severson, "The Demand for Medical Care," *Report of the Commission on the Cost of Medical Care*, Vol. 1 (Chicago: American Medical Association, 1964): pp. 56–76; F. Goldman and M. Grossman, "The Demand for Pediatric Care: An Hedonic Approach," *Journal of Political Economy* (April 1978); W. G. Manning et al., "A Two-Part Model of the Demand for Medical Care: Preliminary Results from the Health Insurance Study," in J. Van Der Gaag and M. Perlman, Eds., *Health, Economics, and Health Economics* (Amsterdam: North-Holland, 1981); J. Newhouse and C. Phelps, "New Estimates of Price and Income Elasticities for Medical Services," in R. Rosett, Ed., *The Role of Health Insurance in the Health Services Sector* (New York: National Bureau of Economic Research, 1976); J.P. Newhouse, C.E. Phelps, and S. Marquis, "On Having Your Cake and Eating It Too: Econometric Problems in Estimating Demand for Health Services," *Journal of Econometrics* (August 1980); C. Phelps, "The Effects of Insurance on Demand for Medical Care," in R. Anderson et al., Eds., *Equity in Health Services: Empirical Analysis in Social Policy* (Cambridge, Mass.: Ballinger, 1975); C. Phelps and J. Newhouse, "Coinsurance, The Price of Time, and the Demand for Medical Services," *Review of Economics and Statistics* (August 1974); G. Rosenthal, "Price Elasticity of Demand for Short-Terms General Hospital Services," in H. Klarman, Ed., *Empirical Studies in Health Economics* (Baltimore: Johns Hopkins University Press, 1970); R. Rosett and Lien-fu Huang, "The Effect of Health Insurance on the Demand for Medical Care," *Journal of Political Economy* (March–April 1973).

TABLE 5-2. Time–Price Elasticities for Physician Services

Travel Time	Total Physician Visits
J. Acton (1976)	
To public Outpatient Dept.	−.6 to −1.0
To private physician's office	−.25 to −.37
F. Goldman and M. Grossman (1978)	−.06 to −.07

Waiting Time	
J. Acton (1976)	
To public Outpatient Dept.	−.12
To private physician's office	−.05
C. Phelps (1975)	−.07

Sources: J. Acton, "Demand for Health Care Among the Urban Poor with Special Emphasis on the Role of Time," in R. Rosett, Ed., *The Role of Health Insurance in the Health Services Sector* (New York: National Bureau of Economic Research, 1976); F. Goldman and M. Grossman, "The Demand for Pediatric Care: An Hedonic Approach," *Journal of Political Economy* (April 1978); C. Phelps, "The Effects of Insurance on Demand for Medical Care," in R. Anderson et al., Eds., *Equity in Health Services: Empirical Analysis in Social Policy* (Cambridge, Mass.: Ballinger, 1975).

by third-party payors. The growth in insurance coverage, both as a percentage of the bill paid and in terms of the type of medical services covered, is income related. As the out-of-pocket price for medical services becomes smaller and smaller, the importance of income declines and time costs become an important determinant of medical use. The estimates of elasticity of demand with respect to time are surprisingly high: −.6 to −1 with respect to travel time to a public outpatient department and −.2 to −.3 to a private physician's office.

Insurance coverage for hospital services is currently quite high, approximately 90 percent of the hospital bill is paid for by private or public insurance. It is therefore unlikely that hospital use will increase rapidly if the remaining out-of-pocket prices were to be paid for under any form of comprehensive national health insurance plan.

Physician in-hospital services also have a relatively high degree of insurance coverage. Physician office visits, however, have less-complete coverage. Any policies that would lower the price of physician office visits could result in a substantial increase in demand for physician services. Several years ago it was conservatively estimated that a 75 percent increase in demand for physician services could occur (20).

The demand for nursing home care appears to be price inelastic, approximately −.2. Thus policies to include nursing home care under national health insurance could result in large increases in use and, consequently, expenditures on such care.

To date, too little is known of the effect on hospital use of a decrease in the price of substitute sources of care. One way in which the cost of medical services can be reduced is to provide insurance coverage (thereby lowering the out-of-pocket price) for lower cost substitutes, e.g., outpatient services and nursing home care. How successful such a policy will be depends, in part, on the cross-elasticity of demand of hospital care to the price of such lower cost substitutes.

TABLE 5-3. Estimated Income Elasticities of Demand for Medical Services

Study	Physician Services	Medical Care Expenditure	Nursing Home Care
F. Goldman and M. Grossman (1978)	1.32 (pediatric visits)		
B. Chiswick (1976)			0.8
C. Phelps (1975)	.11		
R. Rosett and L. Huang (1973)		.25 to .45	
V. Fuchs and M. Kramer (1973)	.57		
R. Anderson and L. Benham (1970)	.63		
M. Silver (1970)	.85	1.2	
P. Feldstein and J. Carr (1964)		1.0	
P. Feldstein and R. Severson (1964)	.56	.6	

Sources: R. Anderson and L. Benham, "Factors Affecting the Relationship Between Family Income and Medical Care Consumption," in H. Klarman, Ed., *Empirical Studies in Health Economics* (Baltimore: Johns Hopkins University Press, 1970); B. Chiswick, "The Demand for Nursing Home Care: An Analysis of the Substitution Between Institutional and Noninstitutional Care," *Journal of Human Resources* (Summer 1976); P. Feldstein and J. Carr, "The Effect of Income on Medical Care Spending," *Proceeding of the Social Statistics Section of the American Statistical Association* (1964); P. Feldstein and R. Severson, "The Demand for Medical Care," *Report of the Commission on the Cost of Medical Care*, Vol. 1 (Chicago: American Medical Association, 1964): pp. 56–76; V. Fuchs and M. Kramer, *Determinants of Expenditures for Physicians Services in the United States, 1948–1968* (New York: National Bureau of Economic Research, Occasional Paper 117, 1973); C. Phelps; "The Effects of Insurance on Demand for Medical Care," in R. Anderson et al., Eds., *Equity in Health Services: Empirical Analysis in Social Policy* (Cambridge, Mass.: Ballinger, 1975); R. Rosett and L. Huang, "The Effect of Health Insurance on the Demand for Medical Care," *Journal of Political Economy* (March–April, 1973); M. Silver, "An Economic Analysis of Variations in Medical Expenses and Work Loss Rates," in H. Klarman, Ed., *Empirical Studies in Health Economics* (Baltimore: Johns Hopkins University Press, 1970).

While our knowledge of price elasticities of demand is increasing, we still do not have adequate knowledge of a number of areas, such as the effect of deductibles and income-related copayments (21). However as additional data become available from the RAND study and from other large population surveys of families in their use of medical services, estimates of these factors as well as of time elasticities will become more accurate. Economists will then become more confident in forecasting the effect on utilization of changes in prices and co-payments. Such estimates should be particularly useful in the design and evaluation of alternative national health insurance programs.

APPLICATIONS OF DEMAND ANALYSIS

THE ALLOCATION OF HOSPITAL BEDS

Since 1948 the Hill-Burton program, a federal act, has subsidized the construction of thousands of hospital beds, costing billions of dollars. The Hill-Burton criterion for supporting hospital bed construction was that 4.5 hospital beds should be available per thousand population in areas with more than 12 persons per square mile; that 5.0 beds per thousand should exist in areas with between 6 and 12 persons per square mile; and that 5.5 beds per thousand should exist in areas with fewer than 6 persons per square mile. According to the Hill-Burton formula, population density is the sole determinant of beds per thousand population.

In one of the earliest hospital demand studies, Gerald Rosenthal contrasted the Hill-Burton standard with a demand-based approach to determining the number of hospital beds in an area (22). Rosenthal first constructed a model of the demand for hospital utilization. He included both economic (price, insurance, and income) and noneconomic (age, marital status, sex, percent urbanization, race, education, and number of persons per dwelling unit) variables in the demand model. The data were based on state averages for 1950 and 1960. His dependent variables, by state, were patient days, admissions per thousand population, and average length of stay. Separate regressions were estimated for each of the dependent variables for 1950 and then again for 1960. To calculate the expected number of beds per thousand population in any state based on demand factors, Rosenthal inserted the average value for each of the independent variables in each state into the regression model. The number of patient days was estimated for each state on the basis of that state's demand characteristics. The average-sized hospital in a state was used in conjunction with the probability (uniform across states) that it would be filled when translating the estimate of patient days into the number of beds for that state. To make sure that the pressure on facilities in each state was uniform, the same probability of being full (one day in 100) was used; further, since the average-sized hospital varies between states, the substitution of one state's size for another's was avoided.*

Based on each state's demand characteristics, the average size of its hospitals, and the same probability of being full, the number of beds per thousand population was estimated for each state for 1950 and 1960. The number of beds per thousand varied from less than two to more than four, with each state having the same pressure on its facilities. The results of this demand-oriented approach were then compared state-by-state with those yielded by the Hill-Burton formula. Since the Hill-Burton formula does not consider any demand characteristics, only population density, the pressure on facilities varied greatly between states: those with low demand factors had lower occupancy rates and excess

---

*If admissions to a hospital have a Poisson distribution, then, given the same probability of being full, smaller hospitals will have a lower average occupancy rate than larger hospitals. For example, if it is estimated that on any given day in a community there will be a demand for 400 patient days, then these patient days may be translated into beds in the following manner:

The mean is equal to the variance in a Poisson distribution. Thus $\bar{x} = 400$, $\bar{x} = \sigma^2$, therefore the standard deviation (σ) = 20. If it is desired to have a bed available 99 times out of 100, then that would encompass three standard deviations of the distribution. Thus, the number of beds is determined by

$$\bar{x} + 3 (\sigma) \text{ or } 400 + 3(20) = 460 \text{ beds}$$

and the average occupancy would be 86 percent (400/460).

If the estimate of demand were to be equally shared among 10 independent hospitals, then the number of beds required would be $40 + 3(6) = 58$ multiplied by 10 hospitals, for a total of 580 beds. Each 58-bed hospital would have an average occupancy rate of approximately 68 percent (40/58).

hospital beds; those with high demand factors had greater pressure on their facilities through higher occupancy rates, and consequently a greater likelihood of their not having a bed when needed. To equalize out the pressure on facilities, Rosenthal recommended using a demand model to allocate beds among areas.

Rosenthal also demonstrated how the demand model could be used for social policy. If a state desired to increase its utilization, it could lower the price of care and increase insurance coverage in the population. (The number of beds necessary to meet this higher estimate can then be calculated in the same way as previously described.) Manipulating demand factors to bring about a change in utilization was shown to be a more efficient policy instrument than relying on a set number of beds to satisfy legitimate needs for care.

Proponents of the thesis that the bed supply creates a bed demand implicitly assume that the pressure on facilities (not necessarily the occupancy rate) will be the same across all facilities. To test this hypothesis, Rosenthal calculated a pressure index for each state, which was the actual occupancy rate as a percentage of its maximum occupancy. This pressure index varied from a low of 80 to more than 100. The fact that different facilities had different pressures as well as occupancy rates suggests that supply does not create demand. In addition, high pressure indices correlated positively with demand variables and correlated negatively with supply variables. Rosenthal concluded that high demand led to greater pressure on facilities, while an increased bed supply led to lower pressure on facilities.

This additional evidence that demand factors affect hospital utilization suggests that bed allocation should be based upon relative demands in an area rather than upon an arbitrary standard.* If a change in utilization for a particular population group is desired, it can be brought about more directly and efficiently by changing demand factors rather than by simply changing the number of beds.

USING A DEMAND MODEL TO EXPLAIN ANNUAL CHANGES IN PERSONAL HEALTH CARE EXPENDITURES

Personal health care expenditures have increased from $10.9 billion in 1950 to $255.0 billion in 1981. The average annual rates of increase have, however, varied from 8.1 percent and 10.0 percent per year during 1950–1960 and 1960–1968 to more rapid annual percentage increases after the introduction of Medicare and Medicaid in 1966, 12.4 percent per year during 1968–1972, 12.8 percent during 1972–1976, and 14.1 percent during 1976–1981.

The rapid increases in medical care expenditures during these various periods have been the result of increased demands for medical care, the increasingly large involvement of government in the financing of medical care, and increases in the costs of providing such services. Together, these changes in demand and

---

*The Rosenthal study should be considered illustrative of the type of demand study to be undertaken for purposes of policy and planning. For actual planning of facilities in an area, a less aggregative demand model would be needed. Estimates of the demand for beds by service—obstetrics, pediatrics, medical-surgery—would also be more useful. Inclusion of substitutes for hospital care and greater stability of the parameters of the model would provide greater confidence in the application of such a model.

supply have resulted in increased prices and quantities for medical services, both of which constitute a part of the increases in expenditures for medical care.

Although many of the factors affecting both demand and supply during these periods have changed, most factors have been changing gradually. The price of medical services is perhaps the most important factor that has sharply changed. In addition to increases in the price of medical care, there have been increases in the population, changes in its age distribution, and increases in personal incomes that have led to increased demands for medical care. A more detailed analysis of changes in medical care expenditures would examine additional demand factors, but the changes in prices, incomes, and population can be used to provide a rough approximation of the importance of these demand factors in contributing to increases in medical care expenditures during these periods (23).

As shown in Table 5-4, the rise in the price of medical care as measured by the Medical Care Price Index, which is part of the Consumer Price Index, substantially contributed to each period's increase in medical care expenditures. For each of the periods examined, medical price increases represent approximately one-half of the annual percentage increase in medical expenditures. Before 1968, medical prices contributed slightly less than one-half of the annual percentage increase, but in the post-1968 period the increase in medical prices contributed more than one-half of the annual percentage increase in medical expenditures. When the rate of increase in medical prices is subtracted from the rate of increase in medical expenditures, the result is the average annual percentage increase in the *real* quantity of medical care purchased.

To explain changes in the quantity of medical care purchased during this period, we must first adjust for changes in the population, which will give us the annual percentage increase in the quantity of medical care per person. Subtracting the rate of increase in population from the rate of increase in real medical output yields the annual percentage increase in quantity of medical care per person during this period. As shown in Table 5-4, population changes explain only a small percentage of the overall rate of increase in medical expenditures, particularly in the post-1968 period. During this latter period, population had been increasing at a smaller annual rate while the overall rate of increase in medical expenditures had been increasing more rapidly than in the past.

Per capita incomes were rising (although at different annual rates of increase) during the different periods examined. If an income elasticity of 1.0 is assumed—that is, the increase in consumer demand for medical care will increase at the same rate as the increase in income—then part of the annual percentage increase in medical care can be accounted for by increased per capita incomes.

Medical care prices have been increasing at a faster rate than prices in the rest of the economy. Thus, in addition to the use of the annual rate of increase in medical prices to determine the rate of increase in *real* medical care purchases, the rate of increase in medical prices relative to the prices of other consumer goods and services can be used to represent an increase in the price of real medical care services. With an increase in the price of a service we would expect a decrease in demand for that service; the size of the decrease in demand for medical care would depend upon the price elasticity of demand for medical care. Assuming that the price elasticity of demand for medical services is −.2, which means that the demand for medical care is relatively price inelastic, a 1 percent

TABLE 5-4. Factors Affecting Changes in Personal Health Care Expenditures

Factor	Average Annual Rates of Change (%)					
	1950–1960	1960–1968	1966–1981	1968–1972	1972–1976	1976–1981
Personal health care expenditures	8.1	10.0	13.2	12.4	13.2	14.1
Accounted for by						
Rise in price of medical care (CPI Medical Care)	4.0	3.7	8.0	5.7	8.7	9.8
Population increase (resident population)	1.7	1.3	1.1	1.2	1.0	1.1
Rise in real personal income per capita, increasing medical expenditures by an equal percentage (income elasticity = 1.00)	1.9	3.5	1.5	2.2	1.1	.5
Decline in quantity demanded because of rise in relative price of medical care (price elasticity = −.2)	−.4	−.4	−.3	−.2	−.1	−.3
Total accounted for	7.2	8.1	10.3	8.9	10.7	11.1
Unexplained residual	.9	1.9	2.9	3.5	2.5	3.0

Sources: Robert Gibson and Daniel Waldo, "National Health Expenditures, 1980," *Health Care Financing Review* 3 (September 1980): 36, Table 3; U.S. Department of Health, Education and Welfare, *Social Security Bulletin* 40 (April 1977): 88–91, Tables M39–M40; U.S. Bureau of the Census, *Statistical Abstract of the United States, 1981*, 102 ed. (Washington, D.C.: U.S. Government Printing Office, 1981), p. 9, Table 8; "Estimates of the Population of the United States to April 1, 1982": *Current Population Reports*, Series P-25, No. 914 (June 1982); U.S. Bureau of Labor Statistics, *CPI Detailed Report* (January 1982), p. 80, Table 1A; p. 88, Table 5A; U.S. Department of Commerce, Bureau of Economic Analysis, *Survey of Current Business* 62 (April 1982): 10, Table 1.7.

increase in price would lead to a .2 percent decrease in quantity demanded. With reference to Table 5-4, the rate of increase in the quantity of medical care will decline by .2 multiplied by the relative rate of increase in the price of medical care.

When these factors affecting demand are summed up for the different periods, most of the annual percentage increase in medical expenditures can be accounted for. The amount of the unexplained residual is smaller for the pre-1968 periods than for the more recent periods—0.9 and 1.9 percent for 1950–1960 and 1960–1968, respectively; 3.5 and 2.5 percent for 1968–1972 and for 1972–1976, respectively; and 3.0 percent for 1976–1981.

It is likely that the larger unexplained residual, from 1968 to 1972, which is the percentage increase in real medical care output that cannot be explained by the demand factors we have described, represents changes in the *type* of medical services produced. When medical prices were used to adjust expenditures to determine real output increases, it was assumed that the output produced was similar over time. After Medicare was introduced, the age distribution of hospital patients changed; the aged constituted a larger proportion of the patients. The aged require more costly types of service than the nonaged. Also, after Medicare, hospitals increased their service quality by adding more facilities and services and increasing ratios of personnel per patient, both of which would contribute to an increase in real expenditures per person in the post-Medicare period. It is likely that if the foregoing analysis included these factors, the size of the unexplained residual would be much lower.

THE DEMAND FOR MEDICAL CARE FACED BY THE FIRM

Up to this point we have discussed the determinants of demand for medical services. The demands for hospital care, physician services, nursing and home care are derived from the demand for a treatment. Based upon estimates derived from empirical studies, the demand for hospital and physician services was determined to be relatively inelastic with respect to price. However, it is important to distinguish between the overall market demand for a service such as hospital care, and the demand facing an individual provider. While the overall demand for hospital care may be relatively inelastic with respect to price, the demand facing an individual hospital, especially in a community with several hospitals, is likely to be more price elastic, since any one hospital is a possible substitute for another.

Hospitals are aware that they must compete with other hospitals. The way in which they attempt to increase their share of the market in an area is to compete for physicians. Because patients are hospitalized where their physicians have staff appointments, if hospitals can increase their number of staff physicians, the derived demand for that hospital will increase. To attract and retain physicians, hospitals attempt to acquire facilities and services that their staff physicians may require for treatment so that they do not have to refer their patients to other hospitals and other physicians. If the hospital is currently operating at, or near, capacity, then it will invest in additional beds. If physicians have to ration beds and facilities among themselves, they may decide to affiliate with hospitals that are willing to provide the necessary resources to increase their productivity.

Although the overall demand for hospital care may be relatively price inelastic, the demand facing any individual hospital is more elastic, particularly when physicians in an area have multiple staff appointments. This distinction between the overall patient demand for hospital care and the demand facing any individual hospital is important when examining the market structure of hospitals to determine whether they have the characteristics of a natural public utility.

APPENDIX: THE EFFECT OF COINSURANCE ON THE DEMAND FOR MEDICAL CARE

A diagram may clarify the effect of coinsurance on the demand for medical care. Figure 5-4 shows the relationship between the price of medical care and the quantity demanded, with all of the other determinants of demand being held constant. When the price is P_1, the quantity demanded will be Q_1. If insurance were provided that carried a coinsurance feature, then the person using it would have to pay the remainder of the price. The price paid by the patient would be P_2, which is, for example, 80 percent of P_1; the third-party payor would pay the remainder of the price, $P_1 - P_2$. As a result of the 20 percent price reduction, the patient will now demand Q_2 of medical services. (The actual increase in quantity demanded as a result of the decrease in price due to coinsurance will depend upon the size of the coinsurance and the price elasticity of demand.) As long as there is some responsiveness of price to quantity demanded, coinsurance will increase demand by lowering the price the patient will pay for medical care.

Although insurance coverage represents a *movement* down an individual's demand curve, the aggregate effect of an increase in coverage is to cause a *shift* in the demand for medical care. For example, according to the demand curve represented by D_1 in Figure 5-5, an individual would demand Q_1 units of medical care if the price he or she had to pay were $10 per unit. If the individual were now provided insurance with a coinsurance feature requiring that only 80 percent of the total price be paid, then at a price of $10 per unit the individual need only pay $8. Therefore, the individual would move down his demand curve and consume Q_2 units at a price of $8 per unit. The actual price of Q_2 units is not $8 per unit but $10 per unit; the third-party payor pays 20 percent, or $2 per unit. Thus, the actual demand curve for medical care has shifted to the right. Similarly, if the initial price were $14, the patient with demand curve D_1 would consume Q_3 units of medical care. With the introduction of an 80 percent coinsurance program, the patient would have to pay only 80 percent of $14, or $11.20 per unit. The patient would move down his demand curve and consume Q_4 units at a price of $11.20 per unit. The total price per unit at Q_4 is, however, $14 per unit. Each of the points on the original demand curve (D_1) now represents only 80 percent of the total price. The new demand curve (D_2) represents the relationship between the total price per unit (80 percent of which is paid for by the patient and 20 percent by the third-party payor) and the quantities demanded at these different prices.

The analysis of the effect of insurance on the market for medical care be-

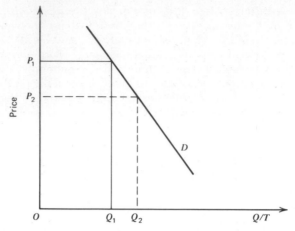

Figure 5-4. The effect of coinsurance on the demand for medical care.

comes more complicated when there is a coinsurance provision and a rising supply curve for medical care. For example, according to Figure 5-6, the patient's original demand curve is D_1. The provision of health insurance with a coinsurance feature (for simplicity, it is assumed to be 50 percent, with the remainder being paid by the government) will result in a shift in demand for care to D_2, which represents the amount that both the patients and the government will pay for medical care. Every point on demand curve D_2 represents a doubling of the price for a given quantity over D_1, since it is a 50 percent coinsurance program. So far the analysis is similar to the previous example. However, since the new demand curve (D_2) intersects the supply curve at a higher price than previously, a new equilibrium price and quantity of medical care, P_2 and Q_2, will

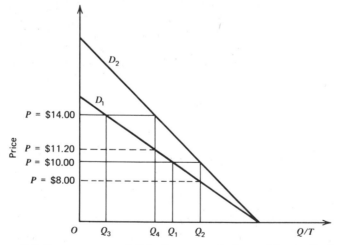

Figure 5-5. Insurance as a shift in the aggregate demand for medical care.

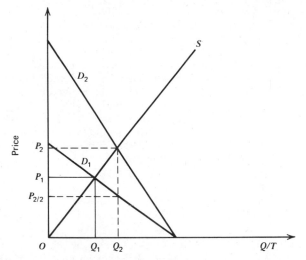

Figure 5-6. The effect of coinsurance on the aggregate demand for medical care with a rising supply curve.

be established. Q_2 is thus the only level of quantity at which the public pays one-half the price of medical care ($P_2/2$) that is also an equilibrium position. Thus, the price the consumer will pay with a 50 percent coinsurance is greater than 50 percent of the original market price ($P_1/2$). The introduction of a percentage copayment feature does not mean that the consumer's price will be a similar percentage of the original market price. Nor does it mean that the amount of care used will increase by that same proportion. The greater the coinsurance paid for by the government (or other third party), the greater the consumer's use of medical services will be, but the actual price the consumer must pay and the amount actually consumed will depend upon the elasticity of both demand and supply. The more elastic demand and supply are, the greater the increase in quantity and the less the rise in price will be.

REFERENCES

1. Roger Lee and Lewis Jones, *The Fundamentals of Good Medical Care* (Chicago: The University of Chicago Press, 1933).

2. Kevin J. Lancaster, "A New Approach to Consumer Theory," *Journal of Political Economy,* April 1966.

3. Michael Grossman, "On the Concept of Health Capital and the Demand for Health," *Journal of Political Economy,* March–April 1972.

4. Two valuable reviews of the early literature in this area are: Martin S. Feldstein, "Econometric Studies of Health Economics," in M.D. Intriligator and D.A. Kendrick, Eds., *Frontiers of Quantitative Economics,* Vol. II. (Amsterdam: North-Holland, 1974), and Herbert E. Klarman, *The Economics of Health* (New York: Columbia University Press, 1965).

5. A number of surveys have collected data on family income and expenditures on medical care. A few of the better-known surveys are those conducted by the National Center for Health Statistics as part of the Health Interview Survey and published in Series 10, *Vital and Health Statistics* (Washington, D.C.: U.S. DHEW, various years.) The National Opinion Research Center, University of Chicago, has also conducted national surveys on medical expenditures. These surveys, which have been conducted at five-year intervals beginning in 1953, have been presented in various publications, such as Odin W. Anderson, Patricia Collette, and Jacob Feldman, *Changes in Family Medical Care Expenditures: A Five Year Resurvey* (Cambridge, Mass.: Harvard University Press, 1963). A more recent national survey (1977) of medical care expenditures was undertaken by the National Center for Health Services Research, and is referred to as the National Medical Care Expenditure Survey.

6. The distinction between permanent and transitory components of income and their relationship to consumption are discussed by Friedman in terms of his permanent income theory of consumption in Milton Friedman, *A Theory of the Consumption Function* (Princeton, N.J.: Princeton University Press, 1957).

7. For a more complete discussion of the role of time in the demand for medical care, see Charles E. Phelps and Joseph P. Newhouse, "Coinsurance, the Price of Time, and the Demand for Medical Services," *Review of Economics and Statistics*, August 1974: Also see, Jan P. Acton, "Demand for Health Care Among the Urban Poor, with Special Emphasis on the Role of Time," in Richard Rosett, Ed., *The Role of Health Insurance in the Health Services Sector* (New York: National Bureau of Economic Research, 1976).

8. The same data were analyzed by Anne A. Scitovsky and Nelda M. Snyder, "Effect of Coinsurance on Use of Physician Services," and Charles E. Phelps and Joseph P. Newhouse, "Effect of Coinsurance: A Multivariate Analysis," in *Social Security Bulletin,* June 1972.

9. Scitovsky and Snyder, "Effect of Coinsurance on the Use of Physician Services," p. 15.

10. Anne A. Scitovsky and Nelda McCall, "Coinsurance and the Demand for Physician Services: Four Years Later," *Social Security Bulletin* (May 1977).

11. Several articles have discussed the role of the physician in the manner described above. Several of the earlier ones are Robert Rice, "Analysis of the Hospital As An Economic Organism," *Modern Hospital 106(4)* (April 1966); Paul J. Feldstein, "Research on the Demand for Health Services," *Milbank Memorial Fund Quarterly* (July 1966), and Martin S. Feldstein, "Econometric Studies of Health Economics," *op. cit.*

12. Victor Fuchs, "The Growing Demand for Medical Care," *The New England Journal of Medicine* (July 25, 1968): 192.

13. Max Shain and Milton Roemer, "Hospital Costs Relate to the Supply of Beds," *Modern Hospital*, April 1959, and Milton Roemer, "Bed Supply and Hospital Utilization: A Natural Experiment," *Hospitals* (November 1, 1961).

14. The discussion that follows is based on the article by George Monsma, "Marginal Revenue and Demand for Physicians' Services," in H. Klarman, Ed., *Empirical Studies In Health Economics* (Baltimore: Johns Hopkins University Press, 1970), and the article by Mark Pauly and Mark Satterthwaite, "The Pricing of Primary Care Physicians' Services: A Test of the Role of Consumer Information," *The Bell Journal of Economics* (Autumn 1981).

15. For a more complete discussion of the above studies and their sources, see the article by Monsma, *op. cit.*

16. M. Pauly and M. Satterthwaite, *op. cit.*

17. Hirsch S. Ruchlin et al., "The Efficacy of Second-Opinion Consultation Programs: A Cost-Benefit Perspective," *Medical Care* (January 1982).

18. For a comprehensive review of demand studies up to the mid-1970s see Larry J. Kimbell and Donald E. Yett, *An Evaluation of Policy Related Research on the Effects of Alternative Health Care Reimbursement Systems* (Human Resources Research Center, University of Southern California, undated) (Mimeographed). Also see, Joseph P. Newhouse, "Insurance Benefits, Out-of-Pocket Payments, and the Demand for Medical Care: A Review of the Recent Literature," *Health and Medical Care Services Review* (July–August 1978) and Joseph P. Newhouse, "The Demand for Medical Care Services: A Retrospect and Prospect," in Jacques Van Der Gaag and Mark Perlman, Eds., *Health, Economics, and Health Economics* (Amsterdam: North-Holland, 1981).

19. For a more complete discussion, as well as a description of the study, see Joseph P. Newhouse et al., "Some Interim Results From a Controlled Trial of Cost Sharing in Health Insurance," *New England Journal of Medicine* 305(25) (December 17, 1981).

20. Joseph P. Newhouse, Charles E. Phelps, and William B. Schwartz, "Policy Options and the Impact of National Health Insurance," *New England Journal of Medicine* (June 13, 1974).

21. See, however, Joseph P. Newhouse et al., "The Effect of Deductibles on the Demand for Medical Care Services," *Journal of the American Statistical Association* (September 1980).

22. Gerald Rosenthal, *The Demand for General Hospital Facilities*, Monograph No. 14 (Chicago: American Hospital Association, 1964).

23. The discussion in this section is similar to that presented in an earlier article by Victor Fuchs, "The Growing Demand for Medical Care," *The New England Journal of Medicine* 192 (July 25, 1968).

CHAPTER 6

The Demand for Health Insurance

Although the number of services covered and the percentage of the bill paid by health insurance have been increasing over time, insurance coverage still varies greatly by population group, by services covered, and by percentage of the medical bill covered. In pointing to the percentage of the medical bill covered by insurance as a measure of its "adequacy," anything less than 100 percent coverage (or at least a "high" percentage) is deemed by some to be "inadequate." The policy recommendations that follow from such a normative judgment are based either upon the assumption that inadequacy is a result of insufficient financial means on the part of consumers for purchasing the appropriate amount of insurance, or that the inadequacy is a result of the health insurance industry's failure to provide more appropriate coverage. The recommendations based upon this normative judgment of inadequate health insurance are that the government should either provide comprehensive coverage under its own auspices or subsidize the purchase of health insurance.

To determine the "appropriateness" of health insurance coverage in the United States, appropriateness in an economic sense must be defined. It is also important to determine whether there are market conditions that distort the consumer's ability to select the economically appropriate quantity of health insurance coverage. This chapter, therefore, examines the determinants of the demand for health insurance. A subsequent chapter examines the economic efficiency of the health insurance market to determine whether there are (or have been) distortions on the demand or supply side of that market that result in either "too much" or "too little" (or insufficient varieties) of health insurance being offered. The conclusions with respect to the supply side of that market should indicate the appropriate role of government, if any, as a provider of health insurance.

110

HEALTH INSURANCE TERMINOLOGY

As a preface to the analysis of the demand for health insurance, a brief discussion of a number of concepts used in health insurance is in order.

DEDUCTIBLES

When consumers pay a flat dollar amount for medical services before their insurance picks up all or part of the remainder of the price of that service, this is referred to as a deductible. Deductibles may be set in a number of ways: they may apply to each unit of service, or they may be cumulative—for example, once $100 has been paid by the consumer for physician services within a year, the third-party payor will contribute to the price of additional visits. Deductibles may also be established either on a family basis or for each individual. Deductibles may also be related to family income, with higher deductibles being required of persons with higher family incomes, as has been proposed under certain national health insurance schemes.

There are several reasons for using deductibles. One is that it lowers the administrative costs of claims processing in a situation where there are many small claims and the cost of handling these claims is high. In such a situation, the transaction costs might exceed the amount the people are willing to pay for insurance; a deductible provision lowers the transaction costs and enables consumers to purchase insurance for the remainder of their medical expenses at an amount that they are willing to pay that is greater than the transaction costs. Another reason that is offered by proponents for having deductibles is that in the distribution of medical expenses, both in the aggregate and by component of care (physician services, drugs, hospital care), a large percentage of families incur little or no medical expenditures within a year, whereas a smaller percentage of families incur very large expenditures. This phenomenon is illustrated in Figure 6-1A. The insurance cost of covering medical expenditures would obviously be lowered if a deductible were placed at the low end of the expenditure spectrum, as indicated by line A in Figure 6-1A. A third reason is that if the deductible is greater than the price of the service, an incentive is provided for the consumer to shop around.

The case against deductibles is generally made on the grounds that the deductible, no matter how small, may be a deterrent to needed care. Further, a flat deductible, irrespective of family income, represents a greater burden to low-income families than to high-income families.

The effect of the deductible on use of services is complex. If there is a deductible, once the deductible is exceeded and additional services are free, the deductible will have no effect on decreasing the use of services. Once the deductible has been paid, the patient will use the services as though their price were "zero." If the deductible has not been exceeded, then the price of the services will determine (other things being held constant) how much they will be used. A deductible by itself, therefore, will either tend to result in greater use of services (similar to a zero price) when a low deductible is used, or if the deductible is high, it will tend to make insurance coverage irrelevant to many

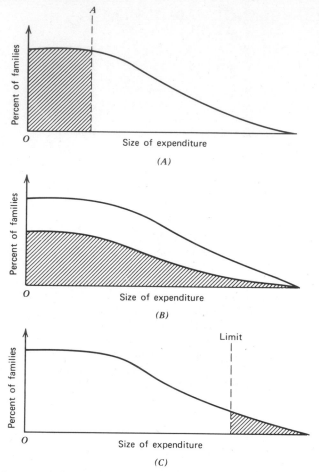

Figure 6-1. The expected distribution of family medical expenses with different types of copayments: (A) the imposition of a deductible, (B) a coinsurance provision, (C) a maximum or limit to coverage.

users of care. How effective a deductible will be will depend upon the size of the deductible, the expected medical expenditures of the family (if on a family basis), and on family income.

COINSURANCE

When the third-party payor reimburses the patient for a certain fraction of the price of the service, the arrangement is termed coinsurance. A coinsurance level of 20 percent in effect lowers the price to the patient of those covered services by 20 percent. If the price of the services should rise, then the insurance would pay 20 percent of the new, higher price. Coinsurance levels can also vary by service covered and by family income. The advantage of coinsurance is that it reduces the price of the service and still provides the patient with an incentive to seek out less costly providers. The effectiveness of a coinsurance feature will depend upon how responsive utilization is to lower prices, which is the price elasticity of demand. If use is very unresponsive to price, then coinsurance will merely be a way of reducing the cost of the insurance package to the consumer. Depending upon the level of coinsurance and the price elasticity of demand, coinsurance can change the distribution of medical expenditures, as shown in Figure 6-1B. Coinsurance would result in the consumer's paying for the shaded portion of Figure 6-1B, while the third-party payor would pay for the remainder of the medical expenses.

LIMITS AND MAXIMUMS

One method of reducing the cost of providing insurance coverage to the consumer is to reimburse patients for medical expenses up to a maximum dollar amount or a maximum amount of services; any expenditures above that limit become the responsibility of the patient. This approach shifts the cost of large expenditures, generally considered to be catastrophic, to the patient incurring them instead of distributing them among all insured persons. Limits have been used in the past by Blue Cross, such as when it covered hospital services up to a maximum of 30 days spent in the hospital. The part of medical expenditures that is excluded by limits and maximums is generally the tail of the distribution, as shown in Figure 6-1C. Large expenditures, incurred by a small percentage of families, are generally not responsive to prices; to exclude this part of the distribution from coverage appears to be particularly unwise, since large, unexpected losses to a small percentage of the population meet the criteria defining insurance risks. If the objective of using limits is to enable the insurance company to lower its insurance premium to consumers, then an alternative approach would be to use a small deductible for the many families that have small expenditures. This front-end deductible, when applied to many families, would be less of a financial hardship than would a catastrophic expense befalling a small percentage of the population.

Insurance coverage for the tail of the distribution, i.e., the large expenditures incurred by a small percentage of the population, is generally referred to as major medical or catastrophic insurance. Major medical coverage was an innovation introduced by the commercial insurance companies in the late 1940s to compete with Blue Cross, which until that time was the dominant third-party underwriter, and which sold hospitalization insurance only up to a maximum limit.

OTHER FORMS OF COVERAGE

Insurance contracts may include any or all of the above in various combinations of deductibles, coinsurance, and limits. Other aspects of insurance coverage also should be briefly mentioned. Some coverage may specifically exclude certain diseases that are preexisting conditions of illness in a potential insurance purchaser. Allowing such purchases would be like allowing a person who knew that his house was going to be burned to buy insurance to cover his loss. Other kinds of insurance coverage may include continuation of salary if a person becomes ill, or disability benefits if the person is unable to be fully rehabilitated once an illness has been incurred.

INDEMNITY VERSUS SERVICE BENEFITS

When Blue Cross was started in the 1930s, it provided a "service" benefit for hospital care, which meant that the price to the patient for the stay in the hospital (up to a maximum period) was reimbursed in full to the hospital. There were no cost-sharing provisions, deductibles, or coinsurance features for the patient. An indemnity benefit, which was offered by commercial insurance carriers, differed from a service benefit in that it reimbursed the patient, not the hospital, for medical costs the patient incurred. The amount of reimbursement was often a fixed dollar amount or a percentage of the price. Naturally, the hospitals that had founded Blue Cross preferred the service-benefit approach, since it meant that they would be reimbursed for all their services and there would be no incentive for the patient to shop around for the least expensive hospital. The hospitals would also incur lower collection costs if they could bill Blue Cross for all of their patients rather than have to collect from each patient. A more detailed discussion of the Blue Cross service benefit policy and a comparison between it and an indemnity policy is found in Appendix 1 of this chapter.

THE THEORY OF DEMAND FOR HEALTH INSURANCE

The consumer's demand for health insurance represents the amount of insurance coverage he or she is willing to buy at different prices (premiums) for health insurance. Additional insurance coverage will be purchased if the insurance premium (price) declines; once the consumer has *some* insurance, the marginal benefit of increasing the comprehensiveness of the insurance declines the more coverage he or she has. When the marginal benefit to the consumer of additional coverage equals the cost of buying that insurance, then, other things being equal, the "appropriate" amount of insurance will have been purchased. Appropriateness, in the economic sense, is defined as occurring when the marginal benefit of additional insurance to the consumer equals the marginal cost of purchasing that increased coverage.

According to this definition, 100 percent coverage of all medical expenses would be demanded only when the administrative price that was added onto the price paid by the consumer for that coverage was free. At positive administrative prices for insurance, the consumer would demand less than 100 percent coverage. This is because the marginal benefit of the last unit of insurance coverage would be purchased only if the price of that additional coverage to the consumer were small. Adding an administrative price above the pure premium would cause the total price of those last units to be greater than their marginal benefits. The consumer would purchase additional coverage only to the point where the benefit of additional coverage equaled the total price of additional coverage.

Keeping in mind that the appropriateness of the amount of insurance coverage consumers will buy will be related to their perception of the value of additional coverage compared with the additional cost of that coverage, we will examine the demand for health insurance under two conditions. In the first situation there is no "moral hazard": the demand for medical care is completely price inelastic in that patients cannot control the size of the loss once they are ill (1). In the second situation the effect on the demand for insurance coverage when moral hazard does exist will be considered.

To understand the factors that affect the demand for health insurance, it is necessary to be familiar with the economic theory underlying the purchase of insurance. This discussion should clarify why people buy insurance for some risks and not others. The economic theory of insurance is then used to predict the type of insurance expected to be most prevalent in the health field.*

To explain the demand for insurance, one must assume that an individual wishes to maximize his or her utility, which is the usual assumption that is made in demand analysis. Since a person does not know that he or she will be affected by an illness requiring a loss of wealth to pay for it, the individual who seeks to maximize his or her utility when subject to uncertain events seeks to maximize his or her *expected* utility. That is, the person can choose between two alternative courses of action:

1. He or she can purchase insurance and thereby incur a small loss in the form of the insurance premium, or,
2. He or she can self-insure, which means facing the small possibility of a large loss in the event that the illness occurs, or the large possibility that the medical loss will not occur.

To determine whether consumers will purchase insurance for an unexpected medical event or self-insure and bear the risk themselves, it is necessary to compare courses 1 and 2 to determine which choice provides them with a higher level of utility.

The use of expected utility, as discussed by M. Friedman and L. Savage in their classic article, "The Utility Analysis of Choices Involving Risk" (2), assumes that the consumer selects among alternative choices according to whether one choice is preferred to the others, and ranks these choices according to how much one choice is preferred over another (i.e., cardinal rankings). Although one can think of the utility function as having no unique origin or unit of measure, once some unit of measure and a point of origin are accepted, the utility function of an individual can be described for all levels of wealth. Further, for an individual to purchase insurance, he or she must believe that the marginal utility of wealth is decreasing; although the preference is for more wealth rather than less wealth, the additional wealth has a lower marginal utility. The relationship between total utility and wealth is shown in Figure 6-2A; as will be shown, unless the utility function exhibits this relationship to wealth, the "rational" individual will not purchase insurance.

---

*Throughout this analysis, for the sake of simplicity, it is assumed that utility functions are independent, i.e., the degree to which others have insurance to cover their medical loss does not affect an individual's desire to subsidize another person's purchase of insurance.

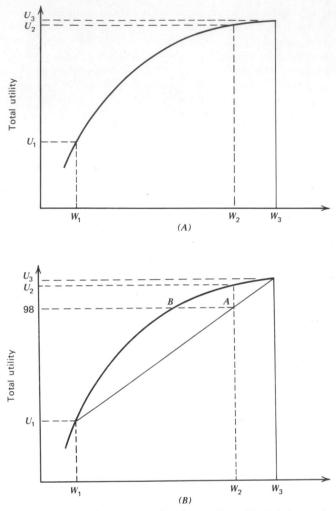

Figure 6-2. The relationship between total utility and wealth: (A) diminishing marginal utility with increased wealth, (B) expected utility.

To illustrate the choices an individual has who is trying to decide whether or not to purchase health insurance, we will assume that if an illness occurs it will cost $8,000. If the individual is currently at W_3, meaning that his or her wealth is $10,000, then if the event occurs, $8,000 must be paid out, thereby moving the individual to wealth position W_1. (The corresponding utility levels at W_3 and W_1 are U_3 and U_1, respectively.) Let us assume that the probability of the individual's requiring medical services costing $8,000 is .025—that is, 2½ percent. The "pure premium" of the insurance that would cover the actuarial value of the expected loss would therefore be:

$$.025 \times \$8,000 = \$200$$

If the person were to buy insurance at the actuarial value of the loss, then he or she would pay $200, thereby reducing the level of his or her wealth position to point W_2 on Figure 6-2A, which represents $9,800. Let us further assume that the decrease in wealth to $9,800 as a result of purchasing insurance places the individual at U_2, which is equivalent to a utility level of 99, U_3 being 100 and U_1 being 20. The choices facing the individual therefore are:

a. To purchase insurance for $200 and move to a lower level of utility, 99, or
b. Not to purchase insurance and have a 2.5 percent chance that he or she will incur an $8,000 loss and thereby move to a utility level of 20 (U_1), which is associated with a wealth position of $2,000, or face a high probability of 97.5 (100 − 2.5 percent) that a loss will not be incurred and thereby remain at a wealth position of $10,000 with an associated utility level of 100.

To compare choices a and b, we must use expected utility. The expected utility of choice b is the weighted sum of the utilities of each outcome, with the weights being the probabilities of each outcome. Therefore, the expected utility of choice b is

$$P(U_1) + (1 - P)(U_3) = .025(20) + 97.5(100) = 98$$

To determine whether a person would buy health insurance, we compare the utility level of choice a, which represents purchasing insurance and thereby leaves the person at utility level $U = 99$, with the expected utility level of choice b, which represents not purchasing insurance and thereby results in an expected utility level $U = 98$. Since the utility level of choice a is greater than that of choice b, we predict that the person would purchase insurance. In this example it is assumed that the insurance is sold at the actuarially fair premium and that the utility function with respect to wealth is similar to the one described in Figure 6-2A—namely, diminishing marginal utility with respect to increased wealth.

The expected utility of choice b, $U = 98$, is shown in Figure 6-2B, by the straight line drawn on the utility curve extending from U_3, W_3, to U_1, W_1. The straight line represents expected utility for different probabilities that the illness will occur. The lower the probability that the event will occur, the closer the expected utility will be to the point furthest to the right on the utility curve. As the probability that the loss will occur increases, the expected utility value moves down to the left on the straight line, closer to the point represented by U_1 on the curve. In other words, if the loss is certain to occur, then the individual will be at W_1 ($2,000) with a corresponding utility level of U_1 (= 20). Since the calculation of expected utility is based on the weighted sum of the probabilities of being at the different utility levels, as the probability of being at U_1 increases, the expected utility estimate declines in a linear fashion.

Because the actual utility curve (decreasing marginal utility with respect to wealth) is always above the expected utility line (constant marginal utility with respect to wealth), we hypothesize that this individual will always buy insurance, if it is sold at its actuarially fair value. However, insurance is never sold at its actuarially fair value because there are administrative, claims processing, and marketing costs. To determine whether or not an individual, as represented in

Figure 6-2B, will buy insurance when there are these additional costs above the pure premium, we must calculate the maximum amount above the pure premium he or she would be willing to pay for insurance.

Referring back to Figure 6-2B, $W_3 - W_2$ represents the dollar amount of the pure premium for an $8,000 loss that has a 2.5 percent probability of occurring. Since the utility level with insurance is greater than the expected utility level (99 versus 98), the person purchasing insurance will be willing to pay an amount above the pure premium that makes the actual utility level *after* the additional payment equal to the expected utility level. When the actual utility level is equal to the expected utility level (at $U = 98$), then the person will be indifferent as to whether he purchases insurance or he self-insures. Any amount of additional payment that places the actual utility level lower than the expected utility level will result in a person's deciding to self-insure; that is, he or she will be at a higher expected utility level with no insurance than with insurance.

This discussion is illustrated in Figure 6-2B. Point A is the expected utility without insurance. If one draws a straight line from point A to where it crosses the actual utility curve, then at this point, B, a person's actual utility level and expected utility level are the same, $U = 98$. The distance from A to B on the wealth axis is the additional amount above the pure premium that a person would be willing to pay for that insurance. At every point along the expected utility line, which represents a different probability of the event's occurring, there is an additional amount above the pure premium that a person would be willing to pay for insurance. At points close to W_1, which represent a high probability that a person will incur a large enough loss to leave him or her at wealth position W_1, a person would be willing to pay a smaller amount above the pure premium; the distance between the expected utility line and the actual utility curve, which would leave him or her at the same level of utility, is closer at that point.

As shown in Figure 6-3A, with an expected utility level at point E, the pure premium would be $W_3 - W_4$, which is a fairly large amount, since the probability of the loss's occurring is quite high. A person would be willing to pay an additional amount above the pure premium equal to the distance EF, since at point F expected utility is equal to actual utility. Any amount greater than EF would place a person at a lower point on his or her actual utility curve. Actual utility would then be less than the expected utility of not buying insurance. The amount above the pure premium which is equal to the distance EF, is smaller than at another part of the graph, for example, CD. At point C a person is willing to pay an additional amount equal to CD, which would make the actual utility level indicated by D equal to the expected utility level indicated by C. CD is greater than EF because the probability of the loss's occurring is larger at point E. As the loss becomes almost certain to occur, the person can save for the event instead of paying the same amount (equal to the pure premium) to an insurance company *plus* an additional amount to cover other insurance company costs. In the case of near-certain events such as annual medical or dental checkups (probabilities approximately 1.0), it would be cheaper to self-insure. At large probabilities and at very small probabilities (very rare events) a person is willing to pay less over the pure premium than at other, more intermediate probabilities.

Another factor that influences how much over the pure premium the person is willing to pay for insurance is the magnitude of the expected loss. When the

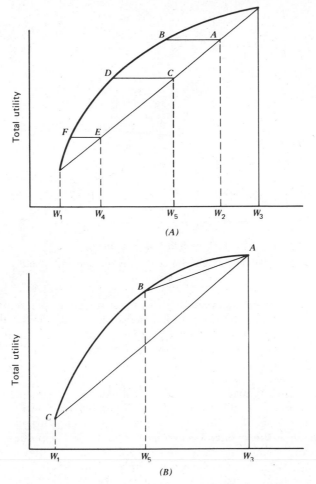

Figure 6-3. The amount above the pure premium an individual is willing to pay for health insurance: (A) according to different probabilities of the event occurring, (B) according to different magnitudes of the expected loss.

expected loss is relatively large, as shown in Figure 6-3B, a person can lose $W_3 - W_1$ ($8,000) without insurance if the illness occurs. If, on the other hand, the loss is relatively small, as for a visit to the dentist for a filling, then this loss will be represented by a smaller possible loss in wealth if it occurs, $W_3 - W_5$. The expected utility line for the large loss is AC; for the small loss it is AB. The distances $W_3 - W_1$ (expected utility line AC) and $W_3 - W_5$ (expected utility line AB) represent different-sized losses with the same probabilities of occurrence. The area between the actual utility curve and the expected utility line is much greater for the large loss than for the small one. Given the same probabilities that either the large or the small loss will occur, a person is willing to pay a larger amount above the pure premium for the large loss than for the small one.

To determine the demand for health insurance, we must now combine the

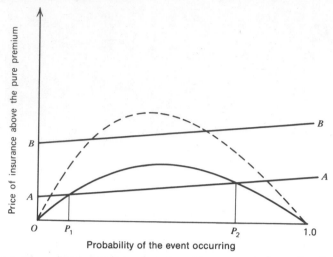

Figure 6-4. The relationship between price of insurance and quantity demanded.

preceding discussion of risk aversion (the total utility curve of the individual that increases but at a decreasing rate), the probability that a loss will occur, the magnitude of that loss if it should occur, and information on the price of insurance—that is, the amount charged above the pure premium. To illustrate the price-quantity relationship of the demand for health insurance, reference is made to Figure 6-4.

The price of insurance along the vertical axis in Figure 6-4 is the amount *above* the pure premium that the person must pay for insurance; along the horizontal axis is the probability that the event will occur. The curved line starting at "0" probability of the event's occurring and ending at a probability of "1.0" (certainty) is the amount above the pure premium that the person is willing to pay for insurance. This area is taken from the previous figures and is merely the distance between the actual utility curve and the expected utility line. Since insurance is never sold at a price just equalling the pure premium (included are costs for marketing, administration, and claims processing), the price of insurance is represented by line AA in Figure 6-4. The reason it increases as the probability of the event's occurring increases is that there are greater administrative costs, such as record keeping and verification, when claims are more frequent (have a higher probability of occurring). Since line AA intersects the solid curved line representing the amount above the pure premium the person is willing to pay for insurance, the person will buy insurance for events that fall between P_1 and P_2. Between those two points the price the person has to pay for insurance is *less* than the amount he or she would be willing to pay, meaning that he or she would be better off (at a higher level of utility) if the insurance were purchased. The price of insurance is *greater* than the amount he or she is willing to pay for events that have either a very small probability of occurring (the area 0 − P_1) or a very high probability of occurring (to the right of P_2. Based upon Figure 6-4, we would predict that illnesses having both a very small probability of occurrence as well as those that have a high probability of occurrence, namely, routine care, would be unlikely to be insured against by individuals. An individual if required to purchase insurance for these two events would be worse off, since the marginal benefits to be derived from that coverage would be smaller than the costs of insurance!

If the price of insurance were to rise to line *BB*, we would expect the individual represented by the solid curved line to self-insure—that is, to demand *less* insurance coverage. With a higher price of insurance, the new price will now *exceed* the additional amount above the pure premium the individual is willing to pay. Regardless of the probability of the event's occurrence, the individual would be worse off if more had to be paid for insurance than he or she was willing to pay. Only if the magnitude of the loss, as shown by the dashed curved line, were greater than price line *BB* would the individual purchase insurance for that probable loss. Thus, as the price of insurance rises, the individual will be less likely to insure for certain events. This inverse relationship between the price of insurance and the quantity of insurance demanded is the demand schedule for insurance.*

Another aspect of Figure 6-4 is that given the price of insurance (line *BB*), a person is more likely to insure against events that have a greater magnitude of loss than against events with smaller possible losses. This aspect of the demand for health insurance can be seen with reference to the price of insurance (*BB*) and the two curved lines representing different possible losses. Referring back to Figure 6-3, we saw that the amount above the pure premium that a person was willing to pay was less for small losses than for large losses, given the same probability of the event's occurring. One interesting implication of this relationship between the price of insurance and the size of the loss is that as the cost of medical care rises, the size of the probable loss increases, and this by itself should result in an increase (a shift) in the demand for health insurance.

In summarizing this theory of the demand for health insurance, attention should be drawn to two areas: (1) the factors which affect the demand for health insurance, and (2) the welfare implications (is the person better or worse off?) of requiring an individual to purchase health insurance against all types of medical illness, the routine as well as the low-cost services. The following factors would affect the demand for health insurance:

1. How risk averse the individual is. If he or she has a utility curve that is increasing but at a decreasing rate (i.e., diminishing marginal utility with respect to increased income), then the individual is willing to pay an amount above the pure premium for insurance coverage.

---

*In a recent study using state-level cross-sectional data for fiscal year 1977, Roehrig estimated the elasticity of demand for health insurance with respect to the price of health insurance to be in the neighborhood of -1.0. Demand was measured as the proportion of total private health care spending (hospital, physician, and dentist services) paid by Blue Cross–Blue Shield and other private health insurers. The price of insurance was taken to be proportional to the load factor (the premium-benefit ratio) and was corrected for the tax deductibility of health insurance using state-specific estimates of the marginal income tax rates (including social security taxes, federal income taxes, and state income taxes). The estimated elasticities with respect to income and the hospital semiprivate room rate were small and not statistically significant while the elasticity with respect to the price of physician services was estimated to be $-.60$. Charles S. Roehrig, *The Impact of Technology on the Demand for Hospital and Medical Care*, Chapter 4, Final Report to the Division of Health Professions Analysis, HRA, DHHS, 1982, Contract Number HRA-232-80-0041.

2. The probability of the event's occurring. As shown in Figure 6-3, for those events that have a very low or a very high probability of occurring, a person is willing to pay less above the pure premium than for events that have a more intermediate probability of occurring.

3. The magnitude of the loss. The larger the magnitude of the loss, as in Figure 6-3, the greater will be the amount above the pure premium that the individual is willing to pay for insurance.

4. The price of insurance. The higher the price of insurance (the amount above the pure premium), the fewer will be the events the individual will insure against.

5. The income of the individual. Income has two effects on the demand for health insurance. First, at higher levels of income, health insurance is likely to be provided as a fringe benefit. If health insurance is purchased by the employer for the employees, then the employer can purchase more health insurance for the same amount of money than if the employer paid the employees the equivalent amount to purchase it themselves. This is because the employees would have to pay income taxes on that money if the employer gave the money directly to them. As employees' incomes rise, they move into a higher marginal tax bracket. The price of health insurance to the employees, when purchased by their employer, becomes sufficiently reduced so that it may actually be *less* than the actuarial value of the expected loss, i.e., the pure premium. In this manner the income tax system encourages the purchase of a greater-than-optimal amount of health insurance. The second effect that income has on the demand for insurance might counteract this situation. The size of a person's income and wealth will affect the amount above the pure premium he or she is willing to pay for health insurance. At both low and high incomes the marginal utility of income is either relatively high or low, so that such persons might prefer to self-insure (3); the distance between the expected and actual utility curve is less at high and low incomes than for intermediate income levels.

The demand for health insurance is thus affected by economic variables, price and income, the tastes of the individual toward risk aversion, and the size of the probable loss. The next section will apply this theory of the demand for health insurance to determine how well it predicts the type of medical costs that the population will insure against.

It is interesting to speculate on the welfare implications of this theory of the demand for insurance. In attempting to maximize their utility, consumers will allocate their income so that the marginal benefit from each of the goods and services they consume equals the prices they must pay for those different goods and services. If the price (which represents the marginal cost of producing those goods and services) exceeds the marginal benefits to them, then they will be worse off by purchasing those goods and services. They can increase their utility by cutting back on those goods and services for which the marginal benefit is less than the price that must be paid and using the funds saved to purchase other goods and services whose marginal benefits (per dollar) are greater. In this manner they will achieve a higher level of utility than by any other allocation process. If, however, consumers are *forced* to purchase a good whose price is greater than its marginal benefit, then they clearly end up worse off than before. Forcing consumers to pay a price for a good that is higher than its marginal benefit is a situation that can occur in the health field if all consumers are required to have complete comprehensive insurance coverage against all of their medical expenses.

As shown in Figure 6-4, there are two situations in which the price of insurance will exceed the amount above the pure premium that the consumer is willing to pay. The first is for medical losses that have either a very high or a very low probability of occurring. In Figure 6-4, the area to the right of P_2 represents medical losses that have a high probability of occurring; these routine medical expenses are for such purchases as Band-Aids, a dental visit, and over-the-counter drugs. Comprehensive insurance coverage to include such routine medical expenses would necessitate a price, perhaps in the form of a tax on the consumer, that would have to exceed what they would be willing to pay above the actuarial value of those losses; requiring consumers to pay that price by law clearly leaves them worse off than if they could self-insure for those losses.

A second situation in which a consumer is made worse off by being required to purchase complete insurance coverage is where there are small medical losses. The price of insurance for that coverage (line BB) is greater than the amount above the pure premium (the solid curved line) the consumer would be willing to pay.

It might be argued that since the price of insurance is less than the aggregate amount consumers would be willing to pay in all situations, requiring insurance coverage for even those medical expenses that they would prefer not to insure against would, on an aggregate basis, still leave them better off with insurance than without. As long as the different forms of coverage are divisible and do not have to be sold together, consumers would be better off with *some* coverage than with either complete coverage or none at all. The welfare implication of mandatory insurance coverage that covers all medical losses, no matter how small or routine and expected they may be, is that some consumers will be worse off than if they had a choice and could self-insure in those situations.

AN APPLICATION OF THE THEORY
OF THE DEMAND FOR HEALTH INSURANCE

The theory of the demand for health insurance can now be used to explain why we observe some people insuring against certain types of medical loss (e.g., hospital care) and not others (e.g., dental care). (When we later introduce the concept of moral hazard, we will see that although people may buy insurance for hospital services, they still may not insure against all hospital expenses, preferring to bear some of the costs themselves.) Also, since not everyone is a "risk averter" (their expected utility curve may be equal to or greater than their actual utility curve with respect to wealth), we would expect some people not to buy *any* health insurance. They would do so, not out of ignorance or irrationality, but because they are not risk averters—i.e., for the same reason as that some people gamble. Before the price of health insurance was greatly reduced as a result of being widely available as a fringe benefit, a sizable percentage of the uninsured,

37 percent, according to a survey conducted in the mid-1950s, indicated that they felt they were just as well off without health insurance (4). The potential market for health insurance at that time was less than 100 percent of the population. As the price of medical care increases over time, i.e., the size of the potential loss is increased if an illness occurs, and also personal income increases, the demand for health insurance is expected to change. (In 1974, only 10 percent of the uninsured believed they were just as well off without health insurance; the percentage of persons believing this increased with higher incomes: 15 percent of those with incomes greater than $15,000 were in this category (5).) Thus, at any point in time, the potential market for health insurance depends on the various factors which affect the demand for health insurance.

To determine how well the model of the demand for health insurance predicts the type of health insurance found in the population, we will examine the purchase of insurance coverage by type of medical expense. Costs for hospitalization and for surgery would seem far more likely to qualify as high expected losses, with a relatively low probability of occurrence, than would medical losses such as physician visits, in the home or office, optometric services, drugs, and dental care, all of which involve relatively smaller medical expenses and are considered by families to be more routine and budgetable.

In examining older rather than more recent data,* we find that the economic theory of the demand for health insurance is able to explain the type of health insurance observed in the population quite well. Using data from a 1957–1958 household survey of the U.S. population, medical expenses by type of service were classified according to whether they had a high or low probability of occurring and whether they had a high or low potential loss if they did occur. Low probability of occurrence was arbitrarily defined by whether 20 percent of the population incurred an expense for that medical service during the past year; high potential loss was also arbitrarily defined by whether the average cost incurred by persons using that medical service was greater than $40. These data are shown in Table 6-1, together with the actual percentage of expenditures covered by insurance for each of the medical services examined. According to the data, the prevalence of insurance is generally consistent with what the economic theory of the demand for health insurance would lead us to expect. Those medical services that have a low probability of occurrence and a high expected loss are more likely to be covered by insurance than those expenses with either a high or low probability of occurrence and a low expected loss.

Although the percentage of medical expenditures covered by insurance has greatly increased since the period covered by the above data, we would still expect a difference in the distribution of medical expenses covered by health insurance: those medical services with a lower probability of occurrence and a high potential loss are likely to have more of their expenses covered by insurance than those services that are considered routine and/or have a relatively lower potential loss. The same relationship holds for more recent data as well. Consumer out-of-pocket expenditures for short-term hospital care are approximately 11 percent of total hospital expenditures, with the remainder being paid

---

*The demand for insurance in recent years has been distorted by the increased availability of health insurance as a fringe benefit, thereby sufficiently lowering the price of insurance in some cases to where it is now lower than the actuarial value of the pure premium.

TABLE 6-1. Classification of Medical Services by Probability of Occurrence, Potential Loss, and Insurance Benefits, 1957–1958

Type of Medical Service	Probability of Occurrence	Magnitude of Expense	Percent of Expenditures Covered by Insurance	Expenditures on This Type of Service as a Percent of Total Medical Expenditures
Hospital care	Low	High	58	23
Physician charges for:				
Surgery	Low	High ⎱	48	7
In-hospital visits	Low	High ⎰		
Office visits	High	Low ⎱	7	24
House calls	High	Low ⎰		
Drugs and medicines	High	Low	1	20
Other medical services	Low	Low	1	8
Dental care	High	Low	—[a]	15

Sources: R. G. Rice, "Some Health Insurance Implications of the Economics of Uncertainty," unpublished paper presented before The American Public Health Association, October 6, 1964. Tables 1 and 2 based on data published in O. W. Anderson, P. Collete, and J. J. Feldman, *Changes in Family Medical Care Expenditures and Voluntary Health Insurance: A Five Year Resurvey* (Cambridge, Mass.: Harvard University Press, 1963).

[a]Less than one-half of 1 percent.

for by private insurance and government programs. For physician services, approximately 38 percent of the total expenditures are out-of-pocket; the out-of-pocket percentage is 71 percent for dental care, 82 percent for eyeglasses, and 80 percent for drugs (6).

In summary, then, the model of the demand for health insurance suggests that a measure of the adequacy of health insurance should *not* be the percentage of aggregate medical expenses covered by health insurance, with anything less than 100 percent being considered inadequate. Instead, the adequacy of health insurance coverage should be examined separately for each type of medical service. Even if everyone were a risk averter, we would not expect people to buy insurance for all of their medical expenses. The price of insurance (i.e., the amount above the pure premium) for some medical expenses would exceed the amount some people were willing to pay. Requiring everyone under such circumstances to purchase health insurance for *all* of their medical expenses would make people *worse off*, since the costs of the coverage for some expenses would exceed the benefits.

THE DEMAND FOR HEALTH INSURANCE UNDER CONDITIONS OF MORAL HAZARD

We have shown that if the demand for medical care were completely price inelastic and therefore involved no moral hazard, people would still not demand

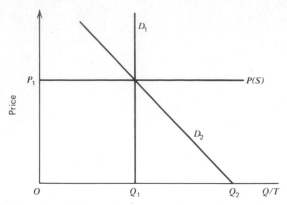

Figure 6-5. The demand for medical care under conditions of moral hazard.

completely comprehensive health insurance because of selling and transactions costs. This section introduces the concept of moral hazard in order to show that its existence also would result in a demand for health insurance coverage which would cover less than 100 percent of a person's medical expenses (7).

If demand for medical care were inelastic with respect to price, then the individual's demand curve in the event of illness would look like D_1 in Figure 6-5; that is, the individual would demand Q_1 units of medical care. In the case of moral hazard, it is possible for the patient to affect the size of their loss. If an individual became ill, the quantity of medical care that he or she would demand would depend, in part, on the price that had to be paid for that care. If insurance covered the entire cost of the illness episode, then the individual represented by demand curve D_2 would demand Q_2 units of medical care. The presence of some elasticity in the individual's demand curve indicates that the individual will demand different quantities of medical care depending upon how much must be paid for that care. Since insurance lowers the price of medical care to individuals, they will consume more care than if they had to pay the entire price themselves. It is this behavior of individuals that is termed "moral hazard." To the individual consuming medical care under these circumstances, it is perfectly rational behavior—he or she is equating the marginal cost of purchasing that care with the marginal benefit of additional units. Since the marginal benefit of additional units of medical care decreases as the quantity of medical care consumed increases, the individual will continue to consume additional units as long as the marginal benefit of those additional units exceeds their additional cost. Insurance coverage that reduces the price of care to zero under these circumstances results in an inefficient use of medical resources. Since the individual with insurance consumes medical care until the marginal benefits and marginal costs of the last units are equal, this will be at a point where the "true" marginal costs (the costs of *producing* those units) are greater than the marginal benefits. "Too much" medical care will be consumed, and the value of those additional units will be less than the costs of their production. This is illustrated in Figure 6-5 at the point where Q_2 units of medical care are consumed by an individual with 100 percent insurance coverage, with the costs of producing each unit indicated by the supply curve (S).

Another implication of the existence of moral hazard is that although individuals with insurance will consume Q_2 units of medical care if they become ill, they may be unwilling to purchase an insurance policy that provides such extensive coverage. As both consumers of medical care and purchasers of insurance, individuals are expected to consider the price involved in both cases: as consumers of medical services, greater utilization resulting from having insurance will result in their having to pay a higher premium for it. Instead of paying that higher premium, an individual may well prefer to self-insure or to purchase a less comprehensive insurance policy. For example, with reference to Figure 6-5, assume that an individual has both a .5 probability of not incurring any medical illness during the year, in which case his or her demand for medical care would be zero units, and a .5 probability of requiring medical care for an illness during that year. If the individual required medical care, with a corresponding demand curve of D_1, the individual would consume Q_1 units (which represents 100 units) at a cost of $10 per unit. The pure premium in this situation would be .5(0) + .5($1,000) = $500 per year. If, however, the individual's demand curve were D_2 (where Q_2 represents 200 units of medical care), then the pure premium under these circumstances would be .5(0) + .5($2,000) = $1,000 per year.

These differences in premiums resulting from the price elasticity of the demand curve may be great enough for some individuals to prefer self-insurance, in which case the expected loss to them would be $500 per year [.5(0) + .5($1,000)]. They would consume Q_1 units of medical care if they became ill because, even though their demand curve may be represented by D_2, they would have to pay P_1 dollars per unit (which is the intersection of D_2 and S) and would consequently consume Q_1 units of care.

Individuals differ in their demands for medical care. If Figure 6-5 represents different demands for medical care, and one individual's demand is D_1 while the average demand among the rest of the population is D_2, then a premium for comprehensive insurance to the individual represented by demand curve D_1 would be based upon a utilization level indicated by Q_2, multiplied by a price of P_1. Under these circumstances an individual may well prefer self-insurance, which would mean a .5 probability (as in the previous case) of being ill and, if so, paying a price P_1 multiplied by Q_1 units of medical care. In both of these examples, *requiring* the individual to purchase comprehensive insurance that is the same as that which is purchased by the rest of the population will make the individual worse off (the marginal costs of the premium for the comprehensive coverage will exceed the marginal benefits of that insurance).

As a result of the effect of moral hazard on the use of medical care, several approaches have been suggested to limit utilization. One approach is to rely on medical providers by providing physicians with incentives to decrease utilization or by instituting utilization review committees. Alternatively, some persons, when purchasing insurance, might prefer intermediate choices between the extremes of comprehensive coverage or self-insurance. Deductibles and coinsurance enable consumers to bear some of the risk themselves and pay a smaller premium than if all their medical costs were covered by insurance.

In Figure 6-6 (A), the cost of comprehensive insurance would be represented by utilization level Q_2, multiplied by price P_1 (multiplied by the probability of .5). The cost of self-insurance would be P_1 multiplied by Q_1 (.5). The cost of an insurance policy with a coinsurance feature that lowered the price to the

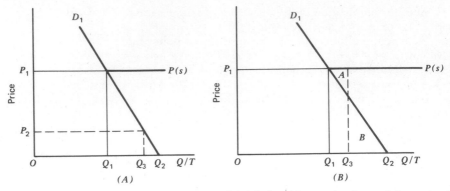

Figure 6-6. The effect of (A) coinsurance and (B) deductibles on the demand for medical care.

patient from P_1 to P_2 would cost $P_1 - P_2$ multiplied by a utilization level of Q_3 (.5). The premium cost of a policy with a coinsurance feature would be between the costs of the other two alternatives. The availability of coinsurance would make insurance more attractive to some people who would prefer no insurance if their only other choice were comprehensive insurance.

In his article on the economics of moral hazard, Pauly also discusses the use of deductibles to reduce the cost of insurance premiums. Using only deductibles results either in the consumption of the same amount of care as in the case of no insurance, or conversely, in consumption of the same amount of care as in the situation of complete insurance coverage. This effect of deductibles on utilization is illustrated in Figure 6-6 (B). Without insurance, the individual represented by demand curve D_1 would, in the event of illness, consume Q_1 units of medical care; with complete insurance coverage the same individual would consume Q_2 units of medical care. If a deductible were instituted for the individual with complete coverage, then before the insurance would pay the medical costs the individual would have to use and pay for Q_3 units of medical care at a cost of P_1 times Q_3. After that amount had been paid, the price of additional care (assuming no coinsurance feature) would be zero and he or she would consume Q_2 units of care. If the individual decides not to consume up to the deductible, which is P_1 times Q_3 units of medical care, then he or she will merely act as though he or she has no insurance and use Q_1 units of care. Whether or not the individual will pay the deductible ($P_1 \times Q_3$) and then consume up to Q_2 units of medical care depends upon whether the excess amount that must be paid for the deductible, area A in Figure 6-6, which is above the individual's demand curve, is less than the "consumers surplus," represented by area B. The "consumers surplus" is the area under the demand curve that consumers would be willing to spend, but do not have to, since it would be at no cost if they first bought Q_3 units of care. If area B exceeds area A, consumers will then pay the deductible and consume Q_2 units of medical care.

Just as the effect on utilization of the coinsurance feature will depend upon the price elasticity of demand and the amount of the coinsurance, the effect the deductible has will also depend upon its size and the price elasticity of demand.

In our discussion of deductibles and coinsurance, differences in income have been ignored; it is obvious that any copayment feature that is unrelated to income levels will have a more important effect on lower-income persons than on higher-income persons.

The conclusion to be drawn from the discussion of the demand for health insurance, whether moral hazard is assumed to exist or not, is that even if all individuals were risk averters, insurance coverage for 100 percent of all of their medical expenses should not be required for all persons. When there are transactions costs for administering claims, and when people have different demands for medical care, no single insurance policy is best for everyone. Some persons will prefer to have only some types of medical expense covered; because of the existence of moral hazard, others will prefer to have some cost-sharing features.

ADDITIONAL FACTORS AFFECTING THE DEMAND FOR HEALTH INSURANCE

We have seen that the demand for health insurance is affected by the price of that insurance, the probability of loss, the magnitude of the potential loss, income, and the consumer's "tastes," meaning how risk averse the individual is. The existence of moral hazard was shown to result both in an increase in the price of health insurance by increasing utilization and in a decrease in the demand for health insurance through its effect on the price variable.

Another factor which affects the price of insurance is whether the individual is part of a large group when purchasing insurance. Group policies are sold at substantially lower prices. In part the reduced price reflects lower administrative costs per individual; some of the administrative costs are handled by the group itself. Another reason for lower prices to group members is that there is less likelihood of adverse selection. Individuals seeking to purchase health insurance may be doing so because they believe they will be using such coverage in the near future. To guard against such self-selection and the possibly higher risks associated with it, the price of the policy will be higher to an individual than to a person who is part of a large group, where such adverse selection is less likely. The higher price of insurance to persons who are not part of a group leads to a smaller demand for health insurance.

Another important factor affecting the demand for health insurance is the tax deductibility of health insurance premiums. As incomes increase and people move into higher tax brackets, there is greater incentive for them to demand fringe benefits rather than increases in their cash incomes. Health insurance premiums paid by the employer are excluded from the taxable income of the employee (not just federal taxes, but state and social security taxes as well). In addition, half of the health insurance premiums paid by the employee are deductible from federal income taxes. This tax treatment lowers the price of health insurance and has led to a much greater demand for it than would have occurred otherwise. It has been estimated that these tax policies result in a loss in excess of $10.6 billion a year to the government (8). The tax treatment of health insurance coverage is, in effect, a subsidy for the purchase of health insurance and is greater for higher-income persons in higher tax brackets. One reason for the increasing comprehensiveness of health insurance coverage for small claims ("first dollar coverage") is that the premium for such losses is *less* than the actuarial value of such losses as the individual moves into higher and higher tax brackets. These government tax policies thereby stimulate the demand for health insurance and influence the comprehensiveness of the coverage.

A third factor affecting the demand for health insurance is the method used for reimbursing the provider. Cost-based reimbursement and the use of service benefit policies remove any incentives that may exist either for the patient to shop around or for the provider to provide care more efficiently. If the provider's costs are reimbursed in full, regardless of what other hospitals may charge, and if the patient is not required to pay any portion of the hospital's bill, as is the case under a service benefit policy, then any incentives for cost constraint on either the demander or the supplier have been removed. This method of provider reimbursement, preferred by hospitals and accepted by Blue Cross, has increased hospital costs, increased the magnitude of the probable loss due to a hospital episode, and thereby resulted in a further *increase* in the demand for protection against such large losses. The greater the probable loss, the greater will be the demand for health insurance.

SUMMARY AND CONCLUDING COMMENTS

The preceding discussion on the demand for health insurance offers an approach to answering the following questions: how much health insurance should the population have (i.e., what percent of total health expenditures should be covered by insurance), and what components of medical services should health insurance cover? The answers would indicate the degree to which the provision of health insurance in the population is economically efficient. Government intervention to increase or to change the type of health insurance in the population can then be evaluated in terms of whether such action moves the population closer to or further from what would be an optimal quantity and type of health insurance.*

To discuss the efficient amount and type of health insurance in the population, it is necessary to have some criteria to evaluate what is efficient and what is inefficient in the purchase of health insurance. Assuming competition in the provision (supply) of health insurance, the price at which health insurance is sold will equal the marginal costs of providing it. In a competitive market, the suppliers will also respond to demands for different types of health insurance coverage and provide such coverage at a price that reflects the cost of producing it. (These two assumptions are discussed in Chapter 8, "The Market for Health Insurance.") The condition for economic efficiency on the demand side is that

---

*This discussion assumes no redistribution of medical services; when national health insurance proposals are discussed later, this assumption will be changed. Another assumption, which will subsequently be discussed, is that there are no externalities in the provision of personal medical services. Since redistribution of medical care to low-income persons may in fact have external effects, the efficient distribution of health insurance coverage may necessitate a different amount and type of insurance to low-income groups.

consumers would purchase the type and quantity of health insurance coverage to the point where its price equals the marginal benefit to them from additional insurance coverage. Since the demand curve indicates the marginal benefit to be derived from the purchase of health insurance, if the cost of additional insurance exceeds its marginal benefit, then consumers will be better off purchasing less coverage. When the quantity of health insurance demanded is equal to the cost of providing that insurance, then the individual will purchase the appropriate quantity; that is, the conditions of economic efficiency are met. At that point, the marginal cost of producing health insurance equals the marginal benefit to the consumer of that additional coverage.

The demand for health insurance was analyzed under two assumptions: first, that no moral hazard existed, in that the price of medical care did not affect its utilization or the quality of the care demanded; and, second, that moral hazard did exist, meaning that there is some price elasticity with resect to the demand for quantity and quality of medical care. In the first situation it was shown that individuals would *not* want to insure against all events. Insurance would be more likely for those medical services where the expected loss is greater and where the probability of the event's occurring is neither extremely high nor rare. Requiring insurance for all losses and all probabilities of their occurring, as well as for all individuals, would be economically inefficient; the cost of the insurance would exceed the marginal benefits to the consumer of additional coverage.

Based on this discussion, what percentage of the distribution of health expenditures should be covered by health insurance? The distribution of health expenditures is skewed, as described earlier in Figure 6-1: many people have relatively small expenditures, a smaller percentage of the population have larger expenditures. We would expect the large expenses with a low probability of occurrence to be covered by insurance, which suggests that the curve shown in Figure 6-1 should be modified. At a *minimum*, the tail of the distribution (relatively large expenditures for a small percentage of the families) should be covered by insurance, through major medical or catastrophic insurance, as shown in Figure 6-7.

When the demand for health insurance under conditions of moral hazard was discussed, it was shown that, given the differences in preferences among people in their demands for medical care, it would be preferable to offer people more than an all-or-nothing choice. Some persons might prefer some insurance to either no insurance or complete coverage. What this suggests with regard to the distribution of medical expenditures is that the curve might be modified still further, as shown in Figure 6-7. Since the administrative costs of handling small claims are likely to exceed the amount above the pure premium people are willing to pay for relatively routine, smaller expenses, a deductible might be included for such expenses, as represented by the shaded portion of the curve in Figure 6-7.* Since there is moral hazard, people might prefer some copayment to

---

*It has been claimed that deductibles and coinsurance provisions in health insurance will result in a decline in the demand for preventive services, which are lower-cost, more predictable medical services. Evidence of this alleged adverse effect is difficult to find. One can make the case that if preventive services have an effect on future medical demand, then presumably insurance companies should be willing to subsidize the purchase of such services. Most, if not all, health insurance actually precludes such services from coverage. Similarly, HMOs and PPGPs have cut back on their use of

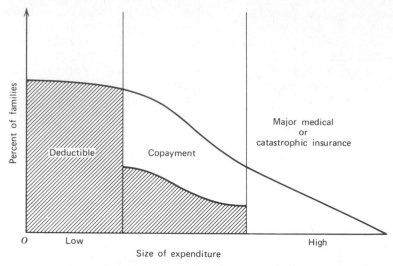

Figure 6-7. The effect of health insurance on the expected distribution of medical expenses among families.

reduce the size of their premium. Thus, a coinsurance feature would reduce the size of the medical expenses in the middle area. Insurance, in this instance, would cover less than 100 percent of medical expenditures (different parts of the distribution of medical expenses would be covered at different percentages), and the premium for such insurance would be much lower than if it covered the entire distribution of medical expenses.

In discussing other factors affecting the demand for health insurance, we dealt with the tax deductibility of premiums; as incomes increase and people move into higher tax brackets, they have a greater incentive to purchase insurance against more, though smaller, medical expenses. The effect of the tax deductibility of health insurance premiums is a movement *away* from economic efficiency in the demand for health insurance. The "true" cost of health insurance has not been lowered, but its price to higher-income consumers has been. They will, therefore, be purchasing "too much" health insurance. The tax treatment of health insurance premiums has reduced the price of insurance against smaller, more predictable medical expenses to higher-income people to a point that may be *below* the actuarial value of those expenses. If the tax deductibility of health insurance premiums were no longer allowed, there would be less distortion in the purchase of health insurance, because the decision to purchase would more closely correspond to the cost of the insurance and the perceived marginal benefits to the consumer of that additional coverage.

An important question raised by the discussion of the demand for health insurance is which components of medical care should be covered by health

---

preventive services, again presumably indicating that the costs of such services are greater than their potential savings. Thus, if copayments actually reduce the demand for preventive care, it is not clear that increased demand for such services would have favorable cost/benefit ratios.

insurance. When only one component of medical care, such as hospital services, is covered by insurance, then the price of hospital care to the consumer relative to the prices of other forms of care has been distorted. The decision to use the different forms of care is based, in part, on the relative prices the patient must pay for such care. Inasmuch as these relative prices will not reflect the relative costs of care, moving toward greater economic efficiency in the use of medical care will require the patient to face prices proportional to the costs of such care. An example of insurance coverage which distorts the use of medical components by distorting the relative prices of medical care faced by the consumer is the Blue Cross service benefit policy. Service benefit coverage provided very complete coverage for just hospital care and excluded nonhospital care from coverage; this led to an inefficient (more costly) form of treatment when services which could be performed on an outpatient basis were instead performed in a hospital. This policy has been changing.

Another aspect of the service benefit policy that leads to inefficiency, albeit in the production of hospital services, is that by covering the entire cost of a hospital episode regardless of the hospital that the patient enters, it provides no incentive for the patient to seek less expensive hospitals; instead the incentive is the opposite: it is in the patient's interest to seek the highest-quality services he or she can, regardless of price.

There are certain types of health insurance which do not distort the relative prices faced by the patient when seeking care. An example is indemnity insurance, which reimburses the patient a dollar amount. Patients and/or their physicians, therefore, have an incentive to minimize the cost of a medical treatment, and the relative prices of the different components of medical services will not be artificially distorted.

Another approach to achieving allocative efficiency in the use of medical services is the use of capitation payments to cover the use of all medical services. Under these arrangements, someone, presumably a physician, prescribes the optimal combination of resources such that the relative costs of different medical services used by the patient equal their relative marginal benefits. Prepaid group practices and health maintenance organizations (to be discussed more completely later) are organizational arrangements whereby the patient is covered by a capitation payment system.

A final aspect affecting the economic efficiency of the demand for health insurance is the method of provider reimbursement, which will be discussed subsequently in greater detail. Certain methods of reimbursement, such as cost-based payments to hospitals, result in higher health care costs than other methods. These higher costs—presumably reflecting greater provider inefficiency under this method of reimbursement—increase the size of the probable loss, thereby resulting in a greater demand for health insurance than would occur if other, more efficiency-oriented payment mechanisms were used.

An important reason for understanding the demand for medical care, as well as the demand for health insurance, is to be able to determine whether or not the quantity (and quality) of medical care consumed is optimal. The optimal rate of output of medical care will be achieved when the price of that care (which is presumed to equal the costs of producing that care under a competitive system) is equal to the marginal benefit of that care to the consumer, which is reflected in the price the consumer is willing to pay. As has been shown, the type of insurance coverage that exists (service benefit coverage) and the tax treatment of health insurance premiums are two reasons why prices in medical care to consumers are distorted, thereby resulting in consumption of a nonoptimal amount of medical care.

To determine whether the price of medical care to the patient reflects the minimum cost of producing that care, it is necessary to turn to an analysis of the supply side of the medical care market.

APPENDIX 1:
THE ALLOCATIVE INEFFICIENCY OF
BLUE CROSS'S SERVICE BENEFIT POLICY

The type of insurance coverage offered by Blue Cross, both when it was started and currently as well, is primarily for hospital care. A person with Blue Cross would not have to pay any of the charges for hospital care, but he or she would generally have to pay the full price for any other forms of medical services, such as physician services or nursing home care, used in the treatment of the illness. Blue Cross's service benefit policy caused an "overuse" of hospital care relative to other medical components used in treatment and resulted in a cost of treatment that is higher than if other, less costly, but equally efficacious, forms of care were used. This conclusion is illustrated in Figure 6-8. Assume that treatment for a medical illness can be achieved with varying amounts of hospital and/or physician services. This substitutability in the use of components for treatment is shown by the indifference curves in Figure 6-8. (The shape of the indifference curve indicates the degree of substitutability among components, and it depends upon the particular illness involved and its seriousness.) The budget constraint AB indicates the quantity of physician and hospital services that the patient can purchase without insurance: either OA units of physician services, OB units of hospital care, or some combination of the two within the budget constraint. The slope of the budget constraint indicates the relative prices of physician and hospital services. With no insurance, a patient with a particular illness and with budget constraint AB will consume OC units of physician services and OD units of hospital care. If the patient had indemnity insurance which reimbursed a given amount of money for medical care, then the budget constraint would shift out parallel and become JK. If the patient became ill, then with the indemnity insurance he or she could buy more medical care than previously and the slope of the new budget constraint would remain the same; the relative prices of the components would not change but the patient could buy more of each, thereby moving to a higher indifference curve (III). The effect of the indemnity insurance is similar to an increase in income when the patient is ill.

If, instead of indemnity insurance, however, the patient just had hospitilization coverage with a coinsurance feature, then the price of hospital care to the patient would be reduced, and the budget constraint would rotate to the right and become AG. The effect on the mix and quantity of components used when there is just insurance for hospital care and not for any of the other components is

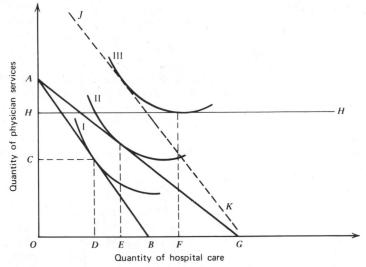

Figure 6-8. The allocative inefficiency of Blue Cross's service benefit policy.

similar to the income and substitution effects of a price change. The patient will use relatively more hospital care, since the price of hospital care relative to out-of-hospital care has been reduced. This is the substitution effect. The income effect will be an increase in the use of both components, as long as they are normal goods.

If the patient were now to receive a service benefit policy, which essentially makes hospital care completely free because there is no out-of-pocket cost to the patient, then the substitution effect would become even greater than in the previous case. Line HH is horizontal to indicate that there is no price constraint on the purchase of additional units of hospital care. (It is lower than point A because, presumably, it would require more of the consumer's income to purchase the policy; hence, less would be available to purchase physician services.) The individual, when ill, will use relatively more hospital care than in any of the previous cases. Because there is some disutility to being in the hospital, the use of the hospital will not increase infinitely. Patients, through their physicians, will substitute hospital care for those forms of medical care that can be provided in a nonhospital setting. Diagnostic testing in the above case would be free to the patient if performed in the hospital, whereas the full price would have to be paid if it were performed outside of the hospital.

Although quality of hospital care is not shown in these diagrams, part of the increase in quantity of hospital care may be viewed as an increase in quality. Since the price of hospital care to the patient has been reduced to zero with a service benefit policy, the patient will also demand higher-quality hospital services, such as requesting the removal of an appendix in a teaching hospital when a smaller, less care-intensive community hospital would be equally satisfactory. This demand for increased quality of hospital services will result in an even greater misallocation of resources. Part of this misallocation is indicated by the budget constraint *JK*, which, since it is tangent to the same indifference curve, would make the patient as well off as the service benefit policy would but represents the use of fewer resources. The slope of line *JK* represents the relative prices of hospital and physician services if the patient had an indemnity type of insurance or had to pay the full price of these services in the event that he or she didn't have insurance. The relative prices of physician and hospital services are presumed to represent the relative marginal costs of physician and hospital care. Producing the quantity of medical care represented by the indifference curve that is tangent to the service benefit policy (line *HH*) can be achieved more efficiently by using the medical components according to their relative prices as well as their relative benefits in treatment. The magnitude of misallocation would be the difference between line *JK* and a line with the same slope intersecting the point of tangency between the indifference curve and line *HH*.

In this discussion, the allocative inefficiency resulting from insurance which provides coverage for just hospital care will depend upon how much the price of hospital care is subsidized relative to the prices of other medical components (the most severe case being the Blue Cross service benefit policy), the degree of substitutability of hospital care for other forms of care, and, lastly, upon the price elasticity of demand both for hospital utilization and for increased hospital quality.

The effects of a hospital service benefit policy have been threefold: one, the hospital has been used when other less expensive but equally effective forms of treatment could have been used, thereby raising the cost of producing medical care; second, hospital use has increased to a point where the additional benefits to the patient of time spent in the hospital are very low. The real cost of resources to produce the additional care was greater than the price faced by the patient, thereby resulting in a situation where the marginal cost of producing that additional care *exceeded* the marginal value to the patient of increased use. Third, there has been a much greater demand for quality of hospital services on the part of patients and their physicians because the price of higher-quality services to the patients is zero under a service benefit policy and quality may be considered a normal good; therefore, they will demand increased quality to the point where the additional benefits derived from it equal the price to them. Since the price of higher-quality hospital services is zero, the amount of quality demanded will be greater than it otherwise would be; the cost of resources used in producing higher-quality care will, at the margin, exceed the additional benefits derived from it by the patients. These, then, are the three misallocative effects of different types of hospital insurance policies, with the greatest misallocation occurring in the case of a service benefit policy.

An approach that has been suggested for remedying these inefficiencies is to mandate the use of utilization review procedures. These review mechanisms attempt to reduce excess utilization instead of changing the distortion in the relative prices of care to the patient, which has brought these inefficiencies about in the first place. An alternative approach for correcting such inefficiencies, when it may not be desirable to reinstitute patient incentives, is to provide incentives to the *physician* to use the least costly mix of components. An example of such an incentive system, to be discussed more fully later, is the development of capitation plans for payment of medical services, such as health maintenance organizations.

APPENDIX 2:
THE EFFECT ON THE INSURANCE PREMIUM
OF EXTENDING COVERAGE TO INCLUDE
ADDITIONAL BENEFITS

As a consequence of Blue Cross's hospital service benefit policy, with its resulting "overutilization" of the hospital, a number of persons have suggested broadening Blue Cross's coverage to include out-of-hospital care. The hoped-for effect of adding additional coverage is that substitution away from the hospital toward lower-cost substitutes will occur and Blue Cross premiums can be reduced.

To determine whether or not adding coverage for a nonhospital benefit will reduce the total costs of care (i.e., the premium), we need the following information:

1. the price elasticity of demand for the newly covered benefit;
2. the copayment factor for the new benefit;
3. the cross-elasticity of demand between hospitalization and the new benefit;
4. the cross-elasticity of demand between the new benefit and any complementary components of care; and
5. the relative prices of hospital care, the new benefit, and any other complementary components affected.

This information would be used in the following manner to determine whether making a service benefit policy more comprehensive would actually lower the total costs of care. (The same approach can be used to examine the mix of medical components for any insurance package.) Assuming that the demand for hospital care is as it appears in Figure 6-9A, then without any insurance, the patient would have to pay the full cost of a hospital episode if he or she became ill; the patient would have to pay P_{H_1}, and according to his or her expected demand, would use Q_{H_1} days of hospital care. The consumer's total expenditures for hospital care would be $(P_{H_1} \times Q_{H_1})$. With a Blue Cross service benefit policy, the price of hospital care to the patient would become "zero," and the expected utilization in the event of illness would be Q_{H_2}. Total expenditure for hospital care in this case would be $(P_{H_1} \times Q_{H_2})$.

Including in the insurance contract physician services in the office with a coinsurance feature will now result in a lower price to the patient, from P_{M_1} to P_{M_2}, and an increase in utilization of physician services, from Q_{M_1} to Q_{M_2} as in Figure 6-9B. The amount of the increase in physician visits will depend upon the price elasticity of demand for physician services and the size of the coinsurance payment. The cost to the insurance company of covering physician services is that part of the actual price that the insurance company will have to pay $(P_{M_1} - P_{M_2})$, multiplied by the number of physician visits, Q_{M_2}. (The patient would pay the remainder, $P_{M_2} \times Q_{M_2}$.)

If physician services act as a partial substitute for hospital care, then with the reduction in the price of physician visits, patients (through their physicians) will demand less hospital care. How much less hospital care will be demanded will depend upon the cross-elasticity of demand between hospital utilization and the

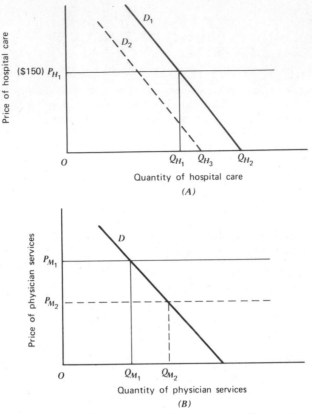

Figure 6-9. The effect on hospital utilization of insuring out-of-hospital services: (A) hospital utilization, (B) physician services.

price of physician visits, which is equal to the percent change in hospital utilization divided by the percent change in the price of physician visits. This is shown in Figure 6-9A by a shift in the demand for hospital care to the left indicated by demand curve D_2. Since the price of hospital care to the patient with a service benefit policy has been assumed to be "zero," the new quantity demanded will be Q_{H_3}. The size of the shift in demand for hospital care will depend upon the magnitude of the cross-elasticity of demand and the size of the reduction in the price to the patient of physician visits.

The savings in hospital expenditures to the insurance company of including coverage for a nonhospital service would be the difference in hospital utilization $(Q_{H_2} - Q_{H_3})$, multiplied by the price of hospital care, P_{H_1}. If the savings in hospital expenditures were greater than the cost to the insurance company of the subsidy for physician services, then total cost (the premium) would be reduced.

In actuality, there might be other services affected by the subsidy for physician visits. If there are medical services that are complementary to the use of physician visits in the office, then there will be an increase in use of these services (a shift to the right in their demand curve). These additional costs may be borne by the patient rather than by the insurance company if they are not for an insured service.

The following is a numerical example of the graph we have been discussing, illustrating whether or not insuring a nonhospital service will reduce the total cost of the premium. Let us assume the following values for each of the data required in our example:

- Hospital utilization (Q_{H_2}) when physician services are not covered by insurance is 800 patient days per 1,000 population.
- The price of hospital care is $150 per day.
- The price of a physician's office visit is $20.
- Physician visits are 600 per 1,000 population.
- The price elasticity of demand for physician visits is -1.0 (a 10 percent decrease in price leads to a 10 percent increase in physician visits).
- The cross-elasticity of demand between hospital patient days and the price of physician visits is $+.2$ (a 10 percent decrease in the price of a physician visit leads to a 2 percent decrease in hospital patient days).
- After physician visits are included in the insurance coverage, the coinsurance rate is 50 percent; i.e., the patient has to pay only 50 percent of the price of physician services. (It is also assumed that the price of physician services remains at its previous level.)

With this information we can now calculate the change in the cost of the premium as a result of including physician visits with a 50 percent coinsurance feature.

The total cost of the premium per 1,000 population before physician services are added to the coverage is

$$\frac{TC}{1,000} = P_{H_1} \times \frac{Q_{H_2}}{1,000}$$

$$\frac{\$120,000}{1,000} = \$150 \times \frac{800}{1,000}$$

or $120 per person. The total cost of the premium *after* physician visits are covered at a 50 percent coinsurance rate is

$$\frac{TC}{1,000} = P_{H_1}\left(\frac{Q_{H_3}}{1,000}\right) + .5P_{M_1}\left(\frac{Q_{M_2}}{1,000}\right)$$

which is

$$\frac{\$117,000}{1,000} = \$150\left(\frac{720}{1,000}\right) + .5(\$20)\left(\frac{900}{1,000}\right)$$

or $117 per person.

The difference is computed as follows:

1. The increased expenditure on physician visits is

$$.5(\$20)\left(\frac{600}{1,000}\right)(1.5) = \left(\frac{\$9,000}{1,000}\right)$$

This is the coinsurance rate (.5), multiplied by the price of physician visits ($20), multiplied by the number of physician visits per 1,000 population (600/1,000), multiplied by the percent increase in physician visits as a result of the 50 percent reduction in physician prices to the patient (a − 1.0 price elasticity multiplied by a 50 percent reduction in price).

2. Subtract the savings on decreased hospital utilization, which is

$$\$150\left(\frac{80}{1,000}\right) = \frac{\$12,000}{1,000}$$

This is the price of hospital care, multiplied by the reduction in patient days as a result of a lower price of physician visits. (The cross-elasticity of +.2 when multiplied by a 50 percent reduction in the price of physician visits is equal to a 10 percent reduction in hospital utilization; this is then multiplied by 800 PD /1,000.)

3. The net effect of the savings on hospital expenditures less the increased physician expenditures is

$$\frac{\$12,000}{1,000} - \frac{\$9,000}{1,000} = \frac{\$3,000}{1,000} \text{ or } \$3 \text{ per person.}$$

Given the data and assumptions used in this example, the effect of insuring physician visits would be a net decrease of $3 per person in the total cost of the premium ($117 versus $120 per person).

In the preceding example, insuring an out-of-hospital service would further reduce the insurance premium if the price of hospital care increased relatively faster than that of the nonhospital service, if the substitutability between the two services (cross-elasticity) increased, and if the price elasticity of demand for the nonhospital service were reduced.

Adding insurance coverage for an out-of-hospital service is more likely to reduce hospital utilization when this service is used *in conjunction with* hospital care in treatment of an illness episode. If physician services are covered by insurance and are not used as part of the treatment for an illness, then there may be a large increase in physician utilization without any consequent lowering of hospital utilization; in fact, additional physician utilization may act as a complementary factor to hospital care in that increased physician office visits might result in increased case finding by the physician. A major medical policy, which covers all the medical services used in treatment (after a sizable deductible has been paid), is more likely to result in substitution away from the more costly components (9).

REFERENCES

1. The discussion in this section borrows heavily from an unpublished article by J. J. German, "A Note on the Economic Theory of Insurance with Implications for Health Insurance," mimeographed (January 1967), and the article by Dennis Lees and Robert Rice, "Uncertainty and the Welfare Economics of Medical Care: Comment," *American Economic Review*, March 1965. The comment by D. Lees and R. Rice (as well as the comment by M. Pauly in the next section of this chapter) were written in response to Kenneth J. Arrow, "Uncertainty and the Welfare Economics of Medical Care," *American Economic Review*, December 1963. Arrow claimed that the market for health insurance requires government intervention because there are gaps in consumer's health insurance coverage, and that this is evidence that the market is not producing certain services that consumers are willing to purchase. Lees and Rice argued that Arrow's claims are not evidence of market imperfections but rather are a result of transactions costs. For example, "[T]he transactions cost to the individual of completing and filing applications and forms, paying premiums, keeping records, etc., as well as possible costs of obtaining information, may be of sufficient magnitude to make insurance policies against certain losses not worthwhile." Arrow replied that individuals who cannot take advantage of the economies of group health insurance will face too high a transactions cost (i.e., the price of insurance is greatly in excess of its pure premium) and thus may not purchase health insurance.

2. M. Friedman and L. Savage, "The Utility Analysis of Choices Involving Risk," *Journal of Political Economy* 56(4) (1948), 279–304.

3. On this last point see the discussion by Jan Mossin, "Aspects of Rational Insurance Purchasing," *Journal of Political Economy*, July/August 1968.

4. E. Friedson and J. Feldman, *Public Attitudes Toward Health Insurance*, Research Series No. 5 (New York: Health Information Foundation, 1958).

5. Based on unpublished data in the 1974 Health Interview Survey and published in *Catastrophic Health Insurance* (Washington: Congressional Budget Office, January 1977), p. 58.

6. Robert Gibson and Daniel Waldo, "National Health Expenditures, 1980" *Health Care Financing Review* 3 (September 1981): 20, Table 2, and Department of Health and Human Services, *HHS News* (newsletter dated July 26, 1982): Table II.

7. The discussion in this section is based on the article by Mark Pauly, "The Economics of Moral Hazard: Comment," *American Economic Review* (June 1968). In Pauly's comment to Arrow's reply to Lees and Rice, he argues that even if there are certain economies in government provision of health insurance that would lower transactions costs, other costs may more than offset such possible savings. In addition to a loss of consumer choice, the existence of "moral hazard" would cause consumers to demand less insurance "at the premium its behavior as a purchaser of insurance and as a demander of medical care under insurance makes necessary." In other words, the existence of moral hazard would result in higher prices for insurance and, consequently, a decreased demand. The lack of complete health insurance coverage in the private market can also be explained by moral hazard, which would not be lessened even if government were somehow able to reduce the transactions costs of insurance to individuals.

8. Nancy Greenspin Thompson and Ronald Vogel, "Taxation and Its Effect Upon Public and Private Health Insurance and Medical Demand," *Health Care Financing Review* 1 (Spring 1980): 40. For an analysis of the effect that the tax subsidy of health insurance premiums has had on the demand for health insurance, see: Martin Feldstein and Bernard Friedman, "Tax Subsidies, The Rational Demand for Insurance and the Health Care Crisis," *Journal of Public Economics*, 7(2), April 1977.

9. The reader is referred to the following articles for a more complete discussion of the issues covered in this section: Mark V. Pauly, "A Measure of the Welfare Cost of Health Insurance," *Health Services Research*, Winter 1969; Karen Davis and Louise B. Russell, "The Substitution of Hospital Outpatient Care for Inpatient Care," *The Review of Economics and Statistics*, May 1972; Martin S. Feldstein, "The Welfare Loss of Excess Health Insurance," *The Journal of Political Economy*, March–April 1973.

CHAPTER 7

The Supply of Medical Care: An Overview

DETERMINANTS OF SUPPLY

CHARACTERISTICS OF PRODUCTION FUNCTIONS

Underlying the supply of any good or service is the production function. The production function describes the technical relation between the output of that good or service and the resources (or inputs) used to produce it. If the output were nursing care per patient, then included in the inputs would be the number of and type of nurses on the nursing unit. This technical relationship between nursing care per patient and the types of nurses may be expressed in the following general form:

$$Q_{npc} = f(\text{RNs, LPNs, ADs, UN})$$

where Q_{npc}, which represents quantity of nursing patient care, is functionally related to the number of registered nurses (RNs), licensed practical nurses (LPNs), nursing aides (ADs), and the type of nursing unit (UN).

Certain characteristics of medical production functions affect the cost and quantity of care provided. The relationship just stated between nursing care per patient and the type of nurses suggests that to some extent the various types of nurses are substitutable for one another in the production of nursing care. The substitutability is not one-to-one, i.e., one LPN cannot substitute for one RN. RNs presumably have more skills as a result of their additional training, and therefore LPNs can substitute for some or most, but perhaps not all, the tasks the RN performs. The degree of substitutability between different types of health

143

workers is important to determine, since it provides information the decision-maker needs if he or she is to minimize the costs of providing nursing care.*

In the health field there are a number of legal restrictions on the tasks that various health professionals can perform. Even if a nurse is capable of perform-ing certain tasks that are reserved solely for the physician, the nurse may not perform them because she would be violating the state practice acts. The effect of these legal restrictions is to limit the degree of substitutability in the produc-tion function. Thus, the decisionmaker is not legally able to combine the inputs at will; the law limits the extent to which inputs may be substituted in producing a given level of output. If legal restrictions prevent substitution from occurring when it would not result in a diminution of the quality of care, then the legal restrictions have increased the cost of producing that care. The "costs" of restric-tive practices, therefore, are the additional resources required to produce a given level of care at a given level of quality.

Another characteristic of the stated production function is that not all the inputs can be varied simultaneously at each point in time. At any time, the decisionmaker can vary the combination of nurses and their numbers on the nursing unit. To change the type of nursing unit itself, by enlarging it or improving it through greater use of monitoring mechanisms, would take longer. The "long run" is that period of time in which the administrator can vary not only the number and type of nurses but also the size and character of the nursing unit. The "short run" is that period of time in which the administrator can vary only the other inputs, not make changes in the nursing unit itself. Another exam-ple of the short versus the long run would be with regard to physician services. In the short run, an increase in physician services can be achieved by having the physician work longer hours or by hiring auxiliary workers. In the long run, medical schools may increase the number of physicians, which are the fixed input in the short run.

These distinctions between the long and short run are important for deter-mining the least costly way of producing nursing and other types of medical care. If there is an increase in the demand for nursing care derived from an increased demand for medical and hospital care, then the administrator can increase the number of nurses on the unit to provide more care. (The combination of nurses used to provide that increased care will depend upon which combination is least costly.) It might be much less costly if the nursing unit itself were changed; therefore, in the long run, all the inputs, including the nursing unit, will be changed to form a combination that will minimize the cost of providing that greater amount of nursing care. (Varying the size of the nursing unit is equivalent to moving along a long-run average-cost curve—i.e., determining the effects of scale of the nursing unit on cost per unit of output.)

One further aspect of the production function is worth mentioning. Techni-cal change has usually been defined as a greater output that is produced with the same or fewer inputs. In medical care, technical change has usually meant that

---

*Various studies have been undertaken to ascertain the degree of substitutability that exists between various health professionals, such as dental auxiliaries and dentists, physician assistants and physi-cians. For an example of a study attempting to estimate the degree of substitutability of nurses, see Richard C. Jelinek, "A Structural Model for the Patient Care Operation," *Health Services Research,* Fall–Winter 1967.

illnesses that formerly could not be treated can now be cared for with a higher probability of a successful outcome. Such technical change, which is really a change in medical care output, usually results in increased rather than decreased use of inputs. An example of technical change that has led to a decrease in input use is the use of new drugs, which has decreased the use of more expensive institutional care. Thus, both types of technical change have occurred in medical care. It is important to hold the effects of such technical change constant when analyzing the production function for medical care.

DETERMINING THE LEAST-COST COMBINATION OF INPUTS

To determine the least costly combination of inputs to be used as output is increased, the following information is required. First, it is necessary to have some knowledge of the marginal increase in nursing care as each type of nursing personnel is increased. If the number of LPNs and ADs is held constant, the increase in patient care corresponding to an increase in the number of RNs is not constant; the law of variable proportions states that after some point the marginal product (contribution) of an additional RN will begin to decline. The same will be true for each of the other categories of nursing personnel. The marginal contribution to increased patient care for each type of input can be empirically determined, and both it and a second type of information are necessary if the decisionmaker is to minimize his costs of increasing patient care. The second type of information needed is the relative prices of the different inputs used in the production function. Even if an RN contributed one and a half times more to patient care than an LPN, increases in patient care should not necessarily be achieved through increases in the number of RNs. If RNs' wages were twice as great as those of LPNs, then it would be less expensive to achieve an increase in nursing care by increasing LPNs rather than RNs, assuming no change in quality. The relative prices (wages) of different inputs, together with knowledge of the relative productivity of the inputs, will determine which combination of inputs to use for producing a given level of output or for meeting an increase in output.

To go from the production function to the supply schedule, it is necessary to combine information on the productivity of the inputs with information on their relative prices. Once prices are used in conjunction with the production function, we can describe the minimum-cost combination (i.e., relative prices and relative marginal products) for each level of output, which is the supply schedule or the amount of output that can be provided at different prices of that output. Supply schedules are rising because in order to provide a greater amount of output, the marginal productivity of inputs eventually declines and marginal costs rise, hence the costs of that additional output increase. Also, to increase the quantity of services, more resources must be drawn into production, and it is necessary to pay higher wages for these resources to bid them away from their current use. (The marginal cost curve shifts to the left.) In the long run, when all the inputs in the production function can be varied, the supply schedule will become more elastic, i.e., it will require less of an increase in cost to increase supply.

Certain assumptions implicit in the foregoing discussion should be made explicit, since they may not prevail, or perhaps are believed not to prevail, in the medical markets. The first is the assumption of substitutability in the use of inputs to produce a given output. In the health field, a great deal of emphasis is placed on the use of ratios of skilled health manpower to the population. If there is substitution between skilled and other types of manpower to provide medical services, then the use of such simple ratios (i.e., fixed coefficients of production) is inappropriate. Another assumption usually made with respect to production functions and supply schedules is that the different combinations of inputs that could be used to provide medical care are all technically efficient; that is, they are the minimum quantities necessary to produce a given level of service. It has been alleged that in certain sectors of the medical market too many inputs are used in producing a given service. It has also been alleged that the most economically efficient combinations of inputs are not used, because the input combinations that are used may be based upon the marginal productivities of the inputs without regard to their relative prices. The assumption that decisionmakers are desirous of minimizing the cost of producing medical services must be examined.

GOALS AND INCENTIVES OF DECISIONMAKERS

Economic efficiency in production requires decisionmakers to use knowledge of the marginal productivity of their inputs and their relative prices to produce the output at minimum cost. In the health field decisionmakers may have goals other than cost minimization; further, the relative prices of the inputs used in production may be distorted. If there are government subsidies for certain inputs, such as hospital capital or educational programs for certain manpower categories, then the relative price of the subsidized input has been lowered and relatively more of it may be used in production because it is cheaper to the decisionmakers.

To the extent that the goals of the decisionmakers differ from cost minimization, and the provider payment mechanisms enable them to pursue these other goals (and to the extent that there are legal restrictions on the use of inputs), the supply curve of medical care will be more inelastic. In other words, it will take larger price increases to produce an increase in services than it would if the objectives and constraints were similar to those of a competitive industry.

The example of the production function used above (nursing care), the information required in order to be able to minimize costs (marginal productivity and relative prices), and the assumptions underlying the behavior of the decisionmakers (a desire to minimize costs) can be applied equally well to other levels of the medical sector. The physician faces a production function in providing treatment for an illness of a particular diagnosis and of a given level of severity. The inputs in this instance would be the different institutional settings, such as a hospital, physician offices, or a nursing home.

The concern with the production function at the aggregate level is usually discussed in terms of the organization for the delivery of medical care—namely, the combinations of institutional settings that are least expensive for producing patient care. To determine which delivery systems (combinations of inputs or institutional settings) in a production function to provide medical care are least expensive, we would need to have information pertaining to marginal productivities and the relative costs of the different institutional settings, and an understanding of the objectives of the decisionmakers who are responsible for combining these inputs to produce patient services.

EVALUATION OF ECONOMIC EFFICIENCY IN PRODUCTION

The concept of economic efficiency is relevant to both the demand and the supply side of an industry. When evaluating economic efficiency, we are concerned that the rate (and type) of output be "optimal." Economic efficiency in demand is related to economic efficiency in supply through prices. In discussing the demand for medical care we saw that it is unlikely that economic efficiency, so defined, would occur in the output of medical care. The reason was that the price of medical care and of its various components is distorted as a result of existing insurance coverage, the tax deductibility of insurance premiums, and the incentives faced by the patient's physician, who may act not to minimize the patient's cost of treatment but rather to minimize the physician's own cost of providing that treatment and/or to maximize the net revenue garnered from the components used in treatment.

In our examination of the supply side of the medical care sector we are also interested in the criterion of economic efficiency. If the various markets within the medical care sector are determined to be economically inefficient, then the cost of medical care is higher than it should be. By examining the reasons for deviations from economic efficiency, we can make policy recommendations that would improve the efficiency of the market and inhibit the rapid rise in the cost of medical care. The "return" to greater economic efficiency in the production of medical care is the discounted present value of the possible cost savings. In an industry in which more than \$250 billion is spent, and in which expenditures are rising at approximately 15 percent per year, a savings of even 2 to 3 percent would result in a return in excess of \$30 billion.

The economic efficiency of the supply side of the medical care sector also has important policy implications. If the supply side of medical care is relatively inelastic, requiring relatively large price increases to bring forth an increase in medical care output (because the providers are not attempting to minimize their costs), then this will influence the type of redistribution programs proposed on the demand side, specifically, the type of national health insurance programs that can be instituted. As shown in Figure 7-1, a relatively inelastic supply curve, represented by S_1, would, with an increase in demand from D_1 to D_2, result in a greater price rise and a smaller increase in services provided than if the supply of medical services were more elastic. A more elastic supply schedule would, for the same increase in demand, provide $Q_2 - Q_1$ more services at a smaller increase in price: P_2 rather than P_1. The total cost of the increase in demand would be $P_1 \times Q_1$ in the inelastic case, versus $P_2 \times Q_2$ in the situation where supply is more elastic. In the latter case more of the increase in total expenditures would go for increased medical services, whereas in the former there would be more rapid price increases with a smaller increase in services. The cost of a national health insurance program would be greater and the availability of services di-

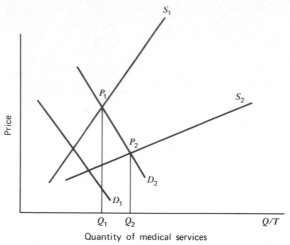

Figure 7-1. The effect of different supply elasticities on the price, quantity, and cost of national health insurance.

minished when supply is more inelastic; because of greater costs, the feasibility of instituting such a program, as well as its comprehensiveness, is reduced.

The economic efficiency of the supply side of medical care will influence decisionmakers as to the type of national health insurance program that is developed, when it will be implemented, and what it will cover. There will also be redistributive effects among different population groups in society depending upon the inelasticity of the supply of medical services. Greater inelasticity will mean greater increases in prices, wages, and incomes of the providers of medical services. The rest of the population will finance such increases from their own incomes and from taxes they pay to support demand shift programs in medical care.

By analyzing the elasticity of the supply of medical services, it is possible to more accurately forecast the effect on prices and expenditures of demand-increasing programs and to evaluate the performance of the providers of medical care. If analysis reveals that the supply of medical services is determined solely by the nature of the production function for producing those services, and further, that the providers are attempting to minimize their costs, then very few changes will be possible to improve the performance of the industry. The increase in medical prices and the type of output being produced could not be altered without serious and harmful effects on the industry and the patients. If, however, the production function is artificially constrained by legal restrictions, and there are few incentives for the providers to minimize their costs of production, then it would be possible to improve the performance of the medical sector.

In evaluating the performance of each of the medical markets, our first step will be to examine the market structure of each of the separate markets, beginning with the institutional settings in which care is provided, proceeding to the manpower markets, and ending with the education markets. Each medical market will be compared with a hypothetically competitive medical market. The competitive market is used as the yardstick for comparison, since it is inclusive of the conditions necessary for economic efficiency. The performance that might be expected under a competitive market will then be compared with what is observed in the particular medical market. Any divergence in performance between what is theoretically expected and what is observed will be analyzed in terms of differences in the structure and assumptions underlying the hypothetically competitive and actual markets. Public policy recommendations to improve the performance of the particular market studied will be made with reference to the differences in the structure and, consequently, the expected performance of the two markets.

Market performance can presumably be improved through alternative approaches: first, the actual market can be restructured to more closely approximate a competitive industry, wherein decisionmaking is decentralized and greater reliance is placed on competitive pressures to achieve the goal of economic efficiency. Alternatively, greater emphasis can be placed on regulation and centralized decisionmaking to achieve the desirable outcomes of a competitive market. Under either of these approaches there needs to be a comparable set of measures by which to evaluate the performance of each market. Unless there is some similarity between the desired outcome measures, differences between the advocates of increased regulation and the proponents of greater use of market pressures will be expressed in terms of value judgments rather than in more measurable terms reflecting the most efficient way to achieve a given outcome. In the health field, proposals for restructuring the delivery of medical services are often based more upon a general set of values that stop short of a clear definition of what the performance outcomes of the industry should be. If the health industry is evaluated using performance measures that are different from those traditionally used in evaluating economic efficiency, then those measures should be clearly enunciated and the implicit values underlying them should also be clearly explained. The two approaches suggested for improving market performance—increased regulation versus greater reliance on market pressures—will also be examined. A theoretical analysis and empirical evidence will be provided to indicate what might be expected to occur under these different approaches toward improving market performance in medical care.

For each of the institutional and educational markets, we are interested in the following aspects of economic efficiency: 1) Is each "firm" (hospitals, physicians' offices, medical schools) minimizing its costs of production? 2) Is the number of firms in the industry the "right" number; i.e., is each firm taking advantage of whatever economies of scale may exist? 3) Are the firms, and the industry as a whole, producing both a type and a quantity of output demanded by the consumers?

Taking each of the above concerns in order, in an industry characterized by pure competition 1) each firm must be efficient, otherwise it will not be able to survive; 2) the number of firms in the industry is determined by both the extent of economies of scale in production, and, in the long run, each firm is operating at that plant size that is most efficient, i.e., the minimum point on the long-run average-cost curve, and patient travel cost; and 3) the suppliers each respond in the short run (and in the long run through the entry of new firms) to changes in demand. To what extent does this performance occur in each of the medical markets? For each of the institutional and educational markets an analysis will be made of firm efficiency, of system efficiency (which determines the number of firms), and of the supply response to changes in demand. To the extent that there are indications of inadequate performance in any particular industry, we will examine several of the assumptions that underlie a competitive industry: is entry permitted into that industry by other firms, what are the goals and objectives of the suppliers, and what are the payment and incentive mechanisms in that industry? Major segments of the medical sector, such as hospitals and medical schools, are dominated by nonprofit firms. Do their objectives, which differ from those of traditional for-profit firms, lead to either desirable or undesirable differences in performance? Do reimbursement methods that have traditionally been cost-based in certain medical markets have any effects on performance? And, finally, what have been the effects on performance of barriers to entry into various medical markets that have been advanced on the grounds of consumer protection?

CHAPTER 8

The Market for
Health Insurance:
Its Performance
and Structure

It is important to determine how efficiently each sector of the medical care market performs. If these separate submarkets do not perform efficiently, then there may be a legitimate role for public intervention to increase the efficiency of the marketplace. Government intervention to increase efficiency is different from, and should be kept separate from, government intervention to redistribute the output of the medical care market. A government policy that attempts to do both simultaneously, either through a government agency or comprehensive regulation, may do neither as well as separate policies, directed toward either efficiency or equity.

Economic efficiency should be judged from both the demand side and the supply side of the market being examined. Economic efficiency with regard to supply usually means two things: that the number of firms in the market is the "right" number—that is, each firm operates at a minimum point on the long-run average-cost curve; and that each firm attempts to minimize its cost of production—that is, achieve internal efficiency. With respect to the demand side, adjudgment of economic efficiency is based on the "optimal" quantity (and varieties) of the product being produced. In discussing the performance of each of the markets being studied, we shall examine economic efficiency in demand as well as in supply. Hypotheses will be offered to explain possible divergence from economic efficiency, since any intervention to improve economic efficiency in this market should be consistent with the reasons for inadequate performance.

THE DEMAND SIDE OF THE HEALTH INSURANCE MARKET

THE MARKET DEMAND FOR HEALTH INSURANCE

The factors affecting the aggregate demand for health insurance, as discussed previously, are the price of insurance, the probability of loss, the magnitude of the loss if it occurs, the income of the consumer, and how risk averse the individual is. With increases in the price of medical care, the size of the potential loss increases, which in turn causes an increase (shift to the right) in the demand for health insurance. Increases in incomes lead to a greater demand for fringe benefits, which in turn also results in an increase in the demand for health insurance. (An increase in the aggregate demand for health insurance represents an increase in the percentage of the population with some insurance, an increase in the portion of the bill covered by insurance, as well as coverage for new benefits.) The price elasticity of the overall market demand for health insurance is considered to be approximately − 1; for each 1 percent increase in the price of insurance there will be a 1 percent decrease in the demand for insurance (1).

THE DEMAND FOR HEALTH INSURANCE FACED BY THE INDIVIDUAL FIRM

Health insurance is provided primarily by Blue Cross and Blue Shield (BCBS) plans, which are nonprofit, and the commercial carriers, which are for-profit. A small but growing portion of the health insurance market are prepaid health plans, such as Kaiser. More recently, a number of larger companies have decided upon self-insurance as an alternative means of providing their employees with health insurance. Smaller companies are also considering this option, together with a reinsurance component, to protect themselves against catastrophic losses. Thus, the increased aggregate demand for health insurance has expressed itself in increased demand for each of these competitive arrangements. Table 8-1 shows the increase in the population covered by hospital insurance both over time and by type of carrier.

What is of interest in this table is the changing market shares by type of insurance company. Since 1970, the share of the market held by commercial carriers has declined, from 56 percent to 50 percent. Blue Cross's share has remained relatively constant over that period at approximately 39 percent. Independent plans, which include prepaid health plans, company self-insurance plans, and administrative service contracts only, have been increasing their share of the market from 4 percent in 1970 to almost 12 percent in 1980. Although the overall market demand for health insurance may not be very responsive to the price of insurance, that portion of the aggregate demand sold by each firm is much more price elastic. The simple reason is that although there are few substitutes for health insurance in general, there are good substitutes available for any one firm selling insurance. The demand curve facing each firm is more elastic than the aggregate demand for insurance; however, each firm is not a perfect substitute for every other firm. Each firm has some leeway in how it sets

TABLE 8-1. Enrollment of Persons with Hospital Expense Protection, 1950–1979

Year	Civilian Population	Net No. of Persons Insured		Gross Number of Persons Insured							
		Total No.[a]	% of Population	All Insurers		Commercial Insurance		Blue Cross–Blue Shield		Independent Plans[b]	
				Total No.	% of Total	No.	% of Total	No.	% of Total	No.	% of Total
1950	150,790	76,639	50.8	81,691	100.0	39,601	48.5	37,645	46.1	4,445	5.4
1955	162,967	101,400	62.2	113,976	100.0	58,507	51.3	48,924	42.9	6,545	5.8
1960	178,140	122,500	68.8	140,055	100.0	76,597	54.7	57,464	41.0	5,994	4.3
1965	191,605	138,671	72.4	160,485	100.0	89,839	56.0	63,662	39.6	6,984	4.4
1970	203,499	154,263	75.8	190,758	100.0	107,163	56.1	75,464	39.6	8,131	4.3
1975	214,957	168,448	78.4	210,976	100.0	112,069	53.1	85,762	40.7	13,145	6.2
1979	224,367	170,791	76.6	220,753	100.0	109,842	49.8	85,409	38.7	25,502	11.6

Sources: Marjorie Smith Mueller, "Private Health Insurance in 1975: Coverage Enrollment, and Financial Experience," *Social Security Bulletin* 40 (June 1977): 6; Marjorie Smith Mueller and Paula A. Piro, "Private Health Insurance in 1974: A Review of Coverage Enrollment and Financial Experience," *Social Security Bulletin* 39 (March 1976): 7; Marjorie Smith Carroll and Ross H. Arnett II, "Private Health Insurance Plans in 1978 and 1979: A Review of Coverage, Enrollment, and Financial Experience," *Health Care Financing Review* 3 (September 1981): 56, 66. The figures for "Net Number of Persons Insured" prior to 1970 come from the Health Insurance Association of America, and are published in *Source Book of Health Insurance Data, 1980–1981* (Washington, D.C.: Health Insurance Institute, 1981), p. 13. Population figures come from the Bureau of the Census's *Current Population Reports*, Series P-25, No. 901, July 1981, and *Statistical Abstract of the United States, 1980* (Washington, D.C.: Government Printing Office, 1980), p. 6.

[a]"Duplicate coverage (i.e., similar coverage by more than one insurer) has been eliminated in this column. No adjustment has been made for duplicate coverage in the other columns.

[b]"Independent Plans" includes those covered by prepaid health plans and self-insured health plans. Persons covered by Minimum Premium Plans and plans using Administrative Service Only Agreements are also included in this category.

its prices, i.e., determines its insurance premium. One of the factors that differentiate one firm from another is the type of benefits provided; not all firms offer the same type of insurance coverage and they differ on the use and extent of copayments. The insurance carriers also differ as to whether the patient is reimbursed by the insurance company after he or she has reimbursed the health care provider, or whether the insurance company pays the provider directly. Insurance companies also have different reputations, and in markets where information on the relative performance of competing firms is not complete, people may be willing to pay a higher price for what they perceive to be a favorable reputation.

The "product," health insurance, differs both according to "real" characteristics, such as type of coverage, patient cosharing arrangements, and methods of payment of claims, and according to perceived differences in product, such as reputation for payment of claims. We would therefore expect to observe price differences between insurance firms in accordance with these product differences. If the prices of insurance differ between firms by a greater amount than what is justified by product differences, then we would expect groups of insured persons to begin to switch their insurance coverage. Thus, insurance companies will compete among themselves for the insured population on the basis of price as well as in terms of product differences. If insured groups move between insurance firms according to the differences in prices and products, the market will perform in an efficient manner. The "product" will be expected to change over time and also to conform more closely to the preferences of the insured group.* If additional firms selling insurance enter the industry, we would expect the resulting price competition to bring the price of insurance relatively close to the pure premium; that is, the cost of administration, claims processing, and marketing functions would be produced efficiently and there would not be any excess profits in the industry. (The more price elastic the demand curve facing the individual firm is, the closer the price will be to average cost and the less likelihood there will be of excess profits in the long run.) The efficient performance of this industry is not contingent upon each consumer's having perfect information regarding all the price and product differences among firms. The costs of acquiring such information are clearly too great for each individual; however, large groups such as unions would be expected to develop such expertise. Also, since approximately 85 percent of insurance is purchased by groups, it is the information acquired by these groups that brings about competition among insurance firms. (Because such information is costly to acquire, we might also expect the product and price differences to be more favorable to large groups that acquire it.)

The price of insurance that we have been referring to is the benefit/premium ratio, which is the percent of the total premium paid out in benefits to each insured group. If, for example, the premium for each member in a group were $1,000 per year and the utilization experience of that group resulted in an average pay-out of benefits equal to $900 per member per year, then the benefit/

---

*Since there are such large differences in the costs of handling a group and an individual, we would expect that most individuals in a group would prefer to forego the benefits of individually tailored policies to take advantage of the lower cost of a single group policy.

premium ratio would be .9. The difference between benefits and total premiums goes to administration, claims processing, marketing, and profit for the insuring firm. When the benefit/premium ratio is close to 1.0, then the group is "experience rated," which means that the premium reflects the expected experience of the group. The more the health insurance industry approximates a competitive industry, the closer we would expect the benefit/premium ratio to be 1.0. Where information is inadequate or where there are monopolies in the sale of health insurance, there is greater divergence from 1.0 in the benefit/premium ratio. In a competitive industry we would expect groups to change insurance companies when their benefit/premium ratio surpasses the amount they are willing to pay for real or perceived product differences between firms. One indication of the performance of the industry would be the variation in benefit/premium ratios when size of group is held constant: the smaller the variation, the more efficient the market. (Because of economies of scale in administering different-sized groups, the larger the size of group, the closer the benefit/premium ratio would be to 1.0.) Not only would price reflect the minimum costs of producing the services of the insurance industry in a competitive market, but also the choice of insurance packages would most closely approximate the preferences of the insured group.

To provide some indication of the competitiveness, hence performance, of the health insurance industry, it is important to examine the pricing of health insurance policies.

Table 8-2 shows the ratios of expenditures (benefits) to premiums by different types of insurance plans for the period 1955–1979. There are two points of interest in this table. First, the benefit/premium ratio for both the Blues and the commercials have increased over time. The relative closeness of these ratios, both between the Blues and commercials and to a benefit/premium ratio of 1, suggest that this is a relatively competitive industry.* Second, the differences in the benefit/premium ratio between group and individual policies indicate the large savings to an individual from participating in a group plan.

A further indication of the competitiveness of the insurance industry was the approach used by Blue Cross for many years to price its insurance coverage (community rating) and how market forces caused a change in that approach.

THE EFFICIENCY AND EQUITY ASPECTS OF COMMUNITY RATING

When Blue Cross was started, the method used for establishing premiums to be paid by subscribers was community rating, whereby premiums were the same to all subscribers regardless of the experience of the group on which the pure

---

*It may be argued that the increasing benefit/premium ratio is the result of more efficient methods of administration. Increased computerization of claims processing has undoubtedly occurred over the time period examined. However, unless there were competition between firms, these decreased administrative costs would not have been passed on to the subscribers; the benefit/premium ratio could have remained the same and the companies would instead have received larger profits. Competition forces these savings to be passed on in either lower premiums or greater benefits, thereby reducing the ratio.

TABLE 8-2. The Ratio of Benefit Expenditures to Premium Income, According to Type of Plan, 1955–1979

Year	All Plans	Blue Cross–Blue Shield			Commercial Insurance Companies			Independent Plans[a]
		Total	Blue Cross	Blue Shield	Total	Group Policies	Individual Policies	
1955	.805	.887	.915	.824	.725	.839	.530	.912
1960	.855	.921	.928	.904	.789	.904	.529	.965
1965	.874	.939	.953	.901	.819	.936	.547	.906
1970	.915	.958	.973	.922	.872	.958	.581	.962
1975	.927	.982	1.001	.939	.886	.984	.511	.867
1979	.898	.926	—[b]	—[b]	.875	.923	.654	.888

Source: This table was developed from data provided in Marjorie Smith Carroll and Ross H. Arnett, "Private Health Insurance Plans in 1978 and 1979: A Review of Coverage, Enrollment and Financial Experience," Health Care Financing Review 3 (September 1981): 75.

[a]"Independent Plans" includes plans that offer health services on a prepaid basis, and self-insured health plans.
[b]Data are not available.

156

premium was based. (Blue Cross initially covered only hospitalization, which is still the dominant form of its coverage.) Aged persons, who would be expected to have much higher hospital use rates than younger persons, were charged the *same premium*.* The benefit/premium ratio for aged persons was, therefore, greater than 1.0; the benefits paid on their behalf exceeded the premiums they paid for insurance. Since the average benefit/premium ratio for all groups in a community rating system had to be close to 1.0, this meant that groups of low users of hospital services had benefit/premium ratios of much less than 1.0.

The effect of community rating, when the expected costs of groups differ, is that a subsidy is provided to high-use groups, financed by a "tax" on the lower-use groups (2). Any such "subsidy-tax" system can be evaluated on the basis of two economic criteria: first, its effect on efficiency—namely, does it affect the quantity of health insurance purchased?—and, second, its equity—does such a redistribution scheme cause the higher-income subscribers of Blue Cross to subsidize the lower-income subscribers?

With regard to the efficiency aspects of community rating, low-user groups are typically low-risk groups. There is a certain amount above the pure premium that the individual is willing to pay for health insurance. Charging low-risk groups an amount above their pure premium much greater than the amount they would be charged if they were experience rated would result in fewer low-user groups' purchasing insurance. Such low-user groups might decide to self-insure rather than pay the Blue Cross community rate. Depending upon the price elasticity of demand for insurance, low-user groups would, under community rating, demand less insurance. Like an excise tax that is placed on some goods and services and hence distorts their relative prices, a community rate is a tax on the insurance premium of a low-risk person. The result of such a "tax" is a decreased demand for health insurance coverage. Changing from a community rating system to one based on experience rating should result in the low-risk group's purchasing more health insurance. For this reason a community rate is considered economically inefficient. (A similar inefficiency occurs when a monopolist charges a price for a service that exceeds its cost of production.) Community rating does not permit the low-risk person to purchase insurance at its costs of production, which is its actuarial value plus administrative cost.

Perhaps the main reason for community rating, according to its advocates, is that it enables persons who would otherwise not be able to afford health insurance to pay the premium. Without government subsidies, Blue Cross, in using community rating, acts as a welfare agency as it subsidizes high-risk/low-income persons by taxing low-risk/higher-income persons.† The redistribution argument in favor of community rating offered by its proponents can be countered by the argument that community rating is an inefficient mechanism for redistributing medical care, and a mechanism that may not have its desired effects.

---

*Even under community rating, however, premiums differed according to whether the individual was married or single and whether or not he or she belonged to a group.

†An additional reason suggested for community rating is that it is insurance with a longer time horizon. Since everyone grows old, the young (low-risk) who subsidize the aged eventually receive such a subsidy themselves. Still another reason offered is that the administrative costs for determining the necessary information to experience-rate each group may outweigh the possible savings to different groups receiving a lower premium.

Using risk as a basis for determining a subsidy for medical insurance involved the assumption that all high-risk people have lower incomes than low-risk people. This may be accurate on the average, but there are certainly high-risk aged persons who have higher incomes than low-risk younger persons. The direction of the subsidy, however, goes from the low-risk to the high-risk, regardless of their relative incomes. Further, the actual subsidy goes to the group that *uses* hospital services more, not necessarily to the group that has the highest risk of hospitalization. A study of Michigan Blue Cross revealed that the most heavily subsidized group was the auto workers. The next most heavily subsidized group was comprised of health care professionals—physicians, nurses, and other hospital employees (3). These subsidized groups are *not* the lowest-income groups belonging to Michigan Blue Cross. (One possible reason for the auto workers' being subsidized in their purchase of Blue Cross is that they represent a large group with more market power than many of the other smaller groups that belong to Blue Cross.) What appears to have occurred in practice under community rating is that the subsidy-tax concept operates in reverse: higher-income persons may be subsidized by lower-income persons.

If everyone agreed on the value judgment that subsidies should be provided to lower-income families to purchase health insurance, these values could be realized more efficiently through a system of direct subsidies to those families instead of authorizing Blue Cross to operate the subsidy-tax system. Blue Cross's goals may not include being the most efficient welfare agent. Instead Blue Cross may attempt to increase its enrollment, and, in so doing, it will allocate its taxes and subsidies according to a policy that will facilitate the greatest increase in its growth. This policy would be to charge lower premiums to groups whose demands are more elastic, such as large unions, and higher premiums to groups with less elastic demands instead of matching the subsidy to income level.

The community rating concept used by Blue Cross appears to be inefficient because it raises the price of health insurance to low-user groups, thereby resulting in a lower demand for health insurance by these groups than if they were experience rated. Community rating is also an inefficient method of distributing subsidies for the purchase of health insurance. One also wonders whether it was ever a viable concept; that is, could such a pricing system for health insurance survive in a competitive market?

Unless community rating were legally mandated as the method for pricing premiums among all health insurance companies, competitive forces would cause insurance premiums to become experience rated. Even if Blue Cross used community rating, a competitor could offer to sell health insurance to lower-user groups at a price that would approximate their expected experience rate. For low-user groups the premium would be lower than the Blue Cross premium, and we would expect them to switch their insurance coverage from Blue Cross. As more low-user groups left Blue Cross, the Blue Cross premium to the remaining subscribers would increase, in turn causing additional groups that were subsidizing others to change their insurance coverage. As long as the various groups purchasing health insurance were attempting to maximize their health care benefits per dollar spent, and if they had sufficient information on the different benefit packages, the premiums charged by different companies, and the performance of the insurance company in payment of claims, we would not expect a community rate to survive in a competitive environment. Obviously, not every group has the necessary information or expertise to determine whether it should insure with a company other than Blue Cross. All it takes for the community rating concept to be changed, however, is for a few groups to decide to change their coverage. Some companies (or unions) have a sufficiently large number of employees to provide them with an incentive to develop the expertise and information on alternatives to Blue Cross. All purchasers in the market do not have to be informed for competition in health insurance to work. If only some of them have the necessary information and act on it, the effects of their behavior will be sufficient to produce a more competitive rate structure; price competition among the insurers will result in lower rates to the smaller, less-informed groups.

As we would expect, Blue Cross abandoned its community rating concept as competition from commercial insurance companies increased. (This provides some evidence that competition in the health insurance market causes providers to respond to consumer demands.) Some of the larger Blue Cross plans, which are subject to less competition, have not gone all the way to experience rating. They have what is called "merit rating," which is a modified experience rate that allows for some subsidies and taxes to different groups. It is doubtful, however, that these subsidies and taxes are based on the incomes of the group; they are more likely related to the size of the group and the likelihood of its switching to another insurance company.

It is doubtful that even legally mandating community rating among all insurance carriers would be a workable system. The major health insurance benefit offered by Blue Cross under community rating was service benefit coverage for hospital care: Blue Cross paid each hospital on the basis of the hospital's own costs or charges; the patient was not responsible for any hospitalization costs and was entitled to a semiprivate accommodation while in the hospital. If subscribers have different preferences regarding the benefits for which they would like to purchase insurance and the amount of copayment desired (both of which determine their premium), then it would be very difficult to maintain a series of community rates that would accommodate such preferences. Maintaining a community rate for the single set of benefits provided by Blue Cross, when subscribers differ in their utilization experience and in their preference for benefits and cost sharing, is highly inefficient. Diversity in consumer preferences can be dealt with most efficiently by a health insurance system that offers a variety of benefits, cost-sharing arrangements, and rate structures. If it is determined that certain groups have incomes that are inadequate to purchase a "minimum" level of health insurance, and if it is society's desire to provide them with at least a minimum level of health insurance, subsidies can be provided directly to those groups instead of mandating a similar insurance scheme for all persons that would be administered by a company that would use an internal subsidy and tax system.

THE SUPPLY SIDE OF THE HEALTH INSURANCE MARKET

Based on the above discussion, it appears that the demand side of the insurance market is quite competitive. The supply side is examined next to determine the efficiency with which health insurance is produced. Efficiency in production concerns both the number of firms selling health insurance, that is, the extent to which there are economies of scale among health insurance firms, and whether each firm is itself operating in the most efficient manner. The determination of economies of scale would indicate how many firms could compete in the sale of insurance and whether or not the insurance business is a "natural" monopoly, that is, can the functions performed by insurance companies be performed less expensively by just one firm.

The health insurance industry also has several characteristics which distinguish it from other industries. Certain firms in this industry receive advantages over other firms. These competitive advantages are believed to enable BCBS to achieve greater market shares than they would otherwise. Since BCBS are nonprofit organizations, there is the issue of what BCBS do with their increased market power. To whom do the competitive advantages of BCBS accrue? Are the consumers the beneficiaries, in terms of lower health care costs? Or, alternatively, are the beneficiaries the providers, hospitals and physicians, and the Blues themselves, in terms of higher salaries and internal "slack" within the organization?

The following sections discuss the competitive advantages that the Blues have over the commercials, the extent of economies of scale in the production of health insurance, and the consequences of the Blues' greater market power.

There are certain financial requirements for becoming a supplier of health insurance such as minimum reserve requirements. These requirements, however, have not been sufficiently restrictive to prevent new firms from entering different regional markets. Because Blue Cross plans are nonprofit, they receive more favorable tax treatment than do commercial companies. In return for such treatment, they are subject to greater regulation by the insurance commissioners in each state, who must approve their premiums.

> Typically, the Blue Cross and Blue Shield plans pay no premium tax while the commercial insurers pay 2 percent or so. As a percentage of the insurance firms' costs, this 2 percent represents an enormous advantage for the Blues. For example, only 5 percent of Blue Cross premiums are kept to pay expenses. Thus, the typical tax advantage lowers Blue Cross costs by more than 30 percent. Blue Shield expenses are a larger percentage of premiums, but even for Blue Cross and Blue Shield combined, only about 8 percent of premium income pays expenses, so that the premium tax break alone lowers costs by more than 20 percent.
>
> Furthermore, many states exempt the Blues from other taxes that commercial insurers must pay, such as property taxes. Some states regulate the ratio of benefits to premiums for commercial insurance sold to individuals. This eliminates sales of certain types of commercial policies with high selling costs or administrative costs or both. (4)*

---

* In a study on *The Regulation of Health Insurance* (unpublished doctoral dissertation, Department of Economics, University of California, Santa Barbara, 1974) H.E. Frech states that "Most states charge no premium taxes on Blue Cross while charging between 0.5 percent and 4.0 percent of premium for domestic and foreign (out of state) commercial insurers" (p. 59). In his empirical findings, Frech finds that "regulation of rates or prices of health insurance leads to a higher Blue Cross market share, more extensive insurance purchases and higher prices and quantities in the hospital market." He concludes: "An examination of the actual regulation of health insurance and of the legal status of Blue Cross hospital insurance plans, which are controlled by hospitals, shows that health insurance regulation provides competitive advantages for Blue Cross over commercial insurers" (p. xii).

Frech conducted an empirical study to determine the effect that the 2 percent tax advantage had on Blue Cross's market share. It was estimated that Blue Cross was able to increase its market share, on average, by 6.7 percent.

A second competitive advantage that the Blues have over the commercials is that the Blues do not compete with one another. Blue Cross is a loose federation of approximately 69 independently operating plans joined together by an interplan system for handling claims incurred in other areas. The national Blue Cross organization provides certain important functions, such as representing all Blue Cross plans in their relations with the federal government and testifying on legislation affecting the health insurance industry. Each Blue Cross and Blue Shield plan has a monopoly within its market over its type of service; if one Blue Cross firm is more efficient and wishes to expand its market, it cannot enter another Blue Cross plan's area. Each Blue Cross plan benefits by being the designated representative of Blue Cross's reputation and by being the only one to offer the Blue Cross insurance package to subscribers. Commercial companies, on the other hand, compete with one another as well as with Blue Cross.

A third competitive advantage of Blue Cross is that because it was started by hospitals and is favored by hospitals, Blue Cross receives a discount compared with the charges that commercial companies pay to hospitals for the same care in the same institution. This discount may be as high as 20 percent in some cases.*

It is difficult to empirically estimate the extent of economies of scale among different health insurance carriers. Determining the reasons for differences in costs between companies for performing the administrative function requires the assumption that each company performs the same tasks and does them equally well. In fact, however, the administrative function varies between firms. The range of functions includes marketing and selling policies, processing applications and policies, maintaining the policy file, processing claims, reviewing claims, and paying claims. The variety of contracts offered, each entailing a different cost, and the extent to which the company has group or individual policies (it is more costly to handle individual policies) will also differ among firms; taxes may be included in the commercial companies' expenses but not in those of Blue Cross. It is difficult to compare the differences in costs, taking care to separate differences that are due to differences in scale from differences in efficiency and differences in functions performed.

One investigation that attempted to analyze the effect on administrative cost of differences in the size of health insurance carriers, while holding constant the effect of other factors, involved several separate studies. One study examined economies of scale for just commercial health insurance companies, since their output mix (e.g., variety of contracts, percentage of nongroup policies, etc.) is so different from that of Blue Cross. The authors, Vogel and Blair, found that economies of scale do exist and that the administrative cost ratio declines with increased size of operation (5). When economies of scale were investigated sepa-

---

*The Blue Cross discount is believed to be related to both the presumably lower costs incurred by hospitals for billing Blue Cross and to the market power of the particular Blue Cross plan in an area. Although a recent study was unable to verify this last point, the authors found that the discount resulted in an increase in Blue Cross's market share. Roger Feldman and Warren Greenberg, "The Relation Between Blue Cross Market Share and the Blue Cross Discount on Hospital Charges," *The Journal of Risk Insurance* 48 (June 1981).

rately for Blue Cross and for Blue Shield (in their non-Medicare business), no economies of scale were found. The authors then included in their analysis BCBS plans that had merged. They observed lower administrative costs for these merged, larger firms. Based on these studies, the authors concluded that economies of scale do exist in the nonprofit sector, although the gains from such economies are offset by internal inefficiency ("x-inefficiency") because they are nonprofit firms (6).

In a follow-up study, Blair and Vogel undertook a "survivors" analysis to test for economies of scale among health insurers (7). In this type of analysis, firms are assigned to different categories according to their size. The growth of firms in each size category is studied over time. If substantial economies of scale exist, then firms in the largest size classes will grow rapidly at the expense of firms in the smaller size categories. Smaller firms will either have to expand their scale of operation (and/or merge) or they will be forced to leave the industry. The authors found that all but the smallest size categories expanded over the period 1958–1973. They concluded that economies of scale existed but that they were not as large as originally believed, since other size categories also grew.

Vogel and Blair also attempted to determine whether economies of scale exist in the administration of Medicare Part A (hospital claims payment). They found results opposite of what they expected. Administrative costs per claim increased with the size of the firm. The interpretation of this finding was that the method of Medicare reimbursement of intermediaries, which was cost-based, encouraged higher administrative costs (8). In an analysis of Medicare Part B (physician claims) it was found that commercial companies had lower administrative costs than Blue Shield plans (9).

If one type of firm in a competitive market has a cost advantage, it could undercut the prices of other firms and drive them from the market. The cost advantage could provide the firm with a monopoly position. If this were to occur, the public would receive the benefits of that cost reduction in terms of lower prices. However, when Blue Cross plans with a tax advantage are analyzed, it appears that they have been able to increase their market shares but not to the extent thought possible by researchers investigating this issue. This finding has led researchers to develop several hypotheses as to how BCBS use their competitive advantage. Frech argues that since the Blues are nonprofit and their governing boards are often controlled by hospital and physician representatives, the Blues use their competitive advantages to benefit both the providers of care and those working for the Blues (10). For example, hospitals favor complete coverage for hospital care; such coverage increases the demand for hospitals and removes the patient's incentive to shop around. By having Blue Cross use their cost advantage to subsidize the sale of this type of coverage, hospitals benefit. Therefore the Blues benefit the providers by offering their subscribers more complete insurance plans, such as paying a higher percentage of the hospital bill than commercial carriers and not having copayments or deductibles. With lower out-of-pocket costs, the subscribers will increase their demand for medical care. The consequence of this type of coverage is that providers are able to raise their prices and hospital costs increase faster than they would otherwise.

Because the Blues were controlled by the providers, it was in the interest of providers that the Blues had competitive cost advantages. When viewed in this manner, it was also in hospitals' interests to provide Blue Cross with a discount. The Blue Cross discount is a competitive advantage Blue Cross has over the commercials. Several reasons have been mentioned why hospitals gave Blue Cross a discount (i.e., cost savings and market power). Another reason is that hospitals used the discount as a way of providing Blue Cross with additional competitive advantages; the price of Blue Cross coverage is lowered relative to commercial insurance. Hospitals thereby benefited by assisting the expansion of a preferred type of hospital coverage. Weller distinguishes between discounts that are procompetitive, i.e., a firm is a tough bargainer and tries to get the lowest price possible from their suppliers, and discounts that are anticompetitive, i.e., a supplier gives a favored purchaser a preferential price. Based on the findings that Blue Cross plans were started and controlled by hospitals and that those Blue Cross plans with relatively high market shares are also in areas where hospital costs are relatively high, Weller concludes that the hospital discount can be more adequately explained in terms of anticompetitive behavior on the part of hospitals (11).

Anticompetitive measures have also been used by medical societies and physician-controlled Blue Shield plans to make it difficult for certain insurers to compete. Assume that Blue Shield plans do not have any cost advantages over other insurers. A commercial insurer could increase its market share by reducing its premium through the use of cost-saving measures such as copayments, preauthorization of services, utilization review, and preferred providers. To prevent the growth of such plans, medical societies have both boycotted and threatened to boycott patients with this type of insurance coverage. In this manner, providers have precluded certain types of coverage from being offered in the insurance market.*

The cost advantage of the Blues can also be used to benefit their management and employees. They can pay themselves higher salaries, work in more pleasant surroundings, and have a larger staff than necessary.

As a test of the hypotheses that the Blues use their competitive position to benefit both the providers of care and those working for the Blues, Frech and Ginsburg conducted an empirical study and found that Blue Cross plans with

---

*Goldberg and Greenberg describe how early (1930s–1940s) insurance companies in Oregon placed restraints on physician utilization. Preauthorization of services and monitoring of claims were used. When they were faced with competition, the insurance companies acted to lower their costs. Physicians accepted such constraints on their behavior since it was during the depression; physicians did not have as many patients and were not sure of their ability to collect from those they did have. Consumers benefitted from the utilization review and the lower insurance premiums. The response to this situation by the medical societies in Oregon was twofold: first, to threaten expulsion from the medical society of physicians that participated in such insurance plans. Second, the medical societies started their own insurance plans. These plans did not use aggressive utilization review procedures. With the growth of their own insurance plan, physicians were encouraged to boycott the other insurance plans. The effect of these policies was to increase the growth of the insurance plan sponsored by organized medicine and to cause a decline in the other insurance plans. To receive the participation of physicians, these other plans also had to become less aggressive in their cost containment efforts. Lawrence G. Goldberg and Warren Greenberg, "The Emergence of Physician-Sponsored Health Insurance: A Historical Perspective," in Warren Greenberg, ed., Competition in the Health Care Sector (Germantown, Md.: Aspen Systems Corporation, 1978).

greater market power, namely those with a larger market share, offered more complete insurance coverage (12). Frech and Ginsburg also attempted to estimate the effect that increased market power has on the Blues' efficiency. Since Blue plans are nonprofit, it was hypothesized that the managers and employees also share in the Blues' competitive advantage. Frech and Ginsburg found that Blue Cross and Blue Shield plans with lower taxes, hence a competitive advantage, had higher administrative costs per enrollee (13).

Eisenstat and Kennedy studied the relationship between physician control of Blue Shield plans and the efficiency of that plan. The hypothesis of the authors was that greater physician control of Blue Shield plans should result in an increase in the efficiency of the plan; greater plan efficiency would result in more funds being available to increase reimbursement to the providers. In their empirical work, the authors found that for Blue Shield plans having a tax, hence competitive, advantage over commercial insurers, their administrative costs decreased as the percentage of physicians on the Blue Shield board increased. However, for those Blue Shield plans without a tax advantage, hence less market power, the composition of the board had no significant effect on the plan's administrative costs (14). The authors concluded that in markets where the Blues had a competitive advantage the providers act as residual claimants and reduce inefficient operations. Among plans that have no competitive advantage, market competition acts to reduce any plan inefficiency.

Whether physician control over Blue Shield plans causes their fees to be higher or lower has been the subject of several studies, including an investigation by the Federal Trade Commission. Sloan concluded that in physician-controlled Blue Shield plans, reimbursement levels and the number of services provided will be greater than in those plans not controlled by physicians (15). Lynk's study reaches the opposite conclusion (16). He argues that if Blue Shield is acting in the physician's interest, it will set its maximum allowable charge equal to the median charge in the market area. If it were above the median charge, then physicians whose charges were below that level—the majority of physicians—would benefit by a reduction of the maximum allowable charge. The majority of physicians would benefit because they would receive the patients that shift away from those physicians with higher fees that are no longer fully reimbursed by Blue Shield. When the maximum allowable charge equals the median fee in the market area, a majority of physicians will be satisfied, and the market will be stable. Thus physician controlled Blue Shield boards should result in lower, not higher, average levels of payment for insured procedures.* However, regardless of whether physician control of Blue Shield plans increase or decrease physician fees, the authors agree that physician control will be used to benefit the physicians.

---

*In a discussion on whether physician-controlled Blue Shield plans are anticompetitive, which was the subject of the Federal Trade Commission inquiry, Watts claims the results from both the Sloan and Lynk studies are inadequate on this point. Both studies focus on input prices (the fees paid to participating physicians), rather than on the policy premiums, which are more appropriate indicators of market competition. As long as there are no entry barriers, then premiums for similar policies should be comparable. Thus the competitiveness of the insurance market cannot be determined by whether physician reimbursement levels are high or low. Carolyn A. Watts, "FTC Sings the Blues: A Comment," *Journal of Health Politics, Policy, and Law* (Fall 1980).

CONCLUDING COMMENTS

Blue Cross was established and grew at a rapid rate because it was able to see the vast potential demand for coverage of health care costs. The commercial insurance companies entering the market after Blue Cross also grew, because of their innovations in offering a benefit coverage (major medical insurance) that was different from what was offered by Blue Cross, their different reimbursement methods (indemnity payments), and experience rating. Unless competition had been possible, it is unlikely that consumers would have been offered a greater choice in benefits, cost-sharing arrangements, and rates to match their own experience.

The overall conclusion that appears to emerge from the above studies is that the Blues have certain competitive advantages over the commercials. To the extent that individual Blue plans have been able to benefit from these advantages, they have been able to increase their market shares. As a result of their increased market power, the Blues have been able to sell more comprehensive health insurance, which has benefited the providers and led to increased health care costs. The Blues themselves have also benefited from these competitive advantages. The internal efficiency of the firm is affected by the objectives of the firm and the extent to which it is subject to competitive pressures. Their increased market power has enabled the Blues to have greater organizational slack than would have been possible in a competitive market. With regard to the studies on economies of scale, it appears that economies of scale do exist in the administrative function in health insurance companies. However, large Blue Cross and Blue Shield companies, which are less subject to competitive pressures, appear to have internal "slack," which more than offsets gains resulting from economies of scale. Therefore, if monopolies were created to administer any national health insurance scheme, either at a national or regional level, in order to take advantage of economies of scale, the lack of competitive pressures as a result of having a monopoly (such as allowing the Social Security Administration to perform this function) might cause administrative costs to be higher than if more firms competed against one another.*

Maintaining a competitive market structure for Blue Cross and commercial companies would force them to respond to consumer demands for different types of insurance coverage and minimize their administrative costs. In such a situation, health insurance will be produced at the lowest cost and the type of services available will approximate the demands of the insured group. The incentives inherent in such competition are more effective for achieving economic efficiency in the demand and supply of health insurance than having one large

---

*Hsiao attempted to determine whether competitive pressures resulted in lower administrative costs. For the years 1971 and 1972, he compared the administrative costs under the Medicare program, which was administered by the Social Security Administration, with that of the Federal Employees Health Benefit Program (FEBP). The FEBP was administered by a consortium of private carriers, which included both profit and nonprofit firms. After adjusting for some differences in the functions performed in administration of the two programs, he found that administrative costs per claim were lower under the FEBP. Hsiao concluded that the greater efficiency of the private firms was due to the competition among those firms. William Hsiao, "Public Versus Private Administration of Health Insurance: A Study in Relative Economic Efficiency," *Inquiry* 15 (December 1978).

firm administer a standard insurance policy for everyone. Innovations in benefit packages and in cost minimization are more likely to occur when there are strong competitive pressures than when firms, whether they are for-profit or nonprofit, are protected from such competition.

Given the above, admittedly brief, description of the supply side of the health insurance market, what changes, if any, should be made? In the administration of health insurance under public programs (Medicare and Medicaid), it appears that cost-based reimbursement to intermediaries provides them with no incentives to perform their functions at minimum cost. Reimbursement of intermediaries might be changed to a fixed-rate reimbursement and/or a competitive-bid basis; the performance of the intermediaries should be monitored to insure that all administrative functions contracted for are carried out.

There is a great lack of consumer information on performance of private health insurance companies, and it is costly for consumers or insured groups to gather this information. It would be desirable if such information on costs and measures of performance could be made more readily available.

Blue Cross and Blue Shield plans currently enjoy a competitive tax advantage over commercial firms. It is not clear why the different health insurance plans should not be on an equal footing.

The health insurance industry is becoming very competitive. As shown earlier in Table 8-1, although the population is slowly increasing, the percentage of the population with hospital insurance is remaining relatively stable at approximately 77 percent. The implication of this for health insurers is that it is becoming more difficult for them to increase their enrollments. The growth of independent plans, such as prepaid, company self-insurance, and administrative services only, are experiencing the largest percentage growth, greater than 100 percent since 1970. If the insurance carriers are to increase their enrollments, it will have to be at the expense of their competitors.

Continued large increases in their insurance premiums have made business firms aware of the impact this has on the firms' labor costs, and consequently on the prices of their goods and services. Labor leaders are also aware that to merely maintain the same health benefits, their members will have to forego wage increases. It is therefore likely that the trend toward self-insurance by large companies and experimentation with prepaid health plans will continue to remain an important alternative to the traditional carriers (17).

Increased competition among health insurers is likely to have adverse effects upon hospitals. To keep their premiums competitive with other insurance companies, as well as with prepaid health plans, insurance companies will have to reduce their expenditures for hospital care. Hospital expenditures are a major portion of the insurance premium, representing 93 percent of Blue Cross expenditures (18). First, insurance companies are likely to place greater pressure on hospitals to hold down the rate of increase in hospital costs. Second, the insurers will attempt to reduce hospital utilization of their subscribers through stronger utilization review mechanisms and by insuring less costly substitutes to hospital care. The effect of these policies should be to reduce the portion of the insurance premium that is spent on hospitals.

Competitive pressures and the high portion of their premium represented by hospital expenditures provides Blue Cross with an incentive to control hospital expenditures. However, important to understanding the limited and generally ineffective approach used by Blue Cross in the past, namely, controls on increases in the number of beds, was the fact that Blue Cross was started, supported, and controlled by hospitals. Hospitals viewed Blue Cross as a means of increasing the demand for hospital care and of insuring payment to hospitals for their services. As such, it was not in the interests of hospitals to have Blue Cross provide any coverage to patients other than for hospitalization. Out-of-hospital coverage could serve only to decrease hospital utilization. Similarly, it was not in the interests of hospitals to have Blue Cross include any copayments such as coinsurance, because this would provide patients with an incentive to shop around for the least costly hospital. To compete with Blue Cross, commercial companies offered lower-priced coverage by including patient cost-sharing and coverage for out-of-hospital care. Blue Cross, whose benefits were entirely for hospital care, could have kept its premiums from rising rapidly by introducing patient cost-sharing provisions, by monitoring hospital costs, or by decreasing hospital utilization. The first two approaches would have placed Blue Cross in an adversary position with the hospitals that controlled it. Therefore, the only other approach was to control hospital utilization indirectly by decreasing the availability of hospital beds in an area. Blue Cross was already committed to reimbursing hospitals for all of their beds, whether or not they were filled. If Blue Cross could prevent new hospitals from being built, it would not be in conflict with existing hospital administrators. Controls on hospital beds could limit total hospital utilization; because Blue Cross' premium consisted of a greater portion of hospital costs than did the premiums of commercial companies, Blue Cross' premium would be reduced by a proportionately greater amount. It is likely that more direct and effective cost control approaches, such as utilization review, out-of-hospital coverage, patient incentives, monitoring of hospitals costs, and not paying for empty beds, will be used by the Blues in the future.

Increased competitive pressures are changing Blue Cross's traditional relationship to hospitals. Blue Cross will have to develop a more adversarial relationship with hospitals in order to survive in this new environment.

REFERENCES

1. Charles S. Roehrig, *The Impact of Technology on the Demand for Hospital and Medical Care*, Final Report to the Division of Health Professions Analysis, HRA, Department of Health and Human Services, Contract Number Human Resources Administration (HRA)-232-80-0041 (Rockville, Md.: 1982). Charles Phelps has also estimated the price elasticity of demand for health insurance and found it to be $-.5$. Charles Phelps, *Demand for Health Insurance: A Theoretical and Empirical Investigation* (Santa Monica, Calif.: Rand Corp., 1973).

2. For a more extensive discussion of community rating, see Mark V. Pauly, "The Welfare Economics of Community Rating," *The Journal of Risk and Insurance* (September 1970).

3. *Health Care Insurance Regulation Program: An Assessment of Effectiveness*, Executive Office of the Governor, Lewis Cass Building, Lansing, Michigan, March 1973, p. 11.

4. H.E. Frech III, "Blue Cross, Blue Shield, and Health Care Costs: A Review of the Economic Evidence," in Mark V. Pauly, ed., *National Health Insurance: What Now, What Later, What Never?* (Washington, D.C.: American Enterprise Institute, 1980), pp. 251–252.

5. Ronald J. Vogel and Roger D. Blair, *Health Insurance Administrative Costs*, Social Security Administration, Office of Research and Statistics Staff Paper No. 21, October 1975, p. 56.

6. *Ibid.*, p. 63.

7. Roger D. Blair and Ronald J. Vogel, "A Survivor Analysis of Commercial Insurers," *The Journal of Business* 51 (July 1978).

8. Ronald J. Vogel and Roger D. Blair, *The Journal of Business* (October 1975): 92–93. Also, in another study of the performance of Medicare (Part A) processing costs, H.E. Frech found lower cost per dollar processed, lower average processing time (in days), and fewer errors per $1,000 processed in for-profit as compared to not-for-profit firms. H.E. Frech III, "The Property Rights Theory of the Firm: Empirical Results from a Natural Experiment," *Journal of Political Economy* (February 1976).

9. *Ibid.*, p. 91.

10. H.E. Frech III, "Blue Cross, Blue Shield, and Health Care Costs: A Review of the Economic Evidence," in Mark Pauly, ed., *National Health Insurance: What Now, What Later, What Never?* (Washington, D.C.: American Enterprise Institute, 1980).

11. Charles D. Weller, "On 'FTC Sings the Blues' and its Respondents," *Journal of Health Politics, Policy and Law* (Summer 1982).

12. H.E. Frech III and Paul Ginsburg, "Competition Among Health Insurers," in Warren Greenburg, ed., *Competition in the Health Care Sector: Past, Present, and Future* (Germantown, Md.: Aspen Systems Corporation, 1978).

13. *Ibid.*

14. David Eisenstat and Thomas Kennedy, "Control and Behavior of Non-Profit Firms: The Case of Blue Shield," *Southern Economic Journal* 48 (July 1981).

15. Frank A. Sloan, "Physicians and Blue Shield: A Study of the Effects of Physician Control on Blue Shield Reimbursements," in *Conference Proceedings, Issues in Physician Reimbursement* (Washington, D.C.: Health Care Financing Administration, Department of Health and Human Services, 1980).

16. William J. Lynk, "Regulatory Control of the Membership of Corporate Boards of Directors: The Blue Shield Case," *The Journal of Law and Economics* (April 1981).

17. For a more complete discussion on the self-insurance option, see Richard Egdahl and Diana Chapman Walsh, eds., *Containing Health Benefit Costs: The Self-Insurance Option*, Springer Series on Industry and Health Care, No. 6 (New York: Springer-Verlag, 1979).

18. Marjorie Smith Carroll and Ross H. Arnett, "Private Health Insurance Plans in 1978 and 1979: A Review of Coverage, Enrollment, and Financial Experience," *Health Care Financing Review* 3 (September 1981): 79.

CHAPTER 9

The Physician Services Market

INTRODUCTION AND OVERVIEW

Physician services may be provided using different combinations of physicians and other health manpower. Physicians may undertake to perform all of their tasks themselves or they may delegate varying amounts of those tasks to their auxiliaries. With a greater degree of task delegation, physicians will be able to increase their productivity and provide a greater variety of services than do physicians who use fewer auxiliaries. The extent to which physicians delegate their tasks will affect not only the quantity and type of physician services available but also their cost. In evaluating how well the supply side of the physician services market performs, an examination will be made to determine whether physician services could be produced at lower cost and whether a greater variety of services could be provided than is currently the case.

Even if it were determined that physician services are produced at minimum cost, the prices at which they are sold might be greatly in excess of their costs. If such a situation were to exist, then fewer physician services would be purchased than if their prices were lower and closer to the costs of production. Thus, another measure of how well the market for physician services performs is the relationship of prices to costs in that market; because it is often difficult to measure costs directly, this price-cost relationship may be inferred through the method by which physician prices are determined. In relatively competitive markets, prices will approximate costs; in monopolistic markets, the seller's price may greatly exceed the cost of providing that service. If, after an examination of the physician services market, it is determined that a greater quantity (and variety) of physician services, at lower prices, is possible in this market, then policies to achieve such an outcome will be proposed.

The emphasis of this chapter is on the efficiency with which physician services are provided rather than on the efficiency with which medical treatments, of which physician services are one important component, are produced and priced. A subsequent chapter will discuss the broader issue, which will have important ramifications for the physician services market itself. To further delineate the subject area included in this chapter, it should be noted that the determination of the optimal number of physicians in the labor market is excluded; the market for medical education is also discussed in a separate chapter. Although these markets are closely related to the market for physician services, the rationale for discussing these subjects and the pricing and provision of physician services separately is that the determinants of the number of physicians are not identical to the factors that determine the quantity of physician services or how they are priced. The interrelationship between these two markets, the determinants of supply and demand in each market, and the different types of public policies that influence these separate markets are more easily visualized with reference to Figure 9-1.

The demand for physician services is determined by factors such as those discussed previously. There are noneconomic factors, such as need and cultural-demographic factors; the economic factors are the patient's income, the price the patient must pay for physician services (as well as the price of substitute and complementary services), the type and comprehensiveness of insurance coverage, and any time costs that are involved in the purchase and use of physician services. The supply of physician services is affected by the price received for physician services and by the cost of producing those services, which depends upon input productivities and input prices. These are affected by the number of physicians, the amount of hours they work, their use of auxiliaries, the capital and equipment available, and other inputs and expenses necessary to the provision of physician services, such as malpractice coverage.

The price of physician services, as shown in Figure 9-1, is determined by the interaction of both supply and demand factors; in turn, it influences patient demand and the amount of services providers are willing to provide. How the physician services market differs from the traditional demand and supply models will be discussed also.

On the supply side of the market, the number of physicians combined with other inputs determines the available supply of such services. In the short run, all of the inputs except physicians can be varied. Physician hours, which can also be varied, are determined by the labor–leisure trade-off; what happens to the physician's hours of work as both the price received per hour of work and his or her income increases? Namely, do physicians reduce their hours of work as their prices increase? The long run is that period of time in which there can be an increase in the number of physicians. Changes in the number of physicians result from deaths and retirements, immigration of foreign-trained medical graduates and physicians, and increases in the number of U.S.-trained medical graduates (USMGs). The number of USMGs is determined by the demand for and supply of medical education. The demand for a medical education is influenced by a number of factors, among which is the relative rate of return to such an education; as shown in Figure 9-1, the price and quantity determined in the physician services market (which is equivalent to gross physician income) is a component of that rate of return.

Government policies have intervened at several points in the physician markets. With respect to the demand for services, Medicare and Medicaid have served to stimulate the demand for services among specific population groups. Further, the imposition of federal price controls between 1971 and 1974 controlled the annual percent increase in physician fees. In addition to the direct

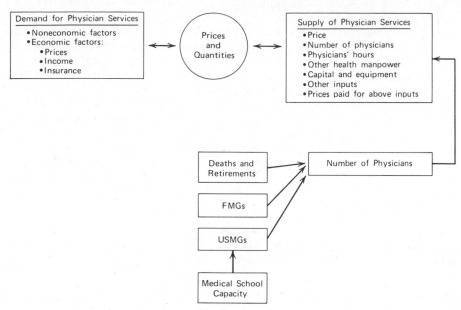

Figure 9-1. The market for physician services.

effects of these two programs, there were also indirect consequences: persons not subsidized by Medicare and Medicaid faced higher prices for physician services; controls on physician prices affected the quantity of those services, the hours the physicians were willing to work, as well as the time patients had to wait to receive such services.

Government policies on the supply side have been directed at increasing the number of physicians by providing subsidies both for the construction of new medical schools and for existing schools to increase their enrollments. Loans and scholarships have also been provided (through the medical schools) to medical students, which influences their demand for a medical education. The government has affected the inflow of foreign-trained medical graduates and physicians by its immigration policies. Of more direct effect on the supply of physician services has been legislation at a state level that places limits on who can practice medicine and defines the tasks that may be performed by various categories of health manpower.

As shown in Figure 9-1, medical education is an important determinant of the number of physicians and, consequently, the supply of physician services. Separate chapters are devoted to an analysis of both physicians' manpower and medical education markets, to include the development of their structural characteristics, their consequent effect on performance, and the relevant public policies within each market.* In this chapter the performance of the physician

---

*Quality-assurance mechanisms are placed, primarily, on medical inputs, such as on the training requirements for physicians, and not on the services provided. The development of such "process" quality measures has had important effects on the structure of health manpower and health education markets. Alternative approaches to achieving quality assurance, and their effect on performance, are, therefore, discussed in chapters dealing with the manpower and education markets.

services market will be evaluated to determine whether physician services are produced in the least costly manner and whether the prices charged for such services are related to their costs of production. A better understanding of costs and the determination of prices in this market will enhance our ability to predict physician prices and expenditures. The consequences of public policy in this market should also be more easily anticipated.

As a basis for evaluating the performance of the market for physician services, observed measures of performance will be compared with what might be expected to occur in a hypothetical competitive market. The reasons for any possible divergence between the observed and hypothetical outcomes will then be analyzed. Policies to improve the performance of the physician services market will be suggested based on the structural characteristics of a competitive market that give rise to desired outcomes.

OBSERVED PERFORMANCE IN THE PHYSICIAN SERVICES MARKET

VARIATIONS IN PHYSICIAN FEES

In a competitive market, prices for similar services would be expected to vary within a relatively narrow range. Prices are unlikely to be identical even for seemingly comparable services for several reasons: some patients may prefer particular physicians because of real or perceived quality differentials. Patients may incur less waiting time when seeing certain physicians and therefore be willing to pay higher physician fees. Finally, there are always search costs involved in finding a particular physician. Since it is costly to gather information on different physicians, some patients who place a high value on their time will do less search and be willing to take a chance on paying higher prices. In fact, identical prices in a market such as physician services would be more indicative of collusion or price fixing rather than competition. If prices for specified services diverge too greatly, however, then some patients will be willing to shift to other providers. As the price differential increases, it will eventually exceed the value the patient places on particular providers and on perceived quality differences. Although prices for the same physician services are unlikely to be exactly the same, they would be expected to vary only within a small range.

Physician fees for similar services have shown substantial variation, both between geographical areas and within an area. For example, the median fee for obstetrical care varied from $350 in Chicago to $650 in New York City; among moderate-sized cities, the median fee for an appendectomy varied between $250 in Des Moines, Iowa, to $480 in Stockton, California (1).

Within the Washington, D.C. area the physician fee for a tonsillectomy varies between $113 and $325. An appendectomy in the same area varies between $250 and $450 (2). Although the range in fees within a locality is usually smaller than the range between cities, fees vary, on the average, by 25 percent for similar services within a city (3). Variations in prices are reduced as patients seek lower prices. Even in competitive markets, search costs, time costs, and quality differentials among physicians would be expected to result in price differences. But it is questionable whether these factors can explain the relatively large price differences for similar services within a city. Also contributing to price variation, particularly between cities and regions of the country, are differences in wage rates and in costs of living. However, even when physician fees are adjusted for differences in costs between cities, fees for similar surgical procedures are still almost twice as great between cities. Based on these data, it would appear that the range in fees for similar services is greater than would be expected in a competitive market.

INCREASES IN PHYSICIAN FEES

In a competitive system the level at which physician fees are established over time is determined by the cost of providing the service. One would expect increased prices to occur in the short run to ration demand; in the long run, however, one would expect increased prices to reflect the costs of the output provided. When the actual trend in physician fees is examined, it appears that until recently fees have increased more rapidly than the costs of providing physician services. As shown in Table 9-1, physician fees have generally risen more rapidly than either the Consumer Price Index (CPI) (all items less medical care) or the All Services component of the Consumer Price Index. Prior to 1965, physician fees rose at a higher annual rate of increase than the CPI. When Medicare and Medicaid were passed in 1966, physician fees increased at an even faster annual rate. In 1966 and 1967, the CPI increased by 3.0 percent and 2.4 percent, respectively. In those same years, physician fees increased by 5.8 and 7.1 percent, which was more than twice the annual rate of increase in physician fees for the previous five years. Price controls were imposed on the U.S. economy in mid-1971 and remained in effect for the medical care sector until April 1974. During that period, physician fees increased at a little over 3 percent per year. After the removal of price controls, physician fees rose sharply from 3.3 percent in 1973 to 9.2 percent in 1974, reaching 12.3 percent in 1975. In 1976 physician fees rose twice as fast as the CPI and their annual rate of increase remained above the CPI for the next several years. In 1979 and 1980, however, the CPI increased more rapidly than physician fees. By 1981 physician fee increases exceeded the CPI, but only slightly. The All Services component of the CPI has shown a closer relationship to physician fee increases. Between 1978 and 1981 physician fees have been rising less rapidly than the All Services Index. Thus, until recently, physician fee increases appear to have risen faster than the costs of providing those services.*

Physician expenditures (expenditures on physician services) have also been increasing rapidly, even when adjusted for population changes, as shown in Table 9-2. Just before the imposition of price controls in 1971 and immediately

---

*During the period physician fees were controlled, it appears that utilization of services increased. There are several possible explanations for this phenomenon: the expenditure data, which were the basis for the calculation of utilization changes, may be inaccurate; physicians may have actually provided additional services; or physicians may have redefined existing services as a means of achieving a higher price increase. This latter view appears to be supported by recent research. Dyckman (1), p. 57.

TABLE 9-1. Annual Rate of Change in the CPI and in Physician Fees, 1955–1981

Year	CPI All Items Less Medical Care	CPI All Services Less Medical Care	CPI Physician Fees
1955–1960	2.0	3.5	3.3
1960–1965	1.2	1.8	2.8
1966	3.0	3.4	5.8
1967	2.4	3.7	7.1
1968	4.1	4.9	5.6
1969	5.4	6.8	6.9
1970	5.8	8.3	7.5
1971	4.1	5.3	6.9
1972	3.3	3.8	3.1
1973	6.4	4.3	3.3
1974	11.1	9.2	9.2
1975	8.9	9.1	12.3
1976	5.5	7.9	11.3
1977	6.2	7.3	9.3
1978	7.6	8.6	8.3
1979	11.4	11.2	9.2
1980	13.6	15.9	11.7
1981	10.3	13.4	11.0

Source: Bureau of Labor Statistics, *CPI Detailed Report*, various issues.

Note: The rates of change are based on the change in the annual average of each index listed in the table.

The "All Urban Consumers" index is used for 1978–1981. Prior to 1978 the only available index was for urban wage earners and clerical workers.

following the removal of those controls in 1974, physician expenditures increased sharply. The recent annual increases in physician expenditures of 12.2 percent (1978), 13.7 percent (1979), and 14.5 percent (1980) appear to be, in large part, a result of price increases rather than increases in physician visits. Since the population has increased at less than 1 percent per year over that period, the major portion of the increase in expenditures must be attributed to increases in physician prices.* Table 9-3 shows the trend in visits per person, which increased at the start of the price control program in 1971, declined after price controls were ended, and has remained relatively constant in the last four years. Also of interest in Table 9-3 is the trend in weekly visits per physician, which increased from 118 in 1966 to a high of 138 in 1973, and to a low of 112 in 1980. In the late 1960s, demand for physician services increased, in part because of Medicare and Medicaid. (During this same period of time physician fees and expenditures began to increase rapidly.) In the early 1970s, price controls provided physicians with an incentive to increase their services as a means of increasing

---

*It is also possible that there has been an important change in the definition of a visit in the last three years. For example, an increase in the number of services per visit would be reflected in a higher price per visit but not as an increase in the number of visits. If there has been a large increase in the number of services per visit, then it must be determined whether these additional services were in fact demanded by patients or whether it is a means whereby physicians can increase their revenues.

TABLE 9-2. Total Expenditures on Physicians' Services by Source of Funds, 1950–1980

Calendar Year	Total Physician Expenditures (Billions of Dollars)	Annual Increase in Total Expenditures (%)	Per Capita Physician Expenditures	Distribution of Physician Expenditures			Third-Party Payments[a] (%)	
				Total (%)	Direct Consumer Payment (%)	Total	Private Insurance	Public Insurance
1950	$ 2.7	—	$ 17.76	100	83.2	16.8	11.4	5.2
1955	3.7	6.5	21.91	100	69.8	30.2	23.2	6.7
1960	5.7	9.0	30.92	100	65.4	34.6	28.0	6.4
1965	8.5	8.3	42.82	100	61.4	38.6	31.7	6.9
1970	14.3	11.0	68.74	100	45.1	54.9	33.9	20.9
1971	15.9	11.2	75.35	100	44.9	55.1	33.3	21.7
1972	17.2	8.2	80.36	100	42.4	57.6	34.8	22.8
1973	19.1	11.1	88.45	100	41.8	58.2	34.9	23.2
1974	21.2	11.0	97.60	100	37.9	62.1	37.0	25.0
1975	24.9	17.5	113.38	100	36.2	63.8	37.6	26.2
1976	27.6	10.8	124.17	100	31.5	64.9	39.1	25.8
1977	31.9	15.6	142.05	100	35.7	64.3	39.0	25.2
1978	35.8	12.2	158.03	100	36.6	63.4	37.7	25.7
1979	40.7	13.7	177.65	100	37.7	62.3	36.1	26.2
1980	46.6	14.5	201.18	100	37.3	62.7	36.3	26.4

Source: Robert M. Gibson and Daniel R. Waldo, "National Health Expenditures, 1980," *Health Care Financing Review*, 3 (1981): 32–35, Table 3; 40, Table 5.

[a]"Total" third-party payments minus the sum of "Private Insurance" and "Public Insurance" equals other forms of third-party payments, namely, philanthropic and industrial in-plant expenditures.

TABLE 9-3. Number of Physician Visits Per Person Per Year and Number of Visits Per Physician Per Week

Calendar Year	Number of Visits Per Person Per Year	Number of Visits Per MD Per Week
1958–1959	4.7	—
1963–1964	4.5	—
1966–1967	4.3	124.1
1969	4.3	126.9
1970	4.6	132.5
1971	4.9	135.8
1972	5.0	—
1973	5.0	137.7
1974	4.9	125.8
1975	5.1	126.5
1976	4.9	128.5
1977	4.8	—
1978	4.8	130.6
1979	4.7	122.7
1980	4.8	112.0

Sources: The data for number of visits per person per year came from the National Center for Health Statistics, "Current Estimates of Health Interview Surveys," *Vital and Health Statistics*, Series 10 (Washington, D.C.: Department of Health, Education and Welfare, various years); and Marcus Goldstein, *Income of Physicians, Osteopaths, and Dentists From Professional Practice 1965–1969* (Washington, D.C.: Department of Health, Education and Welfare Publication No. (55A) 73-11852, 1972), p. 49. The data for number of visits per MD per week came from Marcus Goldstein, *op. cit.*, p. 48; Judith Warner and Phil Aherne, eds., *Profile of Medical Practice*, 1974 ed. (Chicago: American Medical Association, 1974), p. 179, Table 56; and David Goldfarb, ed., *Profile of Medical Practice, 1981* (Monroe, Wisconsin: AMA, 1981), p. 156, Table 14.

their incomes. A possible explanation for the decline in visits per physician in more recent years is the limited increases in patient demand (constant over the last several years) and the increasing supply of physicians (see Table 13-2) to compete for that limited demand. Such an explanation might also account for the more limited increases, relative to the CPI, in physician fees in the last several years.

Further evidence that the rapid increase in physician fees has been unrelated to the costs of providing physician services is the trend in a government index of physician expenses. Over the period for which data are available, physician fees increased more rapidly than the index of physician expenses (4). These years include the period when physician fees were under price controls (while their expenses were not) and when malpractice premiums were increasing rapidly. During the more recent periods, the increase in malpractice premiums has been leveling off, while the annual increase in physician fees is still large.

When physician fees were increasing faster than the costs of providing those services and visits per physician were also increasing, physician incomes would also be expected to increase rapidly. This is apparently what occurred since 1965 after Medicare and Medicaid were passed. Between 1965 and 1975, physician incomes increased by more than 100 percent, which was a more rapid rate of increase than that of dentists, lawyers, and most likely, any other profession. It

TABLE 9-4. Average Net Income From Medical Practice by Specialty, 1970–1980

Specialty	1970	1975	1970–1975 Annual Percent Change	1976[b]	Percent Change	1977	Percent Change	1978	Percent Change	1979	Percent Change	1980[b]	Percent Change	1975–1980 Annual Percent Change	1970–1980 Annual Percent Change
General practice	$33,900	$45,400	6.0	$47,400	4.4	$51,200	8.0	$54,600	6.6	$62,000	13.6	$63,300	2.1	6.9	6.4
Internal medicine	40,300	57,000	7.2	60,500	6.1	61,500	1.7	63,800	3.7	76,200	19.4	79,100	3.8	6.8	7.0
Surgery	50,700	68,200	6.1	73,200	7.3	74,000	1.1	82,600	11.6	96,000	16.2	98,600	2.7	7.7	6.9
Pediatrics	34,800	44,300	5.0	47,000	6.1	48,200	2.6	51,200	6.2	60,400	18.0	63,300	4.8	7.4	6.2
Obstetrics/gynecology	47,100	63,300	6.1	65,800	4.0	69,900	6.2	70,300	0.6	91,800	30.6	92,500	0.8	7.9	7.0
Psychiatry	39,900	44,800	2.3	47,600	6.3	48,200	1.3	50,200	4.2	62,600	24.7	65,100	4.0	7.8	5.0
Anesthesiology	39,400	57,100	7.7	60,100	5.3	65,500	9.0	74,200	13.3	91,400	23.2	94,900	3.8	10.7	9.2
All specialties[a]	41,800	56,400	6.2	59,500	5.5	61,200	2.9	65,500	7.0	78,400	19.7	80,900	3.2	7.5	6.8
CPI All Items[c]	116.3	161.2	6.8	170.5	5.8	181.5	6.5	195.4	7.7	217.4	11.3	246.8	13.5	8.9	7.8

Sources: David Goldfarb, "Trends in Physicians Incomes, Expenses, and Fees: 1970–1980," in David Goldfarb, ed., *Profile of Medical Practice* (Monroe, Wis.: American Medical Association, 1981), p. 114, Table 1. *Bureau of the Census, Statistical Abstract of the United States 1981*, 102 ed. (Washington, D.C.: U.S. Government Printing Office, 1981), p. 467, Table 779.

[a]This category includes the specialties listed and other specialties which are not listed.

[b]The figures in these columns were estimates given by the physicians in the preceding year.

[c]The figures recorded are index levels and percentage changes in these levels.

was estimated that by 1976 physician incomes were twice as large as those of dentists or lawyers (5). Particularly since the mid-1970s, however, physician incomes have not kept up with the rate of inflation. As shown in Table 9-4, for all physician specialties, except anesthesiology, physician "real" incomes have fallen since 1975.

The data on physician fees, visits per physician, and physician real incomes appear to be consistent with each other in showing that a change occurred in the physician services market in the late 1970s.*

THE PRODUCTION OF PHYSICIAN SERVICES AT MINIMUM COST

If physician services were produced in a competitive market, cost-minimizing behavior would result in physicians hiring the optimal number and mix of auxiliaries, and the size of the physician's practice would be determined by the extent of economies of scale in providing services.

As a first step in determining whether physicians are minimizing the cost of providing their services, it is necessary to estimate a production function for physician services. Estimates of the productivity of each of the inputs used in producing physician services and the extent of economies of scale can then be made. An important problem in specifying and estimating a production function is the definition and measurement of outputs and inputs. Unless outputs and inputs are measured accurately, the results of the studies will be questionable.

The output—physician services—consists of examinations, treatment, tests, history-taking as well as health education, recordkeeping, and patient billing. Detailed information on the quantity and mix of each of the services provided in a physician's office is generally unavailable. Empirical studies must therefore use proxy measures for physician services. One often-used proxy for the output of a physician's practice is the weekly number of office visits. When office visits are used, it is implicitly assumed that quality differences, if any, will not bias the results of the study. In physician productivity studies it is also generally assumed that the mix of patient visits among different physician practices is similar.† Over

---

*Also indicative of this change in the physician market during the late 1970s is the changing geographic distribution of physicians. With the increase in the supply of physicians during the 1970s, there has been an increase in the number of physicians locating in small communities. "The percentage of small cities and towns with specialists grew appreciably during the period 1970 to 1979. In general, the specialties that grew the most (in percentage terms) also moved in the largest numbers into previously unserved towns" (p. 2393). This diffusion of physicians into smaller communities is contrary to the views of those who believe that physicians can create their own demand so as to locate where they prefer. Instead, these changes in the geographic distribution of physicians are believed to be the result of competitive market forces. As the supply of physicians continues to increase, these trends in location patterns of physicians should continue during the 1980s. Joseph P. Newhouse, Albert P. Williams, Bruce Bennett, and William B. Schwartz, "Where Have All The Doctors Gone?," *Journal of the American Medical Association* (May 7, 1982). See also William B. Schwartz, Joseph P. Newhouse, Bruce Bennett, and Albert P. Williams, "The Changing Geographic Distribution of Board-Certified Physicians," *New England Journal of Medicine* (October 30, 1980).

†If physician practices are being compared and some of those practices have different specialists or use a greater number of auxiliaries, then the output mix and the productivity estimates may be systematically biased.

time, however, there have been important changes in the physician output mix. Since the 1930s there has been a large decline in the number of home visits, with a corresponding increase in the number of office and hospital visits and telephone consultations. For example, between 1930 and 1965, home visits declined from 45 percent of total outpatient visits to only 4 percent. Since the time spent by a physician on an office visit is approximately half that of a home visit, this change in output mix over time contributed to a large increase in physician productivity (6).

Another output proxy used is annual gross patient billings. While this measure may reflect differences in quality and service mix among practices, it contains a serious problem in that higher patient billings may not reflect differences in output but may result from higher prices being charged for similar services.

The measurement of manpower inputs in production function studies is also troublesome. In addition to quality differences among manpower of a given type, which affect their relative productivities, the categories of health manpower employed in physicians' offices vary. Physician extenders, such as physician assistants and pediatric nurse practitioners, are the closest substitutes for the physician and are more productive than allied health workers (e.g., registered nurses), medical technicians (e.g., x-ray and lab technicians), and nonmedical assistants (e.g., clerical and administrative persons). Productivity estimates of auxiliaries are likely to fall within a wide range and thereby bias the results unless these different manpower categories are separately measured.

A number of studies have attempted to estimate the optimal use of inputs and the extent of economies of scale in physician practices. Based on his studies, Uwe Reinhardt concluded that the average solo physician could profitably employ twice as many auxiliaries as he or she currently does. Employing four rather than two auxiliaries, which is the current average, would result in a 25 percent increase in the number of patient visits per physician (7). As shown in Table 9-5, Reinhardt has calculated the optimal number of aides for a solo physician to hire based on the price received per visit and the weekly wage of the aide. Based on estimates of the marginal productivity of aides, the table indicates that the employment of aides should increase as the price of the visit increases; as the cost of the aide increases, the optimal number of aides decreases.

Other studies on the productivity of aides have reached similar conclusions. Kehrer and Zaretsky concluded that a doubling of allied health personnel in physicians' offices would result in a 20–25 percent increase in total patient visits per physician (8). These authors also found that internal medicine and general practice were more likely to be able to absorb additional auxiliaries. Kimbell and Lorant also found in their study that additional aides would add significantly to the productivity of physicians (9).

Golladay, Smith, and Miller used activity analysis to develop a normative model of how a primary care practice should be organized (10). Their procedure consisted of enumerating 263 tasks in eight major categories of activity that fully describe a typical primary care practice. Five medical school students then acted as observers in a sample of primary care practices for two-week periods and collected data on the frequency with which tasks were performed and who performed them. From this they developed a model of optimal input mix at given levels of output. They estimated that introduction of a physician assistant (PA) increases physician productivity by 49–74 percent. That is, a physician usually producing 147 office visits per week may increase that number up to 265 visits

TABLE 9-5. Estimated Optimal Levels of Aide Input at Various Weekly Salaries and Net Proceeds Per Visit (Solo General Practitioners)

Net Proceeds Per Visit	Weekly Cost Per Aide		
	$70	$100	$160
$ 5	3.7	3.2	1.6
7	4.0	3.7	2.9
10	4.2	4.0	3.5

Source: Uwe Reinhardt. Reprinted with permission from *Physician Productivity and the Demand for Health Manpower* (Cambridge, Mass.: Ballinger, 1974), p. 184, Table 6-14.

per week simply by hiring a PA. Pondy, in a similar study, obtained results that were much the same as those of Golladay et al. He estimated that a physician assistant could raise physician productivity by 40–70 percent (11).

With regard to economies of scale in physicians' practices, Reinhardt concluded that physicians in groups generate between 4.5 and 5.1 percent more patient visits and about 5.6 percent more patient billings than those in solo practice. These results suggest that there are slight economies of scale in the production of physician services. Reinhardt also found that productivity of physicians increased with group size because of greater manpower substitution in groups (12).

As shown in Table 9-6, taken from Reinhardt's study, the average number of weekly patient visits for GPs in groups was 16 percent higher than that for solo GPs. But the group practitioners also seemed to work more hours per week and employ more aides per physician; therefore, mode of practice accounted for about a 5 percent increase in patient visits.

In another study, Frech and Ginsburg tried to determine optimal size of practice by conducting a "survivor test." This technique assumes that over time the size distribution of medical practices will tend toward the optimum. Until the optimum is reached, the fastest growing size is identified as the most efficient. By use of this type of analysis, Frech and Ginsburg conclude that solo practice is very inefficient, and very small practices (3–7 physicians) and very large practices (greater than 26 physicians) are most efficient (13). Hence, there are economies of scale in the production of physicians services.

TABLE 9-6. Average Weekly Patient Visits, Practice Hours, and Number of Aides Per Physician

Practice Mode	Average Weekly Patient Visits	Average Number of Practice Hours	Average Number of Aides Per Physician
Solo	183	60	1.81
Group	213	64	2.12
Group as percent of solo	116	107	117

Source: Uwe Reinhardt, "A Production Function for Physician Services," *The Review of Economics and Statistics* (February 1972): 60.

TABLE 9-7. Distribution of Patient Care Physicians by Group Affiliation, 1980

Type of Practice	Number of Physicians	Percent of Physicians According to Type of Practice	Number of Group Practices	Average Size of Physician Group
Total office-based				
physicians (nonfederal)	271,268	100	—	—
Individual practice[a]	182,978	67.5	—	—
Group practice[a]	88,290	32.5	10,762	8.2
Prepaid group				
practice	20,441	7.5	1,884	10.8
Nonprepaid group				
practice	67,849	25.0	8,878	7.6

Source: Sharon Henderson, Richard Odem, and Karen Ginsburg, *Medical Groups in the U.S., 1980* (Chicago: American Medical Association, 1982), pp. 6–12.

[a]Group practice is defined as a joint practice of three or more physicians. Physicians not in a group are classified as in individual practice.

These studies suggest that there are at least modest economies of scale in physician practices. When the size distribution of physician practices is examined, however, it is clear that physician practices are smaller than would be suggested by the findings on economies of scale. As shown in Table 9-7, the majority of office-based physicians are in individual practice, 67.5 percent (this represents a decline from 76 percent in 1975); the remainder are either affiliated with a prepaid group practice (5 percent) or belong to a nonprepaid group practice (19 percent) where there are, on the average, 7.6 physicians in the group.

Physician practices employ less than the optimal number of aides and their practice size is smaller than what the data suggest is optimal. Yet physician practices are able to survive and even prosper. This evidence is inconsistent with cost-minimizing behavior in a competitive market.

Physician fees, expenditures, and income could not have increased as rapidly as they have until the late 1970s if the physician services market were competitive. The rapid rise in physician fees cannot be explained by increases in physician expenses; nor can differences in costs provide the explanation for differences between cities in prices for the same service. A competitive model of physician pricing, which relies on differences in costs to explain differences in prices, does not appear consistent with observed data.

DETERMINATION OF PHYSICIAN PRICES

A MONOPOLY MODEL OF PHYSICIAN PRICING

When a competitive model, which relies on costs to explain the level of prices, is not able to explain changes in prices and quantities in a market, then a monopoly framework is used to explain the observed phenomenon. To show where monopoly elements are likely to have their impact, the probable effects of an increase in demand are analyzed. With an increase in demand for physician services, prices would increase as existing providers ration the increased demand. As profits increase, an increase in supply would also be expected; with an increase in supply, prices would begin to fall (what would actually be observed is that prices would not rise as rapidly as demand continues to increase). An increase in supply of physician services would be expected from two sources. In the short run, existing physicians can increase their productivity by hiring more auxiliaries and/or increasing their own hours of work. In the long run, additional physicians can be trained and will enter the practice of medicine. Entry barriers are one possible source of monopoly power. A discussion of the long-run supply of physicians and whether or not there are barriers to entry in that market is reserved for Chapter 14, "The Market for Physician Manpower." In the short run, however, the number of currently practicing physicians is large enough so that if physicians were to increase their productivity to the level that is technically feasible, the increased supply of services would inhibit the rise in physician prices. Physicians, however, are not likely to encourage unlimited increases in physician productivity. If physicians were allowed to expand the size of their practices to whatever size is technically feasible, the increased capacity for providing medical services might exceed the increased demand for such services. In that event, competitive pressures on physicians could increase, which would adversely affect their incomes. Thus, under a monopoly model of physician pricing, only gradual increases in productivity would be expected as demands for physician services increased; the purpose would be to insure that increased supply would not outstrip increases in demand. The mechanism whereby productivity increases are limited is the State Practice Acts. Such acts, which are usually proposed to the State Legislature and controlled in their implementation by the medical profession, specify the tasks that different professionals can perform and often the number of physician assistants that can be hired. The consequence of such supply-restricting behavior would be a greater increase in physician fees than would otherwise occur.

The application of a monopoly model to explain physician pricing behavior would not necessarily end with an explanation of restrictions on increased supplies of physician services. Physician prices in excess of costs can occur even though there may be no increases in demand. A decrease in the price elasticity of demand for physician services would be expected to result in an increase in physician fees. This effect on physician fees of a less elastic demand curve for physician services is shown in Figure 9-2. The initial demand and marginal revenue curves are D_1 and MR_1. The physician's marginal cost curve is MC, which is assumed to be constant. The resulting price is P_1. As the demand curve becomes less elastic, e.g., as a result of increased insurance coverage, the demand curve shifts from D_1 to D_2, becoming less elastic. The marginal revenue curve also shifts rightward. Thus, even though marginal costs have not changed, the intersection of the steeper MR_2 with MC results in a higher price, P_2, on the demand curve. Economic theory would therefore suggest that a second possible explanation for the rapid increase in physician fees has been a change in the price elasticity of demand for physician services. Evidence to test this hypothesis is examined next.

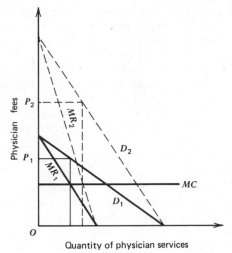

Figure 9-2. The impact of insurance on physician fees.

The method of reimbursement preferred by physicians is fee-for-service, according to their "usual, customary, and reasonable" (UCR) fees. Such a pricing strategy enables the physician to set what he or she believes is the profit-maximizing price. With the growth in private insurance for physician services, the amount the patient had to pay out-of-pocket for such services was reduced; however, patients were still responsible for the major portion of their bill. It was not until 1966, when Medicare and Medicaid were passed, that third-party payors, private insurance, and government became the predominant payors of physician services. As shown in Table 9-2, public payments for physician services increased from 6.9 percent in 1965 to 26.4 percent in 1980. Together with private insurance, all third-party payors now pay 62.7 percent of total physician expenditures. When physician fees are adjusted both for inflation and by the decline in the out-of-pocket price as a result of third-party coverage, the physician fee, in constant dollars faced by the average patient, has actually declined since 1950 (14). As the patients' responsibility for payment of physician fees declined and physicians charged third-party payors according to their UCR fee, physician fees increased rapidly. As more of a physician's fees were reimbursed by a third party, the constraints holding down physician fees were removed.

Insurance coverage for payment of physician fees has not been uniform among all physician specialties. The hospital-based specialties, such as radiology and anesthesiology, has the largest percent of their revenues (approximately 80 percent) covered by third-party payors; surgeons also received a majority of their revenues from third-party payors. The decline in the patient's sensitivity to prices lowers the price elasticity of demand; rapidly increasing prices would be expected in such a situation. Those specialties of medicine that require less use of the hospital, such as pediatrics and psychiatry, had the smallest percent of their revenues covered by third-party payors (approximately 20 percent and 33 percent, respectively) (15). Not surprisingly, members of those specialties with the largest percent of their revenues paid by third-party payors also have the

*This could
also be true
due to higher
productivity
associ. with hosp.
but need cont.
to
barriers by
entry
specialty.*

highest incomes. The usual market constraints, such as patients' seeking lower prices, have been disappearing in the physician services market as more of the physicians' fees are being reimbursed by third-party payors. However, for those physician specialties whose patients have most, if not all, of their bill covered by insurance, their fee increases are being limited by third-party payors. Medicare, Medicaid, and some third-party payors each place different limits on how much physician fees are permitted to increase.

When patients are uninformed about the prices charged by physicians, it is costly for them to seek out this information. Physicians about whom the patient has little knowledge are poor substitutes for the patient's own physician. The poorer the substitute that other physicians are for a patient's own physician, the less elastic the individual physician's demand curve will be. It is for these reasons that the medical profession has opposed advertising among physicians. State medical societies have had prohibitions against advertising in their codes of ethics; if physicians were found guilty of such "unethical" behavior, they could be subject to severe sanctions. Prohibitions against advertising were also included in state medical practice acts. In 1975, The Federal Trade Commission (FTC) charged The American Medical Association, The Connecticut State Medical Association, and The New Haven County Medical Association with attempting to prevent their members from advertising, engaging in price competition, and other competitive practices. The finding by the FTC administrative law judge that the AMA and two medical societies had attempted to limit competition among physicians was upheld by the FTC commissioners, The Court of Appeals, and in 1982 by a tie vote, the Supreme Court. The less information available to patients on physicians' prices, their qualifications, and their availability, the more likely it is that variations in fees (for comparable services) will persist; it becomes too costly, in terms of a patient's time, to search for lower fees and for the type of physician he or she prefers. With little or no information available on physicians' fees and services and as more of the physicians' charges are covered by private insurance or public payments, the potential savings to the patient from searching for a lower fee declines.*

THE TARGET-INCOME HYPOTHESIS

The uncertainty that patients have regarding their medical needs and their reduced sensitivity to physician prices have given rise to the idea that physicians can both induce their own demand and set their own prices. It has been suggested by some economists that the extent of the demand the physician will "create" and the price that will be established are based upon what target income the physician desires (16). The target-income hypothesis of physician pricing suggests that with an increase in the number of physicians, physicians will increase both their prices and their demand to provide themselves with a target income. The target income is said to be determined by the local income distribution, particularly with respect to the incomes of other physicians and profession-

---

*A more complete discussion of the effect on prices of advertising, together with a review of empirical evidence, is contained in Chapter 12.

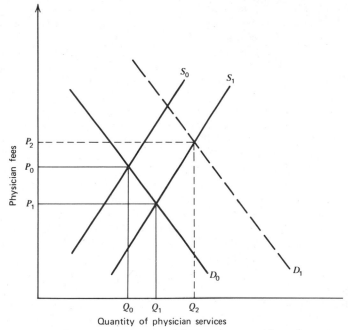

Figure 9-3. An illustration of the target income hypothesis.

als, such as dentists and lawyers, in the area. The prediction of the target-income hypothesis—namely, that an increase in the supply of physicians will result in *higher* prices and/or greater demand—is contrary to traditional economic theory, which suggests that increased supplies will lead to *lower* prices.

Figure 9-3 shows the effect on physician fees of an increase in the number of physicians using traditional economic theory as well as the target-income hypothesis. If market demand and supply were originally D_0 and quantity S_0, respectively, equilibrium will be at price P_0 and quantity Q_0. An increase in the number of physicians in an area would shift supply to the right, to S_1, which would, under traditional economic theory, result in a *lower* equilibrium price, P_1. Under the target-income hypothesis, with an increase in the number of physicians in the community, physicians induce an increase in their demand to D_1. The effect is an increase rather than a decrease in physician fees.

The major evidence upon which the target-income hypothesis is based is the finding that physician-to-population ratios are positively related to physician fees, after adjusting for other variables.* Critics of the target-income hypothesis find fault with both the logic and the empirical work on which it is based. For

---

*Robert Evans concludes that "the market for physicians' services is not self-equilibrating in the usual sense, that price does not serve primarily to balance supply and demand . . . (but that) the primary role of price is instead as an input to supplier incomes, which are not themselves the product of explicit maximizing behavior, but rather of target-seeking through the manipulation of several control variables." Evans (16), p. 173.

example, why should the target income vary among physicians? Further, how does the physician decide on the trade-off between increased fees and increased visits to achieve the target income? The empirical finding of a positive association between physician fees and physician-population ratios is believed to be a result of not adequately adjusting for changes in patient time and quality of a physician visit (17). As the number of physicians in an area increases, there are decreased travel and waiting times to see physicians; this would result in an increase in patient demand as the patient's time costs are lowered. Similarly, as the quality aspects of a physician visit are increased, as measured by the amount of physician time per visit and the length of the visit, the patient would be willing to pay a higher price for a physician visit.

As it becomes possible to more adequately adjust physician prices for such differences, particularly quality and amenity differences among physicians, it should be possible to determine a negative relationship between physician fees and physician/population ratios, which is what would be predicted using traditional economic theory. However, in his study on the effect of increased numbers of surgeons on operations, V. Fuchs argues that time costs are likely to be less relevant when it comes to in-hospital operations, "because the psychic costs of surgery and the time costs of hospitalization are likely to be large relative to the time costs of search, travel and waiting." Fuchs finds that a 10 percent increase in the surgeon to population ratio results in a 3 percent increase in per capita utilization. Also, opposite to what would be expected using traditional economic analysis, he finds that prices are also increased in this situation of induced demand. Thus, although the average surgeon's workload decreased by 7 percent, income per surgeon declined by a much smaller amount. The extent of demand inducement, even among surgeons, is, however, limited, since "the average number of operations per surgeon . . . is far below the level that surgeons consider a full workload . . . and below the quantity that surgeons would be willing and able to perform at the going price" (18).

In a recent article on this subject, Pauly and Satterthwaite examine the situation among primary care physicians, where the patient's insurance coverage is less than for surgeons and therefore price incentives still exist (19). They attempt to explain the observed relationship between an increase in the number of physicians and fees and a decline in consumer information. In choosing a physician, consumers depend on the recommendations of others rather than shopping as they typically do in other markets. When there are few physicians in an area, then each physician's reputation is known throughout the community. Consumers are likely to know people who have gone to each physician. However, when there are a large number of physicians in a metropolitan area the consumer's knowledge of each physician's reputation is less. There is also less information on each physician's qualifications and prices. An increase in the number of physicians in an area, therefore, increases the consumer's difficulty in finding out about each physician. As this occurs, the consumer becomes less price sensitive and the physician's demand curve becomes less elastic. Physicians (or firms in monopolistically competitive markets) will then raise their prices.

While the above model and the target-income hypothesis both predict that an increase in the number of physicians in an area leads to an increase in physician fees, the theories differ in their concepts of physician and consumer behavior. In the target-income theory there is a trade-off between a physician's income and diagnostic accuracy. Physicians are believed to be able to manipulate demand by reducing the accuracy of information they provide to their patients. There is presumably a limit to the extent to which physicians can create demand since they incur a psychic cost from demand manipulation. At some point this disutility to the physician exceeds the value of the additional income they earn. In the Pauly and Satterthwaite model, it is the increased cost of search to consumers as the number of physicians increase that results in higher fees. It has little to do with physicians manipulating demand.

The policy implications of these theories differ. Providing consumers with comparative information on physicians will enhance their ability to select among physicians. As physicians are viewed as better substitutes to one another, their elasticity of demand increases; consequently fees should be reduced.

In reply to critics of the target-income hypothesis, Uwe Reinhardt suggests that physicians may also increase their revenues by prescribing additional ancillary services rather than by increasing their own time. Increased laboratory tests and x-rays may be prescribed by physicians in the belief that quality of care is increased and that the possibility of a malpractice suit is reduced. Reinhardt observed that in West Germany, where the physician/population ratio has increased rapidly in the last decade, the incomes of physicians have not decreased; rather they have continued to increase. Reinhardt believes that increases in fees accounted for only a small part of the growth in physicians' incomes. The bulk of the increase has come from increased delivery of minor medical, x-ray, and diagnostic procedures per patient treated. German physicians have shifted away from time-consuming procedures toward laboratory and diagnostic procedures. There has been a 90 percent increase in x-rays between 1965 and 1974 per patient treated by a physician as more and more physicians in private practice have begun to equip their offices with technical equipment or have joined with colleagues in the establishment of profit-making, physician-owned laboratory co-ops (20).

As insurance coverage for physician and ancillary services becomes more widespread, it becomes relatively easy for the physician to increase fees and to prescribe more ancillary services. If the patient perceives that there is some benefit from such tests, no matter how small, and the price to the patient is zero because of insurance, then an increase in ancillary services would be expected. Such behavior is also consistent with physicians maximizing their incomes.

If the target-income hypothesis of physician pricing behavior is correct, then there are important implications for public policy. With the recent increase in the number of physicians as a result of federal subsidies to medical schools, physician fees would be expected to rise even faster than in the past, as more physicians attempt to attain their target income. Increased expenditures on physician services (with doubtful effects on health status) will not be the only cost to society of such pricing behavior. It has also been claimed that each physician generates between $200,000 and $300,000 in other medical expenses each year. Thus, with an increase in the number of physicians, expenditures on physician and medical services would be expected to increase rapidly. The policy prescription for inhibiting these price and expenditures increases is likely to be the establishment of arbitrary limits on expenditures for physician services and on the number of physicians, as opposed to inducing increases in the supply of physician services. However, before such regulatory approaches are implemented in the physician services market, it should be clear whether or not this market responds to traditional economic incentives. While there appears to be evidence of some demand inducement among certain groups of specialized physicians, there appears to be sufficient doubt about the extent of such a phenomenon to suggest caution in use of this hypothesis as a rationale for certain types of public policy.

PROPOSED CHANGES IN THE PHYSICIAN SERVICES MARKET

The divergence between what was observed in the physician services market and what would be expected if this market were relatively competitive includes a wide range in prices for similar procedures, both between and within cities, that appear to be greater than differences in costs between those locations; a more rapid increase in prices for physician services than in the costs of performing those services; and a more costly mix of manpower (relatively high physician/auxiliary ratios) for providing physician services than is technically or economically feasible. It was hypothesized that these differences from what might be expected if the market were competitive were a result of a lack of information on which patients can base their choice of physicians; uncertainty by patients as to their medical needs and treatment requirements; reduced patient incentives for being concerned with physician prices because of increasing third-party payment for physician services; and reimbursement of physician services under private insurance and government programs on a fee-for-service basis according to the physician's usual, customary, and reasonable fee.

Proposals to achieve greater efficiency in the delivery of physician services, such as increased use of auxiliaries, to have increases in physician fees reflect increases in the minimum costs necessary to provide those services, and to reduce any unnecessary use of services, such as through induced physician demand, should be made with reference to the reasons for the differences between observed and desired performance. In this regard, the following proposals are offered for improving the performance of the physician services market.

AN INCREASE IN PATIENT INFORMATION

Removing prohibitions against advertising among physicians, as proposed by the FTC and upheld by the recent Supreme Court decision, should provide patients with the opportunity to have greater information on physician prices, availability of services, and qualifications of physicians and their staff. The availability of such information should reduce the patient's costs of search. If the ability of the physician to "create" demand is related to the ignorance of patients as to their needs for additional services, then more complete information should result in a reduction of this phenomenon. It is, however, difficult to develop proposals that would fully resolve this problem. One approach by which the patient's knowledge may be improved is to make additional information available on treatment requirements. The trend toward use of "second opinions" for surgery is one such example (21). Not all patients will use information on physicians and on their treatment requirements; however, those patients who do will be better off than they were previously. (It is difficult to imagine that patients will be worse off compared with when they had no information.) Additional information is unlikely, by itself, to be sufficient to resolve all problems of uncertainty in patients regarding treatment requirements. Institutional review mechanisms of surgical procedures, such as through utilization review committees, would also be of use in decreasing the amount of unnecessary demand creation. Changes in the reimbursement mechanism to provide incentives to decrease unnecessary utilization, such as through the use of capitation payments for medical services, will also be useful; this latter approach is discussed in a subsequent chapter.

INCREASED EFFICIENCY IN THE PROVISION OF PHYSICIAN SERVICES

The degree to which physicians can delegate tasks and use physician extenders in their practices is often limited on grounds generally unrelated to issues of quality. In many states, medical licensing boards retain control over the introduction and use of such personnel. To produce physician services at minimum cost, it is first necessary to be able to *legally* employ the quantity of health manpower that is desired and to be able to delegate such tasks to them as they are trained to perform. Any restrictions limiting the physician's use of such persons should be removed; continuing to hold the physician responsible for maintaining quality should provide the same assurance as today that quality is not diminished.

The number of tasks that any physician will delegate will depend, in part, on the size of the physician's practice. In small practices, physicians might prefer an auxiliary to undertake a variety of tasks; in larger practices there would presumably be a greater division of labor. Delegating tasks to be performed according to which profession is licensed to perform those tasks, as is the case today, rather than on the basis of training and experience, can only raise the costs of providing physician services.

One way to increase efficiency in the provision of physician services would be to have the person who is both qualified and has the least amount of training perform any given task. This would be similar to a competitive market in which the price for a given service approximates the least costly methods of producing that service. An incentive for moving in this direction would be reimbursing physician fees at a level equivalent to the level of reimbursement for the individual with the lowest level of training who can perform the particular task (22). If the time of a less-skilled individual—a nurse or physician assistant, for example—can be substituted for a physician's time, the allocation of resources is improved. In the short run, the physician's time is freed for more complex tasks; in the longer run, if lesser-trained manpower takes over some of the tasks now performed by physicians, a smaller supply of physicians will be required. An important feature of a system designed to promote delegation is that it would provide greater financial rewards to a physician who did delegate tasks than to one who did not. Under a fee-for-service reimbursement system, this would occur if the same payment were made for a particular task regardless of whether it was performed by a physician or an aide (assuming quality to be the same in each case). (This would also occur automatically under a capitation system of payment, since physicians or groups of physicians who delegated tasks efficiently would be able to treat a larger number of patients and would end up with more net revenue after covering practice expenses.)*

Reimbursement for physician services according to the task performed rather than the level of training of the person performing it might also affect the specialty distribution of physicians. If a particular procedure can be performed equally well by a family practitioner, a surgeon should not receive a higher fee for performing it. If surgeons are not as busy as they would like to be, and they use their excess time performing services that nonsurgeons can perform equally well, reimbursing surgeons at a higher rate will provide them with a higher income than they would otherwise have. Applying the same principle of reimbursement to performing anesthesia services should result either in more procedures being performed by nurse anesthetists or in anesthesiologists receiving lower incomes.† All physicians do not base their decisions as to which specialty to enter solely on financial considerations; however, for some physicians, income differentials do play a more important role, and in this manner changes in the specialty distribution can occur.‡

Although conceptually satisfying, a "one-fee, one-task" rule would be difficult to establish and implement. Physicians are likely to oppose any changes in the UCR fee system. A change from the current reimbursement system could occur only if a new fee structure were "imposed" on physicians, or if there were greater competition in the delivery of medical services. Given the lack of patient information and the importance of third-party payors, including government, in paying physicians' fees, it is unlikely that in the short run strong incentives can be instituted in the physician services market. Even if it were possible to institute fee schedules through third-party and government payors, a number of problems must be resolved. How is the payment agency to determine the fee for a particular task? How are fees to vary according to different tasks? If the difference in fees for performing different tasks is not proportional to the costs of each task, then an incentive will have been created to perform too many of some tasks and too few of others. Establishing and updating the basic fee around which the

---

*The relationship between the salary method of payment and task delegation is not very clear. Since a salaried physician is rewarded financially for the time spent working, but not necessarily for the efficient use of that time, salary payment does not inherently promote efficient task delegation. A salaried physician might conceivably go too far in either direction—overusing a staff of auxiliaries in order to minimize his or her own work effort, or refusing to make full use of a staff because the physician finds personally caring for a small number of patients to be more satisfying than supervising the care of a larger number. This is not to suggest that a salaried physician will never use auxiliaries efficiently, but without a strong financial incentive, efficient task delegation would have to be promoted by educating physicians as to what style of practice is efficient, and by monitoring their performance in some way to determine how well they approach the standard.

†For hospitals to increase their use of nurse anesthetists, an incentive should be provided, such as allowing the hospital to bill for those services as would a physician.

‡If specialists such as surgeons were able to create their own demand, then a "one-fee, one-task" reimbursement rule might result in an increase in expensive procedures rather than increasing efficiency in the delegation of tasks. The extent to which different specialties can induce their own demand has important consequences for this reimbursement method.

other fees will be related is also a difficult problem (23). The basic fee that is established will determine the incomes of primary care physicians; the relative incomes of the different specialists in medicine will then be determined by their fee schedules relative to the fees of primary care physicians.

The control of physician fees, like any system of price controls, will not only be costly and difficult to administer, but also may not achieve the intended objective, particularly if increased utilization occurs. Before instituting controls, or other basic changes in the physician services market, we should recall that any policy prescriptions in this market should not conflict with the broader goal of achieving economic efficiency in the provision of medical treatments. The changes necessary to achieve efficiency in the delivery of all medical services, which are discussed in a subsequent chapter, should also result in improved performance in each of the submarkets, such as physician services.

INCREASED PATIENT COST-SHARING

The patient's incentive to use information, particularly with regard to physician fees, is related both to the high variability of prices among physicians and to the amount of the physician's bill that the patient is responsible for. Although large price variations increase the return to search, the growth in third-party coverage, both private and public, has lessened patient concern with physician fees and prescribing of tests and services. As the patient becomes responsible for a smaller portion of the physician's fees the patient also has limited incentive to search for the lowest priced health care provider. Price competition among providers tends to decline as insurance becomes more widespread (24). Instead, providers will compete with each other on a nonprice basis. The only incentive consumers have to search is to receive the highest nonprice qualities available from providers.

Approaches that increase consumers' price sensitivity, such as cost-sharing, would restore price competition. As insurance premiums continue to increase, pressures are created by both business and labor to hold down such premium increases. Thus cost-sharing may be reinstituted as a means of limiting the rise in health insurance premiums. Eliminating or reducing the tax subsidy for the purchase of health insurance is also a public policy approach to correcting the problem of "overinsurance." This approach will be discussed more fully in Chapter 20 on national health insurance.

PHYSICIAN ASSIGNMENT UNDER MEDICARE

Under Medicare's Part B Program, physicians have the option of accepting or rejecting assignment for payment of a beneficiary's claim. If a physician accepts assignment, then he or she accepts as full payment the amount that Medicare reimburses; in addition, the patient is responsible for a 20 percent copayment, which must be paid directly to the physician. When the physician does not accept assignment, the patient is then responsible not only for the copayment but also for the difference between what Medicare reimburses and what the physician charges. The beneficiary also has the increased burden of submitting the claim for payment before being reimbursed by Medicare for 80 percent of the physician's reasonable charge. A physician may accept or reject assignment on a claim basis; that is, for the same Medicare-eligible patient, the physician may accept assignment for one claim while rejecting assignment for another claim.

When physicians do not accept assignment, Medicare beneficiaries have an increased financial liability for their medical care. Particularly for the low-income aged, increased copayments result in a decrease in use of physician services. The aged's access to medical care becomes more restricted.

In 1969 the physician assignment rate (assigned claims as a percent of total claims) was 61.5 percent. By 1978, the net assignment rate had declined to 50.6 percent (25). The assignment rate varies both according to region of the country and by physician specialty. Oregon had the lowest percent of services assigned, 18.0 percent, while Rhode Island had the highest, 80.6 percent (as of 1975) (26). When assignment rates are examined by physician specialties, pathologists and radiologists had the highest percent of services assigned, 67.1 and 59.0 percent, respectively, while internists had 44.1 percent. One factor that appears to be important in determining whether a physician accepts assignment is the size of a beneficiary's total charges.

> For persons with annual charges under $100, only 38.2 percent were assigned.
> For persons with annual charges of $2,500 or more, 60.8 percent of the charges were assigned. (27)

Assignment by physicians in these circumstances may be a means of minimizing the risk of nonpayment. Surgeons, who have larger total charges, would therefore, be more likely to accept assignment than primary care physicians.

If the Medicare program is to be effective in increasing access by its beneficiaries, it is important that the physician assignment rate be increased. The following is an analysis of the effect that economic factors, including Medicare reimbursement rates, have on physician assignment. For purposes of this analysis it is assumed that a physician has the following types of patients: private pay patients, which includes those with private insurance as well as Medicare nonassigned patients; Medicare-assigned patients; and Medicaid patients. It is further assumed that the physician's fee is highest for the private pay patients, lower for Medicare-assigned patients, and lowest for Medicaid patients. To maximize his or her income, the physician will serve patients paying the highest fees first, before serving other patients. How many patients in each category will be served by the physician will depend on the size of those markets and the physician's marginal cost schedule.

The Medicare assignment problem can be described with reference to Figure 9-4 (28). The demand curve for physician services is D_1. The marginal revenue curve associated with that demand curve is MR_1. The downward sloping demand curve assumes that physicians have some monopoly power. For private pay patients the physician is a "price setter." The Medicare price is a horizontal line at P_M. The physician is thus a "price taker" in the Medicare (and Medicaid) markets. The physician will start by serving the private market. If the physician's marginal cost curve (MC) intersects the downward sloping MR curve at a point above P_M, such as A, then this will determine the quantity of physician services to be produced and the price charged (the price charged will be that point on the

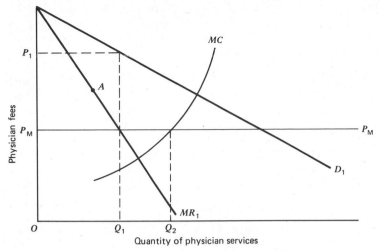

Figure 9-4. Physician decision whether to accept Medicare assignment.

demand curve directly above point A, which is where $MR = MC$). A physician in such a situation would not serve any Medicare-assigned patients. If, however, the physician's MC curve intersected MR at a point below the Medicare price (P_M), then the physician would serve that number of private patients given by the intersection of MR and P_M (shown by Q_1). The physician would also serve Medicare-assigned patients up to the point where MC equals P_M. As shown in Figure 9-4, the physician would serve OQ_1 private patients and Q_1Q_2 Medicare-assigned patients. The price for private patients would be P_1 while the Medicare price would be P_M. The physician's MR curve is changed so it becomes MR up to the point of intersection with P_M and then it is horizontal (P_M). (In this example the physician would not serve Medicaid patients, assuming Medicaid pays a price less than P_M.) A physician would enter the Medicaid market if the number of both private and Medicare patients is relatively small so that the physician's MC curve intersects the Medicaid price, which would be horizontal, as is the Medicare price, but presumably at a lower level.)

Several important factors affect the physician's assignment rate. These may be classified as demand factors, supply factors, and Medicare policies. For example, if there is an increase in incomes or private insurance so that the private demand for physicians' services increases, then the demand and MR curves would shift to the right. If MC is unchanged, then MC would intersect MR at a point to the right of Q_1. The physician would serve more private patients and fewer assigned patients. The reverse would occur if there were a decrease in private demand. A change in the factors affecting the physician's MC curve, such as increased wages for personnel working in the physician's office, would also affect the assignment rate. With an increase in MC, the new MC curve would intersect P_M to the left of Q_2. There would thus be a decrease in the acceptance of assigned patients. Similarly, a decrease in MC should result in an increase in assignment. Medicare policies also have an effect on assignment. An increase in Medicare's price would raise P_M. The higher P_M would intersect the MR curve at a point to the left and higher than the previous point. Assuming that the higher P_M intersected MR at point A, then there would be a decrease in private pay patients served (as well as an increase in their price) and an increase in the number of assigned patients. Other Medicare policies may have an effect on P_M without explicitly changing it. For example, if Medicare makes it more (less) difficult for physicians to collect their fees for assigned patients, such as by delaying (speeding up) payment then this would be similar to a decrease (increase) in Medicare's net price. The consequence would be an increase (decrease) in the number of private patients served and a decrease (increase) in the number of assigned patients.

The above factors affecting assignment rates suggest alternative policies that may be used to increase assignment. Medicare reimbursement rates can be increased, physicians accepting assignment could be reimbursed faster, and policies to lower the physician's MC curve could be instituted. Each of these policies would increase assignment. The costs of these policies would, however, vary greatly. Another alternative, in addition to the above, is to eliminate the physician's option of participating on a claim by claim basis in Medicare. Physicians would face an all-or-nothing choice of either accepting assignment for all their Medicare patients or not participating in Medicare. Undoubtedly, a number of physicians would decide not to participate. However, to many physicians Medicare patients represent a significant portion of their total practice. The increasing supply of physicians and the growing competition among physicians for patients will lead many physicians to decide it is in their economic interest to accept assignment, if offered such an all-or-nothing choice. The above policy alternatives should not be considered as mutually exclusive. Instead, the costs of each of these alternatives (both to the Medicare program, to the beneficiaries, and to private patients) should be considered along with the increase in assignment rates that they would achieve.

CONCLUDING COMMENTS

What is the economic outlook for the physician services market? If one believes that physicians can create their own demand, particularly when insurance becomes widespread, then an increasing supply of physicians suggests more rapidly rising physician fees and expenditures in the years ahead. In such a scenario there are no market forces to prevent an increasing share of our resources from being devoted to physician services.

Alternatively, certain trends in this market suggest that market forces do operate. In the years ahead these market forces are likely to become stronger and inhibit rapid increases in fees and expenditures. First, the FTC's victory over the American Medical Association, thus permitting advertising, should result in increased information to consumers about physicians' fees, qualifications, accessibility, and so forth. The consumer's cost of search should be lowered as physicians begin advertising. Second, the increase in the number of physicians should continue through the 1980s. Physicians will strive to increase their workloads to maintain their real incomes. Although there is evidence of some demand inducement among certain specialized physicians, physician visits per capita have been constant for the last several years; when examined on a per physician basis, visits have been declining. Thus, incentives have been created for increased competition among physicians for patients and referrals. Whether and how physicians compete depends on the role of insurance. As more of the physicians' charges are covered by insurance, the patient has little incentive to search for lower-priced physicians. Instead, the patient's incentive is to use additional physician services and to search for higher-quality physicians. Thus whether advertising and the increasing supply of physicians results in price competition depends on the insurance sector.

Medicare has already placed limits on how much the physician will be reimbursed. Physician fees under Medicaid are typically set below Medicare levels. Although these two large payors act as a constraint on physician fee increases, their success depends on what happens to the nongovernment sector. Private insurance does not reimburse all physician services at a uniformly high level. For some services the amount paid out of pocket by the patient is much larger than for other types of services. Thus an important constraint on the increase in physician fees is the limited coverage for certain types of services. Also, when the patient is responsible for the full amount above the physician's allowable charge, as in the case of Medicare patients and those privately insured patients whose physicians do not take assignment, price incentives are reintroduced into the market. Even in the current market, price incentives still exist and serve to limit fee increases. This is particularly the case for those physician services where there is little or no insurance coverage and for those insured patients who are responsible for all or a large part of the fee above a certain limit.

Another important market force affecting the physician services market is increased competition among health insurers. Insurers compete according to premiums, as well as other factors. If an insurance company merely reimburses the physician in full regardless of his or her fee, the insurance company's premiums will increase sharply. As premiums increase, two things will occur. There will be a decrease in demand for such coverage, and new insurance companies will enter the market. (One such entrant might be a company offering its employees their own self-insurance plan.) As long as some purchasers are willing to buy less comprehensive insurance, i.e., deductibles, copayments, and perhaps restrictions on which physicians they can use, insurance companies will respond to these demands. The remaining insurance companies will suffer losses in their market shares. With the increase in the supply of physicians there should be a sufficient number of physicians willing to participate under more restrictive agreements, at lower fee levels, or to perhaps become "preferred providers." To maintain their market shares, the other insurance companies will be forced to hold down their premiums. This might be accomplished by setting more stringent fee schedules (if the insurance company offers service benefit policies) and/or increased patient copayments. Whether physicians participate in different insurance programs will depend, in part, on what their competitors—other physicians—are willing to do.

The slow growth in the size of the population, the increased supply of physicians, the ability of physicians to advertise, a market where the patient is still responsible for a sizable portion of the bill, and (even if there were 100 percent insurance coverage) competition among health insurers, should serve to stimulate market forces so that price competition begins to play its traditional role in the physician services market.

REFERENCES

1. Median physician fees are those in the 50th percentile. Zackary Y. Dyckman, *A Study of Physician Fees* (Washington, D.C.: Council on Wage and Price Stability, Executive Office of the President, March 1978), pp. 95–103.

2. 1976 physician fees were collected and published by the Health Research Group as reported by B.D. Cohen, "Fees for Same Surgery Found to Vary Widely," *Washington Post* 102:1 (March 30, 1979).

3. Dyckman, *op. cit.*, p. 89.

4. *Ibid.*, p. 89. For more recent years, see Benson L. Dutton and Peter McMenamin, "The Medicare Economic index: Its Background and Beginnings," *Health Care Financing Review* (September 1981).

5. Dyckman, *op. cit.*, p. 74.

6. Uwe E. Reinhardt, *Physician Productivity and the Demand for Health Manpower* (Cambridge, Mass.: Ballinger, 1975), p. 82.

7. Uwe Reinhardt, "A Production Function for Physician Services," *The Review of Economics and Statistics* (February 1972): 63.

8. B. Kehrer and H. Zaretsky, "A Preliminary Analysis of Allied Health Personnel in Primary Medical Practice," Working Paper, Center for Health Services Research and Development (Chicago: American Medical Association, 1972): 95.

9. L. Kimbell and J. Lorant, "Production Functions for Physicians' Services," Working Paper submitted by Human Resources Research Center to Economic Analysis Branch under Contract No. 110–70–354 (Rockville, Md.: Health Services and Mental Health Administration, Department of Health, Education and Welfare, 1972).

10. Kenneth R. Smith, Marriene Miller, and Frederick L. Golladay, "An Analysis of the Optimal Use of Inputs in Production of Medical Services," *Journal of Human Resources* 7 (Spring 1972): 208–224.

11. Lewis R. Pondy, "Physician Assistants' Productivity: An Interim Report," unpublished paper, Duke University School of Business Administration, January 1971.

12. Uwe Reinhardt, "A Production Function for Physician Services."

13. H.E. Frech III and P. Ginsburg, "Optimal Scale in Medical Practice: A Survivor Analysis," *Journal of Business* (Chicago: University of Chicago, January 1974).

14. James R. Cantwell, "Copayment and Consumer Search: Increasing Competition in Medicare and Other Insured Markets," *Health Care Financing Review* (December 1981).

15. Steve G. Vahovich, ed., *Profile of Medical Practice* (Chicago: American Medical Association, 1973), p. 146.

16. Examples of empirical studies lending support to the target-income hypothesis are: Martin S. Feldstein, "The Rising Price of Physicians' Services," *The Review of Economics and Statistics* 52 (May 1970): 121–133; and Robert G. Evans, "Supplier Induced Demand: Some Empirical Evidence and Implications," in Mark Perlman, ed., *The Economics of Health and Medical Care* (New York: Halstead Press, 1974), pp. 162–173. For an excellent review of the target-income hypothesis and a reply to its critics, see Uwe E. Reinhardt, "Comment on 'Competition Among Physicians' by Frank Sloan and Roger Feldman," in Warren Greenberg, ed., *Competition in the Health Care Sector: Past, Present, and Future,* Proceedings of a Conference, Sponsored by the Bureau of Economics, Federal Trade Commission, March 1978. (Germantown, Md.: Aspen Systems Corporation, 1978).

17. For a critical review of the target-income hypothesis see Frank Sloan and Roger Feldman, "Competition Among Physicians," in Warren Greenberg, ed., *Competition in the*

Health Care Sector: Past, Present, and Future, Proceedings of a Conference, Sponsored by the Bureau of Economics, Federal Trade Commission, March, 1978. (Germantown, Md.: Aspen Systems Corporation, 1978).

18. Victor R. Fuchs, "The Supply of Surgeons and the Demand for Operations," *Journal of Human Resources* (Supplement) (1978): (*XIII*), 35–36, 38.

19. Mark V. Pauly and Mark A. Satterthwaite, "The Pricing of Primary Care Physicians' Services: A Test of the Role of Consumer Information," *The Bell Journal of Economics* (Autumn 1981).

20. Uwe Reinhardt, "Proposed Changes in the Organization of Health Care Delivery: An Overview and Critique," *Milbank Memorial Fund Quarterly* 51 (Spring 1973): 169–222.

21. One of the findings in a study of over 11,000 consultations scheduled during a 7½ year period "consistently show that roughly one-third of those voluntarily seeking a second-opinion consultation and roughly 18 percent of those required to seek a second-opinion consultation were not confirmed for surgery by a board-certified panel consultant." Those that were initially recommended for knee surgery, bunionectomies, hysterectomies, and prostatectomies had the highest rate of nonconfirmation. Eugene McCarthy, Madelon Finkle, and Hirsch Ruchlin, *Second Opinion Elective Surgery* (Boston: Auburn House Publishing, 1981), For a different perspective on unnecessary surgery, see Mark Pauly, "What Is Unnecessary Surgery," *Milbank Memorial Fund Quarterly* (Winter 1979).

22. This concept is discussed more completely in S.O. Schweitzer and J.O. Record, "Third Party Payments for New Health Professionals: An Alternative to Fractional Reimbursement in Outpatient Care," *Public Health Reports* 92 (November–December 1977): 518–526.

23. For a more complete discussion of this issue see Uwe Reinhardt, "Alternative Methods of Reimbursing Non-Institutional Providers of Health Services," in *Controls on Health Care* (Washington, D.C.: National Academy of Sciences, 1975).

24. Joseph Newhouse, "The Structure of Health Insurance and the Erosion of Competition in the Medical Marketplace," in Warren Greenberg, ed., *Competition in the Health Care Sector: Past, Present, and Future*, Proceedings of a Conference, Sponsored by the Bureau of Economics, Federal Trade Commission, March 1978. (Germantown, Md.: Aspen Systems Corporation, 1978).

25. Thomas P. Ferry, Marian Gornick, Marilyn Newton, and Carl Hackerman, "Physician Charges Under Medicare: Assignment Rates and Beneficiary Responsibility," *Health Care Financing Review* (Winter 1980): 50.

26. *Ibid.*, p. 52.

27. *Ibid.*, p. 57.

28. The discussion in this section is based on Lynn Paringer, "Medicare Assignment Rates of Physicians: Their Responses to Changes in Reimbursement Policy," *Health Care Financing Review* (Winter 1980). Also see Donald E. Yett, William Der, Richard L. Ernst, and Joel Hay, "Blue Shield Plan Physician Participation," *Health Care Financing Review* (Spring 1981); Frank Sloan, Janet Mitchell, and Jerry Cromwell, "Physician Participation in State Medicaid Programs," *Journal of Human Resources* (Supplement) (1978) (*XIII*); and Frank Sloan and Bruce Steinwald, "Physician Participation in Health Insurance Plans: Evidence on Blue Shield," *Journal of Human Resources* (Spring 1978). The above articles also contain empirical estimates for the different factors affecting physician participation rates.

CHAPTER 10

The Market for Hospital Services

BACKGROUND

The most important institutional setting to be analyzed is that of hospitals. In 1980, hospital expenditures totaled more than $100 billion, or 40 percent of the total expenditures for health care. Hospital expenditures constitute the largest single health care expenditure category and are rising at a rate of 15 percent per year (1). The hospital is also the most expensive setting on a per unit of service basis, and it has been both the object and the beneficiary of much federal and state legislation. A great deal more emphasis will, therefore, be devoted to hospitals than to the other institutional settings.

Hospitals are classified according to the major type of service delivered, length of stay, and control or ownership. A short-term hospital is one in which its patients, on average, have lengths of stay of less than 30 days. Hospitals with lengths of stay in excess of 30 days are referred to as long-term hospitals. Of the 6,965 hospitals listed by the American Hospital Association, 6,407 are classified as short-term hospitals. The major types of services by which hospitals are classified are psychiatric, tuberculosis and other respiratory diseases, and general and other special. The predominant type of hospital is the general and other special; 6,396 hospitals have this service classification. Hospital control or ownership can be categorized as either governmental, i.e., federal, state, and local; nonprofit, i.e., voluntary or community; or for-profit.

Mental, tuberculosis, and long-term hospitals have generally been public institutions, probably both for reasons of welfare and because of externalities such as the contagiousness of tuberculosis, which led the state to provide care for such persons to protect the rest of the population. The demand for such public institutions, however, has been declining. From 1955 to 1980, the average daily census declined 99 percent in tuberculosis hospitals, 73 percent in psychiatric hospitals, and 61 percent in long-term hospitals. The decline in demand for tuberculosis hospitals has been the result of improved environmental conditions, widespread testing and earlier discovery, and improved treatment techniques to reduce the length of stay. New treatment techniques for mental illness, specifically drug and shock therapy, have changed the demand for incarceration in a psychiatric hospital to a demand for qualified personnel, facilities for treatment, and a shorter length of stay. The short-term general hospitals have developed substitute facilities in the form of psychiatric units; these, together with community mental health centers, provide services that have left only the poor, the senile, and the incurable to the care of mental hospitals, which provide care of a different quality at much lower cost. The decline in demand for long-term hospitals is partly attributable to the development of substitute facilities, i.e., nursing homes, along with increased patient incomes and insurance coverage to pay for such care.

The demand for care in short-term general and other special hospitals during this same period (1955–1980), however, increased 84 percent in its average daily census. The rapid increase in demand for these facilities has resulted partly from the change in medical technology as well as from various economic and demographic factors.

The analysis to follow of the market for hospital services will concentrate on the performance of the short-term general hospital, and within that type of hospital, the voluntary, nonprofit institution. The predominant form of control and organization of the short-term general and other special hospitals is nongovernmental nonprofit; these hospitals number 3,248. State and local governmental are next in predominance, numbering 1,816; then come the for-profit hospitals with 700, and finally federal hospitals, 324. When one examines the data in Table 10-1 on admissions and the number of beds and employees, the voluntary nonprofit short-term general hospital is even more predominant as the major institution involved in the delivery of hospital services. These institutions have almost two-thirds of the short-term general beds, admit 67 percent of the patients, and employ more than 67 percent of all hospital employees.

The same table reveals that the large majority of short-term general hospitals have less than 200 beds, with more than one-third of the voluntary hospitals having less than 100 beds. From Table 10-2, which shows the distribution of community hospitals by bed size, it is clear that the average size of hospitals has been increasing over the past decade. The number of hospitals in the smaller bed size categories has been declining as the number of hospitals in the larger bed size categories has been increasing. This change has occurred through the expansion of the smaller hospitals.

The growth in short-term general hospitals in the period 1965 to 1980, which saw the passage of Medicare and Medicaid legislation to finance hospital care, is shown more vividly in Table 10-3. The growth in the number of hospitals was very small over this period: 1.6 percent. To accommodate the increase in utilization represented by a 32.7 percent increase in patient days, there was a 33.3 percent increase in the number of beds in these hospitals. Since the growth in beds exceeded the increase in utilization, there was a slight decline in occupancy rates, from 76 percent in 1965 to 75 percent in 1980. This table also gives evidence of the growth in hospital outpatient visits. The reasons for this increased role of the hospital in ambulatory care are varied. The hospital has served as a substitute for the physician's office. An increased demand for physician services has been generated by rising incomes, insurance coverage, and federal financing. Although the number of physicians has increased greatly over

TABLE 10-1. Selected Data on U.S. Hospitals, 1980

Type of Hospital	Number of Hospitals	Beds	Admissions	Total Patient Days (Thousands)	Employees
Short-term					
General	6,088	1,066,473	37,732,778	294,758	3,069,614
State and local					
government	1,816	209,502	7,419,378	54,074	590,608
100 beds	1,261	62,976	2,141,395	13,461	127,802
100–199 beds	293	40,864	1,502,568	10,631	97,761
200–499 beds	202	61,959	2,372,343	17,274	202,438
500+ beds	60	43,703	1,403,072	12,708	162,607
Voluntary	3,248	684,012	25,281,387	195,418	2,054,696
100 beds	1,121	63,667	2,205,304	14,552	142,171
100–199 beds	821	116,552	4,369,163	31,178	309,514
200–499 beds	1,052	331,029	12,649,804	97,444	1,010,312
500+ beds	254	172,764	6,057,116	52,242	592,699
Proprietary	700	85,316	3,097,854	20,344	186,024
100 beds	345	19,173	691,705	4,134	39,790
100–199 beds	225	31,258	1,136,257	7,359	66,911
200–299 beds	95	22,086	805,664	5,590	50,474
300+ beds	35	12,799	464,228	3,261	28,849
Federal	324	87,643	1,934,159	24,921	238,286
Long-term[a]	558	266,064	536,786	83,278	341,132

Source: © American Hospital Association, *Hospital Statistics*, 1981 ed. (Chicago: American Hospital Association, 1981), pp. 8–11.

[a]Includes general, psychiatric, tuberculosis, and other respiratory diseases, and all other.

TABLE 10-2. Distribution of Community Hospitals, By Bed Size Category, 1965 and 1980

Bed Size Category	Number of Hospitals		Percent Change
	1965	1980	
6–24 beds	562	259	−53.9
25–49	1,445	1,029	−28.8
50–99	1,482	1,462	−1.3
100–199	1,108	1,370	23.6
200–299	541	715	32.2
300–399	306	412	34.6
400–499	129	266	106.2
500 or more	163	317	94.5

Source: © American Hospital Association, *Hospital Statistics*, 1976 ed. (Chicago: American Hospital Association, 1981): p. vii; 1981 ed., p. xv.

TABLE 10-3. Selective Characteristics of Community Hospitals, 1965–1980

Community Hospitals	1965	1980	Percent Change
Number of hospitals	5,736	5,830	1.6
Total beds (thousands)	741	988	33.3
Average number of beds per hospital	129	170	31.8
Total admissions (thousands)	26,463	36,143	36.6
Average daily census (thousands)	563	747	32.7
Average length of stay	7.8	7.6	−2.6
Percent occupancy	76.0	75.6	−0.5
Outpatient visits	92,631	202,310	118.4

Source: © American Hospital Association, *Hospital Statistics*, 1976 ed. (Chicago: American Hospital Association, 1981), p. vi; 1981 ed., p. xiv.

this period the excess demand for physicians has apparently spilled over to the hospital's outpatient department.

Data in Table 10-4 showing the change in hospital finances over the past 15 years support this view of the increased role of the community hospital in the delivery of medical services and the increase in expenditures required to pay for this care. Hospital expenses have grown by more than 700 percent; payroll expenses have also increased, but by a lesser amount (527 percent), suggesting that nonpayroll expenses have increased at a more rapid rate. Part of the increase in total expenses has been a result of increased patient days; when the increase is adjusted for the increase in patient days, total expenses per patient day have increased by 537 percent. In addition to the increase in patient days, there has presumably been a change in the mix of patients as well as a change in what a patient day is today. Suggestive of this change in the medical services delivered by the hospital are the increase in assets per bed (293 percent), which in part represents increased capital and equipment, and an increase in the number of hospital employees per patient day. Additional evidence of the changes that have occurred in the hospital's "product" is the increase in the number of facilities and services offered by hospitals, shown in Table 10-5. Those facilities and services that have shown the largest percentage increase during the 1965–1980 period (based on data collected in both periods by the American Hospital Association) were social work departments, occupational therapy departments, and electroencephalography units. Indicative of the declining birth rate in the United States is the decline in the number of hospitals having premature nurseries: 939 fewer hospitals for a 32.3 percent decrease.

In addition to the changes taking place in the characteristics of individual hospitals, an important trend has been occurring in the industry's structure. It is becoming more concentrated. Hospitals have been affiliating with one another and forming what is referred to as "multihospital systems." The types of multihospital systems varies widely. In some systems, the hospital affiliation agreements are relatively weak. The hospital and its medical staff are able to retain their decision-making authority. The reasons usually given for weak forms of affiliation are the hospital being able to take advantage of economies of scale,

TABLE 10-4. Financial Data for Short-Term General Hospitals, 1980, and Percent Increases from 1965[a]

	Expenses						Assets					
	Payroll (thousands)		Total (thousands)		Total Expenses Per Patient Day		Plant (thousands)		Total (thousands)		Total Assets Per Bed	
Type of Hospital	1980	Percent Change 1965–1980	1980	Percent Change 1965–1980	1980	Percent Change 1965–1980	1980	Percent Change 1965–1980	1980	Percent Change 1965–1980	1980	Percent Change 1965–1980
All short-term general	$41,079,509	527	$82,593,598	703	$277.89	537	$52,347,643	270	$90,684,240	398	$84,696	293
State and local government	7,419,677	473	15,203,975	663	279.77	569	8,801,430	200	15,588,479	349	74,624	285
Nongovernment not-for-profit	27,642,291	576	55,799,821	740	281.73	521	35,624,415	292	64,456,460	416	93,083	285
Investor-owned	2,316,632	792	5,847,350	1,046	282.74	547	2,915,032	863	4,991,790	1,106	57,355	545
Federal government	4,362,937	370	7,086,176	509	258.38	590	5,006,766	166	5,647,511	197	59,009	225

Sources: 1965 data come from © American Hospital Association, *Journal of the American Hospital Association, Guide Issue* Part 2, 40(August 1, 1966): 442–443; Table 2. 1980 expense data come from American Hospital Association, *Hospital Statistics*, 1981 ed. (Chicago: American Hospital Association, 1981), pp. 20–21; Table 5A. 1980 asset data are unpublished data provided by the American Hospital Association.

[a]1965 figures include all short-term hospitals (excluding psychiatric).

TABLE 10-5. Selected Facilities and Services in Community Hospitals, 1965–1980

Facilities and Services	1965 Number of Hospitals	1965 % of Hospitals	1980 Number of Hospitals	1980 % of Hospitals	Change (1965–1980) Number of Hospitals	Change (1965–1980) % of Hospitals
Blood bank	3,168	61.4	4,173	78.2	1,005	27.4[a]
Cardiac catheterizations			868	16.3	41	5.2[a]
CT (computerized axial tomography) scanners			1,196	22.4	274	29.5[a]
Dental services	1,684	32.7	3,008	56.4	1,324	72.5
Diagnostic radioisotope facility			3,465	64.9	574	23.6[b]
Electroencephalography	1,427	27.7	3,504	65.7	2,077	137.2
Emergency department	4,784	92.8	4,350	81.5	−434	−12.2
Family planning service	248	4.8	523	9.8	275	104.2
Hemodialysis (inpatient)			1,273	23.9	557	83.8[b]
Histopathology			3,484	65.3	664	27.5[b]
Home care department	260	5.0	610	11.4	350	128.0
Hospital auxiliary	3,633	70.4	4,303	80.6	670	14.5
Occupational therapy	580	11.2	1,773	33.2	1,193	196.4
Open-heart surgery facility			566	10.6	43	11.6[b]
Pharmacy	3,019	58.5	5,155	96.6	2,136	65.1
Physical therapy	2,669	51.7	4,709	88.2	2,040	70.6
Postoperative recovery room	3,560	69.0	4,977	93.3	1,417	35.2
Premature nursery	3,091	59.5	2,152	40.3	−939	−32.3
Radioactive implements			1,352	25.3	342	33.2[a]
Respiratory therapy			4,966	93.1	678	19.5[b]
Social work department	894	17.3	4,171	78.2	3,277	352.0

Sources: © American Hospital Association, *Hospital Statistics*, 1976 ed. (Chicago: American Hospital Association, 1976), pp. 185–195; 1981 ed., pp. 191–197; and *Hospitals, Journal of the American Hospital Association* 40 (August 1 1966): 466–471.

Note: The percent change is calculated as: (percent of hospitals in 1980 − percent of hospitals in 1965) ÷ percent of hospitals in 1965. Over time, the American Hospital Association (AHA) has changed its selections of facilities and services on which it reports; consequently some services included in the 1980 AHA survey were not included in the 1965 survey.

[a]The change is between 1979 and 1980.
[b]The change is between 1975 and 1980.

TABLE 10-6. Characteristics of Multihospital Systems, 1981

Type of System	Total Number of Units in System	Total Number of Beds in System	Number of Beds Per System	Number of Beds Per Unit	Beds Per System Owned or Leased	Beds Per System Managed
Investor-owned (30)[a]	795	107,765	3,592.2	135.6	2,437.0	1,155.2
Secular nonprofit (64)	421	66,467	1,038.5	157.9	818.3	220.2
Catholic (46)	320	80,737	1,755.2	252.3	1,628.9	126.3
Other religions (21)	162	23,658	1,126.6	146.0	942.4	184.1
Public (11)	44	18,453	1,677.5	419.4	1,519.1	86.5
Total (172)	1,742	297,080	1,726.7	170.5	1,382.0	345.2

Source: Donald Johnson and Linda Punch, "Multi-hospital Systems Survey," *Modern Health Care*, April, 1982, pp. 68–69.

[a]Number of systems reporting in parentheses.

such as in joint purchasing arrangements. At the other extreme, in terms of affiliation agreements, are hospitals that are completely merged into the larger organization. The institution loses its autonomy. The reasons for this type of arrangement are usually to take advantage of large economies of scale, such as lower interest charges on bond issues, improved cash management, lower malpractice premiums—each of which require the institution to be more tightly integrated with the other hospitals in the system, and because of the need for financial survival. Hospitals facing declining occupancy rates and more stringent reimbursement policies are more willing to give up their autonomy to survive.

In 1981, as shown in Table 10-6, 1,742 facilities belonged to 172 multihospital systems. These systems had a total of 279,000 beds, which represented approximately 30 percent of total nonfederal short-term general beds (2). The trend toward hospital affiliations has increased in the last several years. Some members of the hospital industry believe that during the coming decade the unaffiliated community hospital will be the exception rather than the rule.

These descriptive data illustrate the changes that have been occurring in this market. The short-term general hospital has increased in size and in the volume of services delivered; it has changed its product, and in turn there have been very large increases in the cost of its output. The large sums of money being expended in this market, and the continuing rapid increases in its costs, make it important to determine the efficiency with which it performs.

THE EXTENT OF ECONOMIES OF SCALE IN HOSPITALS

THE REASONS FOR DETERMINING ECONOMIES OF SCALE IN HOSPITAL SERVICES

An important determinant of whether hospitals can be competitive is the extent of economies of scale that exist in the production of services in relation to the size of the market. With economies of scale, the larger the firm (or those firms that increase their output), the lower its average costs will be; if there is competition in the industry, firms with higher costs will not be able to survive. In a market of any given size, more firms will be able to exist as the gains from being a facility size that is least costly occur at small levels of production. The larger the size of the plant required to achieve the minimum costs of production, the fewer the number of firms that will be able to compete. An important reason for wanting to determine the extent of economies of scale in the production of hospital services, therefore, is to ascertain whether hospitals are a "natural" monopoly, whereby only very large hospitals are able to achieve the most efficient scale of operation. Or, are hospitals similar to most other industries in that the gains from large-scale production can be achieved in institutions that are small enough to permit many firms to survive in an urban area? Various persons have referred to hospitals as public utilities, necessitating public utility regulation. An analysis of the extent of economies of scale in hospitals would indicate whether such public utility status is justified on economic grounds.

Two other factors are also important in determining whether hospitals could, theoretically, be a competitive industry. The first is the importance of the patients' distance from the hospital. Patients might be willing to go to a smaller, more expensive hospital if the value of their travel cost and time more than offset the lower costs of going to a larger hospital further away. The total price of hospitalization is the relevant price to the patient, not just the hospital portion of that price. (As will be discussed below, the importance of travel cost varies with the particular service being demanded, as, for example, whether it is emergency or elective care.) The other important factor influencing the degree of competition among hospitals is the role of the physician. Patients do not generally purchase hospital care directly; their physician has a staff appointment at certain hospitals, and patients must generally enter the hospital where their physician practices. We will neglect this important role of the physician temporarily; if hospitals are not a "natural" monopoly, competition among hospitals could still exist, though instead of competing for patients directly, hospitals would compete for physicians and, indirectly, for their patients. If physicians faced appropriate incentives and acted to minimize their patients' costs of treatment, then the effects of this competition would be the same.

One important reason for determining the extent of economies of scale in hospital care is to determine whether hospitals in an area can be competitive, given appropriate patient and physician incentives. If, for reasons to be discussed, hospitals cannot be made into a competitive industry, then knowledge regarding the extent of economies of scale can still be used for planning. Hospital planning has been proposed as a way of efficiently allocating resources for producing hospital care. If economic efficiency in production is to be achieved through planning, then hospital planners will require the same information regarding economies of scale, travel costs, and other costs used in a competitive system to achieve economic efficiency. The concept of regionalization, where of three different levels of hospitals the largest ones serve the population of a region and the smallest serve a community, is based on the belief that there are economies of scale in certain hospital services and that the extent of these economies varies with the particular hospital service. The information that would indicate whether hospital care can be an essentially competitive sector would also be important for planning those same services, if planning were used as an alternative to competition to achieve an efficient production of hospital care.

More recently, attempts to improve hospital performance have included proposals to change the method of hospital reimbursement. Again, knowledge of the extent of economies of scale in hospital services, as well as of the other reasons for the wide variation in costs between hospitals, is necessary for establishing reimbursement systems to improve hospital efficiency. In a system of rate regulation of hospital services, one method for determining which hospitals should be permitted to maintain or add specified facilities and services could be based upon a reimbursement rate that is related to the minimum average cost of providing the specified service. Hospitals able to take advantage of economies of scale in producing that service would be able to cover their costs and would thereby be able to offer that particular service. The rate-setting agency under such a system would have to have knowledge of the extent of economies of scale for the different services for which it was establishing reimbursement rates.

Thus for the purpose of understanding the hospital industry, such as whether such a sector could be competitive, and for purposes of hospital planning and rate regulation, it is important to determine the extent of economies of scale in the provision of hospital services. How the information on hospital costs can be specifically used for each of these purposes will be discussed in a subsequent section dealing with public policy on hospitals.

EMPIRICAL FINDINGS ON THE EXTENT OF ECONOMIES OF SCALE IN HOSPITAL SERVICES

The theoretical relationship between hospital cost and size is U-shaped. As the size of the facility (and its production) is increased, its average cost per unit should decrease, reach a minimum, and then increase. The reasons for this expected relationship are several: with a larger facility there can be greater specialization of labor; further, with the emphasis on licensure as a means of assuring competence of personnel in the health field and the consequent limited flexibility in delegation of tasks, licensed and specialized personnel can be used more fully in a larger institution than in a smaller one. Specialized equipment and facilities can also be used to their capacity in larger institutions. Lastly, larger institutions are more likely to be able to take advantage of quantity discounts in purchasing than are smaller institutions.* Offsetting these advantages is the greater proportion of time and effort required to coordinate and control work in large organizations. In general, for sufficiently small outputs, efficiency increases with size, because the advantages that accrue from the use of specialized labor and equipment far outweigh the increased cost of management. As size increases, however, the reduction in per unit cost afforded by greater and greater specialization begins to decline and is eventually outweighed by increased costs of coordination and control. Other things being equal, average hospital costs thus may be expected to decline initially and then rise as size is increased, as shown by the U-shaped curve in Figure 10-1. How rapidly these gains and losses from scale of operation occur is what determines the shape of the long-run average-cost curve.

This theoretical relationship is not easily determined, however. Hospitals are not homogeneous in size or other characteristics. Hospitals are multiproduct firms. In addition to producing inpatient services, which differ in their quality, the type of patient treated, and the severity of the particular case, hospitals also produce outpatient services, education, training, research, and community services. Hospitals also differ in the amenities they provide. There are further differences among hospitals, such as in the prices they must pay for their labor and nonlabor inputs as well as in hospital efficiency. With all studies that have attempted to estimate the effect of size on average cost, the difficulty has been to adequately measure and to then hold constant all the other factors which affect hospital costs, while estimating the net effect of size alone. The consequence of not being able to hold these other factors constant is that the relationship between size and costs is likely to be biased.

---

*To some extent small hospitals may circumvent the various diseconomies associated with their size by purchasing auxiliary services from outside firms.

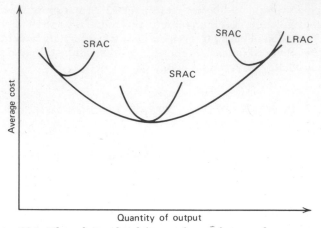

Figure 10-1. The relationship between hospital size and average cost.

For example, if economies of scale exist in larger hospitals, which usually treat patients who are more seriously ill, then unless differences in the type of patient are accounted for, it may seem that the observed relationship between cost and size is that larger hospitals have *higher* per unit costs. The result of failing to hold constant differences in costs between hospitals that are a result of factors other than size (such as seriousness of illness) may be seen in Figure 10-2. The hospital represented by the short-run average-cost curve at point *C* may be on a lower long-run average-cost curve than hospital *B* or *A* because it may provide fewer services. If one were to observe raw data on average cost and size, then one might observe data points which represent the relationship between hospitals *D* and *A*. It would appear that hospital *D*, which is smaller, has lower costs than hospital *A*, and that average costs increase as the size of the hospital is similarly increased. If adjustments are made for the differences between these

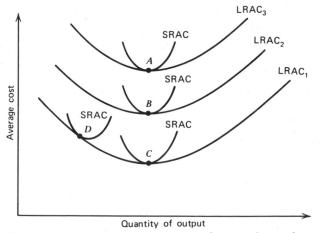

Figure 10-2. Variations in average cost between hospitals.

two hospitals—namely, the reason they are on different average-cost curves—then it can be observed that for the product hospital A is producing (on long-run average-cost curve $LRAC_3$), it is producing its output in the least costly facility (it is operating in a facility which is at the minimum point on its long-run average-cost curve). Hospital D, however, is not only producing a different product (one that is less costly to produce than the one produced by hospital A), but it is also in a facility that is not least costly; it is at point D rather than point C.

In competitive industries it is difficult to empirically estimate a long-run average-cost curve because unless all firms are operating in a least-cost-sized plant, they could not survive. One would not expect to observe data on firms in plant sizes that are on either the declining or rising portion of the long-run average-cost curve. There are several reasons, however, why it should be possible to trace out a long-run average-cost curve for hospitals. Hospitals have been reimbursed, in large part, on the basis of their individual costs; further, patients may have insufficient information to compare prices between hospitals (nor are they likely to have an incentive to do so if their insurance is a service benefit policy), and lastly, since the physician is the manager of the patient's treatment, the physician's staff appointment may be in one of the higher-cost hospitals. The patient would be more concerned with the overall cost of treatment than with the cost of any one component of that treatment. Thus, it is possible to observe data on hospitals whose average costs vary widely, though their survival is not threatened. This somewhat extended discussion points out the necessity for holding all the other factors that affect hospital costs constant if one is to be able to successfully trace out the effect of just size on cost.

Previous investigators who have attempted to estimate the extent of economies of scale in hospitals have not been unaware of these problems. Empirical studies have differed in the approaches used to control for these other factors affecting hospital costs. Early studies on hospital costs tended to use more aggregated data; subsequent studies have used more refined data from groups of hospitals that are more homogeneous, at least with respect to location, and that have more detailed data available on their patient population. For example, to measure differences in the hospitals' product, various investigators have used the number of facilities and services, others have grouped hospitals by comparable facilities and services, while still others have classified facilities and services according to whether they are basic, quality-enhancing, complex, or community services (3). Investigators have also included patient case-mix measures—that is, the proportion of a hospital's patients classified into various diagnostic categories (4). In an attempt to include a quality variable, some investigators have included a measure of the use of hospital inputs or even some measure of the hospital's costs as a proxy for quality. There are still severe data problems involved in adequately controlling for all the variations in hospital output. There are, in addition, the difficulties of measuring the nonpatient care outputs of the hospital, such as teaching programs (and the impact interns and residents have on hospital costs), outpatient services (which may share facilities and equipment with inpatient services in the hospital), and so on.

All of the studies on hospital costs have also found it difficult to adjust for differences in hospital efficiency, making it difficult to separate the effects of efficiency on costs from the effects of differences in hospital size. Additional technical problems include the difficulty of adjusting for differences in prices paid by hospitals for their factor inputs that are unrelated to differences in hospital size. Since larger hospitals are located in large urban areas, where wage rates are often higher, it must be determined how much of the larger hospitals' higher wage costs are paid for the same type of hospital worker as elsewhere and how much for more highly skilled workers. An important limitation of most previous hospital cost studies (pointed out by Pauly) is their failure to adjust hospital costs for differences among hospitals in the contributions of physicians to the hospitals' output. Hospitals differ in their employment of staff physicians. In hospitals without salaried physicians, the physician charges the patient separately for services rendered. Hospitals that employ physicians will have higher costs than hospitals that do not, though there may be no differences in their output. Interns and residents also provide patient care; their costs are included in the costs of those hospitals that have such educational programs, though their (or the patient's physician's) contribution to hospital output is not included in those hospitals that do not have such programs. The foregoing are some of the conceptual and data problems involved in estimating the net effect of hospital size on cost. (See the end of this chapter for a selected bibliography on hospital cost studies.)

The empirical approach used to derive the effect of size on cost, while controlling for other differences between hospitals, is to use some form of multivariate analysis. The general form of such an equation is

$$AC = f(B, S, C, Q, V, P, E, D, O)$$

where AC = the dependent variable, usually average cost per patient day or per admission*

f = a functional relationship, connoting the dependence of AC on the variables on the right side of the equation,

B = the measure of hospital size, usually measured in terms of number of beds

S = the hospital's service capability, usually measured by some enumeration of facilities and services in the hospital

C = a measure of patient case mix, measured by the proportion of patients in a given number of disease classifications

Q = a measure of quality, inadequately measured to date (if included at all) by some variable such as inputs per patient, e.g., lab tests

V = severity of illness within a patient disease classification, possibly measured (inadequately) by the number of surgical procedures

P = an adjustment for differences between hospitals for wages and other factor prices that are unrelated to hospital size

E = differences in hospital efficiency that are unrelated to hospital size

---

*If the dependent variable is in the form of total cost rather than average cost, it is claimed that the variance in total cost between large and small hospitals is not equal; therefore, there is a problem of heteroscedasticity. If the dependent variable is average cost per patient day rather than per admission, then a decrease in the length of stay will increase the average cost per day, because more inputs are used in the early days of admission.

D = educational programs, e.g., number of interns and residents, affiliations with a medical school and a nursing school, as well as representing research and other training programs

O = other variables such as the physicians' contributions, outpatient visits, and so on.

Once the model has been specified in this manner and reasonable proxies have been developed for the various theoretical variables, data are collected on either a time-series or cross-sectional basis, or some combination of the two. That is, yearly data are collected on each of the listed variables for each hospital in a state, a region, or the country as a whole. (The assumption is that each data point for a hospital represents a given-sized facility, i.e., a short-run average-cost curve, which can then be used to trace out a long-run average-cost curve.) The advantage of using a cross-sectional analysis rather than a time-series approach (which would be yearly data from one or more hospitals over a long period) is that technology, medical practice, and illnesses can generally be assumed to be constant for a given period for each of the hospitals in the study. Other problems with conducting a time-series study are that data may be unavailable for long periods or accounting methods may have changed. There may also have been changes in the hospital's management and efficiency over time as well.

The method used to estimate the effects of each of the above factors on costs is multiple regression analysis. This method provides measures of the effects that each variable has on average cost, the significance of that variable, and the variation in average cost that is explained by all the variables in the equation. In order to determine whether there are economies of scale, the output measure is allowed to be curvilinear, i.e., either the variables are transformed into logarithms or a squared term is included for the output measure.*

The foregoing discussion of statistical estimation has been cursory. The interested reader who wishes to pursue it further is referred to several of the review articles that have been written on hospital costs; students with a background in econometrics are referred to the studies themselves, examples of which are referenced at the end of this chapter.

The following is a brief summary of the findings on economies of scale. Because of the conceptual and data limitations in conducting such studies, it is difficult to be precise with regard to exact estimates for the effect of any of the theoretical variables on hospital costs. Economists studying hospital costs disagree as to whether the various studies have been able to hold all the other

---

*For example, if the net effect of beds on average cost per admission is $-.04$ BEDS $+ .0001$ BEDS^2, then the size of hospital with lowest average costs is determined by taking the partial derivative of AC with respect to BEDS, setting it equal to zero, and solving for BEDS.

$$\frac{\delta AC}{\delta \, BEDS} = -.04 + .0002 \, BEDS = 0$$

$$+ .0002 \, BEDS = +.04$$
$$BEDS = 200$$

Average costs per admission would be at a minimum in hospitals with 200 beds.

factors affecting hospital costs constant. Some general findings, however, do appear among the various studies. First, there are some slight economies of scale; hospitals with approximately 200–300 beds appear to have the lowest average costs. The shape of this average-cost curve is shallow, that is, it does not fall sharply nor is the minimum point much below that of hospitals on the ends of the curve. Further, hospitals with greater service capability appear to be subject to larger economies of scale. More recently the emphasis on hospital cost studies has shifted from looking at aggregate hospital costs and their relation to overall hospital size to examining the cost-size relationship by department and examining hospitals with different mixes of facilities and services. Finding economies of scale (or not) for the hospital as a whole does not provide sufficient data for planning, reimbursement, or any other purpose. For example, there are presumably large economies of scale in laundry operation; such information would be useful for a make-or-buy decision. Can a hospital produce its own laundry services more cheaply than it can buy such services from another hospital or from a centralized laundry service? For highly specialized services, the extent of economies of scale can be used to indicate how many such services can be offered in a given area. Which hospitals should be the ones to offer such services is a separate question, but perhaps such information on economies of scale by service can be used to set reimbursement levels, and then any hospital able to provide that service at that price can do so.

Another interesting finding of studies on economies of scale is that the mix of patients in the hospital is an important determinant of hospital costs: in some cases, case mix explains up to 50 percent of the variation in average costs between hospitals. The implication of this finding is that with prospective reimbursement for hospital payment, the hospitals' patient mix and the complexity of the cases are important factors that should be included in the hospitals' reimbursement level.

The finding that small economies of scale exist among hospitals implies that hospitals (with the exception of those in isolated, rural areas) are not natural monopolies in the traditional economic sense.

Many hospitals could exist in a community, possibly competing with one another. Since hospitals appear to add services in a very predictable way as they grow, "basic" hospital services are not subject to large economies of scale. (There are also probably good substitutes available for most of these services in a nonhospital setting, e.g., the physician's office.) In a large community there is little reason why there should not be multiple hospitals, although it is unlikely that each of the hospitals in the community should have all of the same specialized facilities. There would thus tend to be a less competitive market in a particular area as far as more highly specialized services such as open heart surgery are concerned. The demand for such highly specialized services is generally not of an emergency nature; the relevant market for them is likely to be at a state, or even a regional level. Even for these services, it is unlikely that a case can be made for treating them as a natural monopoly.

The purpose of this section was to review the findings on the extent of economies of scale among hospitals in order to determine whether the hospital sector could be a competitive industry, given the proper incentives, and also whether such information can be used for purposes of planning and reimbursement. Based on available empirical information, it appears that the extent of overall economies of scale is small, undoubtedly varying by type of service. A complete understanding of the structure of this industry, however, must go beyond the mere determination of economies of scale. What makes this industry unique, and what affects its performance, are the methods of reimbursement for hospital services and the objectives and incentives of the decisionmakers who control the hospitals. To enlarge our understanding of hospital performance, the next section discusses the objectives and incentives of the hospital decisionmakers.

THEORIES OF HOSPITAL BEHAVIOR

In a competitive system, the simple assumption that firms will attempt to maximize their profits makes it possible to predict what a firm's supply response will be to changes in demand and/or changes in its input prices. With entry into the industry permitted, we would expect firms to minimize their costs and expect prices to reflect the costs of production; there would be no internal cross-subsidization of patients or of users of different services. If prices are not related to costs, then new firms will enter the market and sell the service at a lower price. Because of the assumption of profit maximization and entry, we would expect prices to equal costs (in the long run); the different mix of services provided would reflect what people are willing to pay for those services, which in turn is a reflection of their full costs. The firms competing would all attempt to minimize their costs, and investment decisions would be based on profitability, i.e., demand and cost conditions.

Since hospitals are predominantly nonprofit, what does this difference in objectives imply for the performance of the hospital industry? Does it, as some persons have alleged, result in lower costs of production, since the hospital does not have to earn a profit? Or does it result in poorer performance? We need to develop a model of the nonprofit hospital in order to explain the observed performance of the hospital sector, to predict future performance, and to evaluate whether changes should be made. If changes are to be proposed, then it is important to be able to predict how hospitals will respond to them, and for this we need to understand what motivates the behavior of hospital decisionmakers.

A number of different theories have been developed to explain hospital behavior. These theories will be examined and their predictions summarized. The predictions will be tested by examining their consistency in relation to observed data. The most consistent theories will be examined with respect to their implications for hospital performance and for proposed changes in that performance.

A PROFIT-MAXIMIZING MODEL OF HOSPITAL BEHAVIOR

To begin with our simplest model of hospital behavior, let us examine how a for-profit hospital would determine its price, output, and investment policy. This will pave the way for varying the assumption of for-profit behavior on the part of the hospital. Hospitals are assumed to have a downward-sloping demand curve,

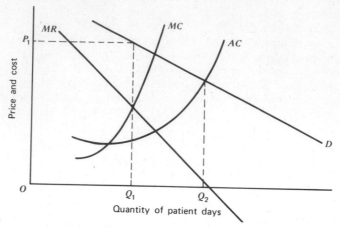

Figure 10-3. Price and output policies of a profit-maximizing hospital.

since there is some product differentiation among hospitals in that their locations differ and any given patient's physician does not have staff appointments (at least in the short run) at all hospitals. To maximize profits, the hospital would select that price on the demand curve where its marginal cost curve intersects the marginal revenue curve; this is shown in Figure 10-3. The profit-maximizing price and output would be P_1 and Q_1, respectively, and the amount of profit would be the difference between P_1 and the average-cost curve at that price, multiplied by Q_1.

Since the hospital is a multiproduct firm with different payors, it will price-discriminate according to the price elasticity of demand for each class of patient and type of service. The hospital's room rate is believed to be more elastic than the demand for ancillary services because patients and/or their physicians may decide to substitute out-of-hospital care or care in a different hospital if the room rate is higher in comparison. Once the patient has been hospitalized, ancillary services are complements to the use of the room, and fewer substitutes are available for those ancillary services. The charges for ancillary services are also generally a small portion of the room charge. Thus, the demand for ancillary services is believed to be relatively price inelastic. If the hospital is interested in maximizing its profits, it will charge higher prices (relative to costs) for those services and that class of patients whose demands are less price elastic.

This simple model of profit-maximizing behavior predicts that hospitals will increase their prices if demand either increases or becomes less elastic, or if the prices of their inputs increase. This behavioral model also predicts that hospitals will attempt to minimize their costs of operation. If hospitals make a profit, then, under this model, they will reinvest those profits on the basis of which investments offer the highest rate of return. Examples of the types of investments they could undertake would be additions to bed capacity, if their occupancy rates were rising, cost-saving technology, or additional facilities and services. New facilities and services could be profitable in their own right or could serve to attract a greater number of physicians to the hospital's staff, thereby increasing the demand for the hospital's beds. An important aspect of this model is that the hospital would set prices as would a profit maximizer, minimize its costs (since higher costs represent foregone profits), and invest only in projects that offer a profitable return.

If there were free entry into the hospital market, then no excess profits would exist in the long run. The performance of the industry would be similar to that of a monopolistically competitive industry where there is price competition, in that though there would still be some product differentiation among hospitals, prices of services and classes of patients would reflect their respective average costs. If there were entry barriers, then excess profits could exist in the long run, as prices exceeded average costs.

How well does this model reflect actual or observed hospital behavior? With regard to hospital pricing policies, there is some evidence that hospitals do price according to their price elasticity of demand. Prices are much greater than average costs for those services believed to be more price inelastic (ancillary services), but are closer to average costs for those services that are more price elastic (room rates and obstetrics) (5). Observed hospital behavior diverges from the profit-maximizing behavior with regard to the assumptions of cost minimization and the profitability of investments. We observe large variations in hospital costs for producing similar outputs. We also observe hospitals making investments in facilities and services about which it is known in advance that they will result in substantial losses; facilities and services are also subsidized by other facilities and services instead of being closed. The main problem with this simple profit-maximizing model of the hospital, however, is that it excludes any important role for the physician. The only role for physicians in this model is that they serve to increase demand for the hospital; however, the model assumes that the hospital will attempt to keep adding physicians to its staff, whereas in reality it appears that the medical staff tightly controls staff appointments and seeks to limit rather than expand physician staff appointments.

There also appear to be barriers to entry or other "peculiar" aspects of the hospital market, since we observe that hospitals are able to survive though they do not minimize their costs and are able to undertake and maintain services that result in losses.

Another behavioral model posits that hospitals act as if they wanted to maximize their output or sales. Under this model, hospitals will attempt to maximize their profits in the short run (by setting prices and output to maximize profits) and invest either in additional capacity, cost-saving technology, or facilities and services that result in the largest increases in their output. The hospitals will still be cost minimizers and profit maximizers, since to do otherwise is to forego revenue, which could be used to increase sales. With reference to Figure 10-3, an output maximizer would increase output to Q_2, which would represent the point on the demand curve where average cost equals price. This does not mean that for every service or class of patients price equals average cost, but it does in the aggregate. This model is similar both in its predictions and in its lack of consistency with observed data in similar areas to the previous model.

UTILITY-MAXIMIZING MODELS OF HOSPITAL BEHAVIOR

The next models to be discussed incorporate some of the observed inconsistencies of the previous models. The first of these models suggests that the manager has objectives other than just profit (which cannot be kept) or being the administrator of the largest hospital. The manager is assumed to have a utility function that includes some measure of the quality of the institution as well as its size. The quality of a hospital is not a well-defined variable; quality may include the type of facilities and services offered in the institution, the quality of its medical staff and the specialists on that staff, as well as the caliber of its labor inputs. Under this "quality–quantity" behavioral model, the hospital will still seek to maximize its profits in the short run through its pricing strategy, but it will then attempt to invest that profit either in increased quantity—increased capacity, cost-saving technology, or facilities and services that result in an increase in quantity of patients—or in prestige/quality investments. Because quantity and quality are to some extent substitutable for one another in the utility function, the manager will have to make a trade-off according to the marginal increase in utility resulting from increased quality or from increased quantity.

The effect of adding quality to the hospital's objective is to cause an increase in hospital costs. This change in costs as a result of increased quality is shown in Figure 10-4. To start, assume that the hospital is operating on average-cost curve AC_1. Since it cannot keep any profits, its long-run price and output will be P_1 and Q_1, respectively. If the hospital invests in increased quality, this results in an increase in its costs; the average-cost curve rises to AC_2, but the increased quality also results in an increase in the hospital's demand, shifting the demand to D_2. The increase in demand may occur as a result of attracting additional physicians to the hospital. After some point, increased expenditures for quality will result in small or negligible increases in demand; at this point the additional cost of increased quality may exceed the additional revenue resulting from the small increments in demand. Additions to quality beyond that point continue to raise the average-cost curve, to AC_3, but do not result in any further shifts in demand. Since funds that are used to increase quality could be used to increase quantity by adding to capacity, the manager has to determine the relative weights to be placed on the quantity–quality trade-off.

The consequences for economic efficiency of a utility model of a hospital attempting to maximize both quantity and quality is that the price of hospital care will be higher than if quality were not continually increased. Continued increases in quality without increased demand will shift the average-cost curve higher, possibly decreasing quantity and raising price. Further, hospitals will be producing a higher-quality product than consumers might be willing to pay for. Such a behavioral model could only be accurate if there were either some barriers to entry, such that lower-cost, lower-quality hospitals could not enter the market, or if consumers had an elastic demand with respect to hospital quality and the price of their care were subsidized. With entry and price competition, consumers would select that combination of price and quality that corresponded to what they were willing to pay for rather than to the quality-quantity preferences of the hospital administrator. Quality in such a case would increase in response to consumer demands for quality. If, on the other hand, barriers to entry existed or consumers did not have to pay the full price for hospital care, then higher levels of quality could exist in the hospital market and would be determined by the preferences of hospital decisionmakers.

How consistent is the quantity–quality model with observed behavior? This model still implies a profit-maximizing pricing strategy and cost-minimizing behavior. It does explain why hospitals might make unprofitable investments or

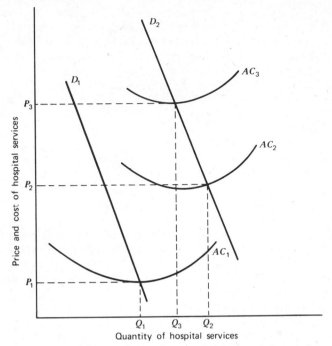

Figure 10-4. The effect on hospital costs of increases in hospital quality.

maintain unprofitable services, as long as these services add prestige to the institution. This model also suggests that a hospital will invest in new technology as soon as it becomes available, not necessarily because of its effect on demand, but because of its effect on the perceived image of the hospital. The quantity—quality model also suggests that hospitals with such objectives will be against the entry of proprietary hospitals into their communities. The nonprofit hospitals would be using internal cross-subsidization of their services to pay for the prestige services, which are money losers. Proprietary hospitals, which do not have a prestige objective and do not have to resort to cross-subsidization of services, will not have to price their services as high as do the nonprofit hospitals. The proprietaries attempt to compete with the nonprofits by lowering the price of the "profitable" services in comparison with the prices charged by the nonprofits. The nonprofits claim that these money-losing services are essential to meet the needs of the community and that the for-profit hospitals are "skimming the cream" by not offering such services.* Others claim that the money-losing

---

*"Skimming" by proprietaries has been investigated in a number of studies. In addition to differences in types of services, such as surgical facilities, differences have been found in the case mix or in severity of illness of patients between proprietaries and nonprofits. One such study, which also contains the references for other studies in this area, is Carson W. Bays, "Case-Mix Differences between Nonprofit and For-Profit Hospitals," *Inquiry*, March 1977. In his conclusion Bays raises the appropriate question: "[W]hy is the pricing structure of nonprofits such that for-profits find it profitable to produce only certain types of care[?]" (p. 21).

services are duplicative in the community and should not be offered by multiple hospitals. The number of hospitals with open heart surgery facilities and their utilization is cited as an example of this duplication. In 1961, 327 facilities reported having such facilities. The percentage breakdown of hospitals with specified cases per year is: 11 percent had *no* cases, 30 percent had 1–9 cases, 36 percent had 10–49 cases, 17 percent had 50 or more cases, and 6 percent were unknown. This survey of hospitals with open heart surgery facilities was repeated in 1969 with similar findings (6). It is difficult to believe that the quality of open heart surgery is the same regardless of the frequency of the surgery performed. To test this hypothesis, a study was conducted of the frequency with which different types of surgery were performed, and resulting mortality rates. In their analysis, the investigators controlled for other factors that might affect mortality, such as the patient's age, sex, and health status. It was found that for complicated types of surgery, the greater the volume of surgery performed, the lower the surgical mortality rates (7).

Though it provides additional explanations on the quality side, this model shares drawbacks with the profit-maximizing and output-maximizing models— namely, the expectation of cost-minimizing behavior, the lack of a clearly defined role of physicians in the decisionmaking process, and the failure to incorporate physician objectives.

The quantity–quality model has been modified to address one of these failings by the inclusion of a "slack" variable in the manager's utility function. Hospital administrators, according to this utility model, are also interested in working in a pleasant environment, as defined by amenities such as thick rugs and higher wages for employees to minimize conflict. This broader utility function of the hospital administrator predicts that hospitals will still price to maximize profits, and then will spend those profits to achieve some combination of quantity, quality, and slack. Again, the survival of hospitals that act in such a manner depends upon a situation of strong barriers to entry, or one where patients are responsible for paying even less of their hospital costs than under the previous models. If entry exists and patients are responsible for payment of their hospitalization expenses, hospitals will have to compete on the basis partly of price as well as of their differentiated product. With the inclusion of slack in the manager's utility function, prices will be even higher than under the previous models. Such a model therefore assumes that patients have become relatively indifferent to the prices charged or that few substitutes are available. Under these circumstances hospitals would compete with one another, but the competition would be to see which hospitals could become the most prestigious, while providing the administrative staff with a pleasant working environment. There would be a great deal of duplication within the industry, excess capacity, high costs, and rapidly rising prices to finance the described behavior.

The foregoing models of hospital behavior, though they apparently explain some observed data in the real world, do not explain other phenomena. For example, why are hospitals nonprofit? If it is because it is immoral to profit from sickness, why then can people profit from hunger and the need for shelter? Also, these models attribute a passive role to physicians. Hospitals, under these models, attempt to attract more physicians to their staffs, yet physicians, according to our observations, attempt to limit additions to their staffs. The decisionmakers in the foregoing models appear to be hospital administrators or an undefined group, but in reality the physicians are in control of the hospital, its pricing policies, and investment behavior. The next model of hospital behavior attempts to rectify these weaknesses.

A PHYSICIAN-CONTROL MODEL OF HOSPITAL BEHAVIOR

As stated earlier, the physician is the manager of the patient's illness, with responsibility for deciding upon the components to be used in providing treatment. As someone with a stake in what inputs are used, the physician might also be expected to combine the treatment inputs in such a manner so as to increase his or her own income and/or productivity. This view of the consumer's demand for medical care is based on the assumption that the total price of medical care is the relevant price to the consumer, not the individual price of specific inputs such as hospital care. (This assumption was more appropriate before there was such widespread insurance for hospital care.) If the consumer is more concerned with the total price of the treatment than with the price of its separate parts, then more of the total price would be left for the physician the less the patient has to pay for any other component, such as hospital care. Conversely, "[T]he greater the supply price of the inputs, the smaller the return to the producer of a given quantity of the final product" (8). That the total price of medical care is the relevant price to the consumer can be illustrated with reference to Figure 10-3. If two inputs are used in providing a medical treatment, hospital and physician services, then, given the patient's demand for medical care and an average-cost curve which represents the cost of hospital care, the difference between the price charged the patient and the amount that goes to pay the hospital is available to the physician. The physician acts as a contractor, retaining the amount left over after all the other inputs have been paid.*

This profit-maximizing model of the physician can be used to explain a number of apparent anomalies in the health field. The medical staff of a hospital is assumed to control the hospital under this model; it is further assumed that the decisions undertaken by the hospital represent the objectives of the staff physicians. If the demand for medical care were to increase, it would be in the physicians' interest that it be met by an increase in hospital capacity, which would increase the physicians' productivity, rather than by an increase in the number of physicians. For example, with reference to Figure 10-5, physician and hospital services are two inputs in a production function. With an increase in the demand for medical care, the increased output, represented by the highest isoquant, can be produced with different quantities of either physician or hospital services. At the initial amount of medical care being produced, isoquant Q_{MC1}, the combination of physicians and hospital care is Q_{MD0} and Q_{H1}, respectively. As the quantity of medical care to be provided increases to isoquant Q_{MC4}, the number of physicians and the amount of hospital care can be increased in the same proportions as previously. It will be more in keeping with the interests of the physi-

---

*Such profit-maximizing behavior on the part of the physician is not necessarily inconsistent with the physician's acting in the patient's economic interest as well. If hospital care is free to the patient (because of insurance coverage), while the patient must pay the full price for use of other components, it may be in both the patient's and the physician's interest to hospitalize the patient.

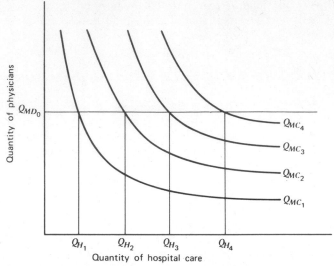

Figure 10-5. A production function for medical care.

cians if their number remains the same while the amount of hospital care is increased. With the same number of physicians, Q_{H4} of hospital care will be required. Since the quantity of medical care produced is greater even though the number of physicians has remained unchanged, the marginal productivity of the physician has increased; correspondingly, the marginal productivity of the hospital has fallen. This is similar to the law of variable proportions, which requires output to be increased by increasing the use of one input while holding constant the quantity of another input; the marginal productivity of the variable input—in this case the hospital—will eventually decline. The higher the physician's productivity, the greater his or her income will be.

This model suggests that physicians would favor increases in the hospital's capacity to provide additional services; increases in the hospital's capacity to handle more physician services as demand increases, such as increasing the number of interns and residents, who provide physician services for which the physician can charge the patient; additional facilities and services, such as an excess of operating rooms and obstetric facilities, so the physician does not have to wait or be inconvenienced; and facilities and services that are available in other community hospitals so that the physician does not have to refer a patient to another hospital and physician, thereby risking the loss of a fee. The staff physicians who do not have staff appointments at other hospitals would thereby favor hospital investment, even though it may be duplicative for the community, because it increases their productivity and income. Physicians would also prefer some hospital slack, enabling them to economize on their own time.

The effect of physician control over hospital investment policies is to cause technical inefficiency in production; too many inputs are used relative to the physician input in meeting increased demands for medical care. The price to the physician for these other inputs is zero, particularly if they are paid in full by some third-party payor or the government. Before a large percentage of the population had coverage for hospitalization, we would have expected the physician to be more concerned with the hospital's costs, since the higher those costs, the lower the payment available to the physician would be. With larger hospitals, however, the effect on any one physician's income of inefficient behavior on the part of the hospital would be small. Only in smaller hospitals, with correspondingly fewer physicians, would the physicians be expected to be concerned with the efficiency of the hospital's operation. As insurance coverage for hospital care became more widespread, however, and as payment to hospitals was based on the hospital's costs, regardless of what they were, increases in hospital prices became less of a concern to the physician. As the price of hospital care to the patient grew smaller, physicians were able to increase their charges to the patient and were unconcerned with the effect on costs of the hospital's investment and efficiency behavior.

The physician-control model also provides some explanation of hospital pricing behavior. The physician would prefer that the hospital assign relatively low prices to services that are complementary to the physician's services, in which case we might expect (prior to the widespread availability of hospital insurance) to find hospital charges for the operating room priced at or below cost. The physicians would also be expected to favor profit-maximizing price policies (when they did not conflict with their own pricing strategies), since such prices would result in greater hospital profits, which could then be invested internally according to their preferences. The hospital's physicians might also want the hospital to provide outpatient departments and preventive care services, which might at first appear to compete with the physicians. The outpatient department, however, is a convenient way of avoiding the financial risk of caring for low-income patients and allows physicians to allocate more of their time to higher-income patients. Physicians are also relieved of providing emergency services, thereby allowing them more time for more remunerative services or for leisure. The same explanations can be offered for having the hospital provide preventive care, in that the physician's time is freed for acute services, which offer a higher return per unit of time.

An interesting aspect of the physician-control model of hospital behavior is that it explains why hospitals are nonprofit. If physicians are in fact the real decisionmakers in the hospitals, then hospitals are nonprofit because this form of control is more profitable for their physicians. The advantages to the physician of nonprofit hospitals are several. First, a nonprofit hospital cannot sell medical services directly to the patient; consumers cannot buy all their medical care from the hospital because they must first go to a physician if they require hospitalization, thereby increasing the demand for physicians. The medical societies have ensured that hospitals will not be able to compete with physicians by having the various states enact legislation prohibiting the corporate practice of medicine. Under such legislation, only physicians can practice medicine, not organizations operated by nonphysicians. Second, if hospitals are nonprofit, then they can receive relief from payment of taxes, become the recipients of philanthropic contributions (which are tax deductible), accept volunteers, who provide services at no charge, and receive substantial government subsidies, such as from the Hill-Burton program. In addition, the physicians can receive the assistance of interns and residents, for whom they do not have to pay salaries, and receive the benefits of their services. The effect of these various subsidies is to cause hospital costs to be lower than what they would otherwise be. If physicians are concerned with the total price of care that the patient pays, then they would favor subsidies to their inputs of production. If physicians were to own (or use) a for-profit hospital, then they would have to pay the market price for the inputs used in production. By having the hospital input subsidized, it becomes relatively cheaper to expand the hospital input when there is an increase in demand for medical care. Further, if the physicians own the hospital, then the larger that hospital becomes, and the greater becomes the number of physicians associated with it (or who share in its ownership), the less incentive each physician has to be concerned with the hospital's costs because the effect of any savings (or profit) on any one physician is so small. The advantages of for-profit ownership decline as the size of hospital and the number of physicians increase (9). Another advantage to the physician is that the nonprofit hospital can only use surplus funds internally. Hospitals would have to use a criterion other than profitability for the investment of their funds. In lieu of profitability, the hospitals (the board of trustees and the managers) would settle upon prestige as a goal, which would also be consistent with the investment objectives of the hospital's staff physicians. The institution would be more willing to invest in duplicative services and facilities than if it were accountable to stockholders.

A last advantage to the physicians of the nonprofit situation is that they will retain a stronger control over the decisionmaking within the hospital. In viewing medical societies as cartels of physicians, it is important to examine the principle that the cartel always has to control the amount of output produced by each of its members. The individual has an incentive to increase output, since the costs of doing so are less than the cartel's profit-maximizing price, and unless the cartel can prevent its members from expanding their output, the monopoly price will fall. Since there are so many physicians, it is relatively costly to monitor the output of individual physicians in their offices (though the cartel can limit inputs contributing to increased production, i.e., which personnel can practice medicine). It is far easier to limit the number of hospital beds per physician, which also acts as a constraint on the physician's productivity. By controlling the number of hospital beds, the medical society limits competition among physicians for patients. Limiting the number of hospital beds, however, makes them a scarce resource. If the physicians were to bid for these scarce inputs, it would transfer income from the physician to the hospital. To retain these monopoly profits for themselves, the physicians, who control the hospital, use a form of nonprice rationing, by seniority or some other standard, to distribute the scarce hospital privileges among themselves (10).

There are a number of important policy implications in a behavioral model of hospitals which states that hospitals are controlled by the physicians to increase their incomes. First, since the payment for hospital services is separated from the payment for physician services, when the hospital was paid on a cost basis the physicians were neither financially responsible nor accountable for their decisions. There were no constraints on how the physician used the hospital or influenced its investment policies. Voluntary planning efforts to reduce unnecessary duplication could not be expected to succeed, since they were contrary to the physicians' interests. Cost-control policies that do not involve the physician can achieve only a limited success, since it is the physician who makes the treatment decisions that determine the hospital's costs (11). Unless reimbursement policies are related to the total price of medical care, with the physicians being held financially responsible and thereby having an incentive to minimize the cost of providing that care, the success of efforts at cost control in hospitals will be limited.

Another implication of the physician-control model is that as the number of physicians increases at a more rapid rate than in the past, less care will be provided in the hospital and more of it will be provided in the physician's office. Referring back to Figure 10-5, on isoquants, it was shown that physician and hospital inputs are somewhat substitutable for each other. Again, if payments for medical care are based on the total price of that care, e.g., a capitation payment per individual, then the physician can retain more of those funds if less is paid to the hospital. Owing both to limits on the increase in hospital beds and an increase in the number of physicians desiring access to hospital beds, physicians will begin substituting more of their own input in the provision of medical care. (This assumes, however, that the total amount to be spent for medical care per patient is limited and what gets spent on other inputs is no longer available to the physician.) Unless reimbursement policies consider the various incentive effects of physicians, their effect may not only be different from but the opposite of what was intended (12).

CONCLUDING COMMENTS

An examination of the behavioral objectives of hospitals was undertaken because of the effects on economic efficiency of different hospital objectives. Some of the hospital and the physician-control models provide consistent explanations of hospital decisionmaking. Because the determination of prices and investment in duplicative facilities are predicted by several models, it is difficult to conclusively determine the accuracy of certain of the models. Assuming that either the utility-maximizing model or the physician-control model is the more accurate representation of hospital behavior, what are the effects of these objectives on hospital efficiency?

It would appear that the output mix of the hospital industry would not be optimal. There is likely to be a bias toward higher "quality," meaning more facilities and services, greater capital intensity, and a tendency to introduce new technology before its benefits have been fully evaluated. The quantity–quality output mix of the hospital is likely to be different from what patients would be willing to pay for if they were to bear a greater share of the costs of hospitalization and had greater choice in this selection. As a result of the hospitals' desire to enhance prestige or the physicians' desire to enhance their income by increasing their productivity, there is also likely to be unnecessary duplication of facilities and services; that is, to the extent that there are economies of scale in operating certain services, more institutions are likely to be operating at higher costs than necessary because of low use of facilities. There will be system inefficiency, meaning that there are too many firms (facilities and services) operating in the industry. There is also likely to be firm inefficiency because of the desire for slack in the manager's utility function (and because the return to each physician declines, the larger the institution is). When a large percentage of the population is covered by hospital insurance, with payment methods based on each hospital's costs, it is less important for the hospital managers to minimize their costs of operation. Finally, there are redistributive effects (both as a result of the methods used to set hospital prices, such as internal cross-subsidization, and the taxes that are raised to pay for the increase in hospital expenditures) in that the income is being redistributed from taxpayers to persons working directly and indirectly in the hospital sector.

Before examining methods whereby the economic efficiency of this sector may be improved, we shall examine data on hospital performance to determine how well the foregoing hospital behavioral models explain the hospital inflation that has been occurring.

INDICATORS OF HOSPITAL PERFORMANCE: HOSPITAL COST INFLATION

Rising costs have been the focus of recent public concern over the performance of the hospital industry. The explosive increase in hospital costs of the past 15 years, however it is measured, is for many prima facie evidence that the industry is performing poorly and that intervention is needed. Various theories have been advanced to explain the rise in hospital costs, each one with different implications for what, if anything, ought to be done to improve future industry performance. In order to select the most accurate of these theories, we must examine closely the evidence available on hospital cost increases. What follows is a look at the components of hospital cost inflation,* and an evaluation of the various theories advanced to explain it.

Even before cost increase became as controversial an issue as it is today, hospital industry performance was often criticized on other grounds, including cost variations among similar hospitals and facility duplication. In its 1967 report, the National Advisory Commission on Health Manpower cited data on two groups of hospitals to indicate the extent of cost variation (13). One group was comprised of community hospitals with from 100 to 400 beds in a single metropolitan area. Costs per patient were found to be distributed almost evenly over a range of $43 to $65. The highest-cost hospital was 50 percent more expensive than the lowest on a per-patient-day basis, despite the fact that it provided fewer services. The second group included 12 hospitals providing excellent services, with a staff of nearly equivalent quality. Costs per patient day ranged from $54 to $110, with such differences remaining even after adjustments for wage and salary differentials were made.

The second feature often criticized, the low use rates of expensive specialized facilities in many hospitals, has frequently been cited as an indication of the hospital industry's poor performance. It is argued that in many cases several hospitals in a community are equipped with the same facility, even though one

---

* As many analysts have noted, the term inflation may be misleading in this context. Inflation normally refers to increases in the price or cost of an unchanged product, but part of the increase in hospital costs has been related to changes in the nature of the product.

or two such facilities would easily accommodate the community's need. Since it is likely that average costs per use fall as a facility goes from low to nearly full utilization, providing a service in a large number of underutilized facilities would be less efficient than providing it in a few facilities operating at a minimum average cost. The extra costs of maintaining underutilized facilities should, of course, be balanced against the advantages of providing the service in more locations; such advantages might be considerable if a facility is used in emergency situations. In spite of these considerations, duplication of facilities and services has raised the cost of hospital care without providing compensating benefits.

Critics often cite the example of open heart surgery when making this argument. In 1969, 23 percent of all hospitals with facilities for open heart surgery performed less than one surgery per month, and 71 percent performed less than one per week (14). Radiation therapy would also seem to be excessively duplicated. A study of radiation therapy in New Hampshire, Massachusetts, and Rhode Island revealed that 20 out of the 67 hospitals equipped to provide radiation therapy in 1969 were providing 93 percent of all the treatments. The authors conclude that five major centers might be adequate to accommodate all the needs for radiation therapy in the three states without seriously inconveniencing patients (15).

This kind of criticism might apply even to maternity care. Survey data collected by the American Hospital Association indicate that on the average, newborn occupancy is only about 40 percent of the rate hospitals are equipped to handle (16). Teh-wei Hu has estimated a cost function for maternity care, based on data from 30 nonprofit hospitals in Pennsylvania (17). He found that most of the hospitals were operating at much smaller outputs than those associated with minimum average costs. His estimated cost function indicated a minimum average cost point at 1,616 deliveries per year, while the average annual number of actual deliveries in the sample hospitals was just under 1,000.

Large cost variations among apparently similar hospitals and the existence of underutilized facilities and services suggest that there may be extensive inefficiency in the hospital industry. It may be that equivalent output could be produced with fewer resources if they were used more efficiently. Part of the cost increase experienced in hospitals may be attributable to increases in the waste of resources. Cost-increasing changes in hospital resource use presumably have improved the quality of care; for example, increases in nurse-patient ratios should increase the attention provided to individual patients. Similarly, adding a new facility to a community's already underutilized facilities provides a quality improvement by increasing a unit's accessibility to nearby residents in emergencies. Still, it is important to ask whether improvements in quality have always justified their high marginal costs. Current methods of financing hospital care lack strong incentives for consumers, doctors, or the hospitals themselves to weigh the true costs of resource allocation decisions for hospital care. Thus, even decisions which improve the quality of hospital care may often reflect less than optimal industry performance.

Although the discussion that follows focuses on the issue of hospital cost inflation, these other aspects of hospital behavior should not be neglected in evaluating alternative theories to explain the industry's performance.

BACKGROUND OF HOSPITAL COST INFLATION

The difficulty of measuring hospital output is well recognized. In order to discuss cost trends, we must focus on the cost of some unit. The units most commonly chosen for cost comparisons are patient days and admissions, i.e., cases. Neither one is in any sense a homogeneous unit; changes in the nature of the average patient day or the average case may have important effects on costs. Still, they are useful measures for some purposes, and they are the only single measures of the quantity of output we have. For other purposes, the size of the population receiving care may be a more useful output measure. Major payors for hospital care are probably more interested in total costs or costs per capita than costs per patient day or per admission, since their total pay-outs depend on total hospital expenses for the covered population.

Table 10-7 presents some basic statistics on several commonly cited measures of hospital costs since 1950. The first of these measures is the hospital semiprivate room charge index calculated as a component of the consumer price index (CPI) by the U.S. Bureau of Labor Statistics. It is a measure of changes over time in the basic daily room rate, without inclusion of charges for ancillary services, based on information from a sample of hospitals.*

The other measures in Table 10-7 are all based on data collected by the American Hospital Association (AHA) in its annual survey of hospitals, and all are expressed in dollars. The figures reported in the table are for nonfederal short-term general and other special hospitals. The first three of these measures—expense per patient day, expense per adjusted patient day, and expense per admission—are often cited as measures of hospital prices or unit costs. Expenses per patient day are merely the total expenses of hospitals divided by the total number of inpatient days provided. Since total expenses include those for outpatient care, expense per patient day gives a somewhat misleading picture of the average cost of a day of hospital care. Therefore, the AHA calculates an adjusted expense per patient day by converting the number of outpatient visits into patient days according to the ratio of the average revenue per outpatient visit to the average revenue per inpatient day. This adjustment has been criticized as arbitrary, since the revenue ratio may not reflect the ratio of the costs of outpatient visits to inpatient days. (An expense per adjusted admission figure can also be calculated that adjusts the number of admissions for outpatient volume in a manner similar to that in which patient days are adjusted in the expense per adjusted patient day calculation.)

The last two measures in Table 10-7 represent the hospitals' total expenses. The first is in per capita terms (dividing by the U.S. civilian population) and the second is merely total hospital expenses. These measures make no attempt to separate quantity from price changes.

Although each of the cost measures in Table 10-7 is somewhat different from the others, all show similar patterns of increase over time. The trends in these measures of hospital costs over time suggest the following:

---

*The BLS began publishing an index of hospital charges based on charges for a larger number of services in 1972. This index was discontinued in 1977 and an even more comprehensive hospital index replaced it.

TABLE 10-7. Measures of Hospital Costs and Percentage Rates of Increase, 1950–1980

Calendar Year	CPI Semiprivate Room Charge Level	CPI Semiprivate Room Charge Annual Percent Increase	Expense Per Patient Day Level	Expense Per Patient Day Annual Percent Increase	Expense Per Adjusted Patient Day[a] Level	Expense Per Adjusted Patient Day[a] Annual Percent Increase	Expense Per Admission Level	Expense Per Admission Annual Percent Increase	Expense Per Capita Level	Expense Per Capita Annual Percent Increase	Total Expenses (in Millions) Level	Total Expenses (in Millions) Annual Percent Increase
1950	30.3		15.62				127.23		14.06		2,120	
1955	42.3	6.9	23.12	8.1			179.79	7.1	21.07	8.4	3,434	10.1
1960	57.3	6.3	32.23	6.8			244.54	6.4	31.53	8.4	5,617	10.3
1965	75.9	5.8	44.48	6.6	40.56		345.65	7.1	47.73	8.7	9,147	10.3
1966	83.5	10.0	48.15	8.3	43.66	7.6	382.05	10.5	53.12	11.3	10,276	12.3
1967	100.0	19.8	54.08	12.3	49.46	13.3	447.64	17.2	61.87	16.5	12,081	17.6
1968	113.6	13.6	61.38	13.5	55.80	12.8	519.21	16.0	71.84	16.1	14,162	16.4
1969	128.8	13.4	70.03	14.1	64.26	15.2	587.99	13.2	83.42	16.1	16,613	17.3
1970	145.4	12.4	81.01	15.7	73.73	14.7	668.67	13.7	96.97	16.2	19,560	17.7
1971	163.1	12.2	92.13	13.9	83.43	13.2	743.15	11.1	109.67	13.1	22,400	14.5
1972	173.9	6.6	105.21	14.0	94.61	13.4	830.13	11.7	123.75	12.8	25,549	14.1
1973	182.1	4.7	114.69	9.0	101.78	7.6	897.20	8.1	136.94	10.7	28,496	11.5
1974	201.5	10.7	128.05	11.6	113.21	11.2	994.17	11.1	156.19	14.1	32,751	14.9
1975	236.1	17.2	151.42	18.3	133.08	17.6	1,166.80	17.4	184.97	18.4	39,110	19.4
1976	268.6	13.8	172.59	14.0	151.28	13.7	1,324.28	13.5	206.61	11.7	45,116	15.4
1977	299.5	11.5	198.06	13.9	173.18	13.6	1,508.81	13.2	237.65	13.0	51,832	14.2
1978	331.6	10.7	222.02	12.1	193.77	11.9	1,687.58	11.9	264.62	11.3	58,348	12.6
1979	370.3	11.7	248.73	12.0	215.61	11.3	1,882.37	11.5	296.79	12.2	66,184	13.4
1980	418.9	13.1	281.92	13.3	244.92	13.6	2,126.36	13.0	341.18	15.0	76,970	16.3

Sources: © American Hospital Association, *Hospital Statistics*, 1981 ed. (Chicago: American Hospital Association, 1981), p. 5; for data on civilian population, U.S. Bureau of Census, *Statistical Abstract of the United States, 1980* (Washington, D.C.: Government Printing Office, 1980), p. 6; and *Current Population Reports*, Series p. 25, No. 901 (July 1981); for CPI data, Bureau of Labor Statistics, *CPI Detailed Report*, various issues.

Note: Definitions of terms are explained in the text. The hospital data are for nonfederal short-term general and other special hospitals.

[a]Unavailable prior to 1963.

1. The phenomenon of rapidly rising hospital costs is not new. Throughout the 1950s, hospital costs rose 6 to 9 percent annually, on the average, depending on which measure you choose to look at. Hospital cost increases were 4 to 5 percent per year greater than the all-items CPI, which is considered the best available general index of the prices of the things that consumers buy.

2. A marked speedup in the rate of increase in hospital costs occurred after 1966. Although rates of cost increase from 1960 to 1965 remained about what they had been in the 1950s, the rates of increase in all measures of hospital costs in Table 10-7 accelerated in 1966, and even more markedly in 1967. This acceleration is also evident when costs are measured in relation to the rest of the economy.

   Concern over rising hospital costs has heightened considerably since 1966. This is understandable both because rates of increase since then have been much larger than they had been previously and because continued rapid increases have produced a tremendous growth in the total number of dollars involved—each percentage increase in costs amounts to a much larger number of dollars than it did in the 1950s. Cost increases also became more visible after 1966 because since then a larger share of hospital expenditures has been financed out of government budgets. The Medicare program, under which the federal government finances hospital care for the aged, was initiated in mid-1966.* The striking association between this event and the acceleration in hospital costs strongly suggests a cause-and-effect relationship.

3. Since 1967, the increase in hospital costs has abated only during the 1972–1974 period. A fall in the rate of increase in hospital costs relative to the rest of the economy occurred in 1973, in response to the price controls imposed by the Economic Stabilization Program (ESP) (18). After 1974, cost increases returned to their more familiar post-1966 rates, and there is as yet little indication of another slowdown.

4. The trend in hospital costs leveled out during the late 1970s. Then, starting in 1981, hospital cost increases resumed their sharp rate of increase. The reasons given for this slowdown in costs was the threat effect of federal controls on hospitals and the subsequent voluntary effort (VE) started by hospitals. The Carter Administration proposed cost controls on hospitals. Fearing the imposition of these controls, hospitals were reluctant to increase their costs. Hospitals also started the VE as a means of limiting hospital cost increases. A voluntary effort, however, can last just so long, and when the Reagan Administration began, it was believed that President Reagan would be opposed to hospital cost controls. As the political threat diminished, hospital costs began to increase. To limit its growing budgetary commitment under Medicare and Medicaid, however, the Reagan Administration, like previous administrations, has proposed limits on hospital cost increases.

   Figure 10-6 provides a graphical representation of the trends in three of the measures of hospital costs relative to the CPI since 1960. The hospital room charge index, the expense per patient day, and the expense per adjusted patient

---

*The Medicaid program, under which the federal government assists the states in financing medical care for the poor, began at about the same time, but became important slowly over the following years.

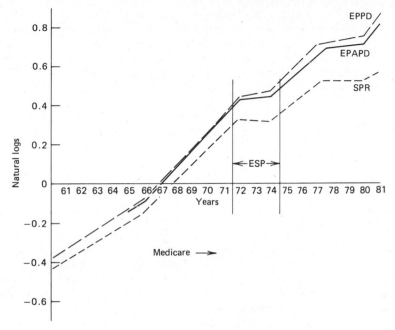

Figure 10-6. Trends in hospital costs 1960–1981. *Preliminary estimates. EPPD, expense per patient day; EPAPD, expense per adjusted patient day; SPR, semiprivate room charge; ESP, Economic Stabilization Program.

day are all deflated by the all-items CPI and scaled to equal one in 1967. The natural logarithm of each of these three series is then plotted as a function of time. The transformation of logarithms is carried out because it allows a constant rate of growth to show up as a linear trend. The figure clearly points out how similar the trends in these cost measures have been since 1960. It also shows how closely major changes in the growth rate of hospital costs have been associated with the beginning of the Medicare program and with the ESP. A plotting of the expense-per-admission series would look very similar to those series included in the figure.

THE COMPONENTS OF HOSPITAL COST INFLATION

We now take a closer look at how the components of hospital costs have increased over time. It is followed by a summary and evaluation of attempts to explain *why* costs have increased so rapidly, in which particular attention is paid to economists' attempts to model the process of hospital cost inflation using economic theory and empirical data.

Total hospital expenses (TE) equal the size of the population (POP) times the average expenses per capita (EPC). EPC, in turn, equals the average number of patient days per capita (PDCAP) and average expenses per patient day (EPPD). EPPD equals labor expenses per patient day, which is the price of labor

(PL) times quantity of labor (QL), and nonlabor expenses per patient day. The percentage change in TE can be approximated by summing the percentage changes in each of its components. A given percentage change in POP or PDCAP results in an equal percentage change in TE, other things held constant, while changes in the prices and quantities of labor and nonlabor inputs effect TE in relation to the proportion that labor expenses (LE/TE) and nonlabor expenses (NE/TE) have to total expenses. Such an accounting breakdown does not explain *why* expenses change, but it may provide clues to such an explanation.

Table 10-8 shows the average percentage increase in each of the components in total expense over various periods between 1960 and 1980. The remainder of this section reviews the percentage increases in these components and the change in their relative weights. Between the years 1966 and 1980, total expenses in short-term general and other special hospitals increased about 15.5 percent per year. (By 1980, 1 percent of expenses amounted to over $750 million.) Part of this increase in total expenses can be accounted for by increases in population and by increases in per capita utilization. During the 1966–1980 period, the U.S. civilian population grew at about 1.1 percent per year. Per capita utilization of hospitals increased .6 percent per year on the average. In the years immediately following the introduction of Medicare, 1966 and 1967, patient days per capita increased by more than 3 percent per year. However, since then the percent increases have fluctuated and in 1972 actually decreased by 1.4 percent. Overall, increases in inpatient utilization have accounted for a relatively small portion, approximately 13 percent, of the total increase in hospital expenses in the post-Medicare period. Expenses per patient day have increased about 13.5 percent per year from 1966 to 1980, accounting for about 87 percent of the total increase in hospital expenses.

Since the largest contributor to increases in total hospital expenses is expenses per patient day, it is useful to examine the percent changes in each of its components. We will try to separate price increases from input increases, with respect first to labor and then to nonlabor expenses. In the 1966–1980 period, labor expenses per patient day increased 12.9 percent per year on the average.* Wages (per patient day) increased at a rate of 9.8 percent per year, and personnel per 100 census at a rate of 2.8 percent. Some of the increase in personnel must be attributed to the expansion of outpatient activity, which increased about 4.9 percent per year, but personnel per adjusted 100 census still increased by about 2.5 percent per year during this period. After separating wage changes from changes in the quantity of labor, it appears, first, that labor expenses per patient day increased somewhat less rapidly than total expenses per patient day in the 1966–1980 period (12.9 as compared to 13.5 percent per year), and, second, that most of the increases in labor expenses—about three-quarters of it—is accounted for by wage changes.

However, these AHA figures provide an imperfect basis for estimating changes in the price and quantity of labor used by hospitals per patient day. For one thing, the payroll data reported underestimate labor expenses up to 1970 by excluding payments for employee benefits. The AHA payroll figures also ex-

---

*Starting in 1971, the AHA included employee benefits as part of labor expenses. By 1980 employee benefits represented 16 percent of labor expenditures.

TABLE 10-8. Annual Percentage Changes in Hospital Expenses by Component, Selected Periods

							Labor				Nonlabor	
Period	TE	POP	PDCAP	EPPD	LE/TE	LEPPD	PL	QLPPD		NE/TE	NEPPD
1960–1966	10.6	1.4	2.1	6.8	.62	6.5	4.0	2.4		.38	7.4
1966–1980	15.5	1.1	.6	13.5	.59	12.9	9.8	2.8		.41	14.4
1966–1971	16.9	1.3	1.2	14.0	.60	14.9	11.7	2.9		.40	12.6
1971–1974	13.5	1.0	.7	11.5	.62	9.9	6.9	2.8		.38	14.3
1974–1975	19.4	1.0	.0	18.2	.60	15.6	11.4	3.8		.40	22.4
1975–1976	16.1	1.0	.0	15.0	.59	13.0	10.2	2.5		.41	17.8
1976–1977	14.2	1.0	−.8	13.9	.58	12.2	8.2	3.7		.42	16.1
1977–1978	12.6	1.1	−.7	12.1	.57	11.5	8.5	2.7		.43	12.9
1978–1979	13.4	1.1	.1	12.0	.57	11.7	9.0	2.5		.43	12.5
1979–1980	16.3	1.2	1.5	13.3	.57	12.1	10.3	1.6		.43	15.0

Source: © American Hospital Association, *Hospital Statistics*, 1981 ed. (Chicago: American Hospital Association, 1981), p. 5; for data on civilian population, U.S. Bureau of Census, *Statistical Abstract of the United States, 1980* (Washington, D.C.: Government Printing Office, 1980), p. 6; and *Current Population Reports*, Series p. 25, No. 901 (July 1981).

Abbreviations: TE, total hospital expenditures; POP, U.S. civilian population; PDCAP, patient days per capita; EPPD, expenses per patient day; PL, price of labor; QLPPD, quantity of labor per patient day; LE, labor expenses; LEPPD, labor expenditures per patient day; NE, nonlabor expenses; NEPPD, nonlabor expenditures per patient day.

231

clude payments to interns, residents, and other physicians, whose numbers are also excluded from the Full Time Equivalent Personnel (FTE) figures. Payments to all physicians also represent a relatively small fraction of total hospital expenses, perhaps less than 5 percent on the average.

Distinguishing increased wages from increased numbers of personnel makes no allowance for the change in the mix of employees. Hospitals employ many types of workers including administrators, clerical workers, housekeepers, food service workers, orderlies, technicians, and nurses with various levels of skill. Since the average wage may be influenced by changes in the skill mix of labor, it may be misleading to interpret wage changes that have been averaged over all workers as an indication of changes in the price of labor. For example, if a hospital replaced a number of registered nurses (RNs) with a larger number of licensed practical nurses (LPNs), its average wages would fall, though its labor prices would be unchanged. At the same time, its number of FTEs would increase, though it is not clear that the quantity of labor employed—holding skill level constant—has actually increased. In general, if hospital employees' average level of skill has declined over time, average wage data understate the increase in the price of labor, and increases in FTEs overstate the increase in the quantity of labor. Just the opposite is true if the average level of skill is increasing.

Unfortunately, relatively little is known about how the skill mix of hospital employees has changed over time. Martin Feldstein has presented some evidence that employment expanded more in the lower wage categories than in the higher ones during the 1960s and early 1970s (19). The evidence was based on BLS surveys of nongovernmental hospitals in several metropolitan areas. Indices of wages increased faster than the AHA average annual earnings figures from 1960 to 1972. Average earnings for all workers will increase more slowly than the average earnings of any class of workers if the lower-paid classes expand relative to the more highly paid. On the other hand, a skill-mix index calculated by the AHA for a sample of 594 hospitals from 1969 to 1974 showed a slight increase during the period (20). The index was a weighted sum of the proportions of hospital services performed by each of four categories of employees, with the weights being the average wages of each category in 1969.

The increase in nonlabor expenses per patient day must be analyzed even more cautiously. The most commonly cited data on nonlabor expenses of hospitals are the AHA figures on nonpayroll expenses—that is, the difference between total and payroll expenses. As mentioned previously, payments for employee benefits (prior to 1971) and payments to physicians (including interns and residents) are not included in labor expenses, so they must show up in nonpayroll expenses, leading to an overestimate of nonlabor expenses. However, since the early 1970s, it appears that the percentage of hospital expenses going to nonlabor inputs has been growing.

It is also difficult to break down the increase in nonlabor expenses per patient day into increases in quantity of inputs and increases in input prices. Hospital spokesmen have long contended that the mix of inputs they purchase is very different from that purchased by other industries, and that it is therefore unfair to deflate their nonlabor expenses by some general price index such as the CPI or the Wholesale Price Index (WPI) to get an estimate of the increase in the quantity of nonlabor inputs used. It has been suggested that the prices of goods that hospitals buy have generally risen faster than the overall price level.

TABLE 10-9. Estimated Weights and Indices Used for Hospital Nonlabor Expenses, 1977

Expense Category	Weight[a]	Sources
Professional fees: medical	10.85	CPI
Depreciation	9.76	Bureau of Economic Analysis
Interest	4.89	Prime rate and domestic bond yields
Malpractice	4.87	American Hospital Association
Dietary	7.64	CPI and PPI
Fuel	5.14	PPI, Energy Information Administration, American Gas Association
Drugs	6.04	PPI
Surgical, medical instruments, and supplies and other supplies	16.38	PPI
Business services	10.03	CPI
Miscellaneous	24.43	CPI, BLS Employment Cost Index
Total	100.03[a]	

Source: Mark Freeland, Carol Schendler, and Gerard Anderson, "Regional Hospital Input Price Indexes," *Health Care Financing Review* 3 (December 1981): 27–28, Table 1.

Abbreviations: CPI, Consumer Price Index; PPI, Producer Price Index; BLS, Bureau of Labor Statistics. This table is on abridgement of Table 1 cited in the source. Several of the expense categories listed in the source's table were condensed into more general categories for this table. For a more detailed exposition of the components of nonlabor hospital expenses refer to source.

[a]Estimated weight of nonlabor expenses in total expenses = 41.09.

Table 10-9 gives a breakdown of nonlabor expenses by component, based on the weights and the indices used for each component. The weights are only estimates of the percentages of each component in total nonlabor expenses (we estimate the nonlabor expenses to be about 40 percent of total expense, so that if the weights in Table 10-9 are divided by 2.5, they yield the percentages of total expenses). It is interesting to note that if these weights are even approximately correct, they indicate that three frequently cited sources of increased costs— food, fuel, and malpractice insurance—are still rather small portions of the total expenses.* According to these figures, for example, a full 20 percent rise in food prices would, in itself, increase total costs per day by only about .6 percent. A 20 percent rise in fuel prices, disregarding the feedback effects on other prices, would have only two-thirds that effect on total costs per day.

Although they are not definitive, studies attempting to develop nonlabor price indices that specifically apply to hospitals have found little evidence to support the hypothesis that hospital nonlabor input prices have risen substantially faster than prices in the general economy. M. Feldstein, for example, has calculated a nonlabor price index, using as quantity weights, data from the 1963 U.S. input-output table on the purchases of the hospital industry from other industries (21). Indices of the prices of the various components were derived

---

*Good data are not available, but it appears that malpractice insurance premiums paid by hospitals have increased tremendously—perhaps over 400 percent on the average, between 1972 and 1977. It seems unlikely, however, based on data from AHA surveys, that malpractice insurance premiums represented more than about 4 or 5 percent of hospital nonlabor expenses in 1977.

from a number of sources; several were unpublished deflators calculated by the U.S. Department of Commerce for manufacturing industries, others were components of the CPI or WPI. The resulting index was found to track very closely to the all-items CPI during the period under study, 1958–1967. Several other studies of hospital input prices have been conducted to aid particular states in setting hospital reimbursement formulas (22). The AHA has also developed a national index of hospital nonlabor input prices, drawing on the work of these researchers in individual states (23). The Health Care Financing Administration also constructs a National Hospital Input Price Index. Table 10-9 is based on data from this index.

Perhaps it is worthwhile to emphasize that increases in the use of nonlabor inputs per patient day need not take exclusively the form of increases in physical quantities of inputs, such as increases in the quantity of food served, laundry processed, laboratory tests performed, energy consumed, and so on, per patient day. A large portion of what are measured as increases in input intensity are undoubtedly substitutions from a lower to a higher quality of inputs. The kinds of diagnostic tests performed change over time and more expensive (and presumably better) methods replace less expensive ones; for example, new, more expensive drugs replace older ones. The continued insistence of hospital administrators that the prices of the things they purchase have been rising faster than prices in the general economy may reflect in part a lumping together of the marginal costs of changes in the quality of inputs with pure price changes.

When the trend in the proportion of nonlabor expenses to total expenses (NE/TE) is examined in Table 10-8, it is obvious that labor inputs have been declining in importance over time relative to nonlabor inputs. This trend contradicts the hypothesis that rising labor costs are the primary cause of hospital inflation.

It seems evident that increases in the quantity of inputs used have been an important source of increases in hospital expenses per patient day, particularly since 1966. In fact, if there had been no increase in the number of workers employed per patient day, and if nonlabor expense per patient day had increased at the same rate as the CPI, total expense per patient day would have increased only about half as much as it did from 1966 to 1980.* Any attempt to explain why hospitals' costs have increased so rapidly must first explain why input intensity has increased so considerably.

THEORIES OF HOSPITAL COST INFLATION

Wage-Push (or Catching-Up) Hypothesis

The theory that the upward push of wages is an important force behind the overall increase in costs has been prevalent in the hospital literature for some time. This wage-push theory has intuitive appeal for several reasons. Since the hospital industry is labor intensive, changes in average wage levels affect a large portion of total costs. Historically, hospital workers are believed to have been

---

*Using a 60 percent–40 percent breakdown between labor and nonlabor expenses, the actual numbers are a 121 percent hypothetical increase compared with a 217 percent actual increase.

underpaid relative to other workers, and therefore relatively rapid increases in hospital wages are explained as a catching-up with wages in other industries. Further, changes in labor productivity in the hospital industry are thought to lag behind that of most other industries. As hospitals begin to match wage increases granted in other industries in the absence of an offsetting rise in productivity, the net effect is rising hospital costs.

The analysis presented in the previous section indicated that rising wages have by no means been the only contributor to hospital cost increases since 1950. Both the number of employees per patient day and the use of nonlabor inputs have increased throughout the period. Since the rate of hospital cost increase accelerated after 1966, nonlabor expenses have actually increased faster than labor expenses, while the number of employees per patient day has increased even faster than previously. Nonetheless, average wages in hospitals have increased relative to the wages of all private nonagricultural workers throughout the post-1950 period, with the exception of 1971–1974. This phenomenon and the catching-up hypothesis deserve further investigation.

Martin Feldstein has used data collected by the Bureau of Labor Statistics to investigate whether hospital employees were underpaid relative to other workers in the past, and how the situation changed between 1957 and 1972 (24). For types of workers also employed in substantial numbers outside the hospital industry, such as clerical workers and housekeepers, he compared wages of hospital workers with those of nonhospital workers in several metropolitan areas for which data were available. He found that in 1957 hospital employees did in fact receive lower wages—the differential was more than 20 percent in a number of jobs and locations. However, by 1964 hospital personnel were often paid more than nonhospital personnel of the same type. In spite of this, hospital workers from 1969 to 1972 continued to make greater wage gains than other industry workers.

By comparing the rates of wage increase of different types of hospital workers during the 1963–1972 period, M. Feldstein also found that percentage increases in the wages of more highly skilled hospital personnel, such as professional nurses and technical workers (administrative workers were not included in the BLS surveys), were at least as great as those of less skilled personnel. Wage gains were not disproportionately large among the lowest-paid workers. Using a different data base and methodology Victor Fuchs essentially corroborated M. Feldstein's findings. He too found evidence of catching-up during the 1960s and concluded that "health workers, starting at a relatively low wage level in 1954, had risen by 1969 to a point of almost parity with other industries" (25). Hospital workers in particular were found to have made larger gains than health workers in general. In fact, by 1969, registered nurses in hospitals earned on the average 24 percent *more* than other workers of the same sex, color, age, and schooling.

These findings by M. Feldstein and V. Fuchs reveal that hospital workers were generally paid less in the past than workers in other industries with similar functions or apparently similar qualifications, and that hospital workers made substantial relative gains in the 1960s. The catching-up hypothesis does not indicate why these differentials existed to begin with, or why wages of hospital workers increased more rapidly in the 1950s or 1960s. If hospitals had traditionally been able to obtain sufficient manpower while paying relatively low wages, why are they no longer able to do so? The catching-up hypothesis also does not explain why hospital wages have continued to increase more rapidly than wages in other industries—except during the period of the ESP—even though M. Feldstein and V. Fuchs both suggest that they had essentially caught up by 1969.*

Another problem with the catching-up hypothesis is that it does not explain why hospitals have increased their use of labor and nonlabor inputs per patient day so rapidly. Based on the analysis already presented, it seems clear that a large portion of the increases in hospital costs per patient day have been due to increases in input use. Thus, the reasons for increased input use need to be explained if the process of hospital cost inflation is to be understood, and if optimal policies toward the hospital industry are to be developed.

It might be argued that increased input intensity was a result of a change in the type of hospital care demanded. For example, an increase in the number of older people in the population would require a more intensive type of hospital care than that required for younger persons. However, despite the fact that the average age of the population has increased, it seems unlikely that changes in the population mix have been responsible for a very large portion of the increase in input use in hospitals. An index of demographic structure in which the proportions of the population in each of 16 age, sex, and color classes were weighted by hospital admission rates in 1963–1964, changed less than 1 percent between 1950 and 1968 (26). A similar index using six age classes and 1970 admission rates as weights increased about 4.5 percent from 1960 to 1974 (27). The increases would be slightly larger if patient day rates were used as weights, since average length of stay also increases with age, as do admission rates. Patient days and admissions, however, increased more than 20 percent on a per capita basis between 1960 and 1974; this is greater than would be expected on the basis of changes in the structure of the population. Further, given such large increases in utilization, it is difficult to see how small changes in the age structure of the population could have led to much larger increases in the use of inputs per patient day.

A further problem with the catching-up hypothesis as a theory of hospital cost inflation is that it does not provide an explanation for the rapid adoption of medical technology, which has been frequently suggested as an explanation for rising hospital costs. Medical technology has made possible the treatment of illnesses previously considered untreatable, and has provided new and presumably higher-quality treatments for other conditions—often at much higher costs than the methods it has replaced. The diffusion of entirely new technologies does not account for a large portion of the tremendous increase in hospital input

---

*One study attempted to determine the different reasons hospital wages increased between 1960–1975. Separate analyses were conducted for the different occupational categories, such as RNs and LPNs. The explanatory factors were of two types: those factors affecting the supply of employees, such as minimum wage laws, unionization, and licensure requirements; and those factors affecting the demand for employees, such as third-party reimbursement, income levels in the area, and physician availability. The results indicated that both supply and demand factors had positive effects on wages of hospital employees. With respect to unionization, it was estimated that when hospital employee groups unionized, wages increased 6.5 percent for RNs, 16.1 percent for LPNs, and 17.6 percent for aides and orderlies. Frank Sloan and Bruce Steinwald, *Hospital Labor Markets* (Lexington, Mass.: Lexington Books, 1980), Chapter 3.

use. Instead these increases can be explained by increases in nursing time devoted to each patient, more intensive use of basic ancillary services (laboratory tests, x-rays), and efforts to improve hospital ambience. These findings are borne out by Anne Scitovsky and Nelda McCall's study, which found large increases in the average number of laboratory tests for such relatively straightforward cases as appendicitis and maternity care (28). Further, the upward trend in hospital personnel per patient day does not support the hypothesis that increases in input use have resulted primarily from the application of new technologies; hiring has not been disproportionately greater among highly skilled personnel.

Use of intensive care and coronary care units has grown since the late 1950s until, by 1974, it accounted for 4–5 percent of the short-term general hospitals' beds (29). Costs per patient day in these units have been conservatively estimated to be three times the average cost within the entire hospital. Although to some extent the high costs in these units reflect the use of equipment unavailable 20 years ago, such high costs are also related to the very intensive use of technologies which have been available for a long time. An intensive care unit might employ over six persons per bed, for example, half of them nurses, compared with an overall average of 2.5 employees per bed in 1975. It appears that the increase in input use is not simply the result of entirely new technology but the result of more hospitals adopting existing technology or using it more intensively.

Much of the increase in input use has apparently come about independently of important technological developments. Perhaps such general increases in the intensity of care are economically justifiable; perhaps their marginal benefits in terms of improved health outcomes and greater patient comfort exceed their marginal costs, or perhaps they do not. Are there underlying reasons for expecting rapid introduction of new technologies into the hospital industry at this time? What influences their rates of diffusion? Does the supplanting of one technique for treating an illness by another always represent a rational choice based on a cost-benefit comparison of the alternatives? An alternative theory of hospital cost inflation might provide a more satisfactory explanation of the adoption of existing and new technologies by hospitals.

A Demand-Pull Model of Hospital Cost Inflation

Economists have generally rejected the notion that hospital cost inflation can be fully or even largely explained by exogenous increases in input prices, changes in the population distribution, and increases in medical technology. Although economists do not agree on a precise theory or model of hospital cost inflation, they generally do agree that the growth of third-party payment of hospital care (payment for care by some party other than the person receiving it) has drastically changed the financial constraints under which hospitals operate. Explanations for why hospitals respond to changes in reimbursement by increasing their costs are more controversial. Two somewhat different theories of the inflationary process, both emphasizing the growth of third-party coverage, have emerged. Each of these theories, the demand-pull model, and variations on it will be discussed.

The percentages of hospital revenues coming from private insurance, government, and direct consumer payments have changed over time. In 1950, 50 percent of hospital revenues were paid for directly by consumers, but that share had been cut approximately in half by 1963, and more than cut in half again by 1980. Only about 9 cents of every dollar received by short-term general hospitals now comes directly from consumers. Through the 1950s and early 1960s, the growth of private insurance was responsible for the shift away from direct consumer payment, but since then the government's role as a third-party payor has grown relative both to consumer and private insurance. From 1963 to 1980, the government share increased from 18 to 54 percent because of the introduction of Medicare and Medicaid.

Rapid increases in the price of a product, coupled with small increases in the quantity consumed, suggest an obvious explanation: demand increasing along a relatively inelastic supply curve. The growth of demand pulls up prices as consumers bid for the available supply. (Upward shifts in supply along a fixed demand curve could produce rapid price increases, but even if demand were quite inelastic, some decrease in quantity consumed would be expected.) It therefore appears that the combination of rapidly increasing costs per patient day and per admission and slight increases in hospital utilization is a result of demand's increasing more rapidly than supply; hence, the demand-pull hypothesis.

If the demand-pull hypothesis is correct, enormous increases in the demand for hospital care must have been occurring since 1950. Although one can suggest several possible reasons why the demand for hospital care might increase, the most plausible is the spread of third-party coverage.

The experience following the introduction of Medicare in mid-1966 is consistent with a view that hospital utilization responds to changes in net price brought about by third-party coverage. At that time, insurance coverage for the elderly improved dramatically, while that of the rest of the population remained essentially unchanged. Survey data indicate that between the period July 1965– June 1966 and the year 1968, hospital admission rates decreased for every group except the elderly, for whom admission rates increased approximately 25 percent (30).

The early effects of Medicare on hospital use are illustrated in a study by John Rafferty (31). Using data from the 995 hospitals participating in the Professional Activity Study (PAS), he looked at changes in case-mix and length of stay for the 65-and-over and the under-65 groups that took place between the 18 months before and the 18 months after the introduction of Medicare. An index of changes in case mix was calculated for each group based on a weighted sum of the proportions of cases of different types, with the weights being the average lengths of stay in the corresponding case types in the base period. Under the assumption that case types with longer average lengths of stay are more severe and less elective, an increase in such a case-mix index indicates a shift to a more complex or severe mix of cases. Similarly, an index of changes in average length of stay was calculated for each group by weighting average lengths of stay in different case types by the proportions of cases of those types in the base period. In this way, an indication could be gotten of the changes in length of stay that are independent of case-mix changes. Comparing the period just after Medicare was introduced with the period just before, Rafferty found that the case mix became more severe and the (case-mix-adjusted) lengths of stay shorter for the under-65

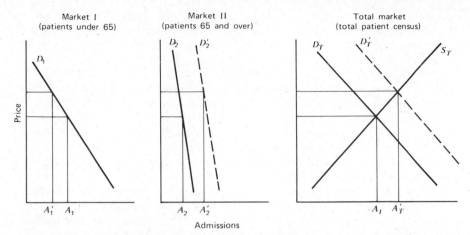

Figure 10-7. The effects of Medicare on hospital use, by age group. [John Rafferty, "Enfranchisement and Rationing Effects of Medicare on Discretionary Hospital Use." Reprinted with permission from *Health Services Research* 10(1) (Spring 1975): 52. Copyright 1975 by the Hospital Research and Educational Trust, 840 N. Lake Shore Drive, Chicago, Ill. 60611.]

population, while case mix remained about the same and length of stay increased for the over-65 group.

These findings are consistent with the following hypothesis, as depicted in Figure 10-7. The total demand for hospital care can be divided into demand by the under-65 group and demand by the 65-and-over group. The older group received a substantial subsidy with the introduction of Medicare, thereby shifting its demand curve from D_2 to D_2', while demand by the younger group remained essentially unchanged. The total demand curve thus shifted up, increasing equilibrium price (particularly if the supply of admissions was relatively inelastic). As price rose, some demand was choked off, and the net effect was an increase in admissions for the 65-and-over group, and a decrease for the younger group. One would expect the elimination of the least serious admissions in the under-65 group and a shortening of length of stay within case types. Rafferty's case-mix and length-of-stay findings suggest that they did act in just this way. While case mix apparently did not change much for the elderly, stays for given case types were lengthened, and this latter phenomenon is consistent with the notion that demand for hospital care increases as net price falls.

An examination of the evidence on hospital utilization before and after Medicare makes a demand-pull model of hospital cost inflation seem plausible. The model is not complete, however, unless it explains why hospitals have responded to demand increases as they have. An industry faced with increasing demand for its product would be expected to increase its output and its price. If the industry were monopolistic, or if increasing output was for some reason impossible, then firms would increase prices to ration demand at or near the existing level of output, thereby earning higher profits. Hospitals' response to increased demand has been somewhat different from either of these predicted outcomes. They have not expanded the number of patient days or admissions to any great extent, but they have adjusted their costs upward with their prices, and have changed the nature of the product they provide, using more inputs and presumably improving the quality of care.

Martin Feldstein, who has formulated and empirically estimated the most explicit demand-pull model of hospital cost inflation to date (32), attributes this response to the dominant role of nonprofit firms in the hospital industry. He asserts that hospital administrators pursue goals such as paying employees generously and equipping their hospital to provide the most advanced scientific medicine, partly in response to pressures from groups within their hospitals, and partly to enhance their own prestige. Owing to financial constraints, none of these goals is ever entirely satisfied. An increase in demand loosens these constraints and thus allows hospitals to go further in the pursuit of their goals. In specifying his model for empirical estimation, M. Feldstein assumes that hospitals will respond to increased demand by doing things which will increase their costs up to the highest level consistent with maintaining a desired level of occupancy.*

The manner of adjusting for an increase in demand in this model is depicted in a simplified way in Figure 10-8. Assume the market is initially in equilibrium at (Q_0, P_0). P_0 is the level of price (and cost) at which quantity demanded just fills the stock of beds to the desired rate of occupancy. Suppose demand shifts to $D'D'$ owing to an increase in insurance coverage. Assuming no further demand shifts and no change in the supply of beds, the new equilibrium point is (Q_0, P_2). But the full adjustment to the new equilibrium level will not be immediate, both because some of the steps that will ultimately increase costs (e.g., adding facilities) take time, and because hospitals may be uncertain about what the new level of demand is. The market may end up in the first year after an increase in demand at a point such as (Q_1, P_1), with hospitals running at a higher than desired level of occupancy. In later years adjustment will continue toward the final equilibrium, though by that time other shifts in demand may have moved the target.

This model of cost inflation has an important policy implication. Controls on particular components of costs can have essentially no effect on total cost increases, since these are determined by changes in demand and the supply of beds.† The rate of increase in input prices merely determines how much of the total increase in costs will go into input prices and how much will go into increasing the quantity of inputs used. Effective wage controls can only lead to a more rapid increase in input intensity than otherwise would have occurred.

Although the demand-pull model of hospital cost inflation appears to explain hospital cost increases in the post-Medicare period fairly well, this is not the case for the more recent cost experience of hospitals. It has been noted that

---

*In theory, hospitals are presumed also to choose the supply of beds within certain constraints. In estimating the model, however, M. Feldstein treats the bed supply as essentially exogenous.

†In the long run, changes in the relative prices of beds and other inputs might influence the choice of bed supply and thus affect the equilibrium cost per patient day. Also, if increases in the quality of care increase demand, input price increases will actually lower the equilibrium level of costs per day by lowering the level of quality that can be produced at any level of costs. See M. Feldstein, "Quality Change and the Demand for Hospital Care," *Econometrica* 45 (October 1977).

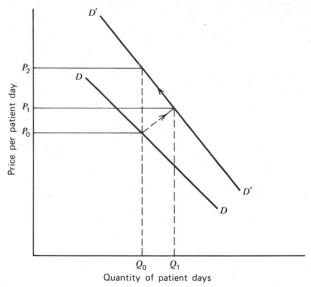

Figure 10-8. A demand-pull model of hospital cost inflation.

because the spread of third-party coverage is held to be primarily responsible for rapid cost increases by demand-pull theorists, a slowdown or halt in the spread of such coverage should similarly lead to a slowdown in cost increases. The percentage of hospital revenues coming from direct consumer payments has changed relatively little since 1971. When rates of cost increase began to slow down somewhat in 1973 and 1974, proponents of the demand-pull theory could argue that this would have occurred anyway and was not the result of the ESP controls. After the controls were lifted, however, this notion was dispelled. The return to very rapid cost increases relative to consumer prices in 1975 and 1976 provides ample evidence that the ESP regulations had done something to control costs. Unless some explanation can be found for a renewed surge of demand in 1975 and 1976, proponents of the demand-pull model must argue that hospitals were still responding to past increases in demand that had been building up during the ESP period. However, it is difficult for the demand-pull model to explain the large increases in hospital costs in the last several years.

But what of hospital occupancy rates? The supply adjustment mechanism posited by M. Feldstein suggests that periods of rapid price increase ought to be preceded by or concurrent with periods of unusually high occupancy. Indeed, hospitals reached their peak occupancy level in 1969 (since 1946), in the midst of the rapid post-Medicare cost increases. Perhaps hospitals did perceive excess demand at this time, to which they responded by increasing costs. But, in that case, the cost increases since 1974 are all the more difficult to understand, since occupancy rates had been dropping since 1969 and by 1975 had fallen to the 1960 level. If hospitals faced heavy excess demand since 1974, it did not show up in occupancy rates. The persistence of rapid cost increases in the face of a leveling off of third-party coverage and rather low occupancy rates casts some doubt on the current relevance of the demand-pull theory of hospital cost inflation.

Variations on the Demand-Pull Model

A variation on the demand-pull model rejects the idea that price and cost increases can be understood as movements toward an equilibrium of supply and demand; instead, it emphasizes not so much the growth of third-party coverage as the level such coverage has reached. This approach is based on the idea that since third-party coverage for hospital care is nearly complete, the fear of choking off demand from individual patients no longer serves as an effective constraint on the growth of hospital costs. This model does not precisely identify the factors that prevent costs from rising even faster than they have. Proponents of this hypothesis generally view hospitals as pursuing the same kinds of objectives assumed by the demand-pull theorists: relatively high wages for employees, the most technically advanced facilities, and high-quality care. Hospitals were believed to have considerable freedom in raising their costs, since third parties generally paid costs on a retrospective basis. The most important constraint facing hospitals may simply have been a fear of eventual rate regulation.

Although this hypothesis may seem similar to the demand-pull model, its implications are different in several important respects. First, there is no particular reason to expect a slowdown in cost increases once the extent of third-party coverage levels off. Costs are not believed to be moving toward some equilibrium determined by demand variables and the bed supply, but are expected to continue rapidly upward as long as retrospective cost reimbursement is used. A second implication is that controls on particular components of hospital costs (e.g., inputs and input prices) may have had an effect on overall rates of cost increase. Third parties are unlikely to seriously question cost increases that are clearly the result of input price increases, but if, for example, wages and non-labor input prices are controlled, hospitals may not feel as free to compensate by overexpanding their use of inputs. The result is that the overall rate of cost increase is lower than it would have been in the absence of controls.

The demand-pull model has strong appeal to economists because it assumes that price and quantity are determined through an interaction of demand and supply. The hypothesis that prices and quantities are determined by an implicit bargaining process between hospitals and third-party payors, and the implications of this hypothesis, are more consistent with the views noneconomists express about hospital cost increases. This hypothesis also more satisfactorily explains the recent rapid increases in hospital costs, which have occurred while the growth in third-party coverage has leveled off and hospitals have experienced falling occupancy levels.

Some mention should be made of still another variant, which might be labeled the cost-reimbursement hypothesis. This theory claims that retrospective reimbursement of costs, as practiced in the past by Medicare and many Blue Cross plans,* imposed weaker constraints on hospitals and was therefore even more inflationary than other forms of third-party reimbursement. This view would seem to be consistent with the sudden jump in expenditure increases at the time of the introduction of Medicare, since it has been estimated that Medicare increased the proportion of patient days reimbursed on a cost basis by 75 percent or more. The post-1966 shift in patient mix toward higher hospitalization

---

*Medicaid programs also reimbursed hospitals on a "reasonable cost" basis, though reimbursements from Medicaid were generally considered less generous than those from Medicare or Blue Cross.

rates for the elderly, which was previously discussed in connection with the demand-pull model, might also indicate hospitals' preference for patients covered by cost reimbursement.

Karen Davis attempted to test the influence of cost reimbursement on hospital costs per admission in a multiple regression study using observations on state averages in 1965, 1967, and 1968 (33). Davis ran individual regressions for each of the years and two pooled regressions using all of the observations; one of the regressions included dummy variables for the years 1967 and 1968 while the other did not. The extent of cost reimbursement was measured by the percentage of total revenues constituted by cost-reimbursed revenues (Medicare, Medicaid, and Blue Cross where it pays on a cost basis). The coefficient on the cost reimbursement variable was significant only in the pooled regression without the year dummy variables, which suggests that it may have served as a proxy for other effects occurring over time (e.g., the general increase in third-party coverage). Davis concluded that the study did not support the notion that cost reimbursement is more inflationary than other forms of third-party reimbursement. A study by David Salkever of southeastern New York hospitals from 1961 to 1967 revealed that when the hospitals' patients were covered by commercial insurance, hospital costs were likely to be higher than when the same proportion of patients were covered by Medicare or Blue Cross (34). In a more recent study, Salkever concludes that the widely accepted demand-oriented view should be broadened to include some inflationary pressures from the supply side (35).

These findings cannot be considered conclusive, of course, but little reason exists on theoretical grounds for expecting cost reimbursements to be any more inflationary than charge reimbursements. If a hospital is free at any time to adjust its charges to cover its costs, and those charges are paid without question by third parties, it is not clear that the effects of charge reimbursement and cost reimbursement would differ. In fact, hospital spokepersons in the past several years have criticized cost payors for not truly paying their full share of costs (because of a refusal to recognize some elements of costs which hospitals regard as legitimate), and they now seem to regard payors who pay full charges as the more generous (36).

Although there is little evidence that cost reimbursement is more inflationary than charge reimbursement by third parties, it does seem clear that the introduction of Medicare allowed hospitals to improve their financial positions. For most hospitals, revenues increased even faster than expenses in the first year after Medicare's introduction, leading to a substantial increase in their net-income-to-total-income ratios (37). A study of a national sample of approximately 250 hospitals indicated that depreciation and interest expenses increased 29.5 percent annually on the average from 1966 through 1968. It appears that hospitals had changed their accounting methods to obtain greater reimbursements from Medicare and other cost payors (38). Evidence of this kind of behavior seems to substantiate further a demand-pull or third-party reimbursement theory of hospital cost inflation. It suggests that in increasing their costs so rapidly after Medicare was introduced, hospitals were not passively reacting to factors entirely beyond their control, i.e., the catching-up hypothesis. Rather, hospitals were taking advantage of loosened financial constraints to accumulate funds to pursue their own objectives.

The process by which hospital costs have increased and the reasons why they have done so are still not fully understood. The evidence does suggest, however, that hospitals have responded to the growth of third-party coverage for hospital care by changing the nature of the product they provide—by increasing their nursing staff per bed, purchasing the most modern equipment, carrying out more diagnostic tests per patient, and so on—and that this process accounts for hospital cost increases far in excess of those experienced generally in the economy. The most recent evidence also seems to indicate that under existing institutional arrangements, there is no inherent tendency for the industry to settle down to rates of cost increase more in line with general inflation rates.

REFERENCES

1. Robert M. Gibson and Daniel R. Waldo, "National Health Expenditures, 1980," *Health Care Financing Review* 3 (September 1981): 9.

2. Donald Johnson and Linda Punch, "Multi-Hospital System Survey," *Modern Health Care* (April 1982): 68–69. For a background discussion on multihospital systems, see Howard Zuckerman and Lewis Weeks, *Multi-Institutional Hospital Systems* (Chicago: Hospital Research and Educational Trust, 1979).

3. For a more complete discussion of hospital outputs, see S.E. Berki, *Hospital Economics* (Lexington, Mass.: Lexington Books, 1972), Chapter 3.

4. For a comprehensive review of the hospital case mix literature, see Mark C. Hornbrook, "Hospital Case Mix: Its Definition, Measurement and Use: Part I. The Conceptual Framework," *Medical Care Review* 30(1) (Spring 1982); and "Hospital Case Mix: Its Definition, Measurement and Use: Part II. Review of Alternative Measures," *Medical Care Review* 39(2) (Summer 1982).

5. W.D. Cleverly, "Input-Output Analysis and the Hospital Budgeting Process," *Health Services Research* (Spring 1975): 41–43.

6. F.C. Spencer and B. Eiseman, "The Occasional Open-Heart Surgeon," *Circulation* (February 1965): 161–162; and Roger D. Platt, "Letter to the Editor," *New England Journal of Medicine* (June 17, 1971): 1386–1387.

7. Harold Luft, John Bunker, and Alain Enthoven, "Should Operations Be Regionalized," *New England Journal of Medicine* 301 (December 20, 1979).

8. Robert Rice, "Analysis of the Hospital as an Economic Organism," *Modern Hospital*, April 1966, p. 91.

9. For a more complete discussion of this point see R. Rosett, "Proprietary Hospitals in the United States," in M. Perlman, ed., *The Economics of Health and Medical Care* (New York: John Wiley & Sons, 1974).

10. For a more complete discussion of this hospital control mechanism by physicians see S. Shalit, "A Doctor–Hospital Cartel Theory," *The Journal of Business*, January 1977.

11. Harris conceptualizes the hospital as two separate firms: a medical staff, which is the demand division, and the administration, which is the supply division. Each of these separate entities are believed to have their own managers, objectives, pricing strategies, and constraints. Cost containment efforts should recognize the role of physicians as demanders of service, rather than being directed solely at the "suppliers" of hospital services. Jeffrey E. Harris, "The Internal Organization of Hospitals: Some Economic Implications," *The Bell Journal of Economics* 8 (Autumn 1977).

12. The following is a representative list of articles dealing with hospital ojectives: K. Davis, "Economic Theories of Behavior in Nonprofit Private Hospitals," *Economic and Business Bulletin*, Temple University, Winter 1972; M.S. Feldstein, "Hospital

Cost Inflation: A Study of Non-Profit Price Dynamics," *American Economic Review*, December 1971; P. Jacobs, "A Survey of Economic Models of Hospitals," *Inquiry*, June 1974; M.L. Lee, "A Conspicuous Production Theory of Hospital Behavior," *Southern Economic Journal*, July 1971; J. P. Newhouse, "Toward a Theory of Non-Profit Institutions: An Economic Model of a Hospital," *American Economic Review*, March 1970; M.V. Pauly and M. Redisch, "The Not-for-Profit Hospital as a Physicians' Cooperative," *American Economic Review*, March 1973. M. Goldfarb, M. Hornbrook, and J. Rafferty, "Behavior of the Multiproduct Firm: A Model of the Nonprofit Hospital System," *Medical Care* 18 (February 1980): 185–201.

13. *Report of the National Advisory Commission on Health Manpower*, Vol. II (Washington, D.C.: U.S. Government Printing Office, 1967), pp. 134–135.

14. Roger Platt, "Utilization of Facilities for Heart Surgery," *New England Journal of Medicine* 284 (June 17, 1971): 1386–1387.

15. Bernard Bloom, Osler Peterson, and Samuel Martin, "Radiation Therapy in New Hampshire, Massachusetts, and Rhode Island," *New England Journal of Medicine* 286 (January 27, 1972): 189–194. It should be noted that, when examining cost data from a small number of the hospitals with radiation therapy facilities, the authors found that costs per patient and per treatment were generally higher in the hospitals which performed a large volume of treatments. This is explained in part by the fact that the major radiation therapy centers treat a more complex mix of cases.

16. James Hauge and Dale Matthews, "Hospital Indicators," *Hospitals* 51 (February 16, 1977): 51–54.

17. Teh-wei Hu, "Hospital Costs and Pricing Behavior: The Maternity Ward," *Inquiry* 8 (December 1971): 19–26.

18. For descriptions of the controls as they applied to hospitals see Stuart Altman and Joseph Eichenholz, "Control of Hospital Costs Under the Economic Stabilization Program," *Federal Register* 39 (January 23, 1974): 2693–2700; Richard Berman, "The Economic Stabilization Program of the United States: August 1971–April 1974," *World Hospitals* 12 (1976); Paul Ginsburg, "Inflation and the Economic Stabilization Program," in Michael Zubkoff, ed., *Health: A Victim or Cause of Inflation?* (New York: PRODIST, 1976), pp. 31–51.

19. M. Feldstein, *The Rising Cost of Hospital Care* (Washington: Information Resources Press, 1971), pp. 53–57.

20. P. Joseph Phillip, James Jeffers, and Abdul Hai, "Indexes of Factor Input Price, Service Intensity, and Productivity of the Hospital Industry," in *The Nature of Hospital Costs: Three Studies* (Chicago: Hospital Research and Educational Trust, 1976), pp. 219–229.

21. M. Feldstein, "The Quality of Hospital Services: An Analysis of Geographic Variation and Intertemporal Change," in Mark Perlman, ed., *The Economics of Health and Medical Care* (London: The MacMillan Press, 1974), pp. 402–419.

22. John Rossman et al., "Report on Upstate Blue Cross Trend Factor 1976," mimeographed (Albany: Hospital Association of New York State, 1976); Michael Gort et al., "Report on the Hospital Price Index of Greater New York," mimeographed (Buffalo, N.Y.: Associated Hospital Services of New York, 1975); and Laurence Berger and Paul Sullivan, *Measuring Hospital Inflation* (Lexington, Mass.: Lexington Books, D.C. Heath Co., 1975).

23. A description of the index can be found in *Guide to the American Hospital Association's Program for Monitoring the Hospital Economy* (Chicago: American Hospital Association, 1974). The AHA has recently developed a new index of hospital input (factor) prices based on a somewhat different approach. Increases in cost per (adjusted) patient day are divided into changes in intensity and changes in factor prices. Changes in intensity are defined as changes in the quantities of various services performed, on

the average, per patient day, with the different services weighted by their base-year unit costs. Changes in factor prices are measured as changes in the unit costs of various services, weighted by their base-year quantities per patient day. See Phillip et al., "Indexes of Factor Input Price, Service Intensity, and Productivity for the Hospital Industry."

24. M. Feldstein, *The Rising Cost of Hospital Care*, Chapter 5, *op. cit.*; and M. Feldstein and Amy Taylor, "The Rapid Rise of Hospital Costs," in *Hospital Costs and Health Insurance*, Martin Feldstein, ed. (Cambridge, Mass.: Harvard University Press, 1981), pp. 19–56.

25. Victor Fuchs, "The Earnings of Allied Health Personnel—Are Health Workers Underpaid," *Explorations in Economic Research* 3 (Summer 1976): 408–431.

26. Martin Feldstein, "Hospital Cost Inflation: A Study of Non-Profit Price Dynamics," *American Economic Review* 61 (December 1971): 861.

27. Calculated from data in National Center for Health Statistics, "Hospital Discharges and Length of Stay: Short-Stay Hospitals, United States—1972," *Vital and Health Statistics*, Series 10, No. 107 (September 1976).

28. Anne Scitovsky and Nelda McCall, "Changes in the Costs of Treatment of Selected Illnesses 1951–1964–1971," Health Policy Discussion Paper, University of California School of Medicine, San Francisco (September 1975).

29. The information on intensive care units is taken from Louise Russell, "The Diffusion of New Hospital Technologies," *International Journal of Health Services* 6(4) (1976): 557–580.

30. National Center for Health Statistics, "Hospital Discharges and Lengths of Stay— 1972" (Washington, D.C.: Government Printing Office).

31. John Rafferty, "Enfranchisement and Rationing Effects of Medicare on Discretionary Hospital Use," *Health Services Research* 10 (Spring 1975): 51–62.

32. M. Feldstein, "Hospital Cost Inflation," *op. cit.* A revised and updated version of the model is "Quality Change and the Demand for Hospital Care," *Econometrica* 45 (October 1977) and is reprinted in *Hospital Costs and Health Insurance (op. cit.).*

33. Karen Davis, "Theories of Hospital Inflation: Some Empirical Evidence," *Journal of Human Resources* 8 (Spring 1973): 181–201.

34. David Salkever, "A Microeconomic Study of Hospital Cost Inflation," *Journal of Political Economy* 80 (November/December 1972): 1144–1166.

35. David S. Salkever, *Hospital-Sector Inflation* (Lexington, Mass.: Lexington Books, 1979).

36. David H. Hitt, "Reimbursement System Must Recognize Real Costs," *Hospitals, Journal of the American Hospital Association*, Parts I and II (January 1 and January 16, 1977).

37. See Paul J. Feldstein and Saul Waldman, "Financial Position of Hospitals in the Early Medicare Period," *Social Security Bulletin* 31 (October 1968): 18–23.

38. See Karen Davis, "Hospital Costs and the Medicare Program," *Social Security Bulletin* 36 (August 1973): 18–36.

SELECTED BIBLIOGRAPHY ON HOSPITAL COST STUDIES

The following list is representative of the large number of studies on hospital costs and patient classification.

Berry, R., "Returns to Scale in the Production of Hospital Services," *Health Services Research* 2, Summer 1967.

Berry, R., "On Grouping Hospitals for Economic Analysis," *Inquiry* 10 (December 1973).

Carr, J., and P. Feldstein, "The Relationship of Cost to Hospital Size," *Inquiry* 4 (June 1967).

Evans, R. G., " 'Behavioral' Cost Functions for Hospitals," *Canadian Journal of Economics* 4 (May 1971).

Feldstein, M., *Economic Analysis for Health Service Efficiency* (Chicago: Markham Publishing Company, 1968).

Francisco, E., "Analysis of Cost Variation Among Short-Term General Hospitals," in H. Klarman, ed., *Empirical Studies in Health Economics* (Baltimore: Johns Hopkins Press, 1970).

Lave, J. R., and L. B. Lave, "Estimated Costs for Pennsylvania Hospitals," *Inquiry* 7 (June 1970).

Lave, J. R., and L. B. Lave, "Hospital Cost Functions," in George Chacko, ed., *Health Handbook 1976* (Amsterdam: North Holland Publishing Co., 1980).

Lee, M. L., and R. L. Wallace, "Classification of Diseases for Hospital Cost Analysis," *Inquiry* 9 (June 1972).

Mann, J., and D. Yett, "The Analysis of Hospital Costs: A Review Article," *Journal of Business* 41 (April 1968).

Pauly, M., "The Behavior of Non-Profit Hospital Monopolies: Alternative Models of the Hospital," in Clark Havighurst, ed., *Regulating Health Facilities Construction* (Washington: American Enterprise Institute, 1974).

Sloan, F., and B. Steinwald, *Insurance, Regulation, and Hospital Costs* (Lexington, Mass.: Lexington Books, 1980).

Watts, C., and T. Klastorian, "The Impact of Care Mix on Hospital Cost: A Comparative Analysis," *Inquiry* 17 (Winter 1980): 357–367.

CHAPTER 11

Relying on Regulation to Improve Hospital Performance

INTRODUCTION

It has been shown that the hospital sector appears to be performing inadequately. The indicators of its poor performance are excessive duplication of expensive facilities and services, rapid inflation of hospital costs, the alleged inefficiency of hospital operation as measured by wide cost variations between hospitals, and the failure to substitute care in less costly settings for hospital care when possible. The following reasons for the industry's poor performance were cited: a service benefit health insurance policy that both removed any incentive for patients to reduce their hospitalization costs and reimbursed the hospital on the basis of its costs; the physician's freedom from fiscal responsibility for the method of patient treatment selected; and the incentives and goals of the hospital physicians and administrative staff to undertake those pricing and investment policies that are to their advantage instead of those that would minimize the community's cost of medical care.

The different approaches that have been suggested for improving the performance of the hospital sector are generally of two basic types. The first places greater reliance on the use of controls and planning through centralized decisionmaking. Under this approach, the decisionmaking authority over the allocation of resources would gradually be removed from physicians and hospital administrators and vested in local and state health planning agencies. Such agencies would ultimately have complete control over all capital expenditure programs and over the setting of hospital rates, and they would have authority to determine which hospitals would be permitted to expand and which should be required to contract. The alternative to increased regulation is to eliminate many of the restrictions that currently prevail in the medical sector and to permit traditional market forces, through competitive pressures, to improve performance. Under the market approach the incentives facing individual decisionmakers would be changed. Any restraints to greater competition among different provider groups would also be removed. An improved allocation of resources would then presumably occur as a result of competition among these provider groups.

It has been difficult to develop a clear dialogue in the health field between these two alternative approaches to improving performance in the medical sector. Differences in opinion occur over the appropriateness of goals, such as what the measures of performance for the hospital system should be, and also over the consumer's ability to choose adequately the appropriate quantity and quality of health care; rarely is the debate simply over which approach—regulation or competition—can achieve a more efficient allocation of medical resources and provide adequate consumer protection. However, unless the debate is clarified so that everyone is debating the same issues, it will remain impossible to separate value differences from differences in methods designed to achieve most efficiently a given set of values.

The following chapters attempt to review the two approaches to improving performance in the medical sector. The first section reviews the methodology for health facility planning, indicating what information is required and how it is to be applied if planning agencies are to ensure the economically efficient use of community resources. The difficulties inherent in planning, such as securing the necessary information, using the appropriate criteria, and then learning the methodology for applying that information and criteria should not be underestimated. The next section discusses the likelihood that planning will improve performance. The experience of regulation in other industries is examined and, based on that experience, the likely consequences of increased regulation in the health field are discussed. The next chapter examines the probable consequences of a greater reliance on market forces to achieve improved performance, and it describes the structural changes in the medical sector that would be required to increase competition.

THE ECONOMICS OF HEALTH FACILITY PLANNING (1)

The cost-based method of payment for care in health facilities together with institutional decisionmakers' desires for prestige and income maximization result in a situation in which each institution acting independently contributes to a misallocation of health resources. There is internal cross-subsidization of services and patients within the hospital, an overinvestment in beds, and an excess of prestige services within a community. Two types of approaches seek to remedy this situation: different payment systems can be established within a system of independently acting units, or a more centralized decisionmaking process can be developed to achieve a more appropriate allocation of resources. This section discusses the latter approach. However, before describing how such a remedy might work, we must specify the criteria to be used and the information needed to determine the optimal number and size of each type of health facility in a community. This theoretical discussion will then be applied to the planning of obstetric facilities for the city of Chicago. Ideally, then, a centralized decision-making agency, such as a local hospital or health planning board, would collect and analyze information according to the method specified in order to achieve the optimal size and configuration of health facilities in a region. This allocation process would be a continuous one, since the information upon which such decisions are based is continuously changing.

A THEORETICAL MODEL FOR DETERMINING THE OPTIMAL SIZE AND LOCATION OF HEALTH FACILITIES

The criterion for determining the optimal size and location of a health facility should be to minimize both the explicit (facility) and the implicit (patient and family) costs of hospitalization. In the past, hospital planners have concentrated primarily on minimizing facility costs; however, when this is the only criterion used, certain costs are shifted to the patient and/or the patient's family. Since they would be willing to pay a certain price not to have to bear these costs, some allowance should be made for such costs in planning the size and number of facilities. Figure 11-1 displays both the explicit (facility) and the implicit costs, as well as their sum, which is referred to as average total cost. To determine a facility's optimal size, it is necessary to find the minimum point on this average-total-cost curve. Each of these cost curves will be briefly discussed.

The average-facility-cost curve shows the relationship between the actual medical costs per case and the size of the facility. This curve is the typical average-cost curve of a firm described in the economics literature. It is U-shaped because of economies of scale; as the size of the facility increases, average costs fall, reach a minimum, and then rise. How rapidly these costs fall and where the minimum point occurs depends on the particular facility in question. For some facilities the minimum point occurs only when the operation is large-scale, while

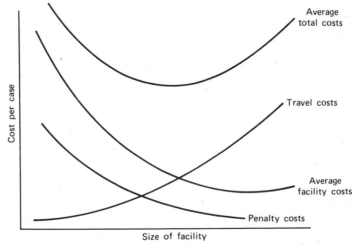

Figure 11-1. Minimizing the costs per case, both explicit and implicit, of inpatient care.

for other facilities the minimum point occurs relatively early; small facilities may be equally, if not more, efficient than larger units. The extent of economies of scale in a health facility will depend upon whether certain minimum quantities of staff and equipment are required for the facility, regardless of its size, and also the extent to which larger units operate at higher occupancy rates than smaller units. (Larger units have higher occupancy rates because the populations they serve are larger; the larger the population, the lower the coefficient of variation of demand. With a lower coefficient of variation, fewer beds, relative to mean size, must be provided to meet peak loads.) Higher occupancy rates make more intensive use of facilities and staff possible, thus reducing the cost per case.

In Figure 11-1, travel costs are shown to rise as units get larger because larger units imply fewer hospitals, requiring patients to travel further for service.* Travel costs include not only the costs of travel but also the value of the patient's time spent in traveling to and from the facility. The third category of costs, penalty costs, is incurred by those who are inconvenienced when the absence of a facility necessitates a departure from regular procedures. If a hospital does not have a bed when a patient needs it, room might be made by crowding existing facilities, minimizing the stay of other patients, delaying elective admissions until a bed is available, or substituting other facilities by sending the patient to a different institution.† How large the penalty cost should be depends upon a number of factors, including the effect on health status of a treatment delay and the inconvenience the delay will cause the patient—inconvenience that the patient would be willing to pay some amount to avoid. As depicted in Figure 11-1, the average penalty cost per case falls as the size of the unit increases, because, as size increases, the number of patients requiring special handling decreases.‡ Needless to say, the penalty cost will vary according to the facility that is being planned and also according to the wealth of the community.

The three cost components—medical costs, travel costs, and penalty costs—together constitute the total costs of an illness episode; it is the sum of these three costs that the community, through its planner, should attempt to minimize.

THE PLANNING OF OBSTETRIC FACILITIES: AN APPLICATION OF THE THEORETICAL MODEL

The preceding discussion of the theoretical relationships between medical, travel, and penalty costs and the size of a health care facility can now be applied to planning a system of obstetric facilities. For several reasons, obstetric facilities

---

*With units of a given size, more travel will be necessary in less densely populated areas. Optimal unit size, therefore, will probably be larger in metropolitan areas. To simplify the drawing of Figure 11-1, a uniform population density has been assumed so that travel costs can be represented by a single function. This means one optimum size for all hospitals in the region.

†Regardless of whether compensation is paid to those inconvenienced, penalty costs should be included in the cost function. Were the solution profit market determined, those who wished to avoid inconvenience could do so by paying a price. With planning, the costs may be allocated differently, but the level of facilities should be the same. See R. Coase, "The Problem of Social Cost," *Journal of Law and Economics*, No. 3, 1960.

‡The number requiring special handling is a function of the coefficient of variation and, therefore, falls as units become larger.

serve as a good example. First, obstetrics is an easier product to define than other types of medical treatment. It is less possible to substitute obstetric services outside the hospital for hospital obstetric services; therefore, only one type of facility must be planned for, rather than several different institutional settings. Also, since more than 96 percent of mothers have their babies in hospitals, demand for obstetric admissions is relatively inelastic with respect to price. Thus, in forecasting demand we need not be greatly concerned with feedbacks between price and demand for obstetrics admissions. (Length of stay for an obstetric admission would be affected by price variables; however, it is easier to adjust for differences in days than for admissions, as will be discussed below.) An additional reason for examining obstetrics is that the statistical characteristics of this demand make it possible to cast the analysis in a rather simple mathematical form. And finally, the problems of low occupancy and duplication of facilities are perhaps greatest in obstetrics.*

Estimating the Demand for Obstetrical Beds

The first step in planning facilities and their location is to estimate the expected demand for such facilities. Perhaps the easiest method of forecasting obstetrical (OB) demand is to collect data on the current number of obstetric admissions. If population data are available, preferably by age and sex for different communities, the number of OB admissions can then be extrapolated using a projection of the population by age and sex category. Population projections, by age, sex, and for different regions, are generally available from city planning agencies and other organizations in the planning region.

For simplicity, the actual numbers of admissions to maternity units in the Chicago region were used.† In this case, the estimates of demand for a recent past period would enable us to evaluate the existing OB system for serving this demand only by comparing it with the costs of alternative OB systems. For planning future OB system requirements, or for determining how the present system should change to meet future OB demand, a projection of OB demand, by area, would be needed.

Owing to seasonality in maternity care, estimates of the demand for OB beds during peak periods of the year are derived from the annual estimate for OB admissions adjusted by a seasonal factor. The adjusted demand for OB admissions thus includes the highest monthly mean demand and the variance in demand during that month.‡

Once we have a demand estimate, we are in a position to translate that

---

*In the Chicago region, where the current study was conducted, the 1965 occupancy rate for obstetrics units was 61 percent, while for pediatrics and medical–surgical units it was 71 and 84 percent, respectively.

†The area covered, as defined by The Hospital Planning Council of Chicago, included Cook, DuPage, Lake, McHenry, Kane, and Will counties in Illinois, and Lake and Porter counties in Indiana. In this area in 1963, 157,000 maternity cases were handled in the obstetrical units of 95 hospitals. The units contained a total of 3,229 beds.

‡To adjust demand for this seasonal factor, monthly data on births for a region (e.g., Chicago) are multiplied by a seasonal index developed from data published by the National Center for Health Statistics, booklets on Vital Statistics, Series 2, No. 9.

demand into the number of OB beds required for different probabilities of being full. The method used for calculating the number of beds required, given different numbers of OB facilities and different probabilities of being full, is the Erlang Loss formula. This formula is a simple queuing-theory model that has been adapted to the present problem. In order to use this model, it has been assumed—and this assumption has been tested against actual admissions and length of stay data for the Chicago region—that obstetric admissions have a Poisson arrival process.* The Erlang Loss formula uses the individual hospital as its basis. The mean daily census for the individual hospital is calculated as follows: the number of OB admissions (157,000) multiplied by the seasonal factor (1.07) equals 168,000; this, multiplied by the average length of stay (4.2), equals 705,000, which is then divided by 365 days, to equal 1,931, which is the mean census (average number of OB days per day) for the system. Because the formula is based on the individual hospital, the mean census must be divided by the number of units in the system before it can be used to solve for the average number of beds for the individual hospital. Therefore, if systems of 45 or 95 hospitals are considered for the region, we divide the mean census of 1,931 by 45 or 95 units to calculate the mean census per hospital in a 45- or 95-unit system; the result is 42.9 or 20.3 patients per day per hospital, respectively.

In using the formula, any two of the following three parameters must be specified. The formula will then solve for the unspecified parameter. The three parameters are 1) the number of beds, 2) the probability of being full (or the percentage of patients turned away), and 3) the mean daily census. Given the mean daily census and the probability of being full, the formula can be solved for the number of beds needed in a 45- or 95-unit system. For the 45-unit system, with a mean census of 42.9 and a probability of .0001 (one in ten thousand) or .001 (one in a thousand), calculations are made for the number of beds in each hospital ($42.9 + 4\sqrt{42.9}$) and then are multiplied by 45 to obtain the total number of beds in a 45-unit system (3,240 beds at probability .0001 and 2,989 beds at probability .001). The process for calculating the number of beds in a system with 95 units is the same.†

Table 11-1 illustrates the principles involved in using this formula. The table is based on a hypothetical system with a number of births equal to that of the Chicago region. The results reported in Table 11-1 show how the number of required beds, cases requiring special handling, and travel times would change for systems composed of various numbers of obstetrical units operating under different rules. The calculations presume that all OB units are of equal size and that they are optimally distributed over the space served. Column 1 shows total bed requirements for a system of independent hospitals, each with sufficient beds to reduce the probability of being full to one in 10,000. Column 2 shows the

---

*While the Poisson arrival assumption is not rejected, a more accurate model seems to be a Poisson process with a shifting parameter. This is because there is a seasonal, monthly, and daily variation in births. In this model, length of stay has been assumed as given. However, if it were to change, then this would result in a change in the mean census, and in this manner the length of stay, or changes in it, would be reflected in the Erlang Loss formula.

† If the OB units are not of equal size, then we cannot simply divide and then multiply the results by 45 or by 95. Instead, the number of beds must be calculated for each hospital separately and the results summed up.

TABLE 11-1. Obstetrical System Characteristics^a by Number of Units

Number of Units	Beds				Number of Patients Requiring Special Handling		Total Travel Time, Hours (Thousands)
	Probability		Penalty	Cost			
	.0001	.001	$500	$250	$500	$250	
	(1)	(2)	(3)	(4)	(5)	(6)	(7)
45	3,240	2,989	2,623	2,430	1,963	5,134	1,422.7
55	3,383	3,102	2,679	2,464	2,198	5,715	1,295.2
65	3,515	3,209	2,729	2,495	2,418	6,264	1,187.3
75	3,635	3,305	2,776	2,523	2,622	6,782	1,108.8
85	3,759	3,407	2,821	2,549	2,810	7,269	1,040.0
95	3,868	3,493	2,859	2,571	2,989	7,724	981.2
105	3,974	3,577	2,896	2,591	3,160	8,164	932.1
115	4,081	3,664	2,930	2,610	3,324	8,588	892.9
125	4,173	3,736	2,963	2,626	3,485	9,012	858.6

Source: Millard F. Long and Paul J. Feldstein, "The Economics of Hospital Systems: Peak Loads and Regional Coordination," *American Economic Review* (May 1967): 123.

^aThe expected number of deliveries in this system is 157,000 per year.

system bed requirements when the probability of being full is one in 1,000.* It is clear that more beds are required if the probability is set low—for a 45-unit system, with each facility having 72 beds, 3,240 beds are needed in the system for a probability of 1/10,000; 2,989 are needed if the probability of being full is only 1/1,000 for the same 45-unit system. Similarly, if the system is composed of many small units—for example, a 125-unit system—the number of beds needed to achieve the same probability of being full is greater than it would be for a system of fewer but larger facilities; that is, a 45-unit system requires 3,240 beds whereas a 125-unit system requires 4,173 beds.†

Calculating the Cost Per Obstetrical Bed

The Erlang Loss formula provides us with a method for calculating the number of beds needed in a hospital system, for a given number of units and a specified

---

*If the probability of being full is 1/10,000, special arrangements would have to be made on average for 15.7 patients per year (since there are 157,000 OB admissions); in the 1/1,000 case, arrangements would be necessary for 157 patients per year.

†Several computer programs were developed for use in solving the Erlang Loss formula. One such program simply specifies the number of beds in a facility and its mean census, and solves for the probability of being full; another specifies some value for the probability of being full, mean census, and an initial value for the number of beds required. The program then compares the initial beds probabilities with the specified probability. For example, to find the number of beds needed, with a given mean census and a specified probability, start with an initial number of beds, e.g., 250. The program then changes beds by increments of 10, e.g., 250, 240, 230. Then, if the probability of being full is between beds equal to 230 and 220, the program changes beds by increments of 1 and then finally by .1. Since the number of beds in a facility will be multiplied by a large number of units to derive the number of beds for the system, the error will be less if the program can find the number of beds in smaller increments, e.g., .1.

probability of being full. It is now necessary to incorporate the additional information on costs per bed, penalty costs, and travel costs (shown in Figure 11-1) to calculate the minimum-cost solution for obstetric care for the Chicago region.

To estimate the extent of economies of scale in obstetric facilities it is important to be able to derive the relationship between costs per OB case and size of the OB facility. Once the cost of an additional bed has been determined, it is possible to examine the trade-off between fewer beds (and the consequent savings in cost per bed) and a higher probability that a patient will not have a bed available when it is needed.*

To derive an estimate of OB costs per bed two obstetrical cost functions were estimated using annual data for the year 1964 and 1965 from 34 Connecticut hospitals. (Data from Chicago hospitals would have been desirable, but they were unavailable.) The results of the cost functions, unfortunately, were not completely reliable and did not indicate economies of scale. (Significant variables have most likely been omitted, such as differences between hospitals in wage rates, and quality of care in the OB units.)† In a subsequent study of economies of scale in maternity units, Teh-wei Hu estimated an average cost function that had the traditional U shape with respect to the number of maternity admissions (2).

Given the foregoing limitations in the regression results, however, the coefficients of these variables are significant and remain stable between the two years. The coefficient of the beds variable in the 1965 regression ($5,613) has been used as the estimate of savings from reducing hospital beds by one, when the number of patients and the average length of stay is held constant.

The Penalty Costs of Not Having a Bed Available

It is difficult to determine the appropriate penalty to assign when facilities are full. In obstetrical cases the options are limited, once the capacity of the unit has been reached. Emergent babies cannot be asked to wait. State laws restrict the use of other facilities within the hospital for obstetrical cases because of the danger of infection. When an obstetrical unit is full, patients must be crowded into existing facilities, they must be sent to another institution, or other patients must be discharged early. In most obstetrical units one or two extra patients can probably be accommodated by crowding at rather small cost; severe crowding or

---

*Beds are the only available measure of facilities, and throughout this study beds are used as the measure of size. A decrease in beds, therefore, represents a decrease in both staff and facilities, though the change in other inputs may not be proportional to the change in beds. In a more sophisticated model of obstetrical care, at least two types of facilities should be considered: delivery facilities and bed facilities. Either type of facility can become a bottleneck. The appropriate relationship between the two types of facilities has been studied by A. Barr, "Computer Simulation of a Maternity Hospital," *British Hospital Journal and Social Science Review*, March 1965; and J. Thompson, R. Fetter, C. McIntosh, and R. Pelletier, "Predicting Requirements for Maternity Facilities," *Hospitals: Journal of the American Hospital Association*, February 1963.

†Since it is likely that the omitted variables are positively correlated with size, their exclusion has probably resulted in upwardly biased estimates of the coefficients on patients, beds, or both. However, M. Feldstein's estimates of obstetrical costs in England show ratios between the fixed costs associated with beds and the variable costs associated with patients that are very similar to those reported in this study. M. Feldstein, *Economic Analysis for Health Service Efficiency* (Amsterdam: North Holland Publishing Co., 1967), Table 5, p. 145.

discharging patients early involves higher costs; the highest costs under present institutional arrangements probably occur when patients are transferred to another hospital. In the case of transfers, the important question is whether the doctor has a staff appointment at another institution where he or she can deliver the mother conveniently; if the doctor does not, the costs of the hospital's being full may be quite high. If only a few patients need to be transferred—and most doctors in metropolitan areas have appointments in at least two hospitals*—it should be possible, even with present institutional arrangements, to find cases that would be transferred at reasonable cost.

For present purposes, we have assumed two values for the penalty cost of failing to have an obstetric bed available when it is needed: $500 and $250 per patient requiring special handling. When calculated more realistically, the penalty-cost function is not linear. For example, if 30 patients in a system have to be inconvenienced, or handled differently, then the penalty cost per patient could be relatively low, e.g., $10. If 20 patients require special handling, then the penalty cost per patient might be $40, and so on to a maximum of perhaps $500 per patient. (If one were planning for emergency facilities in an area, obviously different penalty costs should be assigned by the planners for each emergency patient who is delayed in receiving treatment because of a lack of facilities and staff.) By limiting the range of penalty costs to either $500 or $250 per patient we are able to reflect in the results a sensitivity to different values of penalty costs.

Determining the Optimal Number of Beds Within a Facility

Penalty costs are used in the following way to determine the number of beds within a given facility. One fewer bed in a facility results in a savings of $5,600.† Offsetting this savings is an increase in the number of patients who will not have a bed when it is needed. The increased number of patients who must be handled differently, multiplied by a penalty cost of $500 (or $250), is the cost of having one less bed. The optimal number of beds in a facility is that number of beds at which the additional costs of moving patients (penalty costs) equals the savings from having fewer beds. For example, if the OB facility has 70 beds, then, given its expected mean census, it has a probability of turning away a certain number of patients each year. If the hospital decreases its bed size (and accompanying staff) by one bed, there will be a savings of $5,600. At the same time there will be an increase in the number of patients turned away, given the same expected mean census. As long as the savings of $5,600 is greater than the additional penalty

---

*Our data showed that half the obstetricians in the Chicago region delivered women in more than one hospital in the single month of February 1965. Had data been available for a longer period, they would probably have revealed that more than half the obstetricians in Chicago are connected with several hospitals.

†The costs associated with the number of OB facilities have been assumed to be proportional to the number of beds; i.e., for each bed reduced, costs are decreased by approximately $5,600. However, since the seasonality in demand is predictable, administrators might be able to vary their staffing patterns and thus have less staff in off-peak months. If this is the case, we could have assumed either a lower mean number of beds for the year, since the peak number of beds needed for September is greater than the number needed for the rest of the year, or we could have separately calculated for each month the number of beds needed and their probability of being full. The present assumption of beds and costs being proportional results in a bias against us.

cost, which is the additional number of patients turned away multiplied by the penalty cost per patient, then the hospital should reduce its bed complement. The institution should continue this marginal analysis until it reaches the point where the savings from removing one more bed equals a penalty cost of an equivalent amount.*

Columns 3 and 4 of Table 11-1 give the system bed requirements resulting from these calculations. For a 45-unit system, with a penalty cost of $500 for each patient without an available bed, the total number of beds in such a system would be 2,623, which would mean that each of the 45 units would have an average of 58 beds. If the penalty cost was $250 per patient, then fewer beds, 2,430, would be required. The total number of patients who could not be handled in a routine manner when the penalty cost was $500 is given in column 5; the number who could not be handled with a penalty cost of $250 per patient is given in column 6. For a 45-unit system with a penalty cost of $500 per patient, 1,963 patients would have to be handled in a nonroutine manner; the corresponding number for a penalty of $250 is 5,134 patients. The number of patients in columns 5 and 6 was derived by adding up the numbers who would have to be treated differently *each* time another bed was removed from the facility.

The assignment of an arbitrary penalty cost of either $500 or $250 per patient provides for an interesting observation. When the number of beds in a facility was based upon a probability of .0001 or .001 of being full, the total system requirements for beds was much greater than when a penalty cost of $500 or $250 was used. In effect, using a probability of .0001 or .001 assigns an extremely high penalty cost to the absence of a needed bed. It would, therefore, be preferable to select explicitly a penalty cost per patient rather than to accept implicitly a penalty cost by selecting a probability of being full. Since the penalty cost will vary by type of facility and the particular community involved, and will also change over time, explicit discussion of such penalty costs should provide a more accurate indication of the value the community places on the number and type of facilities it decides to have.

Determining the Optimal Number of Facilities in a Region

At this point it is appropriate to discuss how to determine the optimal number of facilities in a region. As evidenced by Table 11-1, the greater the number of facilities in an area, the greater the total cost for OB care. For the same penalty cost (e.g., $500), a system of 45 independent units handling 157,000 maternity cases a year requires 2,623 beds, whereas a system of 125 independent units requires 2,963 beds. Although the cost in additional beds is greater when facili-

---

*For example, for a given facility assume the beds are decreased by one, which saves $5,600, resulting in five additional patients requiring special handling. Since the cost savings of $5,600 is greater than the additional penalty cost of $2,500 (five patients multiplied by a penalty cost of $500), the calculation continues and another bed is taken away from the facility. Assuming this next bed requires that eight additional patients have special handling, the penalty cost for this next bed is $4,000 (8 × $500). Since the penalty cost is less than the savings of having one less bed, a third bed is reduced. This marginal calculation is made each time. Assuming that now 11 patients require special handling as a result of this last bed reduction, then the savings ($5,600) is approximately equal to the increased penalty cost (11 × $500). If the penalty cost were $500, then there would be no further reductions in beds. At this point three beds have been reduced with a total of 24 patients (5 + 8 + 11) requiring special handling.

ties are more numerous, the greater the number of units serving an area, the lower are the travel costs. In order to determine the appropriate trade-off between travel costs and beds, it is first necessary to discuss the measurement of travel costs.

Travel costs are composed of the time spent in travel and the cost of that time. The cost of time spent in travel has been estimated by H. Mohring at between $1.55 and $2.80 per hour (not including transportation cost) during the approximate time period covered by the data used in this study (3). The amount of time spent in travel can be derived from patient residence surveys or from arbitrary assumptions based on other researcher's work. The relevant travel time should include that of hospital employees and visitors as well as patients. Coughlin found that patients accounted for only 5.9 percent of the total trip miles involved in hospitalization; visitors accounted for over half the travel distance, and employees, outpatients, and physicians made the remainder of the trips (4). If a reduction in the number of units adds one mile to the average travel distance, total travel increases by roughly 17 miles one way (100 ÷ 5.9) or 34 miles round trip per case.

To calculate the amount of patient travel time for different numbers of hospital facilities, we used data that had been collected from a Chicago Area Transportation study on the time and distance between home and hospital for the Chicago region. (The available data were for a sample of Chicago obstetrical patients for the month of February 1965.) Patient travel time was calculated on the basis of the mean travel time to the hospital from each community area. This means that the patients who lived in the community area of their hospital had zero travel time. For other patients, travel time was approximately 12–13 minutes per patient. This mean travel time was then multiplied by the total number of patients, which came to approximately 190,000 minutes or 23,333 hours. When multiplied by 34, to include the round trip time of visitors, employees, and physicians, this equaled 981,000 hours, which represents the travel time under the existing system of 95 OB units serving Chicago. Referring back to Table 11-1, column 7 shows a travel time for 95 units of 981,000 hours. When this travel time is multiplied by $1.55 or $2.80, the result is the total travel cost for the present system. To compare the change in travel times under alternative systems, it is necessary to multiply the existing system travel time by the square root of the number of system units divided by the proposed number of units, e.g.:

$$981,000 \sqrt{\frac{95}{45}} = 1,422,700 \text{ hours for a 45-unit system}$$

To determine a region's optimal number of units, we would try to equate, at the margin, the decrease in costs of having fewer units, hence fewer beds, and the decrease in travel costs of having more units. For example, with 95 units at a penalty cost of $250, the system will have 2,571 beds; the travel hours are 981,000. As the number of units in the system increases to 105, the number of beds increases to 2,591; at approximately $5,000 per bed, costs will increase by $100,000. At 105 units, the travel is 932,000 hours or approximately 50,000 hours less than at 95 units. If travel time is valued at approximately $2 per hour, then an approximate minimum-cost point in terms of number of units in the system has been reached; the increase in hospital costs as a result of having a greater number of beds is approximately equal to the accompanying decrease in travel costs. (This solution should naturally be calculated by moving from 95 to 96 units rather than by using the larger shift from 95 to 105 units.) If different values are used for travel time, cost per bed, and penalty cost, obviously the solution will change. Since each of these costs changes with time, the minimum-cost solution for the community will also change; hence, such estimates should be recalculated every few years.

APPLYING THE MODEL TO THE CHICAGO REGION

In applying the foregoing model to the obstetrics units serving the Chicago region, several separate analyses were undertaken. The first was to examine the probability of being full for each of the obstetrics units in the region. Owing to shifts in the population as well as the population groups predominantly served by certain hospitals, it was found that the existing beds were unequally distributed; i.e., the probability of being full was much higher for some hospitals than for others. (For example, the probability of some hospitals being full was one in 10, while for obstetric units in the older central city hospitals the probability was very small; in essence, they had unneeded beds.) With the existing distribution of beds and units, the expected number of patients who must be specially handled exceeds 2,000 per year. If the same number of beds were redistributed so that the probability of being full was the same for each unit, the number of patients specially handled would be much lower.

The second analysis of the Chicago obstetrics system examined the implicit penalty costs of having a total of 3,229 beds. The number of beds required for each unit was recalculated on the assumption that the penalty cost of not having a bed available was first $500 and then $250. With the existing pattern of demand, and maintaining the same number of units, it would be possible to reduce the number of beds to 2,656 if the penalty costs were $500 per patient, or to 2,412 beds if the penalty costs were $250 per patient. Such a change would raise occupancy rates in obstetric units from 60 percent to 67 percent ($500 penalty cost), or to 75 percent ($250 penalty cost). Most of the contraction would come in the older central city units, while some expansion would be called for in some of the suburban areas. Arrangements of the type suggested would reduce costs of obstetrical services to the Chicago community by about 4 percent of total outlays if the appropriate penalty figure were $500 and 8 percent if it were $250; the reduction in dollar amount would be $1.5 million and $3 million, respectively.*

The third analysis of the model that could be performed but, owing to a lack of time, was not, would examine the number and location of the units in the Chicago region in relation to the travel times of the population. Such an analysis would attempt to show the travel costs associated with different numbers of obstetric units within the existing set of hospitals serving the region.

This section has discussed the type of information needed and the method for its analysis that will result in the optimal size and number of community

---

*These estimates are adjusted for penalty costs. In-hospital savings would be 5 percent and 9 percent in the $500 and $250 cases, respectively.

health facilities. Facilities are optimal in number and size when the sum of all the relevant costs, not just inpatient costs, is minimized. Excluding penalty or travel costs means either assigning a very low value to these factors, or, if arbitrary probabilities of being full such as .0001 or .001 are chosen, implicitly assigning very high penalty costs. (Since inpatient costs are predominantly paid for by the government and third-party payors, and their expenditures often are limited to inpatient costs, it is in their interests to minimize such costs. Such a strategy will shift costs to the patient and others in the health care system.)

The difficulty of the planner's task becomes obvious when we realize that information on medical costs, penalty costs, and travel costs is constantly changing and that these costs also differ for different types of health facilities within an area. Collection of the type of data required by the health planner, particularly the data just discussed on implicit costs, and the planner's continual need to change the number, size, and location of different health facilities, are essentially the tasks that an efficient market would perform. The role of the health facility planner is to substitute for the market mechanism in collecting data, transmitting this information to the various participants, and providing the appropriate incentives to ensure that the correct solution is achieved at minimum cost. This is no easy task. Not only must the health planner be technically trained to do all of the above, but he or she must have the appropriate incentive and the authority to do so. In a subsequent section, the performance of regulatory agencies (including several in the health field) will be evaluated to determine how likely it is that optimal performance by health planning agencies can be expected.

THE THEORY AND PRACTICE OF REGULATION

THE PRESUMED OBJECTIVES OF REGULATION IN THE MEDICAL SECTOR

Proponents of health sector regulation cite different reasons in support of their position. A review of these different arguments will help us to determine whether regulation can (or will) achieve the various objectives they have assigned it, and it will develop a basis for contrasting regulatory and nonregulatory approaches by which regulatory proponents' goals can be achieved.

One set of reasons used to justify increased regulation focuses on inefficiencies in medical care demand. They state that patients are ignorant of the type of treatment an illness requires; that they have neither the information upon which to choose different providers nor the ability to evaluate their competence. Because the costs of incompetent providers can be large, and, in some cases, may be impossible to rectify, consumers need the protection regulation will afford. Another rationalization for regulation is that the type of insurance coverage available provides consumers with no incentive to select lower-cost providers; in fact as patients pay less and less of their medical expenses, their incentive is to select the highest-cost providers in the hopes of receiving high-quality care. The patient thereby also has an incentive to overutilize medical services. Certain persons favoring regulation prefer that professional medical judgment be substituted for consumer judgment in determining medical service use. Such persons would favor using professionally determined need as the determinant of utilization rather than the consumer's willingness to pay, even assuming that the consumer has the means to choose and can afford the medical care chosen.

A second set of reasons used to justify increased medical sector regulation addresses supply inefficiency. The natural-monopoly argument (that large economies of scale exist in the provision of services) is rarely made, except for rural areas and for highly specialized services. The most frequent reasons given for supply regulation are the duplication of services, the excess of beds in communities, and the lack of incentives for the providers to be efficient and to use the least costly combination of services.

A third reason offered for regulation is the need to hold down the large increases in governmental expenditures on medical care. States, as well as the federal government, need to contain the amounts they spend on medical care for the indigent and the aged. The main concern of these governmental entities is not so much efficiency as it is the total dollar amount, which is rapidly increasing each year. Unless the states and the federal government can contain these expenditures, they will either have to raise taxes or else find themselves unable to finance existing or new programs; both alternatives are politically unpalatable to elected administrations.

The last reasons used to justify regulation and planning are that without planning, some persons would not have access to medical care, and scarce medical resources would be improperly distributed. The proponents of this argument claim that reliance on market forces alone to allocate medical care would leave people living in rural or ghetto areas without access to care; who would be willing to serve them?

These reasons for favoring regulation and planning are not exhaustive, but they include the major concerns of the proponents. Demand inefficiencies, particularly the consumer-protection argument, are often used to justify regulation that requires licensure and erects barriers to entry into the profession. Utilization review procedures are also suggested, albeit by a different set of regulation proponents, to improve certain inefficiencies on the demand side. The regulations most often proposed for controlling supply inefficiencies are certificate of need (CON), rate regulation, and other centralized approaches to the allocation of resources. Rate regulation and expenditure limits are usually suggested as methods for containing the total increase in government funds spent on medical care. Certificate of need, which centralizes control over capital expenditures in a planning agency, is also considered by some persons to be a useful means to this end.

For dealing with the equity and maldistribution problem, national health insurance, controls on the location decisions of all providers and professionals, rate regulation, and certificate of need are proposed. National health insurance and control over location decisions are fairly obvious approaches when judged by their intended effects, but the latter two methods may not be. Rate regulation would be used to set prices at a higher level for some services or patients in order to provide a subsidy for other services or persons. CON legislation would prevent the elimination of services or facilities from certain unprofitable areas and would also suggest which areas should be permitted to expand their facilities and services.

As can be seen from the foregoing discussion, the objectives to be achieved by regulation and planning in the medical care field are multiple. It is not possible, nor is it desirable, to compare a market orientation to the delivery of medical services with that of regulation as an alternative means of achieving all of the mentioned objectives. Greater reliance on competitive forces alone will not increase the amount of funds available to improve the poor's access to medical care. Neither will it necessarily improve the distribution of medical resources. Provider competition will not alleviate the concerns of those persons who believe medical care use should be based on professional judgment alone. It is thus inappropriate to fault a market approach to medical services delivery because it fails to meet the objectives sought by the different proponents of regulation. A fairer comparison would be carried out goal by goal. For example, if increased access to medical care is favored, then a government subsidy is required. Given a government subsidy, it is then appropriate to ask which of the two approaches would achieve the goal of increased access more efficiently. If economic efficiency in supply is a desirable objective, then which of the alternative approaches is more likely to achieve that objective? However, the two approaches cannot be comparatively applied to determine whether professional judgment should dictate medical services use. The desire of regulation proponents to base decisions affecting use on professional judgment involves a value judgment and, as such, substitutes a criterion other than economic efficiency in consumption as the objective. It is thus not possible to compare the two approaches with respect to achieving this goal. A market approach would result in economic efficiency on the demand side; professional judgment is a negation of the criteria of economic efficiency in the use of medical services. Therefore, the two approaches cannot be compared.

Thus, in delineating the area in which the two approaches can be compared, we will not address inefficiencies in demand because the basis for comparison would not be acceptable to both sides. We shall also omit, at this point, issues dealing with welfare, equity, or distribution, since we will return to this subject when we discuss medical care financing. At that time, we will discuss alternative approaches to financing medical care, the different values those involve, and the different approaches that may be used to deliver that care. The remaining area in which market competition and regulation can be compared is the achievement of economic efficiency in the supply of medical services. Thus, regardless of what we hold to be the appropriate criteria for evaluating efficiency in demand or for determining how much medical care should be redistributed and to whom, it is still possible to compare the regulatory and market approaches with respect to the supply side of the medical care market.

With this background in the general objectives of medical sector regulation, and with the specific objective of contrasting a market and regulatory approach to achieving efficiency in the provision of medical services, we turn now to an examination of the regulatory approach and its likely consequences.

THE PERFORMANCE OF REGULATORY AGENCIES OUTSIDE THE HEALTH SECTOR

To gain a better understanding of how well regulation is likely to perform in the health sector, it is instructive first to examine the behavior of regulatory agencies outside it. To this end, we shall discuss behavioral models of regulatory agencies and, based upon these models, develop different hypotheses to predict the regulated industry's performance. That performance will then be examined to select the behavioral model that most closely describes the regulatory agency's behavior. In the next section the selected model will be applied to the health field, and its implications and predictive potential for hospitals will be discussed.

The first model of regulatory agency behavior, referred to as the traditional view, assumes that such agencies were established to protect the consumer from the abuses of big business (natural monopolies) and to provide consumer protection in those cases where consumers were unable to judge the quality of the product or service they were purchasing. Under this traditional view of regulation, the regulatory agency, acting in the consumer's interest, should cause the prices of the goods and services produced by the regulated industries to be lower than they would be without such legislation. In this view, the profits of regulated industries would also be expected to be lower than they would be if such regulation did not exist. To protect the public interest, the regulatory agency would exercise tight controls over the regulated industry's prices and profits. Such a comprehensive set of regulatory controls is often referred to as public utility regulation.

Dissatisfaction arose, however, with this traditional view of regulation. It was asked: if public utility regulation was established to protect the consumer from being charged monopoly prices by such natural monopolies as railroads, telephone, and utility companies, why were such competitive industries as trucking, airlines, and taxicabs also regulated? Competitive industries were selectively regulated, a fact that the traditional model could not explain: why was there such extensive regulation of what could be considered a competitive industry?

Another source of dissatisfaction with the traditional view of regulation is the fact that if the regulatory agency's intention was to lower the regulated industry's prices and profits, why would other firms desire to enter the markets served by regulated firms? There should be no reason for unregulated firms to want to compete in regulated markets. Yet in every regulated industry, the regulatory agency strictly limits the entry of unregulated firms into the regulated market. These two dissatisfactions with the traditional view of regulation— namely, the extension of regulation to include industries that could be competitive, and the persistent desire by unregulated firms to enter regulated markets— have resulted in the development of alternative models of the behavior of regulatory agencies.

The view of regulatory agency behavior that directly opposes the traditional view is known as the economic theory of regulation (5). According to this theory, regulatory agencies and their policies are developed for the express purpose of monopolizing the industry. Under the traditional view, the agency regulates the monopolistic firms to achieve the outcome that would occur in a competitive industry. The economic theory of regulation, however, hypothesizes that regulation enables what is or would become a competitive industry to act as though it were in fact a monopoly. The impetus for regulation, or for the capture of the regulatory agency by the industry it is meant to regulate, comes from the industry's desire to use the regulatory process as a vehicle for charging higher prices, restricting its output, raising its profits, and protecting itself from possible competitors.

The economic theory of regulation and legislation suggests that government policies and legislative outcomes can best be understood within a traditional economic framework. Namely, regulation is demanded by groups because of the benefits it confers and is supplied by legislators. The market price equilibrating the demand and supply of regulation is political support. Groups demanding regulatory benefits are willing to pay a price for those benefits, such as providing votes, campaign contributions, and volunteer time. The purpose of regulation under this theory is to use the power of government to transfer wealth from those with little political power to those with more. The suppliers of regulatory benefits, who are ultimately elected officials, require political support to maximize their reelection probabilities (their goal). In attempting to maximize political support, the suppliers of regulation are presumed to calculate the amount of political support gained as a result of providing benefits to one group compared to the political support they would lose by those opposed. Legislators delegate some of their authority since it becomes too costly to constantly legislate each aspect of regulatory behavior. The legislature's preference is to delegate to regulatory agencies rather than the courts. The courts are more insulated from political control since their tenure is for fixed terms and their budgets are less subject to legislative approval.

The success of a group in receiving regulatory benefits depends, not only on whether they are able to recognize what is in their self-interest, but whether they can organize themselves and provide the necessary political support to those who will supply the regulation. Special-interest groups are said to have a "concentrated" interest in regulation; regulation can have a major impact on their livelihood. It is in their economic interest to be informed on regulations affecting their members and to actively promote those interests. The members of such groups are also likely to be more informed as to the positions taken by their legislators at election time. It is for these reasons that Downs concluded, "Democratic governments tend to favor producers more than consumers in their actions" (6). The costs of providing regulatory benefits to a particular group are spread over a large number of people. Consumers are said to have a "diffuse" interest in the outcome of regulation, since the increased prices they have to pay as a result of favorable regulation to an industry has a small effect on the consumer's overall budget. While these costs are relatively small to those who bear them, in the aggregate these losses may be quite large. Given the diffuse nature of the costs of regulation, it is not in the interest of those bearing the costs to become involved in the regulatory process, for consumers to organize other consumers, to gather the necessary information to refute the information provided by the regulated industry, and to become an adversary in the agency's proceedings. Thus because the high information and transactions costs generally exceed the benefits (in terms of defeating the regulation) to an individual, the public generally does not have much input into the regulatory process. The exclusion of the public from most regulatory decisionmaking is particularly true for legislation that is neither publicized nor obvious in its redistributive effects (7). To the regulated industry, which has a concentrated interest, such lobbying efforts before the legislature, its subcommittees, and before the regulatory agency are both worthwhile and necessary.

The economic theory of regulation provides an explanation why industries that would otherwise be competitive demand regulation. Industries that are highly concentrated, that is, that consist of a few large firms, would be more likely to act as a cartel if it were not for the antitrust laws. They could reach agreement on price and output as though they were a single monopoly firm. However, the costs of cartelizing an industry that consists of many small firms, i.e., is an industry that is of low concentration, are relatively large. These costs consist of coordinating agreements among the many firms as to the price that each firm should charge, and establishing output quotas for each firm. It is also costly to monitor the firms to ensure that they do not cheat on price and output. If they do, sanctions must be imposed. Once a price is established that is higher than the price that would prevail under competition, each firm has an incentive to charge a slightly lower price, thereby increasing its own output, hence profit. If this cheating becomes widespread, however, the higher price will fall back to the competitive price. When there are few firms in the industry, it is relatively easy to monitor the prices being charged. However, when there are many firms, it is not only difficult to reach agreement on the optimal price and output for the industry but also to monitor and enforce that minimum price. Because these organizational and enforcement costs are higher for firms in a competitive industry, it is unlikely that they could privately cartelize an industry. To receive the benefits of a cartel, firms in competitive industries must seek regulation. Only through regulation can the minimum price be established, firms prevented from lowering that price to increase their sales, and new firms prevented from entering the industry.

The economic theory of regulation applies to diverse groups that have a concentrated interest in regulation, such as small businesses, labor unions, dairy farmers, and the professions. Unless they were protected by regulation, these groups could not receive the benefits of a cartelized industry. Thus the economic theory of regulation can resolve the two dissatisfactions with the traditional view of regulation. Normally competitive industries demand regulation to provide themselves with the benefits of monopoly power. Unregulated firms continually attempt to enter regulated markets because the prices established by the regulatory agency are higher than those that would prevail in a competitive situation.

At times the economic theory of regulation is similar in its predictions to the "capture" theory, that is, the regulated industry captures the regulatory agency so as to use the regulatory power to its own benefit. The economic theory of regulation is a more satisfactory theory since it provides greater explanatory power in more diverse situations. Groups other than the regulated firms, such as competing industries and labor unions, may also have a concentrated interest in the regulatory outcomes. For example, in the health field the government has developed a concentrated interest in health care cost containment since increased health costs have such a large impact on the federal budget. Since the economic theory of regulation views the regulator as attempting to maximize political support, regulatory benefits will be divided up when there are competing groups, each with a concentrated interest. The division of those benefits, however, is unlikely to be equal.

Another model of regulatory agency behavior, similar in its predictions to the economic theory of regulation, is what Roger Noll refers to as the political–economic theory (8). This theory of regulatory agency behavior gives greater weight to the goals of the regulatory agency itself. The bureaucrats responsible for the regulatory agency wish to increase the size and authority of their agency, thereby justifying higher salaries. To be able to increase its budget, the agency must be able to minimize opposition to its decisions. The agency may thus see itself as serving several different constituencies: the industry to be regulated, the legislators who serve on the subcommittee with responsibility for both the agency's budget and its legislative mandate, and other organized interest groups that might provide vocal opposition to the agency's decisions. When the major interest group concerned with the regulatory agency's decisions is the regulated industry, then this model would be similar in its predictions to those of the capture theory. When several divergent interest groups are affected by the agency's decision, the agency will attempt to prolong the time it takes to reach a decision, thereby increasing the cost to those interest groups participating in the process and delaying the moment when its decision will be appealed. When competing interest groups are involved, the agency will arrive at compromise decisions, which minimize further opposition to the agency and forestall any appeal. Under this theory of agency behavior, when the regulated industry is the main interest group affected by the agency's decision, the agency will produce a decision that is approximate to what the regulated industry desires. As the number of competing interest groups increases, the agency will attempt to minimize its costs by reaching a compromise with the competing groups.

In this view, the regulatory agency will attempt to measure its performance according to fairly obvious indicators. Failure to perform well on these measures could result in opposition to the agency's plans for its budget, its size, and the extent of its legislative authority. Unfortunately, the success indicators will be those that are the most obvious, not necessarily the most important. There are always trade-offs between different measures of performance; however, the agency's decisions will be biased toward the more obvious measures of success, neglecting the less obvious costs inherent in those choices.

These different theories of regulation provide different hypotheses to explain the performance of the regulated industry. Under the traditional view of regulation, the regulated industry would be expected to have lower prices than it would if regulation did not exist. The regulatory agency would also be expected to eliminate inefficiencies inherent in monopolistic markets. Under the economic theory of regulation, the regulatory agency will enable the different firms in the industry to act as a cartel, thereby raising prices, restricting output, and providing regulated firms with higher profits than they would make if regulation did not exist. When there are several competing interest groups, compromises result, and no single group does as well as it would if it were the only group with a concentrated interest.

To date, the empirical evidence indicates that prices of comparable goods and services are *higher* in regulated than in nonregulated industries.* For ex-

---

*There is one exception. Natural gas prices are lower in regulated than in nonregulated competitive markets. The reason for this apparent anomaly is that the buyer of natural gas is the pipeline industry, which is itself regulated by the Federal Power Commission (FPC). The FPC had set the price of natural gas lower than the cost of newly discovered natural gas. This pricing policy by the FPC to benefit the regulated pipelines has not been without certain consequences. Newly discovered natural gas has been sold on an intrastate basis where it is not subject to FPC regulation. This reduction in natural gas in interstate commerce has resulted in shortages in those states relying on interstate pipelines. Paul MacAvoy, "The Regulation-Induced Shortage of Natural Gas," *Journal of Law and Economics* (April 1971). Such shortages were very noticeable during the winter of 1977 when factories, schools, and even residential homes could not receive an adequate supply. Since the price and availability of natural gas is higher in those states where it is sold on an intrastate basis, industry has begun to move to those states in order to ensure receiving an adequate supply, albeit at higher prices.

ample, airlines that flew intrastate only, such as between San Francisco and Los Angeles, were not subject to regulation by the Civil Aeronautics Board (CAB) and were 32 to 47 percent lower in price than airlines that flew comparable distances but were regulated by the CAB (9). Motor carriers that carry agricultural products, and are thereby exempt from Interstate Commerce Commission (ICC) regulation, had rates 41 to 58 percent lower than those charged by carriers subject to ICC regulation (10). "Pipeline tariffs in regulated interstate markets are not only higher than in the unregulated intrastate markets, but apparently in some cases even somewhat higher than an unconstrained monopolist would charge" (11).

The production of electricity, which is generally considered to be characteristic of a natural monopoly, is an interesting illustration of regulators' behavior. In earlier years, not all states regulated the prices at which electricity was sold. Since industrial users of electricity are fewer than residential users and are organized to press their interests, they should be able to exert more influence over the regulatory agency to act in their behalf in the setting of electricity rates. Under the economic theory of regulation we would, therefore, expect industrial users in regulated states to receive more favorable electricity rates than residential users. The price of electricity to industrial and residential users would be expected to differ to reflect actual differences in costs between the two user groups. Therefore, the ratio of the residential to the industrial price of electricity was compared between states that regulate such prices and states that do not. In the two time periods studied, the relative price of electricity was higher for residential users than for industrial users in the regulated states. Thus, the data support the hypothesis that regulation was to the advantage of the more organized interest group and to the disadvantage of residential users (12).

	1917	1937
Regulated states	1.616	2.459
Unregulated states	1.445	2.047

The fact that the regulatory agency restricts entry into regulated industries adds further weight to the evidence that prices are higher in such industries. If regulated prices were comparable to those that would prevail in a competitive industry, then other firms should not find it profitable to enter the regulated market. Yet for all regulated markets an important function of the regulatory agency is to limit entry. This behavior of the regulatory agency is consistent with the hypothesis that the industry seeks regulation in order to establish a cartel. In order to maintain a high price for its member firms' products, the cartel must ensure that production does not exceed that level of output that would be demanded at the cartel's price. To limit the rate of output in the cartelized industry, the cartel must limit the industry's capacity to produce that output; otherwise, firms would find it profitable to increase their output by undercutting the cartel's price.

Regulatory agencies apparently undertake those functions that would normally be assigned to managers of the cartel. To protect its monopoly price, the cartel must limit productive capacity in two ways: first, the regulatory agency must prohibit entry by new firms. For example, since its inception, the CAB had not permitted the establishment of any new trunk line air carrier; entry by existing air carriers into markets served by other air carriers is strictly limited. Second, a well-controlled cartel will attempt to ensure that no excess capacity exists among its current members, lest they be encouraged to produce more than the cartel desires. When cartelization initially occurs in an industry, the industry's output has to be reduced, since the output demanded at the higher monopoly price will be less than it was previously. To ensure that member firms in the cartel do not increase their output, which would undercut and bring pressure on the monopoly price, the cartel must remove the excess capacity that exists among its members, which was appropriate to their previously larger output. As the cartel becomes solidly entrenched, it will be strict in granting permission to its members to expand their capacity so that increased production does not place pressure on the cartel's artificially maintained price. To date, most regulated industries have not been able to assign specific quotas to each regulated firm in each particular market. The consequence of this excess capacity has been intense nonprice competition among the regulated firms to increase their market shares. For example, it has been estimated "that at any given time 40 percent of the trucks on the road are running empty because of government regulations that prevent them from carrying cargo on return trips after making deliveries" (13).

The body of evidence on prices in regulated industries thus appears to support the economic theory regulation and to contradict the traditional view that regulation will lower prices. The empirical evidence, however, indicates that rates of return in regulated industries are not as high as in nonregulated industries; further, the price of common stocks of regulated industries has generally not risen as fast as the stock of nonregulated firms (14).

The lower than expected profitability of regulated industries can be reconciled with both the economic and political-economic theories of regulation. As a political support maximizer, the regulator would allocate the benefits of regulation to competing interest groups. The excess capacity caused by CAB regulation benefited the aircraft manufacturers, airline employees, and suppliers of airline services. For example, establishing a regulated price greater than that which would prevail in a competitive market would cause competition on aspects other than price, thereby benefiting the producers of these other services (15). The higher costs diminish the profitability of the regulated industries' higher prices. The methods by which the regulatory industries' costs are increased are briefly described below.

Cross-Subsidization of Services

Although regulated firms are permitted to charge monopoly prices in some markets, they are always required to use some of those profits to serve other areas or customers by charging prices below the costs of providing the service. Using the profitable markets to subsidize unprofitable markets has been referred to as "taxation by regulation" (16). Regulatory agencies are thus able to bypass state and federal legislatures, whose function it is to levy taxes, by imposing what are in effect taxes on the goods and services of the industries they regulate. The proceeds of such taxes are then spent to maximize the size of the regulated industry. For example, the Civil Aeronautics Board set airline prices that greatly exceeded costs in markets such as New York and Miami, and then required the airlines serving those markets to serve less-profitable cities as well. Passengers flying between New York and Miami paid a monopoly price for that service, part of which was used to subsidize passengers flying between smaller towns, markets for which the airlines might otherwise have discontinued service or sharply raised the price. As a result of this cross-subsidization, overall rates of return to the regulated industry were lower than they might otherwise have been.

The benefits of cross-subsidization are several: influential legislators are able to provide subsidized services to their constituents; the regulated industry is able to enlarge its investment through expansion, thereby increasing absolute profit by earning a fair return on the total investment (including the resources used to service less-profitable areas); and the regulators themselves are able to justify increases in their agency's size and influence. The opponents of this hidden tax are the unorganized users of the service in the monopoly-priced markets.

There is little justification for an indirect tax-subsidy system. Regulatory agencies are not provided with legislative authority to redistribute income among the various users of regulated services, and it is unlikely that the redistribution that occurs is from higher- to lower-income groups. The use of monopoly pricing in one area to generate subsidies to increase use in other areas also results in an inefficient allocation of resources, as too many resources flow into the regulated sector from unregulated sectors in the economy. It has also been suggested that if these subsidies were removed, the communities losing subsidized services would suffer little, as substitute services would expand and replace those lost. If airline service to small communities decreased, other forms of transportation, such as buses, would take its place (17).

Regulation-Induced Inefficiencies

Under regulation price competition is eliminated by the establishment of minimum prices, but other forms of competition are permitted, leading to higher costs. Regulated firms compete among themselves in markets where monopoly prices are established by offering additional services to consumers. In the airline industry, airlines compete on such nonprice aspects as amenities, newer equipment, larger and faster planes, and frequency of schedules. The costs of nonprice competition generally exceed the value consumers place on such services. If consumers had a choice between lower air fares or higher fares that include various additional services, a number of them would prefer to pay lower prices for air travel, arrive a little later at their destination, fly on older planes between some cities, and forego meal service and riding in 747s. Nonprice competition among regulated firms results in excess capacity and in an increase in costs of operation. To ensure that the airlines do not use up all of their profits in nonprice competition (depleting funds to subsidize airline service to less profitable areas), the regulatory agency inevitably places limits on the various aspects of nonprice competition. Thus, the regulatory agency becomes involved in determining what amenities can be offered to airline passengers. The agency governing international air travel (IATA) was forced to define an open-faced sandwich. More and more regulation must be developed to cover services provided to customers as new forms of nonprice competition are generated by the competing regulated firms. The consequences of nonprice competition are an increase in the regulated industry's costs, the creation of excess capacity, and a resource cost that exceeds the value consumers place on such nonprice competition.

Another consequence of regulation that results in higher costs for regulated industries is the removal of incentives for efficient operation. If the price of the regulated service is set high enough to cover the costs of even the highest-cost firm, and if all firms in the industry are able to earn a minimum rate of return, then management has little incentive to be efficient. A more efficient firm cannot keep its savings, because any excess profit will be used to cross-subsidize other services. It is not surprising, therefore, that the caliber of management in regulated firms is lower than in nonregulated industries. The potential rewards for management creativity and efficiency in regulated industries are relatively small.

Regulatory agencies' methods for calculating a regulated firm's rate of return result in certain perverse incentives. The amount of profit allowed in some regulated industries is based on costs incurred, while in other regulated industries it may be based on the size of the firm's investment. In the former case, it is in the regulated firm's interest to increase its costs (hence increase its profits) or to undertake larger investments than necessary. The telephone company's profit increased when it built larger, more elaborate, and longer-lasting buildings.

The method regulatory agencies use to protect regulated firms from potential competition also increases the costs of providing a service in regulated industries. As mentioned earlier, prices in the regulated industry are set high enough to permit the firms with the highest costs to survive. If, for example, a lower-cost method of production is developed as a result of technological change, the regulatory agency will prevent the new, lower-cost industry from driving the regulated, higher-cost producers out of the market in the following ways. First, the regulatory agency will include the new, lower-cost industry (which can become a substitute for the regulated firms) within its regulatory authority. Second, the price of the service will be set high enough to permit the regulated firms to survive and compete (on a nonprice basis) with the lower-cost firms. For example, the ICC initially regulated railroads presumably because they were a monopoly. As trucks, a lower-cost substitute were developed, the ICC regulated them to prevent this new industry from capturing large segments of the markets served by railroads. Barges and other water carriers were brought under ICC regulation in 1940 because of their competition with railroads (18). Rather than allowing the prices of goods shipped in various markets to reflect the costs of shipping, the ICC set minimum rates for goods shipped in interstate commerce that were not reflective of the least-costly method of shipping. Trucking, which could have been a competitive industry, was regulated to prevent railroads from losing some of their markets to lower-cost shippers.

The consequences of extending regulatory authority to include lower-cost producers is that consumers pay prices higher than they would be if competition existed among the different industries and the price reflected the production cost of the lowest-cost industry. Higher-cost industries and inefficient firms are helped to survive in a regulatory environment.

Regulatory Response to Technological Change

Another influence toward higher costs in regulated industries is the regulatory agencies' response to technological change developed outside of the regulated industry. Technological innovations may result in new substitute services or similar services that consumers would be willing to purchase at a lower cost. To prevent the regulated industry from losing its market share and possibly going out of existence, the agency will attempt to retard the introduction of technological innovations. For example, the FCC delayed giving its permission to a firm other than AT&T to put up a domestic communications satellite; the FCC restricted the development of cable television, which would threaten the monopoly of UHF television stations in large cities. The introduction of new technology is stalled because the firms that would profit from it are not those that are regulated.

Another reason why technological change is introduced very slowly in regulated industries is that such change could have an adverse impact on the regulatory agency itself. To minimize criticism of its performance, an agency is unlikely to undertake actions that have a chance of failure. Since the effects of innovation cannot be entirely foreseen, an agency would probably prefer to delay permitting a change until the benefits of the innovation are obvious to all or until the benefits are greatly in excess of the possible costs, according to the agency's determination. The agency's assessment of the possible benefits and costs of innovation is likely to differ from that of consumers, who might be willing to purchase such services were they available on the market. To avoid criticism, the agency is likely to use the most obvious measures of benefits and costs; the less obvious or hidden costs and benefits will be assigned less weight in the agency's deliberations.

In reviewing the empirical evidence on the behavior of regulation in other industries, it appears that the traditional view of regulation, whereby agencies act in the public interest and cause prices to be lower, is an inaccurate description of reality. It appears that a more accurate model is the economic theory of regulation. When there is only one group with a concentrated interest that group will receive the benefits of regulation. When there are competing interest groups compromises are reached and the benefits of regulation are shared. As has been shown, the effect of the regulatory agency's acting in the interest of those whom it is to regulate is that the prices of goods and services in the regulated industry will be higher than if the industry were not regulated. Cross-subsidization of services, inefficiency, a decline in the quality of management, and competition in the areas of amenities and extra services can also be expected in a regulated industry, together with the resulting higher costs. The agency will also impose entry barriers on technologically innovative firms and extend its regulatory authority to include lower-cost substitute providers in order to protect the regulated firms. The extent of regulation will thus increase as the regulatory agency seeks to cover all the gaps that will arise from nonprice competition and from the threat of new firms. Finally, as the scope of its authority and the number of competing interest groups served increases, the regulatory agency will, in order to protect its own interests, resort to using obvious measures of its success. Not only will obvious success measures minimize criticism of the agency's performance but also they will result in the agency's failure to consider trade-offs and other costs that may be involved in its decisions, possibly resulting in a shift of those costs to consumers.

THE PROBABLE CONSEQUENCES OF REGULATION OF HOSPITAL CAPITAL INVESTMENT

Although it is always possible that the consequences of hospital regulation will differ from the regulatory experience of other industries, it is unlikely in the light of the evidence already presented. Hospitals have a great stake in any regulatory process affecting them. Their interests are concentrated, whereas those of consumers concerned about the rapid increase in hospital costs are diffuse. As long as hospitals are the only ones with a concentrated interest, we would expect hospital regulatory agencies to be favorably disposed to the hospitals' interests; in fact, we would expect any hospital regulatory agency to protect the hospitals under its jurisdiction. Contrary to the traditional view of regulation, we would expect hospital prices to continue their upward rise; we would also expect to observe cross-subsidization of services and patients within the hospital. Both the regulatory agency and the hospitals themselves would favor expanding the number of services offered by hospitals. Monopoly pricing of certain hospital services, such as ancillary services, would continue under regulation; the regulatory agency would not become involved in an adversary relationship with the hospitals by requiring them to set prices equal to costs for each hospital service. Since no price competition would exist among the hospitals, nonprice competition to attract customers, namely physicians, would continue in the form of facilities, services, and other inducements. The regulatory agency, in further acting on hospitals' behalf, would inhibit innovations in the delivery of medical care that decrease hospital utilization regardless of its potential cost savings to customers because such innovations would potentially decrease hospital revenues and threaten the survival of some protected hospitals. Similarly, entry into the industry would be sharply curtailed lest a new hospital demonstrate greater efficiency, lower its costs, and render existing hospitals' capacity excessive. Finally, we would not expect hospitals to become more efficient once their survival was assured, nor would the quality of their administrative staff be noteworthy once regulation of hospital operations became pervasive.

The above scenario of the likely consequences of hospital regulation would not obviate any of the reasons for proposing hospital regulation in the first place. The rapid increases in hospital costs, duplication of facilities and services, excess hospital capacity, and the lack of incentives to substitute less costly care when medically possible have been the result of cost-based reimbursement of hospital care, a lack of incentives and information on the part of the patient, and the role of the physician in the use of hospital and other medical resources as a decision-maker without the financial responsibility for those decisions. If the experience with regulation in other industries is any guide to what will occur with respect to hospitals, then these problems will not be resolved through the regulatory process.

A Review of Efforts to Control Hospital Investment

The types of regulation being proposed to alleviate the foregoing causes of inefficiencies in hospital care are worthy of examination. An important regulatory development with respect to hospitals has been the enactment of state certificate-of-need (CON) laws. As a result of such laws, hospitals must secure the approval of planning agencies at several levels of government for all new hospital investment (exceeding a minimum dollar amount, such as $100,000). CON legislation is a natural extension of previous efforts to make the expansion of the health care system more "rational."

Hospital planning on the federal level started with the Hospital Survey and Construction Act (Hill-Burton) in 1946 (19). Federal funds were provided to each state for construction of new beds and for modernization according to a formula based on population and per capita income. In order to receive funds, a hospital (or a prospective hospital) had to obtain the approval of the Hill-Burton agency in its state. The criteria used by the state Hill-Burton agencies for the allocation of funds were relatively simple and considered data only on the number of beds, the population, and the population density in the area. It is difficult to identify the method used by Hill-Burton agencies to allocate Hill-Burton funds for modernization, which eventually became the major use of Hill-Burton funds. To receive these funds, each state had to produce a state plan for its hospital beds, but there is little evidence that such state plans were anything more than inventories of beds and facilities. Under the Hill-Burton program, many small hospitals were started in rural areas that previously did not have a hospital. The Hill-Burton program had the political support of the American Hospital Association (AHA) and the continued endorsement of Congress for 25 years, since each state received a share of the federal hospitals funds. Hill-Burton was responsible for starting many new hospitals, but only in areas where they would not compete with existing hospitals. After several years, the program changed its emphasis to modernizing existing hospitals rather than providing new hospital beds. Hospitals that did not receive Hill-Burton funds were still able to finance new beds from other sources. However, Hill-Burton did little, if anything, to coordinate hospital investment; perhaps for this reason, hospitals have considered it a success.

The next major development in hospital planning came with the development of voluntary planning agencies. In the mid-1960s Congress passed the Comprehensive Health Planning Act. Health planning agencies were set up locally within a state and coordinated by a state-level agency, but they could only attempt to improve hospital planning in a voluntary manner, as they did not have any authority to approve or disapprove hospital investment. When their effectiveness was evaluated, it was determined that planned and unplanned areas had the same amount of unnecessary duplication of facilities and services; also, planned areas experienced a larger percentage increase in their beds, a larger percentage decrease in proprietary hospitals in their area, and no difference in the rate of increase in hospital costs per patient (20). The conclusion would thus appear to be that voluntary hospital planning had no significant influence on hospital costs or investment. Individual hospitals had little incentive to cooperate in hospital planning because it would have frustrated the achievement of their prestige goals. Perhaps as a means of ensuring that planning agencies did not obstruct hospital goals, but instead directed their efforts against potential entrants to the market, planning agencies were made dependent upon hospital contributions for part of their budgets (21).

By the mid-1970s several developments resulted in sufficient pressure for a new and stronger planning law to be passed. Hospital costs had continued to rise rapidly since the passage of Medicare and Medicaid in 1966. Third-party payors, whose premiums were affected by these cost increases, and state and federal governments, whose expenditures under these programs were rising much more rapidly than expected, wanted to contain the increase in hospital expenditures. A stronger planning law was proposed as a solution to the hospital costs problem.

Blue Cross saw capital controls as a way of holding down hospital costs without becoming an adversary of the major hospitals in an area, whose interests Blue Cross served. Hospital associations had by this time also favored stronger controls through planning.

It is interesting to speculate on why hospitals would favor constraints on their capital expenditures. By the mid-1970s, a high percentage of the population had insurance coverage for hospital care, and the demand for hospital care was no longer expected to increase as it had in the past. Further, all hospitals in an area are not equal. Some are already prestigious; they already have a favored competitive position vis-à-vis other hospitals in their area. Continued competition among hospitals presents a threat to the large hospital with many facilities and services and with a large number of staff physicians to keep its beds filled. The larger hospital's interest lay in strengthening local planning efforts to restrict further hospital investment. It would be in the interests of all the hospitals to keep potential competitors out of the industry. With the leveling off of the increases in demand for hospital care, combined with hospitals' fears that more drastic cost-containing measures would be proposed and their desire to retain their favored competitive position, the time was ripe for hospitals to institute local hospital cartels.

The above hypothesis is supported in a recent study by Wendling and Werner (22). This study attempted to explain the passage of state CON laws. The period 1968–1973 was selected for analysis; 22 states passed CON legislation, 16 states defeated such legislation, and 11 states did not undertake any action on this issue. (A change occurred in 1974 which made the years since then less appropriate for analysis. In 1974 the National Health Planning and Resources Development Act was passed which provided incentives and penalties to encourage states to adopt CON.)

The public interest view of CON is that states passed it to control the increase in hospital expenditures, as measured by the percentage change in hospital expenditures per patient day for the 6-year period preceding state action on CON. The economic theory of regulation suggests that hospitals would favor passage of CON in those states in which there is greater competition among hospitals, as measured by the occupancy rate in the state for the preceding 6 years. An increase in competition would lower hospital revenues and make it more difficult for hospitals to expand. Several other variables were also included in the analysis. A measure of industry concentration was used to measure the costs of organizing hospitals to seek regulation. It was also hypothesized that CON was more likely in those states where there was greater competition among the political parties, hence a greater need for political support by the parties; a variable measuring this factor was also included.

The results of the statistical analysis were as expected. There was a greater likelihood of CON passage in those states having lower occupancy rates. The percent change in hospital expenditures per patient day was not related to the passage of state CON laws. Thus where the competitive threat was high (low occupancy rates) and hospitals were highly concentrated, the probability of CON in a state was .76. (The probability of defeat under these conditions was .13.) At the other extreme—hospitals facing little competitive threat and low concentration—the probability of CON in a state was .18; the probability of defeat, since it would be against the hospitals' interests, was .55.

The results of this study support the economic theory of regulation. The probability of CON in a state was highest when the potential benefit to hospitals was greatest and the costs of achieving it were relatively low. This study also suggests that CON is unlikely to have an impact on hospital expenditures because cost containment was not the real purpose of the legislation.

Federal legislation was passed in 1974 providing planning agencies with greater authority over hospital capital expenditures. Hospitals were required to receive planning agency approval for expansion and for investment in new facilities and services. The method proposed for dealing with rising hospital costs was to establish controls on hospital beds and on investment in new facilities and services.

Certificate-of-need legislation is a very conservative approach to containing the rise in hospital costs (23). CON legislation assumes no changes in the method of hospital reimbursement and provides no new incentives to change patient or physician behavior. It is not surprising, therefore, that CON has been unsuccessful in controlling hospital expenditures, which was the problem it was intended to redress. To control the increase in hospital costs, additional regulation had to be developed. As each new set of regulations fails to achieve the desired social goals, stronger regulations are proposed to do the job.

The Likely Consequences of CON Legislation

It is possible to hypothesize how CON legislation will perform in controlling hospital costs and to test those hypotheses against a growing body of data. Based on evidence from other regulated industries we would expect that unless (or until) competing interest groups develop, hospital planning agencies will use their stronger legislative authority to protect the hospitals they are supposed to regulate. The methods used will be to prevent entry by competitors into the markets served by existing hospitals and to preclude innovations that might threaten existing hospitals' revenues.

Entry by potential competitors is a threat to existing hospitals for two reasons: first, a competitor might successfully decrease an existing hospital's market share; and second, a competitor could undercut a hospital's monopoly pricing practices, which generate revenue for cross-subsidization. Cross-subsidization in hospital care occurs in several ways: profitable services such as ancillary services are used to subsidize unprofitable prestige facilities and services for which demand may be insufficient; some patients subsidize other patients who are more severely ill; and patients with commercial insurance subsidize Medicaid patients. Price discrimination is practiced by hospitals by type of service, type of patient, and type of third-party payor. A new hospital in an area could, therefore, threaten the elaborate cross-subsidy schemes by failing to offer certain unprofitable services such as obstetrics and by choosing not to admit severely ill patients, which would enable them to charge lower prices to, for example, commercial carriers. In the health field such pricing practices are referred to as cream skimming. The incentives for new firms to undercut the monopoly prices set by hospitals on certain services are the same as exist in the airline industry and other regulated sectors: new firms are willing to make less profit on services and thus offer to provide them at a lower price. The reason for agency and firm opposition to cream skimming is also similar: if monopoly profits are not made on certain services, patients, and third-party payors, funds would not be available for other uses. In effect, the regulated firm would have to reduce its size.

The objection to cream skimming in health is based on the claim that unless some patients are subsidized they will have to do without such care. These consequences are much more severe than the results of a reduction in airline service to a community. The arguments against cream skimming are based on the premise that charity care is given in significant quantities by hospitals. It is further claimed that the services that would be discontinued if monopoly pricing on other services were no longer possible are sufficiently important for the hospital to continue to provide them. Whatever relevance the charity argument once held for justifying discriminatory pricing has been reduced by the introduction of Medicare and Medicaid. Hospital expenditures that can be attributed to philanthropy were estimated to be less than 1.5 percent of total hospital expenditures in 1970 (24). As third-party coverage for hospital care becomes more comprehensive (as it would if a national health insurance program were enacted), the argument that hospitals need to charge monopoly prices in order to provide charity services becomes more difficult to justify. It has also never been proven that the funds generated by monopoly pricing are used to subsidize those patients who have lower incomes. Many poor patients may not enter the hospital at all or they may go to municipal hospitals. Further, the higher prices charged to patients who are less severely ill are reflected in higher insurance premiums, which fall on lower-income consumers as well.

The argument that without price discrimination a hospital would be forced to discontinue needed facilities and services is also complex. If a facility is costly because it is subject to economies of scale, then all hospitals in a community should not necessarily have this facility. If such a facility is the only one in the community or if more than one hospital should have it, then why should not its costs be reimbursable as part of the hospital costs of those patients requiring its use? The use of costly facilities and services, as well as of hospital care itself, is an insurable risk. Insurance policies that include major medical or catastrophic coverage (rather than those policies that provide front-end, shallow benefits) would reimburse the hospitals for use of such services. If patients cannot afford to pay for such services, then the argument becomes similar to the charity argument. The extent of this occurrence should be determined and a separate subsidy should be provided to low-income patients to pay for their expected hospital expenses (i.e., their insurance coverage can be subsidized). It is likely, however, that the charity argument is not the major justification, nor even an important one, for hospitals' desire to maintain facilities and services that would have to be discontinued if subsidies for their operation could not be provided. It is more likely that hospitals use internal cross-subsidization to bolster prestige services and/or to increase the attending medical staff's productivity than to maintain facilities and services the community considered necessary.

The second argument against permitting entry of a new institution into an area currently served by hospitals is that entry will merely create excess hospital capacity, which the community will end up paying for through increases in insurance premiums. However, the costs of excess capacity will be passed on in the form of higher insurance premiums only if the hospitals are reimbursed on a cost basis. If hospitals were reimbursed as other industries are, the consumer would not bear the costs of hospitals that go into bankruptcy. The hospital and its backers would bear those risks. Hospital proponents would claim that before hospitals would go bankrupt they would fill those excess beds with patients who did not have to be there by extending lengths of stay as well as admitting additional patients. They implicitly threaten that unless the existing hospitals are protected, they will knowingly fill their beds with patients who do not have to be there and the community will end up paying more for its hospital care.

As community demand for hospital care stops increasing, the only requirements for new beds will be replacement of existing ones. It is highly unlikely that a regulatory agency will refuse an existing hospital the right to replace its facilities and award that license to a new organization instead. It would therefore appear that the CON agencies are likely to guarantee the survival of existing hospitals and preclude entry by new competitors, particularly at a time when bed needs in most communities appear to be satisfied. It is interesting to examine evidence of the use of CON legislation to restrict entry. For example, in Kansas City, Missouri, the decision of the planning agency was overturned by the courts on the following grounds:

> The areawide agency had denied the application of Extendicare, Inc., a proprietary institution. The court found that Mid-American CHP had approved all applications by not-for-profit institutions but had denied that of the only investor-owned organization in circumstances that the court described as "arbitrary, capricious, and unreasonable to the extent of being tantamount to fraud." (25)

There is, of course, a fallacy in the argument by the CON legislation proponents who state that the community will have to pay for any excess beds that result from entry into the industry. As long as third-party payors such as Blue Cross and the federal government pay hospitals on the basis of their costs, then the costs of empty beds will be borne by the public. However, this is precisely why certificate-of-need legislation was developed; cost-based reimbursement enabled hospitals to duplicate facilities, resulting in rapid increases in their costs of operation. What other nonregulated industry is reimbursed for its excess capacity? Applying the same logic to the automobile industry would suggest that the government pay for all automobiles that could have been provided in a year and were not, and prohibit importation of foreign cars to reduce the number of unsold U.S. cars it would have to buy up.

An alternative to entry controls for preventing excess capacity would be to establish reimbursement rates for different types of hospital care. If a hospital could not compete with a potential competitor at a given reimbursement rate, then the community would not have to pay for the excess beds or the unnecessary services. A hospital with excess beds and facilities would either have to merge, close those excess beds and facilities, or become efficient enough to compete at a given level of reimbursement. Under such an alternative, the organization and its employees would bear the costs of duplication or inefficiency.

Changing hospital reimbursement methods would more directly solve the problem of excess capacity. The threat that the beds would be filled up with patients who did not require hospital care could be handled either by providing incentives to the hospitals, their patients, the physicians, or the insurance carriers, or through utilization review mechanisms. Guaranteeing a hospital's revenues is too costly a way of preventing unethical behavior.

Whereas competition is a threat to the survival and goals of existing hospitals, barriers to entry guarantee the hospitals' survival. By themselves such barriers will not solve the problem of rapidly increasing hospital costs, which was the justification for their establishment. Therefore, additional, more comprehensive controls will have to be proposed that will once again promise a solution to the problems of excessive and rising costs.

Another major consequence of instituting a cartel over hospital capital investment would be a delay in the introduction of innovation by outside firms and an extension of the cartel's authority over lower-cost producers. Existing members of the cartel would be in favor of introducing technological innovation themselves if it would result in increased prestige for the institution or increased productivity by the hospitals' physicians. The members of the cartel would not be expected to approve of innovational changes in the delivery of medical care that would decrease their revenues. Railroads were protected from competition with trucks when the ICC extended its authority over such low-cost substitutes, thereby regulating their entry and prices to be charged. The health planning agency's treatment of innovation would be expected to be similar. If health planning agencies are viewed as protectors of the hospitals they are meant to regulate, then we would predict that they would want to inhibit the development of any substitute source of care that would decrease the revenues of existing hospitals. Once again, such action would probably be justified as an attempt to prevent substitutes from decreasing the demand for existing hospitals, thereby creating excess capacity. Again the threat would be made that the community would have to pay for this excess capacity through its third-party payors. If, on the other hand, planning agencies are viewed as attempting to minimize the cost of medical care to the community, then they should be seeking to encourage lower-cost substitutes whenever possible. Any excess hospital capacity that results should then be eliminated by the planning agency or not be paid for by third-party payors.

Evidence of delayed innovation in the delivery of medical services supports the hypothesis that CON agencies tend to be more concerned with protecting existing hospitals than with encouraging lower-cost substitutes. A majority of CON laws presently have under their authority free-standing outpatient facilities, which include surgicenters and health maintenance organizations (26). But the justification for placing these areas under CON authority is minimal, since their capacity does not exceed their use, their services are not reimbursed on a cost-plus basis, their incentives or goals are not the same as those of the hospitals, and their costs are not a cause for concern. Therefore, the reasons usually given for CON legislation, such as excess capacity, are lacking in the case of these substitute services. If we wish to encourage the development of lower-cost substitutes for hospital care, then we should exclude these substitutes from regulations that control their entry into the industry and that impose additional requirements on them. Perhaps the only justified requirement to set for such substitutes is to monitor the quality of their services along with a similar requirement for existing health providers.

One can readily imagine how regulating low-cost substitutes for hospitals would hinder their growth. Unregulated, free-standing surgicenters would decrease the demand for short hospital stays associated with relatively simple surgery, and thereby provide a substitute for a service that is priced monopolistically by hospitals. To combat such cream skimming by a lower-cost method of production, hospital associations would try to have it required that all surgi-centers be affiliated with hospitals. This is in fact what has occurred. The reason used to justify this approach is that, whereas the quality of hospital services has already been proven to the planning agency, that of the free-standing surgicenter has not. Through affiliation, hospitals can control the development of potential competitors and avoid revenue loss. Permitting only existing hospitals to establish low-cost substitutes removes any incentives that substitute organizations have to grow at hospitals' expense. The hospitals could limit their use and, by controlling their rates, limit the savings to be achieved by patients and third-party payors. The effect of this approach on hospital revenues, compared to the effect of keeping such substitutes independent and free-standing, is obvious.

The growth of health maintenance organizations (HMOs) could lead to savings by reducing hospitalization. It is estimated that the populations served by HMOs and prepaid group practices use an amount of hospital care half that of patients using a fee-for-service setting. Thus a rapid growth of HMOs would represent a severe threat to existing hospital revenues. Opponents of HMOs have used several approaches to retard the growth of such competitors. Federal HMO legislation, which preempts state laws that do not permit such organizations, mandated that any organization wishing to qualify as a federal HMO had to offer more extensive benefits than were offered by the majority of third-party payors. A larger benefit package raises the premium of the HMO in relation to other health insurance premiums, thereby decreasing its demand. This aspect of the law has been changed. There has also been an attempt, subsequently unsuccessful, to specify input standards for an HMO, such as the ratio of beds and personnel to population served. Specifying sufficiently high inputs limits the possibility for cost reduction and substitution without necessarily assuring quality care.

Placing HMOs under CON authority would limit their growth. HMO organizations such as Kaiser have opposed such moves. They correctly fear that planning agencies will view an HMO's desire to enter an area and build a new hospital as a threat to the existing hospitals, particularly when the community might already have sufficient hospital beds. Group Health Cooperative of Puget Sound and Kaiser, "two of the most substantial and respectable HMOs, have encountered problems in obtaining permission to construct inpatient facilities needed to serve their population in these states. Although they ultimately obtained the requisite approvals after substantial delays, it is fair to ask whether smaller or newer HMOs or HMOs organized under less impeccable auspices could survive a similar encounter" (27).

It is thus easy to understand why the AHA's model bill on CON included such lower-cost substitutes as surgicenters and HMOs under CON authority. Placing constraints other than quality assurance on any innovation expected to lower the costs of medical care is bound to hinder its growth. It is unfortunate that the existing providers of hospital care perceive these issues so much more clearly than the proponents of medical care reform.

Technical Competence and Performance Measures Used by the Regulatory Agency

The degree to which an agency competently fulfills its stated roles can be used to assess the accuracy of models of regulatory agency behavior. It is thus appropriate to review the limited evidence to date on the level of technical competence of health planning agency personnel, the criteria used by the agency for decisionmaking, and the planning agency's effectiveness.

Although health planning agencies are supposed to plan for the health needs of the community, it is readily accepted by all that health planning is a misnomer. The agencies are concerned with facilities planning, primarily with hospitals. Ideally, when developing a plan for community hospital care, agency personnel should understand the factors affecting demands for care, be able to forecast those demands, estimate the costs of providing care in different-sized facilities, and incorporate in their plans the population's preferences as to travel time and cost in receiving care. Because demands, costs, and the community's preferences are always changing, the agency must be able continually to update its master plans. It is difficult to develop technical analyses, and the need to do so has raised many questions. For example, what is the definition of excess capacity in an area? After all, each area requires a standby capacity that will vary by type of facility, location, and population served. In practice, most planning agencies perform technical analyses in reaction to the expansion plans submitted by hospitals. Two U.S. Government Accounting Office (GAO) studies (1972 and 1974) found that very few health planning agencies had any plans for their area (28). A more recent study (1975) concluded that such agencies relied on the hospitals themselves for data, which were at least two years old, and that the techniques used for planning were the old Hill-Burton projections based on obsolete data (29). The technical competence of health planning agencies has apparently not significantly improved upon the rather crude methodologies used by Hill-Burton agencies.

By relying heavily on providers for their data and by using a reactive approach to planning, an agency ensures that its decisions will be heavily influenced by providers. If existing providers wanted to control the planning agency to serve their own interest, they would prefer to have either vague criteria for investment decisions or a sufficiently large number of such criteria to enable the agency to reach and justify any decision the provider desired. Lewin and Associates' findings that planning agencies' criteria were not explicit and that they preferred "full service hospitals"—that is, existing hospitals—and were against proprietary providers support this expectation (30). The importance of controlling information as a means of dominating the decisionmaking process was also demonstrated in the studies cited. A number of agencies were found to rely on provider-dominated primary review committees, and in many instances the agencies' consumer representatives were in the minority at agency advisory meetings. One wonders how effective consumer representatives can be in a situation where they must rely on the providers for the information and presumably the expertise to determine the importance or health need of a certain capital expenditure. (The consumer representatives might also have incentives similar to those of the hospitals to increase investment in and expansion of beds and prestige technology. They can then point with pride to the quality of hospital facilities in their area.) As one might expect, the studies cited found that

[the planning agencies,] efforts to curb unnecessary investment are often not very strenuous. For example, approval rates for investment proposals generally exceeded 90 percent. Also, two thirds of the agencies studied approved additional hospital beds that would raise area bed supplies to more than 105 percent of their future need projections; in fact, half of these agencies approved new beds even though existing supplies already exceeded this level. Most surprising, however, was the finding that fewer than half of all agencies saw cost containment as the primary goal of the investment review programs and one-fifth of the areawide agencies did not consider it a goal at all (31).

Another aspect of regulatory agency behavior observed in such agencies outside the health field is their desire to minimize conflict so as to avoid criticism. With regard to health facilities planning, the existing hospitals form the prime interest group affected by agency decisions; therefore, complaints about these decisions are most likely to come from the existing hospitals, their employees and staff, rather than a new applicant. One might also hypothesize that the quality of an agency's preparation and hence its performance is likely to decline with the number of adversaries questioning its decisions. Related to this issue of minimizing complaints against the agency is the regulatory agencies' attempt to have their own performance judged by the more obvious indicators of industry performance. Innovation and technical change in the delivery of health services in an area might offer huge potential benefits to the consumers. These benefits, however, are not obvious, whereas a hospital's closing as a result of entry by new firms will result in an obvious cost to the community and complaints from the affected hospital and its employees. Thus the health planning agency is likely to go very slowly on innovation, preferring to allow existing providers to introduce innovation if sufficient pressures arise for them to be adopted.

Another example of planning agencies' selecting obvious measures of industry performance as the measure of their own performance is the classic study by Salkever and Bice (32). As pressures increase from third-party payors to hold down hospital capital investment, an agency would be likely to concentrate its efforts on the most obvious measure of hospital investment: beds. Salkever and Bice found that for the study period, 1968–1972, the presence of CON controls in a state resulted in a decrease in changes in the number of beds in that state, an increase in plant assets per bed, and no change in total hospital assets. The authors concluded that controls merely shifted the type of hospital investment. The authors also attempted to determine whether the existence of strong planning agency authority resulted in lower hospital costs. They concluded that there was no evidence to indicate that CON had any effect on hospital costs.

Since the classic study by Salkever and Bice, several other researchers have examined the effect of CON legislation (33). The findings from all these studies are similar. CON does not appear to have any effect on hospital investment nor on the rate of growth in hospital expenditures. Some studies found a shift in hospital investment, from beds to equipment. Other studies found that CON caused an increase in hospital investment; hospitals moved their investment plans along faster in anticipation of CON legislation. Some of the studies measured the "maturity" of CON in a state; it was found that it did not matter how long a state had CON, it was still not effective. Still other studies examined the comprehensiveness of the legislation and the stringency of the CON process in a state. Again the findings are that CON did not have any effect on hospital investment nor on expenditures.

Summary

The evidence on health planning in this country does not support the traditional view of regulation, namely, that regulators will lower the price of the goods and services produced by the regulated industry. Instead, the accumulating evidence on the performance of regulatory agencies in nonhealth fields appears to predict the outcome of regulation in the health field; regulatory agencies are strongly influenced by the industry they are meant to regulate. The methods used by hospitals to influence the health planning agencies have varied from providing them with financial support, data, and technical expertise to functioning as the major participants in the reviews of their own expansion plans. The outcome of health planning regulation should have been predictable in that protection of existing providers should have been anticipated as an objective of the regulatory agencies. Older, established institutions have benefited by being able to continue their operations without being judged in the same manner as new applicants and providers. It was likely that planning agencies would disregard population movements in the awarding of CON certificates, which favors existing hospitals. Not surprisingly, entry, particularly by proprietaries, has been blocked. It was predictable that the development of lower-cost substitutes for hospitals such as free-standing surgicenters and HMOs would be hindered. No incentives have been provided for efficient operations. The problem initially used to justify the CON legislation—to retard the increase in hospital costs and investments—has not been resolved.

Health planning has been a conservative approach to improving hospital performance. It has left unchanged the method used to reimburse hospitals and it has not changed the incentives facing physicians, hospitals, and patients. Moreover, once a hospital receives CON approval of its investment plans (and the probability is very high that it will receive such approval), it has an incentive to undertake the most costly investment, since it will be reimbursed on a cost basis. Health planning agencies have failed to improve the allocation of resources in the delivery of medical care. Even more costly, however, is the regulatory structure that has been created and will be difficult to remove. It is perhaps this latter aspect that will prove to be most costly in the long run.

The failure of health planning agencies to reduce hospital costs is generally attributed to the caliber of persons working in planning agencies, the lack of sufficient representation, and the need for still more comprehensive regulatory controls. The proponents of regulation do not appear to have learned from the experience of other regulated industries or from the past performance of health planning agencies. The additional controls that are being recommended involve regulation of hospitals' charges and budgets. The need for rate regulation is an admission that CON controls have failed to accomplish their tasks; however, the proponents of regulation have not suggested that rate regulation replace CON; instead, complete public utility regulation is being proposed for health providers, with controls on entry, investment, pricing, and services. The likely consequences of these additional controls are not difficult to predict. Hospitals are even suggesting similar proposals themselves to escape more drastic proposals being made by others. The comprehensive controls proposed are likely to guarantee the survival of hospitals at a cost of lost efficiency and innovation for the rest of the community. Perhaps one of the largest costs of health regulation lies in the inevitable trend toward greater regulation as previous regulatory efforts fail. It becomes virtually impossible to undo regulation once it has started; vested interests are established that, in addition to the health facilities, are comprised of the regulatory agencies themselves. Alternative approaches to achieving the goals sought by regulation threaten established interests and thus become more difficult to institute.

AN APPLICATION OF FACILITIES REGULATION: THE ISSUE OF HOSPITAL BED REDUCTION

It has been estimated that there are between 60,000 and 100,000 excess hospital beds in this country (34). At approximately $75,000 a bed, proponents of hospital bed reduction point to the enormous potential savings that could be achieved if excess hospital beds were eliminated (35). These potential savings, however, are not as clear-cut as the proponents of hospital bed reduction would have us believe.

First, what is the definition of excess hospital capacity? Two definitions are generally used. The first, based on the National Health Planning Guidelines, is the number of beds that would be eliminated if the current bed to population ratio were reduced to 4.0 beds per 1,000 population (or lower). The second definition is based on the assumption that an 85 percent occupancy rate would be appropriate for the hospitals in the community. The number of hospital beds in the community should be reduced until an overall 85 percent occupancy rate is achieved.*

Under hospital bed reduction programs, excess hospital capacity can be achieved in one of several ways. Each hospital can reduce its capacity until the community standard of 4.0 beds per 1,000 population is achieved (or until each hospital achieves an 85 percent occupancy rate). Alternatively, the goals of bed reduction can be achieved by targeting certain hospitals for complete closure.

It is important in understanding the bed reduction issue to make explicit the value judgements underlying the use of the above community standards. If the actual bed to population ratio is greater than the 4 beds per 1,000 population standard, it is implicitly assumed that there is "inappropriate" hospital utilization. Therefore, reducing the number of beds will presumably reduce inappropriate utilization. If beds are then rationed, it is assumed that only those most in need of a hospital will be admitted. However, it is not necessarily the case that only inappropriate utilization is reduced when beds are reduced. There are many factors that affect a community's utilization rate. The age of the population, the availability of (and payment for) out-of-hospital substitutes, and whether someone is able to care for the patient at home are just some of the determinants of the demand for hospital care. Placing upper limits on a community's hospital

---

*For purposes of this discussion, excess hospital capacity refers to beds that are either used or for which the hospital has staffs. If a hospital has unused beds, for which it does not staff, then the costs of maintaining those beds are minimal. Most of these costs have been incurred in the past, i.e., capital investment and interest payments, and there would be little if any savings if these beds were eliminated.

use may result in a form of cost shifting; the savings from fewer hospital beds may cause increased costs to patients (and their families) if they have to be treated in a different manner. Even in those situations where there is inappropriate utilization, the hospital and medical staff's admissions policy may not use appropriateness of admission and length of stay as the rationing criteria.

If all hospitals in the community are required to maintain an 85 percent occupancy level, then it is implicitly assumed that the costs of not having a bed available are less than the costs of maintaining those additional beds. Increasing the occupancy rate lowers the probability that a patient will have access to a bed when needed; they may be forced to wait or to enter another hospital. When bed reduction is achieved through closure of a hospital, there are additional travel costs, not just for the patient but also for the patient's visitors. Travel costs should include the value of time spent in travel as well as the transportation costs.

Thus based on the two standards used for defining excess capacity, an appropriate bed to population ratio and/or a desired occupancy level, excess capacity refers to both misused as well as underused beds.

Perhaps the most controversial aspect of hospital bed reduction programs concerns the method used to calculate potential savings. If a hospital is closed, then its total costs are eliminated. (There may be buyout costs which would reduce these savings.) However, that hospital's patients will continue to seek medical care (although some percentage of the patients may no longer seek hospital care). Those patients going to other hospitals will incur costs in those hospitals. Crucial to this whole discussion of hospital bed reduction is the assumption of what the additional costs will be in those hospitals receiving patients from the closed hospital. McClure assumed that 60 percent of a hospital's costs were fixed and 40 percent were variable costs (36). Thus if a hospital were to close and its patients entered another hospital, the receiving hospital would only incur an increase in its costs equal to 40 percent of its average cost per patient. McClure assumed that the hospital's fixed cost would not change; when marginal costs are estimated to be only 40 percent of average costs, average cost per patient would fall as more patients are admitted. If, however, the marginal costs of an additional patient were instead equal to 100 percent of the hospital's average cost per patient, then there would be no savings (assuming all the hospitals had the same average cost and all patients from the closed hospital went to other hospitals). Thus the estimate selected for marginal cost as a percentage of average cost is an important determinant of whether bed reduction programs result in any savings.

A number of studies have estimated the ratio that marginal cost is to average cost. These results, reported in an article by Lipscomb et al. have varied from a low of 21 to a high of 100 percent of average cost (37). The majority of these studies reported marginal cost to average cost ratios, to be quite high. Proponents of hospital closure, however, have used the lower range of estimates to indicate savings from hospital bed reduction programs. While the estimates of the marginal cost to average cost ratio have a wide variation, the results of these studies are not necessarily inconsistent. More important, for purposes of estimating any possible savings due to a bed reduction program, it is more appropriate to use the higher ratio estimates.

Hospitals staff for an expected level of output. However, the very nature of the demand for hospital care is such that while a hospital staffs for an expected output level, there are always unexpected changes in demand. If the number of patient days are either greater or less than the expected level, then the hospital is not able to immediately adjust its staffing pattern. Thus over short periods of time, hospital salaries may be a fixed cost. Short-run marginal costs represent the hospital's response to these unexpected changes in utilization. It is therefore not surprising that short-run marginal costs have been estimated to be between 20 and 40 percent of average costs. Over longer periods of time, however, hospitals are able to make adjustments in their staffing patterns as well as in their other resources, such as capital and equipment. Thus, if a hospital's admissions increase and this increase is expected to be permanent, the hospital will be able to make a complete adjustment to this change over time. Such a process of adaptation is consistent with economic theory. In the long run there are no fixed costs; all factors of production are variable. Higher estimates of the marginal cost/average cost ratio represent more complete adaptation to permanent changes in a hospital's workload. Thus estimates of the ratio of marginal to average costs in the short run are not inconsistent with the higher marginal to average cost ratio found in other studies. In a recent article on this subject, Friedman and Pauly estimate the marginal cost of an unexpected admission to be 35 percent of average costs, while the marginal cost of an expected admission is 98 percent of average cost (38).

Based on the above discussion, it is clear that the use of short-run marginal costs is inappropriate for estimating the savings of hospital closure. If a hospital is closed and its patients are admitted to other hospitals, those other hospitals will anticipate a higher expected patient load. Those hospitals will adjust their resources and staffing patterns accordingly. The closed hospital will produce a savings, which will be its average cost multiplied by its number of patients. However, the marginal costs of that hospital's patients going to other hospitals will be approximately 90–95 percent of those hospitals' average costs.

To calculate whether total hospital costs in the community will be reduced after a hospital closure requires knowledge of the average cost per patient at the hospital targeted for closure, the percent of the hospital's patients that will go to other hospitals, and the long-run marginal cost at those other hospitals.

An important factor in determining which hospitals are targeted for closure is whether or not they are small community institutions. At times, bed reduction policies are used to maintain the viability of the larger hospitals that are suffering from low occupancy rates.

> When the pressures to reduce the community's bed supply become too powerful to resist, the hospitals themselves may coalesce to exercise some control over the process. A common characteristic of such pressure appears to be a predictable squeezing out of smaller, often lower-cost basic institutions by the larger, complex hospitals with the result that there are fewer, larger, more comprehensive service centers usually operating at higher average cost. (39)

Under these circumstances, average cost per admission in the hospital targeted for closure may well be less than the marginal cost of adding patients to the larger institutions. An hypothetical example will clarify this.

As shown in Table 11-2, Hospital X is targeted for closure. Its average costs per patient day are $280.00; it serves 50,000 patient days per year. If the hospital

TABLE 11-2. Estimated Inpatient Savings from Hospital Closure: A Hypothetical Example

	Average Cost Per Patient Day (1)	Total Patient Days (2)	Estimate of Marginal/Average Cost (3)	Marginal Cost of Additional Patient Day (4)	Total Cost of Additional Patient Days (5)	Net Inpatient Savings of Closure (6)
Hospital X (targeted for closure)	$280.00	50,000	—	—	($14,000,000)	—
	300.00	50,000	.85	$255.00	$12,750,000	$1,250,000
			.90	270.00	13,500,000	500,000
			.95	285.00	14,250,000	(250,000)
	325.00	50,000	.85	276.25	13,812,500	187,500
			.90	292.50	14,625,000	(625,000)
			.95	308.75	15,437,500	(1,437,500)
Hospital Y	350.00	50,000	.85	297.50	14,875,000	(875,000)
			.90	315.00	15,750,000	(1,750,000)
			.95	332.50	16,625,000	(2,625,000)

Note: Numbers in parentheses indicate losses.

is closed, $14 million will be saved each year. Hospital Y is typical of the remaining hospitals in the community. Three different estimates of average cost in Hospital Y are provided; three estimates of marginal cost are also assumed for each of the average cost estimates. It is also assumed that all of the patients from Hospital X seek care in the remaining hospitals, and that there is no change in the case mix or number of patients in the receiving hospitals. (It is further assumed that the receiving hospitals care for the additional patients with the same style of medical practice as received by their other patients.)

While the above example is merely illustrative, the results are very sensitive to the following assumptions: the difference in average cost between the hospital targeted for closure and the remaining hospitals; the ratio of marginal to average cost in the remaining hospitals; and (although not shown in Table 11-2) the percentage of the patients from the closed hospital who will continue to seek hospital care. According to the results of the hypothetical example, savings, when they do occur, are relatively small. Any such savings, however, should be considered as gross savings since there are additional costs to be considered.

If a hospital is closed, there is then increased transportation costs and travel time by patients, their visitors, and others to another hospital. The attractiveness of the community to new residents and employers may be decreased. Physicians may leave the area if they are unable to have staff appointments at nearby hospitals. The remaining hospitals will have greater market power since there are fewer competing hospitals. Additional costs are those of the regulatory process itself and the inevitable lawsuits when a hospital is targeted for closure. Part of the hospital savings (i.e., the discounted present value) may be required to pay off obligations incurred by the hospital targeted to be closed. Thus offsetting any possible gross savings are other costs, some direct, others indirect, which are likely to be shifted to patients, their families, and others. These costs, unfortunately, are not always as quantifiable, hence obvious, as the savings in hospital costs; they therefore tend to be neglected or given a smaller weight in the decision process.

One study that attempted to estimate the potential savings from eliminating duplication at a national level concluded that they are "disappointingly small" (40). Net savings from hospital closure are particularly doubtful when the targeted hospitals are small, relatively unsophisticated, community hospitals (41). By the time lawsuits are concluded and the state legislature has had its opportunity to develop political compromises over which hospitals are targeted to be closed, a considerable period of time may pass before bed reduction policies have their effect.

An alternative approach to reducing "misused and underutilized beds" is to strive for policies that decrease the demand for hospital care. Examples of such policies are the inclusion in health benefits of copayments and deductibles for hospital care, coverage of out-of-hospital substitutes such as outpatient surgery, and policies that provide physicians with an incentive not to hospitalize their patients, such as exist in prepaid health plans. The advantage of a demand approach to decreasing utilization is that the patient and/or his or her physician is making the choice of whether to hospitalize, rather than a state planning agency, the patient and physician having perhaps different objectives and valuations of the costs of the various alternatives. A restructuring of patient and physician incentives (as described in Chapter 12) has a greater likelihood of achieving a more efficient use of the hospital.

RATE REGULATION OF HOSPITAL SERVICES

Since CON legislation failed to hold down the large annual increases in hospital costs and expenditures, more direct regulation has been proposed to achieve this goal. Regulation of hospital rates either can be established at a federal level, as occurred under the economic stabilization program from 1971 to 1974, or can be designed and administered at a state level, by a state agency (or commission) or through an intermediary such as Blue Cross. Although the administrative aspects of the sponsorship, composition, and bureaucratic location of the rate regulatory agency are undoubtedly important and may affect the stringency with which rate regulation is applied, this section is concerned with the different objectives underlying rate regulation, alternative methods for hospital reimbursement, their probable consequences, and a review of the experience with different methods of hospital payment.

In order to evaluate the probable effectiveness of different methods of rate regulation, we must 1) review why hospital costs vary and 2) recognize the differing objectives of rate regulation.

Potential and Actual Objectives of Hospital Rate Regulation

The earlier section on the extent of economies of scale in hospitals described the factors, other than size, that affect hospital costs. Those factors will be reviewed here with reference to Figure 11-2. The long-run average-cost curve, represented by $LRAC_1$, shows the relationship between the average cost and the size of a hospital. Different hospital sizes are represented by different short-run average-cost curves (SRAC) along a given LRAC curve. It is assumed that each hospital on $LRAC_1$ is producing the same type of product, by which we mean the same case mix of patients handled in a manner of similar quality. When differences in quality exist between two types of hospitals, they will be on different long-run average-cost curves; for example, if one hospital is a teaching hospital and the other is not, then the teaching hospital will be on $LRAC_2$ and the nonteaching hospital, with lower average costs, will be on $LRAC_1$. Thus, differences in hospital size will be represented by different SRAC curves, while differences in the products that hospitals produce will be represented by different LRAC curves. Further, if two hospitals are identical in size and products, but differ in efficiency, then the more efficient hospital will be represented by a lower SRAC. Finally, since the prices the hospital must pay for its inputs, labor, equipment, supplies, and capital are continually increasing, a group of hospitals represented by $LRAC_1$ will find themselves slowly rising to $LRAC_2$ as the prices of their inputs rise. It will no longer be possible for those same hospitals to remain on $LRAC_1$.

The foregoing brief discussion indicates the issues with which any rate regulation commission must be concerned. The rate regulators must be able to reimburse hospitals while making adjustments for the many ways in which they may differ, including size, products, and efficiency, and they must be able to determine the rate at which hospital input prices are rising, thereby moving hospitals to a higher LRAC. Unless the rate regulators are able to distinguish the sources of cost differences among hospitals and estimate the amount of those differences, the rates that are established may reward some hospitals unfairly

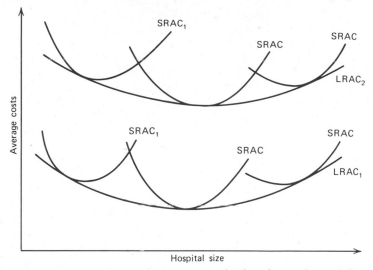

Figure 11-2. Variations in hospital costs as a result of product and size differences.

while penalizing others. Further, unless rate regulators are able to estimate the increase in hospital input prices over time, they will either be rewarding hospitals too generously (if they allow too large a price increase) or they will penalize all the hospitals by granting them too small a rate increase. In this latter case, hospitals will not be able to remain on their original LRAC. Receiving less than the full amount of the price increase (adjusted for input substitution) will require hospitals to move to a lower LRAC, requiring that they produce a less expensive or different product. The task of rate regulators is not easy; unless they are extremely accurate in accounting for differences among hospitals and in estimating increases in hospital input prices, the consequences of their actions will be different from what they intended.

What effect or objective should the rate regulators strive for? Ideally, they should use regulation to achieve an outcome similar to one resulting from a competitive market. If the market for hospital care operated as a perfectly competitive market, then four outcomes would occur, outcomes that regulation should strive to achieve: first, each hospital would be both economically and technically efficient; by being technically efficient it would produce the maximum output for the inputs it used.* To be economically efficient as well, the hospital would have to use the least costly combination of inputs to produce a given level of output (the isoquant is tangent to the isocost line). The resulting internal efficiency (the lowest SRAC curve for a given hospital size and type of output) is desirable, but it cannot be the sole objective of a reimbursement scheme. Internal efficiency results in the hospital's production of output at minimum cost, but it does not identify the types and quantity of output that

---

*If the hospital were technically efficient, then it would be operating on (rather than within) its isoquant for that particular level of output.

should be produced, or whether a particular hospital should be permitted to continue to provide hospital care. A hospital may be doing the best it can, given its size, age, and the facilities it has, but if it is too small or too old to produce its output at as low a cost as other hospitals in the area can, or if some of its facilities are underutilized, the community may be served best by taking away some of its facilities or perhaps phasing out the hospital entirely. Even if all hospitals were internally efficient, total hospital expenditures could be reduced if fewer hospitals were to provide the same quantity and quality of output. Therefore, a second possible objective of rate regulation would be to strive for efficiency in the use of all the hospital resources in the community. Hospital services should be produced at minimum cost as calculated in terms of the entire system of hospitals rather than the individual hospital; in other words, the extent of economies of scale in hospital services should be considered. (Assuming low travel costs, hospitals operating on the SRAC curve that is at the minimum point of the LRAC curve for a given type of product would be preferred.) If one open heart surgery unit can supply the needs of a community, for example, it would be economically inefficient to have duplicate facilities in two or more hospitals.

Achieving efficiency in the use of a community's hospital resources is independent of determining the amount, quality, and type of hospital care to be provided for a given level of medical care demand, which means determining the appropriate LRAC curve the hospital should be on. Determining the quality and type of product to be provided is particularly difficult when inefficiencies of demand exist. The regulators have no market signals or other information on demand preferences to guide their decisions in this matter. Because this issue has been discussed elsewhere, it will be excluded as an objective of the regulatory agency in this discussion. As a third objective, therefore, we will concentrate instead on the issue of how much hospital care should be used relative to other forms of care in providing a treatment at minimum cost. Hospitals are only one setting in which medical treatment can be provided; others include physicians' offices, nursing homes, or a patient's own home. Minimizing the cost of a treatment is likely to require substitution of care away from the hospital to a less costly institutional setting. Reimbursement schemes concerned solely with the rate at which hospitals are paid are unlikely to cause physicians to prescribe nonhospital forms of treatment.

Rate regulatory commissions are generally concerned with hospitals, not with minimizing treatment costs. Hospital rate-setting agencies are also generally unconcerned with issues such as the amount, quality, and type of hospital care the community should receive, concerns which are usually addressed by the CON agency. Once the CON agency approves a hospital's request to add a facility or to undertake a capital expansion program, the rate-setting agency determines a rate for that facility or for the additional beds. It would thus appear that internal hospital efficiency is the rate-setting agency's main objective. The second possible objective, minimizing the cost of hospital care for the community by eliminating unnecessary duplication, is generally a concern of the planning agency. The third possible objective, minimizing the cost of medical treatments, is usually discussed by interested persons; the rate-setting and planning agencies are generally not involved with this broader problem of economic efficiency in the provision of medical care.

A fourth objective is important to several interest groups concerned with the rate-setting process. Some proponents of rate regulation, especially federal and state governments, seek to contain the total amount spent on hospital care. It is important to recognize that success in holding down the rate of increase of hospital expenditures will not necessarily achieve any of the first three objectives. Hospitals may reduce their costs by admitting fewer patients or by releasing patients sooner, thus shifting costs of medical care to other providers or to the consumer. These practices might achieve the third objective if care can be provided adequately and at lower cost in other settings, but they could also lead to undesirable decreases in the amount of care some individuals receive. The objective of merely containing the increase in total hospital expenditures may prevent hospitals from remaining on their original LRAC as their input prices rise. A cost-containment policy that provides hospitals with insufficient funds to move from $LRAC_1$ to $LRAC_2$ as shown in Figure 11-2 (where the difference between the two LRAC curves is a result only of input price increases and not of increased quality or product differences) will force those hospitals to be on a lower LRAC than previously. The lower LRAC would represent a diminution of product in some manner, but not necessarily an increase in hospital efficiency or a desirable reduction in the hospitals' output.

The predominant forms of hospital reimbursement were cost-based, which is retrospective, and billed charges. Under the cost-based payment a share of the hospital's costs, whatever their amount, would be reimbursed by Blue Cross or Medicare. (In calculating its share of the hospital's costs, the third-party payor would, after negotiation with the hospitals, either allow or disallow certain categories of costs.) If the basis of reimbursement was billed charges, then the third-party payor would reimburse the hospital that portion of its costs related to the portion of billed charges paid by the third-party payor. Under Medicare, hospitals had an incentive to raise charges on those services that were used predominantly by the aged, in order to receive governmental reimbursement for a higher portion of the costs of those services. The overall effect of retrospective cost-based reimbursement was to enable each hospital to move to any LRAC curve that it desired and to achieve any size of facility (SRAC) on that LRAC curve. Under a retrospective cost-based reimbursement system, any risks of higher operation costs are shifted to the patients through their third-party payors.

To achieve the objective of internal efficiency (objective 1) and hospital cost containment (objective 4), hospital reimbursement must change from retrospective to prospective payment. Under prospective reimbursement, hospital budgets or rates would be determined in advance; predetermined revenues or rates would limit how much hospital costs could increase and would provide an incentive for hospitals to be internally efficient. The general approach of the proposals offered for prospective reimbursement are discussed below. Within each of these broad classifications considerable variation in rate setting and administration is possible.

Budget Review on a Prospective Basis

Hospitals favor the budget review approach for determining hospital reimbursement. This approach assumes that it is impossible to separate out differences in products, size, and efficiency among hospitals. A representative of the rate-setting agency would review each hospital's budget for the reasonableness of its cost increases.

> Hospitals have an opportunity to explain and defend their budgets, and the rate setting agency or program has an opportunity to question items that appear out of line. Budget review gives the agency more of a chance to influence specific hospital activities and plans before decisions about them are implemented. In short, a detailed, institution by institution examination of costs and cost influencing factors characterizes the budget review method of rate setting. To many, this the attractive feature of this method; to others, its basic drawback. Meaningful budget reviews require considerable expertise—in accounting, economics, finance, and hospital management—which many rate setting agencies and programs do not have. Comprehensive and thorough reviews also require considerable and fairly detailed cost and statistical data; a knowledge of the assumptions, modes of operation, and plans that underlie the figures presented; a knowledge of the need for new programs and services proposed; . . . (typically, the management staffs of a few large hospitals taken together are larger than the entire agency staff), . . . (42).

The proponents of prospective reimbursement on an individual hospital basis stress that it allows for an explicit consideration of differences among hospitals and permits the elimination of waste while treating hospitals fairly. Some variations on this basic approach allow for incentives; if the hospital can keep its costs below the prospectively determined rates, it can keep a portion of the savings; if its costs exceed the rates, it must absorb a portion of the loss. Critics of this approach maintain that it poses no risk for the hospital, and therefore is unlikely to result in cost savings. Because of its familiarity with its own budget, the hospital staff will find it easy to justify any of its expenditures. Further, this system offers little incentive for the hospital to hold down its costs, since it can receive a pass-through for legitimate costs such as wage increases.

What follows is a discussion of the hypothetical effects that prospective reimbursement on an individual hospital basis is likely to have on the various possible objectives of rate regulation.

Impact on Objectives: Internal Efficiency.   The impact on internal efficiency would seem to depend primarily upon the tightness of the rates set in this process. Do they force the hospital to be efficient in order to survive financially? The tightness of the rates depends on the actions of the hospital and the rate-setting (or negotiating) body in the rate-setting process. Peer review boards would seem to have the greatest knowledge of hospital costs, and would therefore be in the best position to determine what rates will promote efficient operation. Such boards, however, may tend to support the recommendations of the hospitals in hopes that their own hospitals will receive similarly favorable treatment in negotiations. Other types of rate-setting bodies may lack the expertise and incentives to determine where rates can be held down to promote efficient operations.

Individuals assigned to regulate costs may be well qualified and highly motivated to promote the public interest, but economists familiar with the performance of regulatory agencies in other industries are skeptical of regulators' ability to promote hospital efficiency. They argue that the information the regulators receive is likely to be biased in the hospitals' favor, and that regulators' fear of having decisions overturned in the courts and of being blamed for financial or service failures of hospitals will make them sympathetic to hospitals' interests. Citing evidence from experience with regulation in other industries, Roger Noll concludes that "whatever regulators do, they apparently do not in general reduce prices below the level that would otherwise prevail due to imperfectly competitive markets" (43).

In addition to how tight the rates are likely to be, the hospitals' likely reaction to those rates must also be considered. It might be argued that regardless of how tight the rates are, once they are set prospectively, hospitals have an incentive to operate efficiently, since the lower actual costs are, the larger the surplus or the smaller the loss that the hospital will absorb. But what could a hospital accomplish with an incentive payment that it could not accomplish by spending right up to the limit allowed it? Administrators might value surpluses for the appearance of efficiency, but this value must be balanced against the cost of offending the medical staff or other groups within the hospital by initiating cost-cutting measures. Surpluses gained through beating the prospective rate in one year might not be worth the price to hospitals if tighter rates were the result in the future. The hospital might be reluctant to reveal the costs involved in truly efficient operation for fear that it would be expected to meet that standard year after year.

If the prospective rate for a hospital is set too tightly, then the hospital might take actions to enable it to live within that rate without necessarily increasing efficiency (44). Some payment unit or units must be chosen to which the prospective rates apply: examples are the total budget, department budgets, the patient day, the admission, or specific services. In each case the hospital might take action to lower its costs without increasing efficiency. If the entire budget is determined prospectively, for example, the hospital can reduce costs by decreasing its volume of services or lowering quality. If reimbursed on a per admission basis, it can admit less complex and costly cases. Similarly, if a hospital wanted to increase its revenues without sacrificing its objectives, it could enlist the cooperation of physicians to do so. For example, a lower occupancy hospital receiving a certain fee per patient day might extend stays unnecessarily or it might perform more tests and procedures per patient if reimbursed a set fee per procedure. Although monitoring procedures such as utilization review might be used to guard against unnecessary hospital utilization, whether such review boards can do so effectively remains to be seen, particularly since they must inevitably rely on physicians' expertise in setting standards.

Efficiency in the Allocation of Resources Among Hospitals.   If the rate-setting body reimburses hospitals for specialized facilities at a rate that would cover costs only when utilization was high, then some hospitals might be forced to phase out underutilized facilities (that is, assuming that marginal cost per use is below average cost until capacity is reached). Setting rates in such detail, however, may require detailed information that is costly to acquire and process, and it may be beyond the competence of the rate-setting body. If a simpler payment unit, such as the patient day or the admission, is used, the excess costs of underutilized facilities might easily be hidden. When prospective reimbursement is on an individual hospital basis, payment for bed expansion or new facilities is tied to approval by a certificate-of-need or health planning agency. Once CON approval is granted, the rate regulatory agency reimburses the hospital for those new facilities regardless of their efficiency of operation or size.

Controlling the Increase in Total Hospital Expenditures.   The preceding discussion of how this mechanism might affect hospital behavior suggests that savings from increased efficiency may be small or nonexistent. Any savings that result from increased efficiency are likely to be offset at least partially by administrative costs, incentive payments made to hospitals, and costs of handling appeals if hospitals are forced to accept rates that they do not consider adequate. If hospitals are allowed to pass-through increases in input prices, if they are allowed to introduce costly, but presumably quality-improving, innovations, or if utilization of services increases, costs may continue to increase at a rapid rate. Even if strict controls are placed on reimbursement per unit (patient days, admissions, specific services), increases in service volume could lead to increases in total hospital expenditures.

Minimizing the Cost of Medical Care Treatments.   Setting hospital budgets or rates prospectively on an individual basis does not by itself provide incentives to substitute less costly forms of medical care for hospital care. As explained above, if the hospital is paid a set fee per patient day, it has some incentive to keep patients longer than necessary (again assuming this does not conflict with other objectives and is not prevented by effective monitoring procedures), since the marginal cost of the extra days during which few services are provided is likely to be less than the additional payment. Similarly, if the hospital is paid a fee per admission, it has an incentive to admit patients who could be treated at less cost in other settings.

Establishing Reimbursement Levels Based on a Hospital's Performance Relative to Other Hospitals

The second basic approach to establishing hospital reimbursement rates is to base the rate upon the particular classification in which a hospital is grouped. Ideally, one would want to be able to classify hospitals according to differences in their products by determining which LRAC curve they are on and then establishing a rate for the output category that reflects the minimum point on the long-run average-cost curve (assuming no travel costs). Hospitals producing similar products would receive one rate per unit of output regardless of their differences in size or efficiency. Presumably those hospitals that are internally efficient and least costly in terms of size of operation will be able to produce their output at a cost at or below the reimbursement rate. Those hospitals that are less efficient and/or not of least-costly size will have to merge, become more efficient, or close down if they cannot produce their output at a cost below or equal to the established rate. Since high-cost hospitals may attempt to change their product line if their costs are greater than the rate established for their group, it is necessary under this approach, more so than under the previous approach, to monitor changes in their outputs, quality, facilities and services. The difficulty is in properly determining each hospital's classification. Critics of this approach, primarily hospital administrators, claim that it is not possible to develop adequate classifications for each hospital. Hospitals vary so greatly in the services and quality of care they provide, and in their case mix of patients, that three or four major groupings will not reflect the differences among them. The result of such inadequate groupings is an unfair system of the rewards and penalties directed to hospitals.

The hospital is under greater risk in this payment system than under the previous one. It is interesting to speculate what the consequences would be were a hospital to claim it could not live within the established rate or were its costs to exceed the allowable reimbursement level. Presumably the hospital would have to cut its costs, but if it refused to do so, what action would the rate-setting agency or its intermediary undertake? Unless strong penalties are used, all the hospitals will revert to retrospective cost reimbursement. Suggested penalties have included auditing the hospital and placing it under a receivership or automatically removing its administrative staff. Two examples of this prospective payment approach are diagnostic-related groupings and current Medicare reimbursement policies.

One method of prospective reimbursement that is receiving increasing attention is diagnostic related groupings (DRGs). This approach has already been instituted in New Jersey, and a variant of it is being considered for hospitalized Medicare patients. The use of DRGs is a recognition that hospitals are multi-product firms; hospitals treat different types of patients. Further, the mix of patients within a hospital also varies among hospitals. Under a DRG approach, hospital reimbursement is tied to the type of patient treated. In its simplest form, a fixed amount is paid to a hospital for each patient within a given DRG. The hospital has a financial incentive to produce care at a cost below the fixed price, since it can retain all or most of the savings. If the hospital's cost exceeds the price for the particular DRG it then loses money.

Conceptually, the DRG approach is appealing. Similar types of patients in different hospitals should use similar quantities of resources. Differences in the costs of producing similar patients are either a result of differences in hospital efficiency and/or style of medical practice. Facing a fixed price, a hospital has an incentive to reduce a patient's length of stay, perhaps treat them as outpatients, and not to use an excessive amount of ancillary services (or other services) in treatment. Hospitals having different patient mixes would be reimbursed accordingly. Commercial insurers are proponents of the DRG approach since different third-party payors are treated similarly; commercial insurers would pay the same prices as Blue Cross and Medicare.

There are, however, problems with DRGs that suggest it is too early to view it as a method that would be instituted for all hospitals. DRGs are empirically determined. In New Jersey, where the DRG approach was phased in and is now used for all hospital payment, patients were first classified according to 83 major diagnostic categories (MDC) (45). Then within each MDC, a number of DRGs were created according to whether the primary and secondary diagnosis, age, and existence of a surgical procedure affected the patient's length of stay. The result was 383 DRGs. It is thus assumed that the resources used for a patient vary according to their length of stay. As experience with the system began to accumulate, the number of DRGs was increased to 467.*

There are wide variations in the costs of patients within a given DRG category. Lengths of stay within a DRG may also vary greatly. Part of the reason for such large variations is the small number of patients within certain DRGs. However, such large variations are also an indication that patients within a DRG are not homogeneous. To the extent that this variation occurs, the problem of windfall gains and losses occur.

A serious concern with the use of DRGs is the classification of patient diagnoses. Often patients have multiple diagnoses. The DRG classification is heavily influenced by the primary diagnosis. The sequence of diagnoses proved to be a major source of error in a study conducted by the Institute of Medicine, which found a 35 percent error rate in the principle discharge diagnosis (46). One study examined the impact on hospital reimbursement if the primary and secondary diagnoses were classified according to which diagnosis maximized the hospital's reimbursement (47). Had such a reclassification actually been used for reimbursement purposes, the hospital's case mix cost would have increased by 14 percent; the hospital would have received a windfall profit.

In many cases the diagnosis sequence may be appropriately switched. However, once DRGs are used for hospital reimbursement, it is not difficult to imagine computer programs being developed to select, in those situations in which either the primary or secondary diagnoses could be appropriately interchanged, the higher-priced diagnosis as the DRG classification. Uncertainty often exists as to the patient's diagnosis. Physicians could be "educated" to select certain DRG classifications rather than others under conditions of such uncertainty. "DRG-creep" could be rationalized as being an appropriate reclassification of diagnoses. However, a financial incentive would also be created for unethical behavior.

Hospitals may decide to classify patients into DRG categories that are reimbursed at higher amounts. To prevent any such potential abuse, utilization review mechanisms must be instituted. In New Jersey, a study found that 26.4 percent of the patients had been misclassified (48). Even if this error rate was unrelated to any financial incentives, such a high percentage of patients incorrectly assigned to DRGs will result in windfall gains and losses to hospitals and payors. Lawsuits would be expected, particularly by self-pay patients, if the error rate remains this high.

Prepaid health plans that do not have their own hospitals have complained about the New Jersey DRG system. If health maintenance organizations (HMOs) undertake preadmission testing that results in a shorter length of stay for their patients, they must still pay the full DRG price. The HMO no longer has an incentive to try and lower the cost of their hospitalized patients.

There are still a number of problems to be worked out with the DRG ap-

---

*One of the most publicized examples of misclassification in the New Jersey experiment was the softball player who had injured his finger. He had to be hospitalized for 2 days so that the bone in his finger could be repaired with a metal pin. The DRG category assigned to this patient was "fracture with major surgery," usually reserved for serious cases such as total hip replacement. While the patient's actual charges would have been less than $1,000, the DRG classification resulted in a bill for $5,000.

proach (49). For example, the DRG approach does not reimburse capital costs; how are these costs to be reimbursed? Further, how are the annual percent increases in DRG prices to be determined? While the DRG approach attempts to set prices for given hospitalized services, this approach provides no incentive for fewer hospitalizations. As the experience with the New Jersey system increases, the feasibility of this approach will become clearer. One aspect of its feasibility that should not be neglected is the administrative costs of such a system, including its method of cost allocation, review mechanism for appropriateness of patient classification, and its need for continual updating.

Medicare reimbursement to hospitals has changed greatly since the time when hospitals were paid their costs plus 2 percent. In 1969 the 2-percent-plus factor was removed. Since 1974 limits have been established for hospitals' routine costs; ancillary service costs were excluded from any limits. Hospitals were grouped according to bed size, urban–rural location, and area per capita income. For each group of hospitals, the 80th percentile of the hospitals' routine per day costs was calculated and 10 percent of the group's median costs was added to that amount. An inflation factor was then used to update these limits (known as Section 223 limits). Hospitals would still be reimbursed for their costs up to the limits in their group. It was estimated that 11.5 percent of hospitals were affected by these limits (50). Certain hospitals were exempt from the limits and hospitals could appeal cost reductions.

Medicare reimbursement policy has continued to become tighter for hospitals. The limit had dropped to 108 percent from 110 percent, and in 1982 the Congress voted to extend the Section 223 limits to ancillary services. The limit for both routine and ancillary services is scheduled to decline from 120 percent in 1983 to 110 percent in 1985. In addition to placing limits on a greater portion of hospital costs for Medicare patients, tighter restrictions were placed on the annual percentage increase in the Section 223 limits.

As the limits on hospitals within a particular grouping become tighter and smaller annual percentage increases are permitted, the attractiveness of Medicare reimbursement to hospitals has declined. Commercial insurers have alleged that hospitals are "cost-shifting," that is, increasing the charges to commercial-pay and self-pay patients as hospitals become more limited in their Medicare reimbursement.

Impact on Objectives: Internal Efficiency.   Proposals to group hospitals imply that cost differences are due to differences in efficiency. It is recognized, however, that differences in hospital costs are also due to differences in location, case mix, and teaching programs. All the proposals attempt to control for some of these factors. Some approaches group hospitals by a small number of criteria, while others, such as the use of DRGs, sacrifice some administrative simplicity for presumably more appropriate groupings. Unfortunately, even careful groupings cannot assure that the remaining cost differences within groups are due to differences in the level of efficiency alone. A hospital with high costs relative to its group may be providing higher-quality care, for example. Most of the proposals recognize this problem and would permit full-cost reimbursement within some range around the group average or predicted cost. However, any inefficient hospitals falling in this range are not given much incentive to become more efficient.

A major weakness of the method that pays hospitals on the basis of a group average is that it never penalizes hospitals that keep their costs in line with their group average. It remains to be seen whether the possibility of receiving a rebate on cost reduction would provide much of an efficiency incentive to a low-cost hospital already confident that its full costs will be reimbursed. If low-cost hospitals are not motivated to become even more efficient by the possibility of earning incentive payments, the average level of efficiency within each group may not change significantly over time. One desirable feature of this approach is that since the individual hospital is judged by a group rather than an individual standard, it need not be concerned that it will be imposing tougher standards on itself in the future by performing well in the present.

Efficiency in the Allocation of Resources Among Hospitals.   If, as many observers suggest, considerable unnecessary duplication of facilities and services exists, then the average costs of providing some hospital services (even if each hospital is *internally* efficient) do not represent the minimum cost at which those services could be provided. Paying hospitals on the basis of group average costs runs a risk of permitting the continuance of too much duplication. Hospitals may seek new facilities or be reluctant to give up existing ones in order to put themselves in a more advantageous group for reimbursement purposes.

Controlling the Increase in Total Hospital Expenditures.   It appears unlikely that a mechanism that merely sets ceilings on hospital reimbursement based on group average costs plus some percentage of the average can do much to stem increases in total hospital expenditures. A careful analysis of the Blue Cross of Western Pennsylvania experience from 1966 to 1968 by Lave, Lave, and Silverman revealed that while the program there apparently put some pressure on high-cost hospitals to move toward the means of their groups, it did not seem to restrict the overall average rate of cost increase in the area (51). Only if this approach is combined with an effective method of limiting the average rate of increase in hospital costs does it appear to have any real chance of limiting the overall rate of increase in expenditures. It remains to be shown that such results are achievable.

Large numbers of appeals are likely to be registered under this approach, as hospitals seek classification for the groups most favorable to themselves. Administrative costs are also involved in determining how hospitals should be grouped, and in cases where a cost function is estimated statistically, considerable data must be gathered and the function must be periodically reestimated. Where patient day is the unit of payment, volume can be manipulated (by extending stays unnecessarily) to increase reimbursement. By making the case the unit of payment and including length of stay and other measures of case mix as determinants of cost, the possibilities of such manipulations are reduced. That is, if the hospital tries to convert outpatients into short-term inpatients, its reimbursement per case will decrease owing to shorter length of stay and easier case mix.

If the mechanism excludes some costs, such as capital and interest, from consideration on the grounds that they cannot be compared validly across hospitals or are uncontrollable, it may be more acceptable to hospitals, but it will also have less potential for controlling overall expenditures.

Minimizing the Cost of Medical Care Treatments.   The classification approach has the same drawback as the previous reimbursement method: it treats hospitals in isolation from the medical care system. Most of the proposals pay hospitals on a per diem or per admissions basis instead of giving them incentives to produce treatments at minimum cost. Paying hospitals according to DRGs is a step toward rewarding them for results rather than processes, and it provides some incentives for minimizing treatment costs. Whether cases can be divided into adequate categories for purposes of this sort of scheme remains to be seen. Nor is it clear that standard costs can be defined in a manner that puts real pressure on hospitals that fail to treat cases at a minimum cost. Finally, the effect of such a mechanism on the quality of care would have to be closely watched.

Setting a Maximum Rate of Increase in Total Hospital Expenditures

In the third basic method of hospital reimbursement, the regulatory authority determines prospectively a maximum allowable rate of increase in community hospital expenditures. Several variations on this basic approach exist. For example, it might be determined that total hospital expenditures in the coming year should not exceed 10 percent. The regulatory authority or its intermediary can then use any number of methods to allocate this 10 percent increase among the hospitals, such as budget review of individual hospitals or a formula approach. The regulatory agency or the intermediary then has an incentive to negotiate harder with the hospitals, since they cannot exceed the maximum allowable increase for all hospitals, referred to as a Maxi-cap. Alternatively, the maximum allowable increase might be established so that each hospital is limited to a 10 percent increase in its preceding year budget. A variation on this method would classify hospitals into several categories and allow a different maximum allowable increase for each classification, with the overall percent increase adding up to 10 percent of total hospital expenditures over the preceding year. This approach can be used by itself or it can be used in conjunction with either of the previous two methods of reimbursement.

The advantage of this approach is that it is relatively simple and straightforward to apply. It can be inexpensive to administer and it is a surer way of placing a limit on how much total hospital expenditures can increase in a year. However, its main disadvantage is that it allows an equal percentage increase both to hospitals that are costly or inefficient and those that have kept their costs down. Classifying hospitals and limiting their percentage increase, as done in New York and currently under Medicare, is an attempt to stimulate efficiency. Another difficulty with this approach is determining the appropriate rate of increase in hospital expenditures. If the market for hospital services were a competitive one, then the percentage increase from one year to the next would represent the effects of shifts in the demand and supply of hospital care, but it would be difficult for a regulatory agency to approximate these demand and supply shifts. Instead, the method used to establish the percentage increase is either a result of negotiations with the hospital associations (it may be arbitrarily determined) or it is related to inflation in the general economy.

Hospital associations have maintained that hospital input prices rather than an economywide measure of inflation should determine the rate of hospital cost inflation. Opponents of this method maintain that, in the long run, hospitals face labor markets similar to other industries', and that allowing the use of hospital input prices reduces any incentive for opposing large hospital wage increases that would affect all hospitals equally. If the percentage increase in hospital costs is arbitrarily determined and set at a low level, then the viability of the hospital system might be threatened; hospitals may be forced to shift costs out of the hospital and on to the patients and/or reduce the quality and intensity of their services.

The annual percentage increase in the hospital's revenues is usually based on an expected level of hospital output, which is usually defined in terms of admissions or patient days. If a hospital's output unexpectedly changes, then adjustments are made to the allowed percentage increase. For example, in the early phases of the Economic Stabilization Program (ESP) a hospital would receive the average revenue per admission for each additional admission; if volume were to increase by 3 percent the hospital's total revenue would also be increased by 3 percent. If admissions were lower than expected, total revenue would be decreased by a similar percentage. Implicit under this approach was the assumption that all costs are variable in the short run, that is, marginal cost equals average cost. Over a longer period of time the hospital is able to vary more of its inputs so that marginal costs should approach average cost.

There are, however, substantial fixed costs in the short run. Hospitals cannot quickly adjust their labor costs as their volume changes; instead hospitals staff for an expected level of output. Unless hospitals are reimbursed at an amount equal to the marginal cost of an additional admission, hospitals will have an incentive to increase their admissions. Similarly, if hospital admissions are less than expected, their loss in revenue should be equal to their savings in marginal cost of having fewer admissions. Otherwise the hospital would be unfairly penalized. This relationship between average and marginal cost per admission and its effect on hospital revenue is shown in Figure 11-3.

The relationship between total hospital inpatient cost and output in the short run is shown by the line TC. The change in TC with changes in output is less than proportionate, indicating substantial fixed costs. Total hospital inpatient revenue (TR) has a steeper slope since it is assumed to vary proportionately with changes in output, i.e., a 3 percent change in output is accompanied by a 3 percent change in total revenue. Point Q_A represents a hospital's expected output level for the period. At point Q_A, the hospital's average revenue (total revenue divided by total output) is equal to average cost (total cost divided by total output). If a hospital has an unexpected (small percentage) increase in its output, from Q_A to Q_b, then its costs increase according to the TC schedule. If the hospital were reimbursed according to its average revenue per admission, then the hospital's revenue would increase according to the TR schedule. The result would be a profit on the additional admissions. Similarly, if output were to decrease, the hospital's TC would decline by a small amount given the large fixed costs in the short run. If, however, the hospital's revenue were decreased according to the TR schedule, the hospital would lose money on its decreased admissions.

In Phase IV of the ESP, the government assumed that the marginal cost of an additional admission was equal to 40 percent of its average cost. Thus if a hospi-

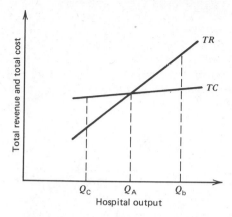

Figure 11-3. The relationship between hospital revenue, cost, and output in the short run.

tal's admissions were increased from Q_A to Q_b, the hospital would receive only 40 percent of its average revenue for those additional admissions. If admissions were lower than expected, the hospital would receive 60 percent of their average revenue for those lost admissions (52). The assumption of marginal cost being 40 percent of average cost was based on a number of empirical studies. These studies indicated that short-run marginal cost (SRMC) varied between .21 and .68. There were many differences between the studies, such as the measure of output used, the statistical techniques employed, and the period of time observed, which would account for the variation in marginal cost estimates.*

The relationship between marginal cost and average cost is important for understanding hospital reactions to certain public policies. Several years ago the State of New York reduced its per diem payment to hospitals for Medicaid patients. Hospitals responded by increasing the length of stay for Medicaid patients (53). As long as the marginal cost of an additional day was approximately .25 of its average costs (and hospitals were being reimbursed at approximately their average costs by Medicaid), hospitals could increase their net revenues by increasing the length of stay of Medicaid patients. If reimbursement policies are not to provide a windfall for some hospitals nor unfairly penalize others, then policymakers must be aware of the marginal cost to average cost relationship.

Impact on Objectives: Internal Efficiency. Proponents of the equal-percentage-increase approach believe that holding allowable rates of expenditure increases below what they otherwise would be forces all hospitals to be more internally efficient. However, those hospitals that are most efficient initially are likely to be hardest pressed by these regulations. If two hospitals are allowed the same rate of expenditure increase, but one is more efficient than the other, the inefficient hospital is allowed not only to remain less efficient than the other but also to increase its costs by a greater absolute amount. Reimbursement formulas in use in New York attempt to deal with this problem by placing ceil-

---

*For example, in one study, when patient days were used as the measure of output, SRMC was estimated to be between .22 and .34; when admissions were the measure of output the estimates of SRMC were higher.

ings on allowable base-year costs. Efficient hospitals may have little incentive to keep cost increases below target levels; instead, they may increase costs to the maximum allowable level each year to assure the largest possible base and least risk of financial difficulty in future years. Even if hospitals whose actual rate of increase was smaller than the target rate were permitted to keep part of the surplus, it is unlikely that such savings would compensate them for tighter future rates.

Efficiency in the Allocation of Resources Among Hospitals.   If a hospital can limit its overall rate of cost increase to the target rate, it has no inducement to give up underutilized facilities. Because this sort of mechanism focuses on rates of cost increase per a simple output measure, such as the patient day or the admission, the potential exists for hospitals to continue hiding the excessive costs of underutilized facilities (although minimum occupancy limits in the New York formulas do make it more difficult for hospitals to continue operating with extensive excess bed capacity). This reimbursement approach does not address the problem of determining when new capital expenditures are justified and how they should be allocated.

Controlling the Increase in Hospital Expenditures.   Although it is desirable to achieve cost savings by increasing efficiency, this approach is primarily concerned with controlling expenditure increases. Its success will depend, of course, on how the target rate of increase is chosen. Any choice of a rate involves political judgments; the proper rate is not objectively observable. For example, the ESP's Phase II choice of 6 percent as a proper rate of cost increase was based on the program's overall goal of cutting the economywide rate of inflation in half. There was no strong evidence that 6 percent was an optimal, or even an achievable, rate of hospital cost increase. Rhode Island set an overall lid on hospital expenditures by holding negotiations between payors and the state hospital association. Other methods of setting an overall maximum increase in expenditures involve somewhat arbitrary choices.

For example, basing the selection of a maximum percentage increase on movements in some index of prices, while seemingly more objective, raises certain questions. For example, what index should be used? If the object is to limit the rate of increase in reimbursement to the rate of increase in input prices, then using a general price index such as the consumer price index or the GNP deflator is probably inappropriate. The market basket of goods and services that hospitals buy is a very special one, and hospitals contend that its price in the recent past has increased at a rate faster than the general prices in the economy. A special hospital price index (HPI) may then be more appropriate. Several recent studies investigating the possibility of developing an HPI have suggested combining existing price indices for different hospital inputs (food, fuels, and so on) into a composite index by weighting the component indices according to the importance of each type of input in hospital budgets (54). This procedure assumes that the prices hospitals pay for inputs should change in the same manner over time as the prices paid by other firms and individuals for similar inputs.

While an HPI constructed in this manner is theoretically superior to a general price index as a measure of hospital input prices, it involves a number of difficulties. Since nurses and medical technicians are employed primarily by hospitals, no adequate external standard may exist by which to judge the appropriateness of their wages. A second problem with the HPI approach is that because of differences between hospitals in their location, size, age, and case mix, they differ in the mix of inputs they use and the prices they pay for them. Even indices calculated at a regional or state level may overlook large variations in input mix. Attempts to classify hospitals into groups and calculate different indices for each group diminish the administrative simplicity of this approach and inevitable lead to additional arbitrary decisions. The extreme solution of using different weights for each hospital will fail to penalize those with an inefficient mix of inputs (e.g., too much capital relative to labor).

Furthermore, it is difficult to forecast movements in input prices. The alternative to penalizing hospitals by setting an incorrectly forecast rate of increase is to adjust the rate retrospectively on the basis of actual price increases. However, this method subjects hospitals and payors to uncertainty about what the final rates of payment will be.

The assumption that the rate of increase in input prices is the proper rate of cost increase is itself open to question. In most industries, if a firm introduces improved production techniques over time, it will use fewer inputs per unit of output, and its costs will increase more slowly than the prices of the inputs it uses. Some innovations do increase hospital productivity in this way, but more often they increase costs by increasing input intensity. Approximately half of the post-Medicare hospital cost increases have been due to increased use of inputs per unit of care (55). Whether or not an intensity factor should be included in the target rate of increase, and how large it should be, was a major issue under ESP and continues to be in New York. The larger such a factor is, of course, the lower the pressure put on hospitals to control costs. Unless the body that sets the lid effectively controls all sources of hospital revenues, hospitals might respond to a tight lid on one revenue source by shifting costs to other payors not covered by the lid.

The apparent simplicity and low cost of administering this target increase approach may be significantly offset by the costs of processing appeals in a manner that promotes hospital efficiency and equity. In New York, the Department of Health received between 150 and 250 individual hospital appeals per year from approximately 330 short-term general hospitals between 1970 and 1973, even before the inclusion of utilization minimums in the formulas (56).

Minimizing the Cost of Medical Care Treatments.   Because this approach, like several others, tends to deal with hospitals in isolation, it does not by itself provide incentives for a more efficient use of all medical care resources. As we have noted, the choice of a unit on which to base volume adjustments may even create undesirable incentives, leading hospitals to take on easier cases that may not actually require hospital care, or to decrease or increase the length of stay, depending on whether the patient day or the admission is the unit of output. Hospitals themselves do not deny this possibility. For example, consider the following critique of the Phase IV regulations by the president of AHA:

> The incentives embodied in the proposed regulations are of the worst kind. They would literally induce hospitals to convert outpatients into short-term inpatients,

in order to reduce the hospital's average per admission charges and expenses. They would encourage hospitals to transfer long-term patients in need of intensive care to referral centers solely for the purpose of improving the average per admission charges and expenses of the transferring hospitals. (57)

EMPIRICAL EVIDENCE ON RATE REGULATION

There is currently some form of rate regulation of hospital expenditures in 27 states. These programs vary greatly according to what percent of the hospitals in the state are included, which third-party payors participate, and according to the method of prospective reimbursement used. In some states a private organization, such as Blue Cross, may use prospective reimbursement, while in other states it is a state agency operating under a legislative mandate. To date, studies have not been able to determine the effect that different types of administrative agencies have had on the control of hospital costs. Several states have mandatory programs in which all hospitals must participate, while for most of the others the program is voluntary. Regulatory programs in which hospital participation is mandatory are likely to have greater influence over hospital cost increases. Generally, the more payors involved in the rate review process, the more effective is the control over cost increases. If just Medicaid or Blue Cross patients are covered by the regulatory process, hospitals can then increase their charges to other payors. Very few of the mandatory programs, only Maryland and Washington State, currently include Medicare patients. The method used by the regulatory agency to control hospital cost increases appears to be crucial to its effectiveness. Those states considered to have a more stringent regulatory program have moved toward a formula approach for determining hospital payment. Classification of hospitals, the use of budget screens, interhospital comparisons, and development of an inflation factor are some of the methods used in the mandatory regulatory programs. Prospective reimbursement programs within a state have changed over time and the length of time a state has had a program varies from one state to the other.

The conclusion reached in recent studies is that mandatory rate regulation appears to have held down hospital cost increases (58).* Biles, Schramm, and Atkinson compared six states with mandatory rate regulation to those states without such regulation over the period 1970–1978. Based on a simple comparison of the annual rate of increase in hospital expense per admission, the authors concluded that while rate regulation did not appear to be effective in the earlier years, between 1975 and 1978 rate review did have an effect on hospital costs. States with mandatory rate review programs had on average, a 3 percent lower rate of increase in their hospital expense per admission. Controlling for other factors and examining a longer time period, Sloan also concludes that in recent years states with mandatory rate regulation have had lower rates of increase in hospital expenditures per admission.

---

*It is not uniformly accepted that rate review is actually the cause for the lower rates of increase in hospital costs. Rate review states have a higher base, i.e., regulated states generally have higher costs per admission. If input cost increases have become more uniform throughout the country then high cost states should show lower annual percentage increases.

Table 11-3 describes the annual percentage increase in total expense per admission for mandatory rate review states and for all other states for the years 1971–1981. Only seven states were classified as mandatory regulatory. Next to each of the regulated states is the date that the regulatory program in that state was initiated. In the early years of rate review, 1971–1975, the federal Economic Stabilization Program (ESP) was also in effect for all hospitals in the country. Although the ESP went through several phases between August 1971 and April 1974, its general approach was to place maximum allowable limits on increases in hospital costs and charges (59). The ESP appeared to be effective in holding down hospital cost increases. This finding is confirmed through studies that used sophisticated statistical techniques as well as a casual examination of the increases in hospital costs both before and after ESP was in effect. (Also see Figure 10-6.) During the period 1971–1975 the annual percentage increase in total expense per admission was similar for both the regulated and nonregulated states. In fact, the nonregulated states had a slightly lower rate of increase in their costs per admission. Starting in 1976, however, the regulated states had a lower rate of increase in their costs. The largest difference between the two groups of states occurred in 1977, a difference of almost 5 percent. In subsequent years the differences between the regulated and nonregulated states began to lessen. By 1980, the difference was only 1.4 percent but for 1981 it increased to 2.9 percent.

The effectiveness of some of the regulated states in holding down hospital cost increases varied year to year. Other regulated states, such as New York, had hospital cost increases that were consistently below the national average. Those regulated states with consistently lower rates of increase in the post-1975 period all used stringent review methodologies. For example, New York has used, and continues to use, a formula approach combined with a maximum annual percentage increase. Hospitals are grouped according to size, type, ownership, and geographic location. Hospitals face a ceiling of 110 percent of the average routine costs for hospitals within each group. Minimum-occupancy limits were also established; 60 percent for maternity, 70 percent for pediatrics, and 80 percent for medical and surgical services. (The effect of this last provision is to penalize low-occupancy hospitals by giving them a lower per diem rate than if their actual patient days were used.) The early New York experience has been analyzed (60). Even in the period covered, 1970–1974, researchers found that rate regulation in New York slowed increases in cost per patient day by about 3 percent per year, and cost per case by about .5 percent per year.

Based on the evidence to date it appears that mandatory rate regulation can reduce the annual rate of increase in hospital expenses regardless of whether it is on a federal level, such as the ESP, or on a state level. However, unless rate regulation programs establish maximum limits on annual percentage increases on hospital expenditures or use a tight-formula approach, rate regulation will not be effective. In the early years of a rate review program, hospitals may not be adversely affected. The requirements placed on hospitals are unlikely to be very stringent and hospitals are likely to have influence over the rate-setting process. As the fiscal constraints on the payors become more severe, as in New York and the federal government under the ESP, and currently under Medicare, tighter controls are placed on hospitals. For a limited time, hospitals may be able to forestall the adverse revenue impacts of such controls by manipulating utiliza-

TABLE 11-3. The Impact of Rate Regulation on the Annual Percentage Increase in Total Expense Per Admission for Community Hospitals, 1971–1981

Regulated States		Years											
		1971	1972	1973	1974	1975	1976	1977	1978	1979	1980	1981	1971–1975	1976–1981
Connecticut[a]	(1974)	13.7	10.1	8.8	7.3	17.0	14.5	11.7	10.7	8.8	12.5	16.0	11.4	12.4
Maryland	(1973)	15.9	9.1	11.5	9.8	17.5	13.8	8.7	9.2	11.9	10.8	15.1	12.7	11.6
Massachusetts	(1971)	14.1	10.3	9.3	12.7	17.4	15.3	14.5	8.7	9.1	15.3	15.8	12.8	13.1
New Jersey	(1971)	14.4	9.8	11.5	10.2	14.8	14.1	10.6	9.1	11.2	10.5	12.2	12.1	11.3
New York	(1969)	9.2	10.5	9.2	10.3	18.7	9.0	7.7	8.9	9.1	11.2	12.6	12.2	9.8
Washington	(1973)	9.8	11.4	10.2	7.8	20.6	17.0	13.7	12.7	10.9	11.5	16.9	12.0	13.8
Wisconsin	(1975)	13.2	10.8	9.2	9.9	16.1	19.9	13.2	13.2	11.4	13.2	18.3	11.8	14.9
Mean percent change regulated states		12.9	10.3	10.0	9.7	17.4	14.8	11.5	10.3	10.3	12.6	15.3	12.2	12.4
Mean percent change all other states		10.8	10.3	8.1	11.5	17.2	16.0	15.4	13.0	12.4	14.0	18.2	11.6	14.8

Source: *Hospital Statistics*, 1972–1982 editions, copyright American Hospital Association.

[a]The numbers in parentheses are the years when rate regulation was initiated.

TABLE 11-4. Patient Revenue and Total Revenue Margins in Community Hospitals, Regulated Vs. Other States, 1975–1981

Year	Patient Revenue Margin (%)[a]		Total Revenue Margin (%)[a]	
	Regulated States	Nonregulated States	Regulated States	Nonregulated States
1975	− 16.2	− 5.3	− 3.57	2.09
1976	− 8.4	− 3.1	.36	3.51
1977	− 10.9	− 3.2	− 1.25	3.22
1978	− 9.9	− 3.5	− 0.2	3.42
1979	− 9.2	− 3.2	− .01	3.75
1980	− 8.6	− 2.9	.50	4.39
1981	− 5.9	− 2.5	1.16	4.54

Source: *Hospital Statistics*, 1972–1982 editions, copyright American Hospital Association.

[a]The net margin was calculated by subtracting total expenses from net patient (in total) revenues and dividing by net patient (total) revenues.

tion, as was the case in New York, and through the use of cost shifting. Eventually, tight controls will affect hospitals' financial position. In New York, an increased number of hospitals closed as rate regulation became more severe (61). Unfortunately a number of these same hospitals also served indigent populations.

An indication of the effect that tight rate regulation has had on hospitals' financial position is the difference in both total revenue and patient revenue margins between the regulated and nonregulated states. [Patient (total) revenue margin is calculated by subtracting total expense from patient (total) revenue and dividing by patient (total) revenues.] As shown in Table 11-4, both patient and total revenue margins were much lower in the regulated states. Hospitals in New York State had negative total revenue margins ranging from .2 to 8.4 percent over the above time period. Continual deficit margins, as in New York, forces hospitals to use up any endowments they may have, reduce the level of their services, and/or decrease the ability of the hospital to serve certain patient populations.

CONCLUDING COMMENTS ON HOSPITAL REGULATION

Various interest groups demand increased regulation of hospitals for several reasons. For some, increased regulation is viewed as a means of assuring access to medical care for all persons, which is the welfare argument; for others, regulation is a means of rationalizing the system of health care delivery, the efficiency argument; for others, regulation is a means of protecting consumers from incompetent providers; for still other groups, regulation is a means whereby the existing providers may be protected from possible threatening changes; and finally, for other interest groups, regulation represents a means for limiting expenditures on hospital care. The relative effectiveness of regulation when compared with alternative approaches can be judged only in terms of a common objective. It is to the advantage of regulation proponents to combine these differing health care goals and objectives and to suggest that only increased regulation can achieve all of them. Proponents claim that alternatives to regulation may be more effective in meeting certain of the desired objectives, but that only regulation can achieve all of the combined goals.

The effectiveness with which regulation is likely to achieve economically efficient medical care delivery was examined in this section. Alternative approaches for achieving the other goals are discussed in other chapters. The consequences of regulation in other industries were examined for purposes of hypothesizing the likely effects of increased regulation in the health field. It was seen that regulation in nonhealth industries led to higher, not lower prices; to cross-subsidization of services; to greater nonprice competition, which in turn led to increased costs in the regulated industry; to protection of the regulated firms, thereby lessening their incentives to strive for efficiency; and to a reluctance to introduce innovation in the delivery of services because such innovation threatens the revenues of the regulated industry. Regulation does not disappear over time; instead, the regulatory agency increases its scope and authority and the number of industries over which its authority is exercised. The degree of regulation also increases: airlines were regulated as to the amenities they can provide; regulated trucks could not travel directly to cities they served and were prohibited from carrying a full load on return trips.

Either proponents of health care regulation are unaware of the experience with regulation in other industries, or else their biases against alternatives to regulation are so strong as to provide them with no alternative. Those proponents with vested interests are very aware of the consequences of regulation in other industries, and they favor it for precisely that reason.

Hospital planning was the first major attempt to regulate hospitals. Voluntary efforts were unsuccessful in achieving the goals of greater efficiency in the allocation of hospital resources, so certificate-of-need legislation was passed. Hospital planning, strengthened by CON, appears to have had some effect, which is predictable from the evidence on regulation in other industries. Proprietary institutions were more likely to be denied CON approval for starting new hospitals or for expansion of their existing facility. Innovations in the delivery of medical services that threatened the revenues of existing hospitals, such as one-day surgery centers and HMOs, were brought under the CON authority of the planning agencies. The growth and development of such free-standing units was retarded. Existing hospitals' expansion plans for new beds in areas that already had excess beds were approved by the CON agency, or else hospital investment was channeled into areas less obvious than beds, but hospital investment did not decline as a result of CON legislation. As hospital costs continued to increase rapidly each year, rather than admitting that CON legislation was a failure, its proponents maintained that the regulatory agencies' staff would improve, and that what was needed instead was still more hospital regulation.

A second regulatory program, which was not discussed but whose effects were similar to what the economic theory of regulation would predict, is utilization review programs. After Medicare and Medicaid had been passed, there was concern that some of the beneficiaries of these programs were receiving unnecessary and/or care of low quality. To rectify this situation, amendments to the Social Security Act were passed in 1972 establishing the Professional Standards

Review Organizations (PSROs). The major emphasis of PSRO programs (over two-thirds of the program's budget) has been on appropriateness of hospital length of stay by Medicare beneficiaries.* Several studies have been conducted to evaluate the effectiveness of the PSRO program. One large study compared the hospital utilization experience of Medicare beneficiaries from 1974 to 1976 in areas with and without an active PSRO (62). The results showed that PSROs had no overall effect on hospital utilization or admissions. Other studies reported similar findings (63).

The effectiveness of PSROs was recently evaluated by the Congressional Budget Office (CBO). Based on 1978 data, CBO reported:

> The 1978 data suggests that a PSRO program in which all Medicare hospital patients are reviewed would reduce Medicare days of hospitalization by about 1.5 percent. . . . The evidence that PSROs reduce Medicare utilization, however, is not firm. Considering the nation as a whole, the program's apparent effect is sufficiently small and variable that it could be an artifact of chance variation in the data. Moreover, in the South, PSRO review seems to increase utilization, a pattern that is difficult to explain and throws all the results into some doubt.
>
> PSROs affect utilization by Medicare patients primarily by shortening hospital stays rather than by preventing admissions. Of the days of care saved in 1978, roughly 90 percent can be attributed to shortened lengths of stay. Since the first days of hospitalization are usually more expensive than subsequent days, this effect does not reduce costs as much as would a comparable change in utilization by means of admissions denials. (64)

With regard to whether the PSRO program saves money, the CBO report states that "the program consumes more resources than it saves society as a whole" (65).

Also important to an analysis of the effectiveness of PSROs is whether their performance is likely to improve over time. Unfortunately, this is not likely. The CBO study found that even though the PSRO agencies matured between 1977 and 1978 their effectiveness did not increase.

The effectiveness of the PSRO program is apparently no different from other utilization review programs. While some studies indicate there may be slight differences in use when a utilization review program is used, a review of these studies by Thomas Bice concludes that there is no conclusive evidence that they reduce per capita use of hospitals or eliminate unnecessary costs. In those cases where a study suggests that utilization review has lowered utilization, Bice states

---

*PSROs generally conduct several types of utilization reviews. Concurrent review determines whether the patient's admission was appropriate and whether the hospital is the appropriate setting for the patient. The patient's length of stay is also reviewed for appropriateness. The extent to which concurrent review is implemented varies among PSROs, some of which have replaced it with retrospective review. If inappropriate utilization is found, reimbursement to the physician and hospital can be denied. Although 203 PSRO areas were designated, by 1978 only 58 percent of those areas had an active PSRO organization. This percentage increased to 95 percent in the last two years. PSROs are physician-sponsored organizations. Physician organizations apply to the government to be designated as that area's PSRO; subsequently, most physicians in an area become members of the PSRO. *The Impact of PSROs on Health-Care Costs: Update of CBO's 1979 Evaluation* (Washington, D.C.: Congressional Budget Office, Congress of the United States, January 1981), p. 7.

that "in nearly all instances these conclusions are questionable on methodological grounds" (66).

Three basic approaches to hospital rate regulation have been discussed. The first was budget review on an individual hospital basis. This approach is the one most preferred by the hospitals because it involves negotiation with each hospital, thereby precluding drastic revisions in a hospital's budget. It offers the smallest possibility for holding down the rise in hospital costs or for promoting greater efficiency within and among hospitals. The negotiators representing the regulatory agency are likely to be more sympathetic in such face-to-face negotiations and less familiar with the hospital's budget than the hospital negotiators. The second approach proposed for hospital reimbursement was to classify hospitals and apply similar rates to those in each classification. This proposal offers a greater possibility than the previous one for increased hospital efficiency, since reimbursement rates are set with less regard for personal factors and are based on more standardized groupings. The problem with this approach is that it is difficult to develop appropriate classifications to allow for the many differences among hospitals. As a result, many hospitals appeal their reimbursement level; some hospitals may be unjustly harmed while others will receive a windfall. The last approach, which can also be used in conjunction with the other ones, is to establish a maximum allowable percentage increase in hospital costs for the coming year. This approach has the same advantages and problems as the preceding one. In addition, placing a limit on the increase in total hospital expenditures that is too low will affect the viability of the hospital system. Each of these approaches and their variations include trade-offs between simplicity in the administration of the reimbursement levels and more numerous hospital appeals, the possibility of unfairness or windfalls, and differing degrees of incentives and effectiveness in achieving the goals of efficiency and cost containment.

None of the foregoing methods of rate regulation has any prospect of success in minimizing the cost of the medical care treatment. No incentives exist for using less costly substitutes for the hospital, nor has the physician's role in the decisionmaking process been explicitly recognized. The approaches proposed for rate regulation are highly conservative; drastic changes in the delivery system are not encouraged. In fact, rate regulation may be viewed as the next-to-last step in making hospitals public utilities, thereby preventing the medical care delivery system from undergoing any major changes in the future. Rate regulation was proposed because CON legislation was ineffective in controlling the increase in hospital costs and in improving the allocation of hospital resources in a community. Instead of doing away with CON regulation, it is to be complemented by rate regulation. However, adequate rate regulation should render CON regulation superfluous. Possible explanations for continuing CON regulation are either that rate regulation by itself is not viewed as able to achieve its objectives or that CON proponents view this additional regulation as the next step before hospitals become public utilities. CON legislation regulates entry and exit in the hospital industry; rate regulation controls hospital revenues and rates, guaranteeing the individual hospital's survival. Perhaps this is why hospital associations are in favor of this trend in hospital regulation. The next regulatory step would be to franchise hospitals. A franchised hospital would be given the responsibility for providing services to certain areas or population groups. If franchising of hospitals were to occur, it will be impossible to promote changes in the delivery of medical care because any such changes will threaten a hospital's monopoly in an area.

THE ECONOMIC OUTLOOK FOR HOSPITALS

For a number of years, hospitals have been considered a growth industry. Revenues have been increasing at better than 13 percent per year, the number of employees and their wages have been increasing relative to other sectors of the economy, and those industries supplying hospitals—firms in the hospital supply and medical technology industries—have been the favorites of Wall Street investors. Even those hospitals that are organized for profit, the investor-owned chains, have been selling at higher price earnings multiples than the stock market as a whole. Is it likely that hospitals and the health care sector will continue to expand? Are hospitals insulated from the economic and demographic factors that effect the growth, maturity, and eventual decline that occur to other industries?

To appreciate how hospitals are likely to change, it is necessary to determine what the trends are that affect both hospital revenues and costs. In addition, which of these trends increases more rapidly will have an effect on whether hospitals will continue to expand the services they offer or whether administrators, attending medical staff, and the Board of Trustees will have to make increasingly difficult choices as resources become scarcer.

As difficult as it is to forecast hospital trends, it is probably easier to anticipate what is likely to happen to hospital costs than to hospital revenues. Cost pressures are likely to continue to increase than decrease. A lower inflation rate over the coming years will lessen some of the cost pressures on hospitals. However, hospital costs have always exceeded the increase in the consumer price index; it is likely it will continue to do so. Health care is basically a service industry in which productivity increases are difficult to achieve. It is also more difficult to substitute capital for labor as in other industries. Continued progress in development of medical technology will also increase costs. In other industries improvements in technology results in greater productivity, hence decreased unit costs. Advances in medical technology, however, result in the use of more technically trained personnel and, consequently, increased unit costs. In addition to a change in its "product"—as a result of improved technology, hospitals are also experiencing a more expensive patient mix—the elderly are becoming an increasing portion of their patients.

Given the continued cost pressures on hospitals, will they be able to pass these cost increases on to the payors of hospital care as they have in the past? Unless they are able to do so, the outlook becomes bleak. It now becomes necessary to examine the forces that effect the trend in hospital revenues.

FORCES AFFECTING HOSPITAL REVENUES

For an industry to be in the growth stage of its life cycle, the factors affecting the demand for its services must be increasing. Important to the demand for hospital care is growth in both the population and in the percentage of the population with hospital insurance. Since population growth in this country is increasing by only 1 percent per year and a large portion of the population currently have some form of third-party (either private or public) coverage for hospital care, the over-all growth in the industry has slowed down. Changes in hospital revenue, there-fore, will come from changes in reimbursement and from changes in utilization rates. Hospital utilization has been increasing at a very slow rate, at less than 1 percent per year between 1975 and 1980. The utilization of hospitals by those under 65 years of age has been declining while utilization by those over 65 has been increasing. The decline in hospital utilization by the nonaged is the result of several reasons which are likely to continue: changes in medical practice, and greater availability of nonhospital coverage. Another important trend is the in-crease in the number of working women, leading to a delay in the age when women have children, and to a smaller number of children.

Although hospital utilization by the aged is increasing, projected revenues from this age group are uncertain; if anything, the rate of increase in reimburse-ment is likely to decline. Hospital reimbursement for the aged depends on gov-ernment policy. When Medicare was introduced in the mid-1960s, government reimbursement was relatively generous; hospitals were reimbursed not only for their costs of caring for the aged but were also given an additional 2 percent. Hospitals' financial positions improved. As government expenditures under Medicare and Medicaid continued to increase, however, the federal government (and state governments with large Medicaid populations) developed a concen-trated interest in holding down the rate of increase in hospital costs. By 1982 it is estimated that the federal government was spending $90 billion on these two programs. And these expenditures were increasing at the rate of 18 percent per year.

There are several ways in which the rate of increase in Medicare expendi-tures can be held down. The first is to change eligibility requirements or benefits. Since Medicare covers the aged, it would be politically difficult for Congress or the current administration to reduce benefits, other than permitting slight increases in deductibles and copayments. A more politically acceptable approach is to increase benefits so as to include less costly out-of-hospital substi-tutes. Examples of such proposals are including home care as a reimbursable benefit as well as providing a Medicare voucher for prepaid health care. Either of these proposals, if enacted, would *decrease* hospital utilization. However, the most immediate way in which government can reduce its expenditures under Medicare is just not to pay the full amount it owes hospitals for care of the aged. This last approach is being used today. Hospitals are increasingly complaining that they are receiving less than their full costs for Medicare patients. Third-party payors, particularly commercial insurance carriers, are concerned about "cost shifting": hospitals charging other payors of care more since the govern-ment is paying less than its share.

Utilization by the aged is increasing and represents a greater portion of hospital utilization. Reimbursement for the aged, however, is less than full cost. Thus with respect to the aged, hospitals' financial positions will deteriorate. And on the horizon are possible changes in benefits that will reduce hospital utiliza-tion by the aged. Further, the higher hospital utilization rate by the aged, a mixed blessing because of the government's reimbursement policies for the aged, may decline in the years ahead if lower-cost substitutes become available to the aged.

Hospitals also face a changing outlook with respect to projected revenues from the nonaged. With the growth in hospital insurance having already occurred, and a relatively stable population base being present, hospitals appear to have entered upon the "mature" stage of their industry life cycle. They cannot count on continued increases in demand by the nonaged as a source of additional revenues. There are of course regional variations in growth in hospital demand. The South and Southwest are growing in population while the Northeast and Midwest are losing population. Thus hospitals located in these regions should face quite different growth prospects.

Insurance companies and Blue Cross Associations are also feeling the effects of limited growth in demand for hospital insurance. Increased enrollment in one insurance company can only come at the expense of another company's market share. The health insurance market has become increasingly competitive. To compete with one another on a premium basis, the insurance carriers and the Blues are placing greater pressures on hospitals to hold down their expenditures. Tighter hospital reimbursement and coverage for less-costly substitutes to hospitals are examples of the approaches being used.

Another source of concern for hospitals are the attempts by business and labor to hold down their health care costs. Rising health costs increase health insurance premiums and, consequently, result in higher labor costs to the firm. These higher costs, in turn, cause the prices of goods and services sold by the industry to increase. As a result, there have been decreases in the demand for those goods and services as well as for the labor used to produce them. To offset the growing cost of their fringe benefit programs, businesses and labor unions are becoming more actively involved in ways to hold down their community's expenditures for health care. Business coalitions are being formed. The purpose of such coalitions is to coordinate the efforts of the payors of care and place greater pressure on the providers to hold down their costs and charges. Business and labor are also experimenting with self-insurance programs, use of lower-cost substitutes to hospitalization, utilization review programs, and are examining alternatives to the fee-for-service system, namely prepaid health care. The effect of all of these efforts will be a decrease in hospital utilization.

The trends in both hospital utilization and reimbursement are likely to be quite different in the 1980s than they were in the 1960s and 1970s.

THE CHANGING MARKET IN WHICH HOSPITALS COMPETE

If a firm has a monopoly position in its area, then even though it may face tighter reimbursement, it does not have to worry about losing its market share to competitors. If, however, a firm is in a very competitive industry, then in addition to worrying about tighter reimbursement and declining utilization, the firm also has to be concerned with competitors and substitute services taking away its market share. An important phenomenon that has been occurring in health care is that more substitutes to hospital care have become available, along with sources of payment for their services.

Three trends have been occurring that are making the hospital industry more competitive.

The Increase in the Supply of Physicians

As a result of mandated enrollment increases to qualify for federal funds, medical schools increased their enrollments throughout the 1970s. New medical schools were also started. The consequence of these capitation grants has been an increasing supply of physicians. The number of physicians has increased 50 percent between 1965 and 1980 and is expected to increase another 40 percent over the coming decade. Such a large increase in both the absolute number of physicians and in the physician to population ratio should have an important impact on the delivery of medical services.

With the increase in supply of physicians, physicians will have an increasingly difficult time maintaining their real incomes. To some extent, physicians will be able to "create" increased demand for their services. It is unlikely, however, that physicians will be able to create sufficient demand to maintain their incomes. Evidence to support this belief is that the number of physician visits per capita over the last few years has not been increasing; on a per physician basis, physician visits are decreasing. Similarly, physician incomes over this period, adjusted for inflation, have been falling. Given the trends in declining government reimbursement for physician service and the growth of health maintenance organizations (HMOs), which "lock-in" their patient populations, physicians will have to develop new approaches if they are to increase their incomes.

Physicians are likely to respond in the following ways to their more competitive environment. First, they will attempt to increase the number of services they provide to their patients. This is likely to include an increase in the number of tests prescribed for each patient as well as an increase in the range of services they offer. Patient counseling and education are examples of a broader mix of patient services. Second, there will be greater competition among physicians for patients. This competition is likely to take the form of physicians making their services more convenient and accessible to patients, for example, by lengthening their office hours, and locating in residential areas so as to be closer to patients. Physicians will also attempt to develop a competitive advantage over other physicians. An example of this type of strategy is attempts by the medical staff to deny hospital staff privileges to new physicians on the grounds that they are not needed. This type of anticompetitive behavior will place the medical staff in conflict with their hospital, since the hospital will need a larger supply of physicians to keep its beds filled. Third, physicians are likely to try to restrict the professional practices of other health professionals through changes in the state practice acts. Increased political competition is likely to occur over which professions are legally permitted to perform certain tasks. Examples of efforts by physicians to limit encroachment on their market demand are the likely conflicts between orthopedic surgeons versus podiatrists, ophthalmologists versus optometrists, and physicians versus nurse practitioners.

As a fourth strategy, physicians are likely to engage in competition with hospitals for patients. Physicians will be more willing to provide emergency services and set up ambulatory care clinics to attract patients away from hospital outpatient departments. Physicians will also perform more outpatient surgery in their offices, which will decrease hospital utilization. The cost per hospitalized patient will consequently increase as the less-costly patients are treated on an ambulatory basis.

Fifth, physicians will be forced to consider forming their own prepaid health plans in order to compete with HMOs and alternative delivery systems. Because of the greater physician supply, prepaid health plans will find it easier to attract physicians. If, as expected, there is an increase in the number of prepaid plans and their coverage of the population increases, physicians may form their own prepaid plans in order to compete on a premium basis. Physicians may also believe that they can keep a greater portion of the premium for themselves if they are able to reduce hospital utilization. These types of competitive responses by physicians have been observed in California and Minnesota, where there has been growth in prepaid health plans. The effect on hospitals of the growth in prepaid health plans has been a reduction in their portion of the premium dollar from 54 percent, which is the national average, to 34 percent in these more competitive environments.

Prepaid Health Plans

Prepaid health plans are currently a small portion of the health care market. Indications are, however, that their growth may increase more rapidly. Both industry and labor now have stronger incentives to experiment with methods that reduce their health care costs. Any federal initiatives in this area, such as a proposed voucher system for the aged, will also serve to stimulate this trend. In the CON process, an incentive has been provided to hospitals by granting them exemptions if they have a high proportion of HMO patients. Another factor that will make it easier for HMOs and prepaid health plans to grow is the increase in the supply of physicians. In the past when the physician to population ratio was much lower, physicians could earn a high rate of return by practicing in the preferred fee-for-service system. Today, younger physicians are more willing to join prepaid health plans rather than incur the expense and uncertainty of starting independent practices.

The growth of prepaid health plans presents hospitals with a major potential threat to their revenues. According to both its proponents and empirical studies, hospital utilization among HMO subscribers is approximately half of that in a non-HMO setting. As more of the population moves into an HMO setting, the effect will be to decrease the demand for inpatient hospital services. The impact on the hospital will not only be a decrease in utilization and revenues but also a higher cost per admission. As the less-costly patients are treated on an ambulatory basis, the average cost of those patients remaining in the hospital will increase.

In areas where prepaid health plans have presented a greater competitive threat to the existing fee-for-service system, the existing health care providers reacted by starting their own prepayment plans. As more of the fee-for-service system is brought under a prepaid arrangement, these new prepaid plans also attempt to lower the hospital utilization of their subscribers. Thus the growth of prepaid plans and the competitive reaction to them by the fee-for-service system should serve to further decrease hospital utilization and revenue.

Multi-institutional Systems

There have always been some hospitals affiliated with one another. The most obvious example is hospitals affiliated with organized religious groups. In more recent years it has been the for-profit hospital chains. An important change that has been occurring recently is the joining together of nonprofit hospitals into what is referred to as multi-institutional systems. What is surprising about such a development is that the medical staff and the nonprofit hospital are willing to surrender some of their autonomy and control in return for the benefits of affiliation. There are various degrees of hospital affiliation. The weakest form is where hospitals share certain "hotel"-type services, such as laundry facilities, or participate in a joint purchasing program. At the other extreme is hospital merger. The stronger the degree of affiliation, the greater is the loss of autonomy by both the hospital and its medical staff. Presumably, the benefits from affiliation are at least equal to the loss in autonomy by the affiliating hospital. Hospitals and their medical staff prefer to be autonomous. Thus they would be willing to trade some autonomy for at least an equivalent amount of benefits.

The structure of the hospital industry is changing; it is becoming more concentrated. As more hospitals enter into affiliation agreements, the share of the hospital market served by such multi-institutional systems has increased. To understand the type of industry in which hospitals will be competing and whether the degree of concentration is likely to become even greater, it is important to analyze the reasons for these changes in the hospital industry. There are two basic reasons why an industry changes its structure: greater economies of scale, and the need for increased revenues.

In past years when demand for hospital care was increasing and hospitals were reimbursed generously, on a cost-plus basis, hospitals were able to increase their revenues and were under less pressure to contain their costs. Currently, the environment in which hospitals compete has changed. For hospitals to grow, and for some to even survive, they need to take advantage of any possible cost savings and of new sources of revenues.

Potential cost savings from affiliation with other hospitals arise in several areas. There are economies of scale in areas such as joint purchasing agreements, data processing systems, and building and equipping hospitals. To benefit from such cost savings requires that the hospital enter into some form of arrangement with other institutions. However, it is not necessary that the hospital give up much of its autonomy in order to benefit from such sharing arrangements. Thus these types of activities will be characterized by the most limited, or weaker, types of affiliation. However, to take advantage of other cost savings requires the hospital to belong to a more tightly affiliated system, with a consequently greater loss of its autonomy. These cost savings are generally financial; for example, in larger hospital systems lower interest charges on bond issues are possible, as is improved cash management through interhospital borrowing; in addition, averaging risks over larger patient populations can reduce malpractice premiums.

The need for additional revenue is also an important reason for restructuring of the hospital industry. In some areas a hospital faces a stable demand for its services, for example, a teaching hospital located in a declining urban area. To increase its revenues and to insure the use of its services, such a hospital may acquire or affiliate with smaller hospitals in surrounding areas. Horizontal integration, that is, hospitals seeking to acquire or affiliate with other hospitals, depends on the part of the country in which the hospital is located. In the South and Southwest, the growth in hospital revenues is generally sufficient to enable hospitals to remain independent. In the Midwest, many hospitals are realizing that unless they are willing to give up part of their autonomy and become part of a larger system, they will not be able to survive.

Hospitals prefer to seek new sources of revenue rather than relinquish their autonomy. There is thus a movement by hospitals to diversify into new lines of business. Hospitals have restructured their organizations so that revenues from new services are kept separate from their inpatient services. As a result of such restructuring, new sources of revenue are not included in calculations for Medicare reimbursement, nor are they subject to state hospital regulations.

The growth in multi-institutional systems has been rapid. The type of hospital affiliation agreements being developed, however, are not uniform. Some hospitals are very tightly controlled by the system to which they belong, while others are not. It is difficult to predict trends in these types of affiliation agreements. Hospitals and medical staffs are unwilling to trade their autonomy unless it is for a compelling reason. Thus we are more likely to observe loose affiliations for the hospital to take advantage of cost savings resulting from economies of scale. Hospitals that are in financial difficulty, either because of falling demand or tighter reimbursement limits, would be more willing to trade their autonomy for survival. Thus the growth of these multisystems depends upon the particular situation in which hospitals find themselves. Indications are that as economies of scale increase, the industry will become more concentrated. Unaffiliated hospitals may find themselves at a competitive disadvantage if they have higher costs.

As the concentration of the hospital industry increases, multihospital systems will have to become more aware of possible antitrust implications of their competitive behavior. Mergers that increase a systems' market share in an area may be attacked by competitors as attempts to monopolize the market. Hospitals will have to become familiar with economic definitions of markets and what constitutes substitute services if they are to be able to successfully defend themselves against antitrust suits.

SUMMARY OF TRENDS IN THE ECONOMIC OUTLOOK FACING HOSPITALS

While the use of the hospital by the aged has been increasing, government reimbursement has become much tighter. As Medicare and Medicaid represent a larger portion of hospital utilization, hospitals are attempting to increase their revenues by seeking higher payments from nongovernment third-party payers. Insurance companies, the Blues, business, and labor, however, are attempting to lower the rate of increase in their premiums by decreasing hospital costs of their subscribers, employees, and union members. Tighter controls on reimbursement, utilization control systems, lower-cost substitutes to hospitalization, and alternative delivery systems are examples of such approaches. The effect of both government and private sector efforts to reduce their health care expenditures is to limit the growth in hospital revenues.

Hospital cost increases, while related to the rate of inflation in the economy, are likely to be difficult to limit. Increases in medical technology will continue to increase the cost of medical equipment; declining younger-age cohorts in the population will result in a smaller supply of nurses and, consequently, higher wages. Government subsidies for capital and health manpower, which in the past have held down hospital cost increases, are being phased out. Hospitals will find it increasingly difficult to increase their revenues to offset increases in their costs.

With respect to the markets in which hospitals compete, hospitals are facing increased competition from the larger supply of physicians, who are seeking to increase their own revenues by performing more hospital services in their own offices. The growth in HMOs will decrease hospital utilization. Multihospital systems, with their cost advantages and their search for additional revenues, will increase the competitive pressures against the free-standing community hospital. Concentration in the hospital sector is likely to increase.

Not all regions of the country nor all hospitals are experiencing the same revenue and competitive pressures. Revenue growth is more difficult in the Northeast and Midwest. As the less severely ill are treated in lower-cost hospitals, teaching hospitals will find they are left with the more expensive cases; their cost per patient will rise even faster, leaving them with the problem of finding additional revenue to continue their patient care, teaching, and research functions. Public hospitals, so dependent on government for their operating funds, will also find it increasingly difficult to survive in the coming decade. In a growing number of regions of the United States, hospitals have become a mature industry. Their growth in utilization is leveling off and may actually decline. New revenue sources are likely to become an increasing concern in the years ahead.

ECONOMIC CHOICES FACING HOSPITALS

Hospitals and other health care providers face three choices in the coming years. Limited increases in hospital revenues, rising costs, and increasing competition will force many institutions to seek a merger with a stronger organization. Becoming part of a larger health care system will be the only option available for many providers. Hospitals and medical staffs will have less autonomy when they make this choice.

Other hospitals, facing the same economic outlook, will use a different strategy for survival; they will seek protection through legislation. Entry controls on new hospitals, to prevent them from entering their markets, and rate regulation, to insure payment for their services, will be proposed to ensure the hospitals' existence. An even stronger legislative mandate would make hospitals equivalent to public utilities; in this case, hospitals would be franchised to serve a given population. Such a franchise would preclude competitors from entering their markets and would guarantee the institution a budget to serve that population.

Protection through legislation will appear to be an attractive alternative to many hospitals. Having a concentrated interest in their institution's budget, hospitals will attempt to influence the state's allocation of funds to hospitals. Based on the evidence of CON programs, hospitals were not adversely affected by such legislation. In fact they were able to turn it to their advantage by precluding entry by proprietary institutions. Hospitals were also not adversely affected by many of the state rate review programs. Similarly, the early hospital reimbursement negotiations under Medicare proved very advantageous to hospitals. However, as is currently the case under Medicare and in stringent rate review states such as New York, some hospitals' financial conditions are deteriorating.

Initially, hospitals receive favorable treatment under a regulatory framework. However, as additional groups with concentrated interests in holding down health care costs develop, such as state governments, business, labor, and insurance companies, compromise decisions are reached by the legislature. And hospitals do not do as well. Their reimbursement becomes tighter and their financial position begins to decline. As other interests begin to dominate the regulatory process, hospitals will find that regulation is being used to freeze the hospital's budget. Rate review, as used in New York State, will become typical for regulated hospitals. As regulation limits hospital revenue, the growth in health care expenditures will occur outside the regulated sector. Other organizations, not subject to regulatory constraints, will be able to innovate and offer profitable services. Regulated hospitals will find themselves in a shrinking market.

Escaping economic competition through legislative protection may guarantee an institution's survival. However, regulation will provide the institution neither with sufficient funds nor with the flexibility to allow it to innovate in health care delivery. Instead, hospitals and other health care providers may realize that the rewards are fairer and the system is more efficient when the outcomes are determined by economic, rather than by political, competition.

Thus the third type of strategy hospitals may adapt to survive and even to grow is to engage in economic competition. To prosper under competition, hospitals must be able to secure new sources of revenue. To do so they must diversify into new services. There are three types of services hospitals should consider diversifying into. The first is to increase the number of feeder systems into the hospital. To keep their occupancy high, hospitals will require a larger patient base. When primary care physicians refer patients to specialists or for hospital utilization, the hospital should try and have those referrals directed to it. To accomplish this, the hospital should increase the number of primary care physicians on its staff and develop free-standing emergency centers and ambulatory care clinics in outlying areas. Such a strategy, however, results in potential conflict for the hospital. If the hospital attempts to add physicians to its staff, the existing medical staff may attempt to retain their competitive advantage over other physicians by denying them hospital privileges. It is important, however, for the hospital to realize that its economic interests on this issue may diverge from those of its existing medical staff. Unless the hospital is able to increase its pool of primary care physicians, it will find it difficult to maintain its occupancy rate in a period when hospital utilization rates will be declining. With the increase in supply of physicians, the relative scarcity of physicians compared to the number of hospitals is changing. Hospitals should be able to set the conditions for staff privileges.

The second type of services hospitals should diversify into are those considered to be substitutes to hospital care. Outpatient surgery decreases the demand for hospital inpatient care. To the extent that there is an increase in the use of outpatient surgery, hospitals will be left with the more costly inpatient surgical cases; and the average cost for surgery in the hospital will increase. To prevent the loss of revenues from outpatient surgery, hospitals should provide this service themselves. If the use of substitute services increases, hospitals will have little choice but to offer these services themselves. Another substitute to hospital care is the HMO. As HMOs attract more subscribers in an area, hospitals will experience decreases in their utilization. (Again, the remaining cost per inpatient admission will increase as the less-costly admissions are cared for on an outpatient basis.) To prevent this loss of revenue, hospitals should consider either starting or affiliating with an HMO. By being part of a HMO not only will the HMO use the hospital for its inpatient services, but the hospital might also share in the noninpatient revenue, which will become an increasing portion of the premium. As government and insurance companies seek to lower their premiums for health care, it is likely that more lower-cost substitutes for hospitalization will become covered insurance benefits. If hospitals are to maintain their revenues, it is essential that they become providers of these substitute services.

The third type of services hospitals should consider as part of their diversification strategy are nonacute care services. Hospitals are primarily involved in the provision of acute care. However, there is a growing demand for many nonacute health-related services, such as wellness and screening programs including hypertension and diabetes control, and vision and hearing programs. Hospitals might find a growing market for these wellness programs in their community as well as for occupational health services that can be sold to industry. Another important set of services for which there is a growing demand are services to the aged. Home health care and retirement centers are examples where hospitals could provide health-related services to the noninstitutionalized aged. The aged population is one of the most rapidly growing population groups in society. There are currently 24 million persons over 65 years of age. At the end of the decade it is estimated there will be 30 million aged. Among the aged, the fastest growing group are those greater than 75 years of age. It is expected that this group will increase by 30 percent, from 9 million currently to 12 million by 1990. As federal and state governments seek to lower their costs for caring for the aged, lower-cost substitutes to inpatient care will become reimbursable. There is also a growing number of aged who will be able to finance such services themselves. The aged will continue to be an important health care market, although not just in terms of inpatient utilization.

The provision of nonacute services, from wellness programs to services for the aged, requires the hospital to develop a different perspective of the industry it is part of. Acute inpatient care should be viewed as only one service in a spectrum of health care services. Viewed from this perspective, hospitals should become vertically integrated organizations, responsible for all of a person's health needs—from the well person to services for the aged. Unless the hospital changes the view of its mission—to that of a health care corporation—it will not be able to perceive the markets, population groups, and services for which it should be competing. A long-term strategy should be based on a clear vision of the organization's mission.

CONCLUSION

All industries have a life cycle. As the industry goes through the stages of growth, maturity, and decline, so do the firms that are part of that industry. Unless firms in an industry have a good appreciation for the changes occurring in the environment in which they compete, they are likely to shrink in size, merge with other firms in a declining industry, or simply go out of business. At times such changes occur slowly. At other times, as when there is a change in legislation affecting an industry, the changes occur very rapidly. The brokerage and airlines industries are examples of industries that have undergone very rapid change as a result of deregulation. New firms have prospered; some older established firms have merged or gone out of business. Whenever an industry faces such changes in its life cycle or in its environment, some firms manage to survive and even prosper. Those hospitals with a clear vision of their mission and the changing environment in which they compete are more likely to survive and prosper in the years ahead.

REFERENCES

1. This section is based upon the article by Millard F. Long and Paul J. Feldstein, "The Economics of Hospital Systems: Peak Loads and Regional Coordination," *American Economic Review*, May 1967.

2. Teh-wei Hu, "Hospital Costs and Pricing Behavior: The Maternity Ward," *Inquiry*, December 1971, p. 23.

3. H. Mohring, "Urban Highway Investments," in R. Dorfman, ed., *Measuring Benefits of Investments* (Washington, D.C.: Brookings Institution, 1965).

4. R. Coughlin, W. Isard, and J. Schneider, "The Activity Structure and Transportation Requirements of a Major University Hospital," *Discussion Paper Series No. 4*, Regional Science Research Institute, Philadelphia, 1964.

5. George J. Stigler, "The Theory of Economic Regulation," *The Bell Journal of Economics and Management Sciences* (Spring 1971). Richard A. Posner, "Theories of Economic Regulation," *The Bell Journal of Economics and Management Sciences* (Autumn 1974). Sam L. Peltzman, "Toward a More General Theory of Regulation," *Journal of Law and Economics* (August 1976).

6. Anthony Downs, *An Economic Theory of Democracy* (New York: Harper and Row, 1957), p. 297.

7. For a more complete discussion of policy typologies, see Michael T. Hayes, "The Semi-Sovereign Pressure Groups: A Critique of Current Theory and An Alternative Typology," *Journal of Politics* (February 1978).

8. The discussion in this section is based upon the article by Roger Noll, "The Consequences of Public Utility Regulation of Hospitals," in *Controls on Health Care*, Papers of the Conference on Regulation in the Health Industry, National Academy of Sciences, Washington, D.C., January 7–9, 1974. For additional references on regulation see the bibliography in Noll's paper.

9. William Jordan, "Producer Protection, Prior Market Structure and the Effects of Government Regulation," *Journal of Law and Economics*, April 1972.

10. Richard Farmer, "The Case for Unregulated Truck Transportation," *Journal of Farm Economics* 46 (1964).

11. Noll, *op. cit.*, p. 32.

12. George Stigler and Clair Friedland, "What Can Regulators Regulate? The Case of Electricity," *Journal of Law and Economics*, October 1962.

13. "The Regulators: Federal Commissions Draw Increasing Fire, Called Inept and Costly," *Wall Street Journal*, p. 1, October 9, 1974.

14. Noll, *op. cit.*, p. 33.

15. C. Vincent Olson and John M. Trapani, "Who Has Benefitted From Regulation of the Airline Industry?" *The Journal of Law and Economics* (April 1981).

16. Richard Posner, "Taxation by Regulation," *The Bell Journal of Economics and Management Science* 2 (1971).

17. George Eads, *The Local Service Airline Experiment* (Washington, D.C.: The Brookings Institution, 1972).

18. Ann F. Friedlander, *The Dilemma of Freight Transport Regulation* (Washington, D.C.: The Brookings Institution, 1969).

19. For a brief discussion of the history of health planning, see Symond Gottlieb, "A Brief History of Health Planning in the United States," in Clark Havighurst, ed., *Regulating Health Facilities Construction* (Washington, D.C.: American Enterprise Institute for Public Policy Research, 1974).

20. Joel May, *Health Planning—Its Past and Potential* (Chicago: Center for Health Administration Studies, University of Chicago, 1967). These findings are also presented in Joel May, "The Planning and Licensing Agencies," in *Regulating Health Facilities Construction*.

21. See P. O'Donoghue, A. Bryant, P. Shaughnessy, *A Descriptive Analysis of CHP "B" Agencies 1973* (Denver: Spectrum Research, Inc., 1974).

22. W. Wendling and J. Werner, "Nonprofit Firms and the Economic Theory of Regulation," *Quarterly Review of Economics and Business* (Fall 1980).

23. For a critical history of certificate of need (CON) legislation, see: Sallyanne Payton and Rhoda M. Powsner, "Regulation Through the Looking Glass: Hospitals, Blue Cross, and Certificate-of-Need," *Michigan Law Review* (December, 1980).

24. J.P. Newhouse and J.P. Acton, "Compulsory Health Planning Laws and National Health Insurance," in *Regulating Health Facilities Construction*, pp. 228–229.

25. William Curran, Richard Steele, and Ellen Ober, "Government Intervention on Increase," *Hospitals: Journal of the American Hospital Association*, May 16, 1974, p. 60.

26. Clark Havighurst, "Regulating Health Facilities and Services by Certificate of Need," *Virginia Law Review*, October 1973, p. 117.

27. *Ibid.*, p. 186. Also see Clark C. Havighurst, *Deregulating the Health Care Industry* (Cambridge, Mass.: Ballinger Publishing Co., 1982), particularly Chapter 8, "HMOs and the Health Planners." This chapter provides a legislative history of health maintenance organization (HMO) development and evidence on the regulatory discrimination against HMOs. This book also contains an excellent comprehensive discussion of a broad range of issues dealing with regulation and competition.

28. Comptroller General of the United States, *Study of Health Facilities Construction Cost* (Washington, D.C.: U.S. General Accounting Office, 1972), and Comptroller General of the United States, *Comprehensive Health Planning as Carved Out by State and Areawide Agencies in Three States* (Washington, D.C.: U.S. General Accounting Office, 1974).

29. Lewin and Associates, Inc., *Evaluation of the Effectiveness and Efficiency of the Section 1122 Review Process* (Washington, D.C.: Lewin and Associates, Inc., September 1975).

30. *Ibid.* Chap. 1, p. 7.

31. David Salkever, "Health Planning and Cost Containment: A Selective Review of the Recent U.S. Experience," Paper presented at the International Conference on Programs for the Containment of Health Care Costs and Expenditures, The Fogarty International Center, National Institutes of Health, Bethesda, Md., June 2–4, 1976, pp. 6–7.

32. David Salkever and Thomas Bice, "Certificate-of-Need Legislation and Hospital Costs," in Michael Zubkoff, Ira Raskin, and Ruth Hanft, eds., *Hospital Cost Containment: Selected Notes for Future Policy* (New York: PRODIST, 1978).

33. *Evaluation of the Effects of Certificate of Need Programs*, Final Report for the Bureau of Health Planning and Resources Development (Brookline, Mass.: Policy Analysis Inc. and Urban Systems Research, 1980). Frank Sloan and Bruce Steinwald, *Insurance, Regulation and Hospital Costs* (Lexington, Mass.: Lexington Books, 1980). F.J. Hellinger, "The Effects of Certificate of Need Legislation on Hospital Investment," *Inquiry* (June, 1976). David S. Salkever and Thomas W. Bice, *Hospital Certificate-of-Need Controls: Impact on Investment, Costs, and Use* (Washington, D.C.: American Enterprise Institute, 1979). Paul L. Joskow, "Alternative Regulatory Mechanisms for Controlling Hospital Costs," in Mancur Olson, ed., *A New Approach to the Economics of Health Care* (Washington, D.C.: American Enterprise Institute, 1981). Bruce Steinwald and Frank A. Sloan, "Regulatory Approaches to Hospital Cost Containment: A Synthesis of the Empirical Evidence," in Mancur Olson, ed., *A New Approach to the Economics of Health Care* (Washington, D.C.: American Enterprise Institute, 1981).

34. Institute of Medicine, *Controlling the Supply of Hospital Beds* (Washington, D.C.: National Academy of Sciences, 1976), pp. 7–9.

35. Total expenditures per bed in nonfederal short-term general hospitals in 1980 were $77,590. American Hospital Association, *Hospital Statistics*, 1981 ed. (Chicago: American Hospital Association, 1981), p. 5, Table 1.

36. Walter McClure, *Reducing Excess Hospital Capacity* (Excelsior, Minn.: Interstudy, 1976), p. 20.

37. Joseph Lipscomb, Ira Raskin, and Joseph Eichenholz, "The Use of Short-Run Marginal Cost Estimates in Hospital Cost Containment Policy," in M. Zubkoff, I. Raskin, and R. Hanft, eds., *Hospital Cost Containment* (New York, PRODIST, 1978).

38. Bernard Friedman and Mark Pauly, "Cost Functions for a Service Firm with Variable Quality and Stochastic Demand: The Case of Hospitals," *Review of Economics and Statistics* (November 1981): 624.

39. Lewin and Associates, *Final Report: Societal Factors and Excess Hospital Beds—An Exploratory Study*, DHEW Publication, No. (HRA) 80-644. (Washington, D.C.: Department of Health, Education and Welfare, 1979), p. 11.

40. William B. Schwartz and Paul L. Joskow, "Duplicated Hospital Facilities: How Much Can We Save By Consolidating Them?" *New England Journal of Medicine* 303 (1980): 1449–1457.

41. In his study on hospital closure in Massachusetts, Shepard found that the most likely result would be "a small *increase* in the area's annual hospital costs, because many patients are referred to more costly teaching hospitals." Donald S. Shepard, "Discontinuation of Hospital Services: When Does It Reduce Areawide Hospital Costs," *Health Services Research* (Spring 1983). Also in a special issue of this journal devoted to hospital closings and financial distress are related articles, such as the one by Alan Sager on the impact on access to care when a community loses its hospital. Hospitals that serve minority and Medicaid populations were more likely to be closed. When the displaced patient populations are moved to more costly teaching hospitals, the result is likely to be higher Medicare and Medicaid costs.

42. William L. Dowling, "Prospective Rate Setting: Concept and Practice," in William L. Dowling, ed., *Prospective Rate Setting* (Germantown, Md.: Aspen Systems Corporation, Winter 1976), p. 32.

43. Noll, "The Consequences of Public Utility Regulation of Hospitals," p. 33.

44. William L. Dowling, "Prospective Reimbursement of Hospitals," *Inquiry*, September 1974.

45. Paul L. Grimaldi, "Equity and Efficiency Implications of Case-Mix Reimbursement in New Jersey," in Gerald L. Glandon and Roberta J. Shapiro, eds., *Profile of Medical Practice 1980* (Chicago: American Medical Association, 1980).

46. *Reliability of Hospital Discharge Abstracts* (Washington, D.C.: Institute of Medicine, National Academy of Science, 1977).

47. Donald W. Simborg, "DRG Creep: A New Hospital-Acquired Disease," *New England Journal of Medicine*, June 25, 1981.

48. Paul L. Grimaldi, *op. cit.*, p. 94.

49. For a critical analysis of the use of DRGs for hospital reimbursement at the present time, see S.E. Berki, "The Design of Case Based Hospital Payment Systems," *Medical Care* (January, 1983).

50. J. Fitzmaurice, *An Evaluation of Alternative Systems of Establishing Hospital Reimbursement Limits Under Medicare* (Washington, D.C.: Health Care Financing Administration, 1976).

51. Judith Lave, Lester Lave, and Lester Silverman, "A Proposal for Incentive Reimbursement of Hospitals," *Medical Care* 11 (March–April 1973): 88.

52. See Paul J. Feldstein, *An Empirical Investigation of the Marginal Costs of Hospital Services* (Chicago: Graduate School of Business, The University of Chicago, June 1961). See also Joseph Lipscomb, Ira Raskin, and Joseph Eichenholz, "The Use of Marginal Cost Estimates in Hospital Cost-Containment Policy," in M. Zubkoff, I. Raskin, and R. Hanft, eds., *Hospital Cost Containment* (New York: PRODIST, 1978), pp. 514–537.

53. Hirsch S. Ruchlin and Harry M. Rosen, "Short-Run Hospital Responses to Reimbursement Rate Changes," *Inquiry* (Spring 1980).

54. See Michael Gort et al., "Report on the Hospital Price Index for Greater New York," mimeographed (Buffalo: Associated Hospital Services of New York, 1975); John Rossman et al., "Report on the Upstate Blue Cross Trend Factor 1976," mimeographed (Albany: Hospital Association of New York State, 1976); and Laurence Berger and Paul Sullivan, *Measuring Hospital Inflation* (Lexington, Mass.: Lexington Books, D. C. Heath & Co., 1975).

55. See Council on Wage and Price Stability, *The Problem of Rising Health Care Costs* (Washington, D.C.: Government Printing Office, 1976), p. 12. There are indications that increases in input prices have accounted for as much as three-fourths of the increase in hospital costs since 1974.

56. Katherine Bauer and Arva Clark, *New York: The Formula Approach to Prospective Reimbursement* (Boston: Harvard Center for Community Health and Medical Care, 1974), p. 47.

57. House Committee on Interstate and Foreign Commerce, Subcommittee on Public Health and the Environment, 93rd Cong., 1st sess., December 19, 1973, statement by John McMahon, p. 43.

58. Brian Biles, Carl Schramm, and Graham Atkinson, "Hospital Cost Inflation Under State Rate-Setting Programs," *New England Journal of Medicine*, September 18, 1980. Craig Coelen and Daniel Sullivan, "An Analysis of the Effects of Prospective Reimbursement Programs on Hospital Expenditures," *Health Care Financing Review* (Winter 1981). Frank Sloan, "Regulation and the Rising Cost of Health Care," *Review of Economics and Statistics* (November 1981). Glenn Melnick, John Wheeler, and Paul Feldstein, "The Effects of Hospital Rate Regulation on Hospital Costs and Utilization, 1975–1979," *Inquiry* (Fall 1981).

59. Information on the application of ESP to hospitals can be found in Stuart Altman and Joseph Eichenholz, "Inflation in the Health Industry: Causes and Cures," in Michael Zubkoff, ed., *Health: A Victim or Cause of Inflation* (New York: PRODIST, 1976), pp. 7–30; Richard Berman, "The Economic Stabilization Program of the United States: August 1971–April 1974," *World Hospitals* 12 (1976).

60. Ralph Berry, "Prospective Reimbursement and Cost Containment: Formula Reimbursement in New York," *Inquiry* (September 1976), and William L. Dowling et al., *Prospective Reimbursement in Downstate New York and Its Impact on Hospitals. A Summary* (Seattle: Department of Health Services, University of Washington, 1976).

61. Hirsch S. Ruchlin and Harry M. Rosen, *op. cit.*

62. A. Dobson et al., "PSROs: Their Current Status and Their Impact to Date," *Inquiry* (June 1978).

63. A brief review of these studies appears in Thomas W. Bice, "Health Planning and Regulation Effects on Hospital Costs," in Lester Breslow, ed., *Annual Review of Public Health*, Vol. 1 (Palo Alto, Calif.: Annual Reviews Inc., 1980).

64. "The Impact of PSROs on Health-Care Costs," A. Dobson, et al., *op. cit.*, p. xii.

65. *Ibid.*, p. xiii.

66. Thomas Bice, *op. cit.*, p. 154.

CHAPTER 12

The Benefits of Competition in Medical Care

AN APPROACH TO INCREASED COMPETITION IN MEDICAL CARE

Increased regulation of the health sector has been suggested as one approach to improving the performance of hospitals and other providers of medical care. The other alternative for restructuring the medical care delivery system is to rely on market competition among providers to achieve greater efficiency in the production of medical care. The traditional belief among medical planners is that competition is wasteful and should be eliminated. Under a system of insurance that provides first-dollar coverage, cost-based reimbursement for hospital care, and an absence of the physician's fiscal responsibility for the resources used in treatment, competition among providers led to duplication of beds and facilities, overutilization of hospitals, and rapidly increasing costs. However, the problem with the current system is not that providers compete but that reimbursement methods and both patient and provider incentives encourage higher costs.

Given the appropriate incentives, competition among medical providers would result in their responsiveness to patient demands as well as their being efficient in producing services and the entire medical treatment. Competition is more likely to stimulate innovation leading to more efficient methods of production and more effective methods of treatment. Opponents of increased competition claim that it will lower the quality of care. However, the current approach toward quality control in medical care, which attempts to ensure the high quality of inputs by imposing high educational requirements and emphasizing the process of providing medical care, has not necessarily protected the consumer from unethical or incompetent providers. Under a competitive system, such as the one to be discussed, the quality of medical care would not be lowered; in fact, as will be shown, there is a greater likelihood that quality will increase.

Under the current system of medical services delivery, providers are reim-

326

bursed separately for their services. The physician, who acts as the manager for the patient's medical treatment, uses hospital resources in providing patient care, but because the patient is generally insured for hospital care as well as for the services of hospital-based specialists, the physician does not have any financial incentives to use such resources efficiently. Owing to the growth in insurance coverage for each provider, physicians do not lose money when unnecessary costs are incurred in treating a hospitalized patient; they are reimbursed their customary fees, and the patient's insurance carrier reimburses the hospital (and hospital-based specialists) separately. Since physicians are the most knowledgeable purchasers in the medical care market, it would appear to make sense to provide them with an incentive to use those resources in the most efficient manner. Such an incentive would be provided if we were to drop the artificial separation between payments to physicians and payments to hospitals and other providers. Instead consumers (or their insurers or government acting on their behalf) should be able to purchase all their medical care from a single organization.

In return for an annual fee per person or per family, the organization would provide the enrollees with comprehensive medical care. The economic rationale behind health maintenance organizations (HMOs), prepaid group practices (PPGP), and prepaid health plans (PHP), as they are variously referred to, is to provide the organization and its physicians with a financial incentive to minimize the cost of medical care to its enrollees by allowing it to retain the difference between the capitation payment and the costs of providing medical services.

These organizations could be structured in a number of ways: they could represent large groups of physicians who would then contract with other medical providers for their services when needed, or they could represent combinations of providers, such as physicians and one or more hospitals. Regardless of how the the particular organization would be structured, it would be responsible for providing all of the medical services required by the patient. The methods used by the organization to reimburse its employees, physicians, and other providers might vary: they could use various combinations of salaried employees, profit sharing (sharing of any residual funds), retainers, or even fee-for-service for participating providers. This approach, using prepayment on a capitation basis and responsibility for delivery of comprehensive medical care, is not new. It was proposed by the Commission on the Cost of Medical Care in the 1930s. Examples of such organizations are the Kaiser Foundation Health Plan and the Group Health Association. More recently, this concept has been used as the basis for the HMO strategy,* which permits a corporate practice of medicine to compete with the current fee-for-service delivery system.

A variation on the prepaid health plan concept was proposed by Ellwood and McClure. They suggested that insurers organize health care alliances (HCAs), which would consist of a set of physicians and hospitals that would be responsible for delivering comprehensive care. Consumers could then shop be-

---

*The originator of the term health maintenance organization is Paul M. Ellwood, Jr. See his "Health Maintenance Strategy," *Medical Care*, May–June 1971.

tween HMOs or HCAs. Communities might have more than one HCA and insurers might set up multiple HCAs.

> [T]o attract consumers, each insurer would attempt to select for participation in his preferred HCAs, providers who could provide good quality care at a reasonable cost, and especially providers who make conservative use of the hospital. To insure competition, no HCA would be permitted to enlist more than half the providers in a community (exceptions would be made in underserved areas). Providers could participate in one or more HCAs if they cared to, but would have to negotiate reimbursement arrangements separately with each HCA. However, the insurer, not the providers, is at risk in an HCA, giving the insurer a strong incentive to select only efficient providers. (1)

An advantage of this proposal is that it puts non-HMO providers in a group, thus making it easier to evaluate the price and quality of that group. The concern with quality would rest not only upon the insurer organizing an HCA, but also on its provider members. They would have a greater incentive to cooperate in monitoring the quality of care practiced by all of the other providers. Quality assurance programs would be more easily developed and monitored for larger organizations than for a large number of smaller, independent providers.

The result of Prepaid Health Plan (PHP) competition to provide medical services for a fixed capitation payment should be the following.

INCENTIVES FOR HOSPITAL EFFICIENCY

Under the system of cost-based reimbursement, in which most of the hospitalized population is covered by some form of hospital insurance, the physician has little or no incentive to be concerned with the cost of hospital care. Under a capitated system of reimbursement for all of a person's medical services, the HMO would either have to operate its own hospitals or purchase hospital care from existing hospitals in the community. The HMO would therefore have an incentive to be more concerned with the costs of their patients' hospital care and would, consequently, select hospitals in the community according to both the hospitals' costs and the services required for their patients. Because they would be the most knowledgeable purchasers in the market, the HMO's physicians would be able to choose those community hospitals with the necessary level of quality of care at the lowest available cost. For example, routine appendectomies need not be performed in high-cost teaching hospitals.

LESS DUPLICATION OF FACILITIES

Facilities and services that currently exist primarily for the convenience of the physician or because they provide prestige to the institution now have a cost associated with their use. If the organization had fewer such facilities, the HMO's premium could be reduced, its benefits increased, or the savings used to reward the HMO's staff. It would not be in the best interests of an HMO to own every type of facility and service. Because some facilities are subject to large economies of scale, it may be financially advantageous for an HMO to purchase such services from other institutions when its patients required them. Since there is now a cost to the HMO and its physicians for having duplicate facilities, we would expect fewer such facilities in the community.

MINIMIZING THE COST OF A MEDICAL TREATMENT

Currently, the use of less-costly substitutes for hospital care is determined by their efficacy in medical treatment, the cost to the patient of care in different institutional settings (e.g., whether the patient's insurance covers out-of-hospital care), and the effect, if any, on the patient's physician of institutionalizing the patient in other than a hospital setting. Under a capitated system of reimbursement, the criteria for use of alternatives to hospitalization will change. The HMO (and the patient's physician) will have an incentive to provide care in the least costly manner. When medically feasible, we would expect to observe greater use of outpatient surgical care in lieu of hospitalization for the same procedure and shorter hospital stays, with the remainder of the patient's convalescence provided for in an extended care facility or even in the patient's home. Not only would we expect physicians to be concerned with the quality and efficiency of each institutional setting but also we would expect them to select the least-costly combination of settings when providing treatment for the HMO's patients. No other reimbursement system provides incentives for minimizing the cost of the patient's entire medical treatment.

INCREASED PHYSICIAN PRODUCTIVITY

Under a capitated system of reimbursement, an HMO's physicians would have an economic incentive to use greater numbers of auxiliary medical personnel in their offices and in the hospital, resulting in an increase in the physician's productivity. As long as the revenue produced by the additional auxiliaries exceeds their cost, it will be in the interests of the physicians and the HMO to add auxiliary personnel. We would thus expect to observe an increase in demand for such personnel from HMOs. HMOs might even develop their own training programs or permit specifically trained registered nurses to perform tasks currently undertaken only by physicians. The medical profession's limit on trained personnel who can substitute for some physicians' services would be changed by the existence of large, economically powerful HMOs. We might thus expect greater delegation in the performance of medical tasks if they were delegated on the basis of training and performance rather than, as under current practice, on the basis of physician status.

INCENTIVES FOR PREVENTIVE CARE
AND HEALTH EDUCATION

To the extent that preventive care delivered to an HMO's enrollees results in decreased future demand for more costly medical services, we would expect the HMO to provide a greater amount of those services than is provided under the current fee-for-service system. Similarly, to the extent that the enrollees' health habits can be improved, thus reducing future demand for medical care, the HMO could be expected to undertake health education programs. To provide them with an even greater incentive to be concerned with their enrollees' health status, HMOs should be encouraged to sell life insurance to their enrolled population (2).

USE OF GENERIC DRUGS

We would expect HMOs to be more concerned with drug prices, as it would be in the economic interests of the physicians and the HMOs to prescribe less costly drugs. The HMO, rather the drug companies' detailmen, would become the main source of drug information for its physicians. The HMO would have an incentive to provide the physician with the option of selecting generic drugs when writing a prescription. Both the source of drug information and the incentives of the prescribing physicians under the HMO approach would be different from those under fee-for-service.

INNOVATIONS IN THE DELIVERY OF MEDICAL CARE

Innovations in the delivery of medical services are potentially threatening to physicians and to other providers of medical care. Innovations may result in substitutes being developed for existing providers. Innovations in types of facilities, treatment methods, and personnel have hitherto been restricted; however, under a capitation system with competition for consumers, HMOs have an incentive to be innovative. Innovations might be found in the diagnostic area, in management techniques, and in delivering services. Greater experimentation with location and accessibility of services to the HMO's enrolled population might occur. HMOs would have an incentive to seek out and quickly adopt (when economically feasible) new techniques with both medical and management applications. Such techniques might enable the HMO to lower its costs or increase its services, thereby enhancing its ability to compete with other HMOs or fee-for-service physicians. One would expect that under a capitated system of reimbursement for medical care, the rate of innovation in medical care delivery methods would be much greater than it has been previously.

THE EFFECT OF ADVERTISING ON THE MARKET FOR MEDICAL SERVICES

An important prerequisite to competition in medical services is advertising. Many people, in addition to medical care providers, are opposed to advertising of medical services. Such opposition is usually based on the fears that consumers will be misled, that they will be induced to purchase unnecessary services, and that the prices of such services will be increased because the cost of advertising will be passed on to the consumer. The argument that consumers will be misled is weak. The Federal Trade Commission (FTC), which seeks to improve market competition, currently polices advertising claims. Existing health providers would be expected to carefully monitor their competitors' claims and provide information to the FTC. Further, it seems unlikely that consumers will be more misled by providers who publish misinformation than they are under a system which suppresses information.

The claim that consumers will be induced to purchase unnecessary services is based on the assumption that providing more information from competing sources will result in greater demand creation than that which occurs when the patient is totally reliant on a single physician for advice. The recent trend toward securing second opinions for recommended surgery contradicts this claim. Surgery is an area where the patient has very little information as to prospective value; two opinions would presumably increase a patient's information and enable him or her to make a more informed choice, thereby resulting in a decrease in the rate of surgery.

Advertising results in lower rather than higher prices. This is difficult to explain to people who believe that advertising would result in an additional cost to the patient. The following discussion will therefore attempt three things: to explain why advertising of medical services should result in lower prices for medical services; to provide some supporting empirical evidence; and, finally, to examine which population groups are likely to benefit from removal of the restrictions on advertising.

Advertising provides price information. In an industry where each firm produces the same product but does not permit advertising of prices, wide variations in prices will exist, since it will be up to the consumer to search out the firms with the lowest prices. Since search is costly, consumers will not keep searching until they find the firm that sells its products at the lowest price. Only when the search costs approach zero will people search until the price differential approaches zero. If information were disseminated through advertising, and no additional expense, such as travel cost to purchase the product, was involved, prices would reflect the costs of producing different products. Differences in quality and variety would exist, but the different prices charged for such products would reflect these additional costs. In a world of perfect information, prices charged for what is perceived to be the same product should be the same.

In the market for medical services, however, information is not only far from perfect, it is almost nonexistent. Because of this, each medical care provider has a relatively inelastic demand curve. A patient is usually unaware of the quality, accessibility, and price of medical services sold by different competitors, which makes these other medical providers poor substitutes for the patient's current provider. Furthermore, even if information on quality and other characteristics of services sold by competitors were made available, if the consumer does not have price information, wide variations in prices of similar products could exist. To determine which services are sold at lower prices, the consumer would have to spend time and money searching (3).

The effect of advertising on prices can be shown with reference to Figure 12-1. With little information available to consumers to be able to judge other physicians, the physician's demand curve is relatively inelastic, shown as D_1. Assuming that the physician-firm wishes to maximize its profits, it will set its price at that point on the demand curve where the marginal revenue (MR_1) and

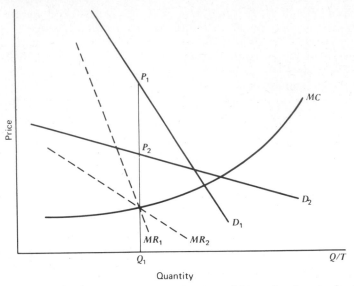

Figure 12-1. The effect of advertising on the elasticity of demand and on the firm's pricing strategy.

marginal cost curves intersect. The resulting price will be P_1. With advertising, consumers have more information by which to evaluate other physicians and health care providers. These other physicians now become better substitutes to one another. As this happens, the physician's demand curve becomes more elastic (the closer the substitute, the more elastic the demand curve). The new, more elastic, demand curve is D_2. For the sake of simplicity, the marginal revenue curves in Figure 12-1 were drawn so that they intersected the marginal cost curve at the same point. With the same marginal cost curve, a more elastic demand curve will result in a reduced price, moving from P_1 to P_2.*

The cost of advertising is not shown in Figure 12-1 since it would be represented by an increase in the firm's average cost curve. Advertising costs may be considered a fixed cost, since they are unrelated to the cost of producing additional quantities of the particular product. Thus, the cost of advertising itself does not affect the price charged by a firm attempting to maximize its profits. The price would be determined by the elasticity of demand and the marginal cost of producing that product. By causing the firm's demand curve to become more elastic, advertising is expected to lower prices.

Advertising of medical services would thus perform two functions. First, it would inform the consumer of those services that are similar and of the differ-

---

*In the nonhealth field, many products are already viewed by consumers as being relatively homogeneous. One firm's soap or aspirin is considered to be a good substitute for the same product produced by another firm. In these cases, advertising is used by a firm to differentiate its product from that of its competitors. As shown in Figure 12-1, if a firm is selling a relatively homogeneous product (demand curve D_2), it advertises to make consumers believe that other products are less substitutable for its own, thereby hoping to change its demand curve to D_1.

ences between services sold by different providers, enabling the consumer to evaluate the degree of substitutability of competing services. The demand curves of the different providers would be made more elastic. As shown in Figure 12-1, with a more elastic demand curve, the price would be reduced from P_1 to P_2. The second advantage of advertising medical services is that it would reduce the consumer's search costs. "Price dispersion is a manifestation of—and indeed it is a measure of—ignorance in the market" (4). Advertising reduces the cost of search, since reading a newspaper or other publication takes less time and money than traveling to different providers to determine the quality, accessibility, and price of the services provided. These search costs are particularly high in medical care. Without provider information, the consumer may first have to purchase the service to determine its attributes as well as its price.* Although advertising is less effective when services are directly experienced, provider information on prices and qualifications will still contribute to the information the consumer needs to make a choice. The consumer might then have to resort to additional sources, such as consumer groups, for information to indicate probable satisfaction with the provider.

These two hypothesized effects of advertising are shown in Figure 12-2. Without advertising, price dispersion would be much greater; as search costs are reduced, price dispersion will decrease. As the demand for lower-priced providers increases, and as medical services are viewed as being more homogeneous, the average price will also decline.

Because of previous restrictions on advertising, it has been difficult to find empirical evidence in medical care to test the hypothesis that advertising leads to lower prices and less price dispersion. Until recently, advertising was prohibited by the state codes that regulate ethics in the health professions. The penalties for violating such codes were severe, including suspension of the practitioner's license. Health institutions are only beginning to advertise. And the Joint Commission on Accreditation of Hospitals does not publicize the findings from their hospital surveys undertaken for accreditation purposes. Evidence on the gains from advertising that can be generalized to the entire medical sector is therefore limited. However, evidence based on a study of one health profession—optometrists—does provide a clear-cut indication of the effects of advertising restrictions and other forms of information control by the profession (5). Based on health interview survey data collected in 1970, Lee Benham and Alexandra Benham related demand factors and a set of variables measuring the degree of information control that the optometric profession maintained in each state to the prices that consumers paid for eyeglasses. The authors then estimated the effect of the prices paid on the likelihood that consumers would purchase eyeglasses. Several measures were used to indicate the degree of control that the optometric profession maintained over the availability of information in a state. One of these was the percentage of optometrists belonging to the state optometric association. A major prerequisite for membership is the willingness of the optometrist to withhold information on prices and services rendered.

---

*Nelson classifies goods into two categories: search goods and experience goods. Search goods are those for which adequate information concerning their desirability exists prior to purchase, e.g., an airplane trip. Experience goods need to be purchased to be assessed, e.g., a dinner in a restaurant. Phillip Nelson, "Advertising as Information," *Journal of Political Economy* (July–August 1974).

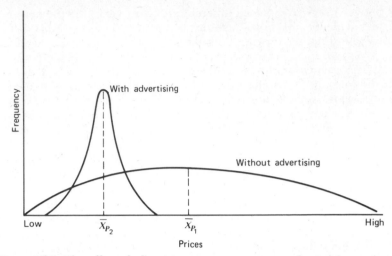

Figure 12-2. The effect of advertising on average prices and price dispersion.

It was therefore believed that the higher the percentage of optometrists belonging to the association, the smaller the amount of information consumers would have on optometric prices and services.

Commercial firms selling optometric services can advertise in certain states. Thus, another measure of the degree of professional control over information was the degree to which commercial firms were restricted or prohibited by a particular state. The third measure was the percentage of eyeglass sales purchased through commercial firms. The larger the market share of commercial firms in a state, the greater was the amount of information presumably available to consumers on optometric services, and the weaker was the optometric association's control over information. These three measures—the percentage of optometrists in a state belonging to the optometric association, the presence or absence of state control over commercial firms' selling of optometric services, and the percentage of total sales by commercial firms—indicated that state's degree of professional control over information on optometric services.

In addition to the professional control variables, the demand equation included the usual factors affecting demand, such as price, family income, race, age, and location (residence in an inner city or rural area). The statistical results of the demand analysis were predictable: the larger the proportion of optometrists belonging to the state association, the higher the price of the product; the price of eyeglasses was increased by $12.18, as membership proportion went from .43 to .91; the elasticity was almost .5: as the membership proportion increased, prices rose by half that percentage increase. The fewer the restrictions on commercial firms, the lower the average price in that state; specifically, $8.46 lower in the less, compared to the more, restrictive states. As the proportion of sales by commercial firms decreased from 79 to 0 percent, the average price increased by $11.71 (6). Thus, the evidence clearly indicates that the greater the degree of professional control over information, the greater the price paid for optometric services.

These results are similar to an earlier study conducted by Benham in 1963, in which he found that states that did not have restrictions on advertising had prices that were on average 20 percent lower ($6.70) than states with such restrictions. In that same study, Benham found that the dispersion of prices, measured by the coefficient of variation, $\sigma/\bar{x}$, was lower in those states that permitted advertising (7). The Benhams found that higher prices had a strong impact on the decision to purchase glasses. "A 30 percent increase in price associated with increased professional control implies a fall in the proportion of people obtaining eyeglasses of between 28.5 and 34.2 percent" (8).

The Benham and Benham study also determined that the effect of professional control was much greater on the less educated: that they are more likely to pay higher prices than those paid by more educated persons in similar situations. The concern that many persons have over the supposedly negative effects of advertising should be reexamined. While it is difficult to generalize about the quality of services the less-educated receive under a system of strong professional information control, it is clear that they are taken greater advantage of than those with higher education, perhaps because the latter are more efficient in the search process.

Benham cites a study that attempted to get at the quality issue. After price advertising began in Florida a survey of retired persons was undertaken. One of the test questions was, "All things considered, the next time you buy eyeglasses or contact lenses, would you return to the same place where you bought your last pair?" The responses were then matched to another question which asked if the place of last purchase advertised prices. The issue, "Are consumers more dissatisfied with opticians who advertise?" was thus answered. "The results show that while 58 percent of the customers of nonadvertising opticians indicated a willingness to give the seller repeat business, 86 percent of the advertisers' customers indicated they would return . . . only 8 percent of the customers of advertising opticians said that they 'probably' or 'definitely' would not go back. A full 25 percent of the customers of nonadvertising opticians gave the same answer. . . . In brief, if there is a quality problem it is not with advertising opticians. Rather it would appear that it lies with those who refuse to advertise their prices." (9) The strong desire health (and other) professions have to maintain codes of ethics that prohibit advertising can be explained by the fact that professional control over information leads to higher prices.

The results of the Benham and Benham studies have been upheld by more recent studies. The FTC found that in cities where advertising was permitted, eye doctors who advertised charged $62.58 for eyeglasses, including an eye examination. In the same city eye doctors who did not advertise charged $74.66. In cities where advertising was prohibited the average price was $94.58. The FTC also found that there were no quality differentials (frequency of incorrect prescriptions and quality of eyeglasses) between those who advertised and those who did not (10).

THE EFFECT OF COMPETITION ON QUALITY OF MEDICAL CARE

It might be useful at this point to comment on permitting for-profit HMOs to deliver medical care. It is believed that for-profit organizations will sacrifice quality for profit. When nonprofit providers do not perform well, it is said that they at least meant well. However, nonprofit status does not ensure high quality. When voluntary hospitals are examined, it is found that their tissue committees do not perform as they should; county nursing homes are not necessarily noted for their high quality of care; state mental institutions and Veterans Administration (VA) hospitals are not centers of excellence. Outside the health field, nonprofit status does not necessarily lead to higher quality, nor does it lead to a sensitivity to the public interest greater than that of for-profit competitors. All public schools are not necessarily of higher quality than private schools; municipal governments are often greater polluters than for-profit firms; and when nonprofit unions manage their own pension funds, they do not often receive a higher rate of return than that received by for-profit mutual funds.

Nonprofit status alone should not relieve us of a concern for quality. Quality should be monitored directly, and if this is done, it should not matter that for-profit providers exist. If only nonprofit providers are permitted, the effort to monitor quality will lessen. The advantage of permitting for-profit providers to compete in the medical market is that, precisely because they are not trusted, a greater incentive will exist to develop and apply strong quality review mechanisms. These quality review mechanisms should then apply equally to *all* providers.

It might be claimed that under a system of capitation payment for medical care, for-profit HMOs in particular, might be tempted to provide minimal medical services so as to retain as much of the capitation fee as possible. Although for several reasons, such a situation is unlikely to occur, several safeguards can be built into the system to ensure that is does not.

CONSUMER CHOICE

One such safeguard would be that no HMO would have a complete monopoly over the delivery of medical services in its area, otherwise it would be subject to the antitrust laws. Most urban areas would be likely to have more than one HMO in addition to the prevailing fee-for-service system. Consumers would choose the HMO they wished to participate in and would renew their choice annually (11). They could also decide not to join an HMO. The various HMOs and alternative delivery systems would have to compete for new subscribers as well as to retain their existing enrollees. Unfortunately, many consumers would never have sufficient information to select the HMO that would provide a given level of care at lowest cost. Other subscribers, however, would be knowledgeable; for example, unions, employers, and other organizations could afford to develop the necessary expertise and information to evaluate the various alternative medical care delivery options available to them. The greater selectivity of these more-informed groups would benefit the less-informed subscribers. If a well-informed group were to switch from one HMO to another HMO, or to fee-for-service under Blue Cross–Blue Shield, then the HMO losing subscribers would have to change in order to accommodate the preferences of the better-informed group if it was to survive. As long as the legislation on truth in advertising is enforced, marketing of HMOs and the competition between them should result in the less-informed benefiting from the actions of better-informed purchasers.

THE PERMANENT NATURE OF THE ORGANIZATION

Large organizations or corporations are usually in business for an indefinite period. The expected long life of such organizations leads them to behave differently than small firms or those in business for a short time. Whereas an individual entrepreneur may go into business, mislead consumers, produce a poor product, and then quickly move on to another area, large corporations cannot afford such behavior. A large corporation cannot undertake those business practices that will maximize its present income at the expense of future business. It cannot afford to purposely produce a poor product. Because HMOs would have their reputations at stake, pocketing the capitation fee and providing little or no service would adversely affect the reputation of the organization and decrease its future business. Poor business practices are therefore more likely to be expected of smaller organizations, for which the costs of moving and entering and leaving business are lower. This would be as true in the medical field as it is for corporations in nonmedical businesses. Kaiser Foundation Health Plan, Health Insurance Plan of Greater New York, and Group Health Association, to name a few, have not been criticized for producing lower-quality health care than their fee-for-service competitors.

SPILLOVER EFFECTS AMONG PHYSICIANS IN THE HMO

Just as the permanence of an organization leads to attempts to maintain or increase quality, so the size of an organization influences its quality. In an HMO or other group practice comprised of a large number of physicians, the quality of care practiced by any one physician in the group affects the reputation, hence the incomes, of the other physicians. This spillover effect helps to ensure that poor medical care is not practiced by any of the participating physicians. We would expect to observe more meaningful utilization review by the participating physicians in such organizations. Under the current system of solo-practice fee-for-service delivery, no economic incentives encourage the enforcement of sanctions against physicians whose performance, when examined by utilization review and tissue committees, is revealed to be unacceptable. Quality of care is thus expected to be higher when physicians practice as part of a group than when they remain economically unaffected by an incompetent or unethical colleague.

EXTERNAL QUALITY REVIEW MECHANISMS

The states could also monitor the health and medical outcomes of all delivery systems, including that of HMOs. Although outcome measures are difficult to determine, emphasizing them in the monitoring process would speed their development and allow greater flexibility in the use of medical inputs to achieve those outcomes (12). Measuring quality in terms of the inputs used or the medical treatment process itself would raise the costs of providing care (hence lessen the competitive advantage of HMOs) and might inhibit innovation in the provision of medical care.*

In addition to continually monitoring the quality of care provided by a state or a federal agency, health officials should publish the results of the quality reviews. Financial penalties and other sanctions should be applied when instances of poor quality were found, but publicizing the result of quality reviews would serve as an additional stimulus to maintaining and increasing the quality of competing organizations.† It is difficult to believe that no quality information is preferable to some, especially when that information is collected and used by the state or federal agency responsible for monitoring quality of care. Although not all consumers will use that information in choosing their delivery system, some large, informed consumer groups will be able to evaluate and use it. Other consumers will then benefit by the actions of the better-informed consumer groups. The development of a broader range of quality measures should improve consumers' ability to choose among delivery systems on the basis of quality, access, and cost.

ADDITIONAL QUALITY ASSURANCE MECHANISMS

Two additional approaches would help to assure that the quality of care provided by HMOs and other delivery systems was at least maintained. The first of these is malpractice suits. Poor quality of care would prove to be too costly to an organization if it resulted in an increase in lawsuits and large awards to the aggrieved parties. One would therefore expect that the threat of malpractice suits would inhibit the provision of poor quality care. Another approach to guard against the deliberate provision of low-quality care to enrollees is to accredit such organizations by a federal quality review organization. In determining minimum criteria for establishing an HMO, the federal agency might consider such factors as minimum financial reserve requirements; capacity to serve a minimum size of population, such as 20,000 persons;‡ and limits on the percentage or number of

---

*Havighurst and Bovbjerg oppose making professional standards review organizations PSROs responsible for the quality of care provided in HMOs on grounds "which range from the danger of inadvertent homogenization of medical practice to the worrisome opportunities presented for anticompetitive or other intentional misuse of PSRO power." Clark C. Havighurst and Randall Bovbjerg, "Professional Standards Review Organizations and Health Maintenance Organizations: Are They Compatible?" *Utah Law Review*, Summer 1975, University of Utah College of Law, p. 411.

†Greater use should be made of financial penalties when instances of poor quality are determined to exist. In the past, strong sanctions for poor quality, such as removal of a license to practice or of the accreditation of a hospital, have been considered so severe that they were rarely used. If less drastic measures such as financial penalties were available, it is likely that they would be applied more frequently to minor infractions of quality which would otherwise have gone unpunished.

‡One reason for establishing a minimum size for the organizations is that there is great variability in a person's medical expenses. A small organization might not be able to absorb the possible losses if certain of their patients required treatment for illnesses considered to be catastrophic. One possible remedy to the problem of size of organization is to require minimum-sized organizations to carry reinsurance.

particular categories of the population served—for example, not more than 50 percent of the Medicaid or Medicare population.*

Contrary to the fears of some, the available empirical evidence, based on well-established HMOs, indicates that their quality of care is higher than that provided under the traditional fee-for-service system (13). Because there is concern that HMOs or other innovative delivery systems would purposely reduce the quality of medical care to their enrolled population either to survive in a competitive atmosphere, or to maximize profits, this should lead to a strong quality assurance program. However, if such quality assurance mechanisms were located at a local or state level, the monitoring agency could be captured by the existing health care providers. The measures proposed by the captured agency would emphasize input and process approaches to quality assurance, to the disadvantage of an innovative organization. Locating the quality assurance agency at a federal level would make its capture by existing providers more difficult; it would also be less costly for all the HMOs to lobby one agency than for each to lobby one or more.

If the emphasis on quality assurance can be shifted from specifying high educational requirements and individual licensure to measurement of the outcome of medical treatment, then much broader latitude would be permitted organizations' use of various personnel to perform specified tasks. The licensing of institutions rather than individuals would enable organizations to be more flexible in their use of personnel. Various health manpower personnel would be assigned tasks that match their training and competence rather than those specified by an individual licensing process under state law, as is the current practice. Institutional licensure should, consequently, result in lower costs for providing medical services, without any diminution in the quality of care (14).

EVIDENCE ON THE PERFORMANCE OF HMOs

The early claims that HMOs perform better than the fee-for-service system were based on data from a few of the larger prepaid group practices, such as Kaiser, Health Insurance Plan of Greater New York, Federal Employees Benefit Program, and Group Health Association. Comparative data on fee-for-service were based on either utilization surveys of the general population or, in several instances, surveys of groups of employees who had a choice between prepaid plans and fee-for-service plans such as Aetna or Blue Cross–Blue Shield. Because of severe data limitations, it has not been possible to isolate the reasons for differ-

---

*If such minimum criteria were developed for the establishment of HMOs (or prepaid health plans), and if these regulations were enforced, then many of the abuses associated with some of the early HMOs that were established in California to serve the Medicaid population, such as questionable marketing techniques and restrictions of access to enrollees, would not have occurred. See, for example, Milton I. Roemer, "Better Weather Ahead for California's Prepaid Health Plans?," *American Medical News*, October 25, 1976, pp. 7–8. See also Paul M. Ellwood, Jr., "Alternatives to Regulation: Improving the Market," in *Controls on Health Care*, Papers of the Conference on Regulation in the Health Industry, National Academy of Sciences, Washington, D.C., January 7–9, 1974, pp. 61–63.

ences in utilization and costs between prepaid health plans and fee-for-service. A major problem in this regard has been subscriber selectivity: if subscribers with low utilization patterns select prepaid health plans, then utilization differences cannot be considered an effect of the plan, nor is it possible to extrapolate the potential savings were prepaid health plans to be mandated for a much larger segment of the population.*

Comparative data from prepaid health plans and fee-for-service are summarized in Table 12-1. Based on a number of studies, it appears that the total cost of medical care (premium plus out-of-pocket expenses) for HMO enrollees is 10–40 percent lower than for persons with comparable insurance coverage using the fee-for-service delivery system (15). The potential gains from prepaid health plans result from first, a lowering of hospitalization rates; and second, on average, lower out-of-pocket expenses for its members. Lower hospitalization is achieved primarily through lower admission rates, although there is some indication of shorter lengths of stay. In general, there are approximately 30 percent fewer hospital days among HMO enrollees as compared to those with fee-for-service coverage (16).

The evidence for the reasons of lower hospitalization rates is mixed. A recent survey of the literature concludes that HMOs do not achieve their lower admission rates as a result of eliminating unnecessary or discretionary procedures; surgical cases are not reduced by a greater proportion than medical cases (17). However, an earlier survey by Donabedian found a lower rate of hospitalization for so-called minor surgical procedures, such as tonsillectomies. In some comparisons, the rate of surgery for tonsillectomies in prepaid group practices (PPGPs) was one-half to one-third of the rate under fee-for-service coverage (18).

Out-of-pocket expense by both HMO enrollees and by those with fee-for-service coverage indicates the completeness of their insurance coverage as well as the utilization by HMO members of services purchased outside of the HMO. Use of outside services by HMO enrollees accounts for 7–14 percent of all of their services received. Rather than being viewed as dissatisfaction with the prepaid plan or as incomplete coverage, a study by Kaiser shows that 14 percent of their enrollees had duplicate coverage (19). Out-of-pocket expenses for HMO enrollees are on average lower than for those with comparable fee-for-service coverage. However, in spite of the lower hospitalization rates among these groups, the annual premium for PPGP is not lower than comparable coverage under fee-for-service; in fact, it is slightly higher. The lower out-of-pocket expenses for their members, however, results in a lower total (premium plus out-of-pocket) annual cost for enrollees in PPGPs (20).

The utilization of physician services is slightly greater among enrollees of prepaid plans. Physician visits per 1,000 enrolled population in the groups

---

*In a recent study, Blumberg attempted to determine whether differential use of health services by prepaid group plan (PGP) members and others was a result of differences in health status. His findings, based upon a sample of persons in California, were that the prepaid plans did not serve a healthier population group: "The percents of those with limitations on activity due to chronic conditions, and of those whose self-appraised health status was 'fair' or 'poor,' were slightly higher among PGP members than among those with other private coverage. The PGP population had somewhat more restricted-activity days and bed-disability days per person (due to both acute and chronic conditions) than those with other private coverage." Mark S. Blumberg, "Health Status and Health Care Use by Type of Private Health Coverage," *Milbank Memorial Fund Quarterly* (Fall 1980): 649.

TABLE 12-1. Comparison of Utilization and Cost Data Between Prepaid Group Practices and Fee-for-Service, Various Studies

Study	Physician Visits Per Year	Hospital Days Per 1,000 Population	Premium Paid Per Enrollee	Out-of-Pocket Expenses Per Enrollee	Total Annual Cost (Premium Plus Out-of-Pocket Expenses)
Michigan study, 1964					
PPGP	4.9	552	$284	$ 89	$373
FFS	4.7	1,155	256	194	450
PPGP/FFS	1.04	.48	1.11	.46	.83
California state employees (multiple choice option), 1970–1971					
PPGP	5.1	533	136	35	176
FFS	4.4	737	161	81	242
PPGP/FFS	1.16	.72	.84	.43	.73
Rochester, New York study, 1978					
PPGP	5.0	388	276	18	294
FFS	5.3	536	241	87	328
PPGP/FFS	.94	.72	1.14	.21	.90

Sources: Michigan study, 1964: Paul J. Feldstein, "Prepaid Group Practice: An Analysis and Review," Bureau of Hospital Administration, School of Public Health, the University of Michigan; California state employees, 1970–1971: Harold S. Luft, *Health Maintenance Organizations: Dimensions of Performance* (New York: John Wiley and Sons, 1981), p. 61, Table 4-1; p. 80, Table 5-1; p. 116, Table 6-1. The PPGP is serviced by Kaiser of Northern and Southern California and the FFS is serviced by Blue Cross/Blue Shield; Rochester, New York study, 1978: Andrew Sorensen et al., "Health Status, Medical Care Utilization, and Cost Experience of Prepaid Group Practice and Fee-for-Service Populations," *The Group Health Journal* 2 (Winter 1981). p.7, Table 7; p.8; p. 11, Table 13. Reprinted by permission of the Group Health Association of America, Inc., 624 9th Street, N.W., 7th Floor, Washington, D.C. 20001. The PPGP is serviced by the Genesee Valley Group Health Association and the FFS is serviced by Blue Cross–Blue Shield.

studied range from 3,880 to 5,190 in PPGPs and from 4,100 to 5,500 in fee-for-service. Kaiser enrollees generally have higher physician visit rates than do members of other PPGPs.

Based on admittedly rough comparisons between PPGPs and the fee-for-service setting, the PPGPs appear to be competitive with alternative delivery systems. Given a fair market test, presumably they would grow and prosper. A study by the Federal Trade Commission appears to lend support to this hypothesis. "An 18-month study by the FTC's bureau of economics found that the creation of health maintenance organizations introduced new awareness of costs on the part of nonparticipating doctors and hospitals. In some cases, doctors or hospitals organized similar groups of their own as a competitive response" (21).

Although relative performance data on PPGPs appear favorable, merely organizing new PPGPs will not necessarily result in comparable gains for the enrolled population. In the last several years, a number of new HMOs have experienced costs that were much higher than expected, particularly those plans sponsored by university medical schools. Before we use these recent experiences to forecast HMO performance and to conclude that they will require vast public subsidies if they are to survive as an alternate delivery system, we must determine whether recent HMO cost data are indicative of their performance. We must also isolate the elements of an HMO that lead to its lower utilization.

Differences in annual medical expenses per enrollee between an HMO and a fee-for-service setting may be a result of the following: differences in their output or products, such as quality or benefits provided; differences in demands for medical care, resulting in differences in per capita utilization rates; and, finally, differences in the per unit costs of providing services. To analyze the reasons for differences in per capita medical costs between the two delivery systems and to determine which system is lower in cost, it is necessary to hold various factors constant. Examples of differences in output between the two delivery systems are those that occur in quality of services (generally very difficult to measure), in the types of services covered by the two alternative systems, in the case mix of their patients, and in their administrative functions, such as marketing and claims processing, that may be performed by an HMO but which are performed by the insurance carrier and included in the premium under a fee-for-service system. To assess differences in the demands for care between the two systems, it is necessary to determine whether differences exist in subscriber population attitudes; for example, do persons who expect to use less care prefer an HMO setting? Patient time requirements may also differentiate the two systems. One system of delivery may require more travel time to fewer providers or greater waiting time than the other.

Per unit costs may vary between alternative delivery systems for several reasons. The per unit costs of hospital care (or any component) may be higher if only teaching hospitals are providing it. Some of the early university health plans suffered from this problem. Such plans subsequently started to use community hospitals to take advantage of the lower costs per day in those settings. Differences in the extent of economies of scale may also exist between the different settings. An HMO probably has to operate at a certain minimum size before it will achieve its lowest costs of operation. It would be misleading to brand a particular delivery system as too costly because it was operating at too small a volume. Finally, differences in operating costs between delivery systems could occur as a result of the quality of management. Unless certain delivery systems are inherently more inefficient, efficiency of operation should also be held constant when making comparisons.

Thus, in making cost comparisons between delivery systems, it is necessary to hold a number of factors constant. Alternatively, one could allow a fair market test to determine relative competitiveness. If one delivery system is more costly than another, we would expect its market share to decline. Since subscribers' tastes also differ, conducting a market test would provide a fairer indication of their choice than would imposing a single mandated system that was based upon inadequate comparative data (and possible faulty criteria).

Although the relative utilization and cost performance of HMOs appears favorable, the reasons for the difference in performance between HMOs and fee-for-service are still unclear. It would therefore be unfortunate to enact legislation restricting the types of institutional and organizational arrangements under which HMOs may develop. For example, many well-meaning persons believe that all physicians participating in HMOs should be salaried. The method of physician reimbursement, however, may turn out to be crucial to the performance of the HMO. Different methods of physician reimbursement provide different incentives: salaried physicians might provide more care per patient, but they have lower productivity when measured by the number of patients seen; physicians reimbursed on some type of sharing arrangement, perhaps in the form of a bonus, may have a greater incentive to reduce hospitalization of the enrollees or to use fewer tests. Previous studies on the comparative performance of HMOs did not control for differences in physician reimbursement. In most of the earlier studies of HMOs, the participating physicians had some financial stake in whatever funds were available at the end of the year (e.g., Kaiser and HIP). Physician interest in developing internal professional control mechanisms is likely to be related to whether physicians are affected, financially or otherwise, by their colleagues' behavior. The possible risks and rewards to the physicians in an HMO may well turn out to be one of the most important factors contributing to an HMO's favorable performance. Until we identify why HMOs favorably perform, it is unwise to restrict legislatively alternative organizational and institutional arrangements in HMOs.

BARRIERS TO THE DEVELOPMENT OF PREPAID HEALTH PLANS

The theoretical and empirical advantages of prepaid health plans would lead one to expect that such plans would have developed in the past and would command a major share of the medical services market. But unfortunately this has not occurred. Until recently, the population enrolled in such plans has represented a very minor portion of the total population with health insurance, and, although it has recently increased, it still represents a small fraction of the potential market. If the medical services market were competitive, a demand for such organizations would exist, particularly if prepaid health plans could provide medical care of a quality comparable to that of the fee-for-service system at lower costs. A favorable cost structure enabling HMOs to be competitive would undoubtedly lead to an increase in the supply of such plans. But since their expected growth has not occurred, we must examine our assumptions about the demand for such plans and possible explanations for the inadequate supply response.

DEMANDS FOR PREPAID HEALTH PLANS

One way to estimate the potential demand for prepaid health plans is to examine what percentage of the population decides to enroll when a prepaid plan is offered in competition with the traditional fee-for-service system.* Several prepaid plans, such as Kaiser, require that potential enrollees have a choice between their plan and an alternative, such as Blue Cross–Blue Shield. Based on studies where consumers have had this dual choice option, 20–60 percent of the subscribers usually chose the prepaid health plan (22). In general, a minority of subscribers choose the prepaid plan, and they do so for a variety of reasons. The advantages of HMOs, as seen by subscribers, are their broad coverage, lower expected costs of utilization, and assured access to care. The major disadvantages of HMOs are the following: first, limitations on the choice of physician; the consumer often desires to retain the current relationship with his or her physician.

> The evidence so far appears to indicate that closed-panel HMOs are most likely to attract enrollees who do not have established patient–physician relationships, and who tend to be members of younger families with a larger number of smaller children. These characteristics are often found in areas with high population mobility. Individuals and families new to a community have not had the opportunity to establish a private patient–physician relationship and they also tend to be younger. The closed-panel HMO offers them assured access without their having to search for sources of routine care in a new and unfamiliar community. Having the option available through the workplace, and having the ability to gain at least some information about the delivery characteristics of the HMO, reduce the burden of searching for sources of care. The open-panel HMO, on the other hand, appears to be most appealing to those who already know the physicians within it and who can enroll and simultaneously maintain an already existing patient–physician relationship.(23)

The second disadvantage of HMOs are that there may be an insufficient supply of the HMO's facilities and physicians in the consumers' area. Third, the prospective subscriber may have insufficient knowledge of how the prepaid plan works. The importance of information on prepaid plans in the selection process is strongly indicated by the relatively high degree of satisfaction among consumers who have joined such plans and by the fact that those consumers have generally remained with those plans. Although it is possible that the type of consumer

---

*It is inappropriate to use present HMO enrollment percentages in the population as an indication of future HMO growth. Currently, large sections of the country do not have access to HMOs. Also large population groups do not have an HMO choice even when it is available; for example, Medicare and Medicaid beneficiaries. In addition, employees in low-wage industries have insufficient employment-related fringe benefits to purchase the more comprehensive health care coverage offered by many HMOs.

who joins prepaid plans is different from the type who does not, which could explain the high degree of satisfaction and the low degree of turnover, a more likely explanation is that a minority of consumers select such plans because they are inadequately informed about the function and performance of prepaid plans.

Based on the percentage of consumers who choose to enroll in prepaid health plans when offered a dual choice, we would expect that the percentage of the population at large demanding prepaid plans would greatly exceed those presently enrolled in such plans. To determine why the growth in such plans has not kept up with the potential demand for them, it is necessary to examine the supply side of this market.

SUPPLY FACTORS AFFECTING THE GROWTH OF PREPAID HEALTH PLANS

One supply factor that would affect the growth of HMOs would be their efficiency relative to alternative delivery systems. A comparison of HMO costs and their capitation premiums with the annual expenditures for medical care in the traditional fee-for-service system indicates that HMOs could compete effectively on a price basis with fee-for-service medicine. The reasons for the very slow growth of HMOs, therefore, must be found in nonmarket barriers that have inhibited their development. The first such barriers were the attempts by state medical associations to deny participating physicians hospital privileges, thereby denying prepaid health plans access to hospitals (24). If a prepaid health plan could not provide its potential subscribers with hospital care when needed, then the plan could not effectively compete with fee-for-service physicians in the community. According to Rueben Kessel, prepaid health plans represented a lower-priced substitute to the fee-for-service physicians because the premium was the same for all persons regardless of their income. Since fee-for-service physicians attempt to price-discriminate according to a patient's income, a plan which charges all patients the same premium is a form of price cutting. In the past, state and county medical associations successfully prevented the growth of many prepaid health plans by revoking the membership of, or refusing to grant membership to, physicians who desired to join them; such memberships had been prerequisites for hospital privileges. Therefore, in order to survive, a prepaid health plan such as Kaiser had to have its own hospitals. Although various medical societies subsequently lost antitrust suits, their actions raised the cost to potential prepaid health plans enough to prevent their large-scale development.

As part of their successful efforts to prevent the growth of prepaid health plans, state medical societies were able to have legislation passed at a state level that placed additional barriers on prepaid health plan development and on their ability to compete with fee-for-service practice.* Restrictive legislation sub-

---

*An examination of the determinants of HMO growth found, "It appears that the developers of the first HMO in a community must focus on the opposition of the established medical community . . . opposition by established physicians decreases the probability that an HMO will be established. . . . Once an HMO has been established, however, the growth of the industry depends on the tastes and preferences of the community." Michael A. Morrisey and Cynthia S. Ashby, "An Empirical Analysis of HMO Market Share," *Inquiry* (Summer 1982): 6.

jected HMOs to strict regulation by the state department of insurance, required physicians to be a majority of the controlling board of an HMO, required HMOs to permit the participation of any physician in the community, required HMOs to be organized on a nonprofit basis, and prohibited HMOs from advertising their benefits and premiums.

Prohibiting an HMO from advertising erects a major barrier to its growth. As discussed above, consumer ignorance of HMOs is probably an important reason why potential subscribers do not join them. HMOs are subject to greater economies of scale than solo practitioners. An HMO must have certain minimum facilities, an organization to enroll members, and possibly its own hospital. Unless an HMO is able to enroll a sufficient number of subscribers, it will be forced to operate at relatively higher premiums, i.e., the declining portion of its long-run average-cost curve. If an HMO were prevented from advertising, it would take longer to reach the number of enrollees required to make its premium competitive with the fee-for-service sector. The time and losses required were too great an obstacle for many HMOs. Restricting the HMO to nonprofit status further removed any incentives that might have existed for nonphysicians to risk their talents and capital to start an HMO.

FEDERAL AND STATE INITIATIVES AFFECTING THE GROWTH OF HMOS

As a result of the aforementioned anticompetitive behavior by local medical societies, the growth of HMOs was largely inhibited. In the early 1970s, the term HMO was coined and President Nixon used the HMO concept as a major federal approach to restructuring the delivery of medical services. Federal policy during this period provided modest support for the development of HMOs and legitimized their existence (25). The growth in the number of HMOs was rapid during this period, increasing almost sevenfold, from 37 in 1969 to 243 in 1981 (26). Although, at approximately 10.3 million persons, the number of subscribers still remained small, HMOs grew in those areas where favorable market conditions such as higher incomes and greater insurance coverage existed.

During 1973 and 1974 a great deal of HMO legislation was passed at a state level; federal legislation was also enacted during this period. Ideally, the legislation should have removed any barriers that prevented HMOs from competing with their fee-for-service competitors, without providing either with any competitive advantages. Unfortunately, while the early legislation did remove some barriers, it imposed greater requirements on HMOs, thereby decreasing their ability to compete. Some legislators may have preferred to allow HMOs to compete with fee-for-service medicine; others, and the interests they represented, wanted to prevent a fair market test of their ability to compete; while still other legislators viewed HMOs as a vehicle for achieving social changes. No matter what the legislative motivation, requirements were placed on HMOs that increased their costs relative to fee-for-service medicine.

The favorable aspects of the HMO legislation exempted federally qualified HMOs from restrictive state laws, allowed the HMOs to advertise their benefits and rates, and provided for a dual-choice option. When a federally qualified HMO was available, employers were required to offer an HMO option to their employees along with the traditional health insurance coverage. To take advantage of these favorable factors, however, federally qualified HMOs had to adopt requirements that would have placed them at a competitive disadvantage. These included: 1) a relatively large financial requirement; 2) placing HMOs under certificate-of-need (CON) laws;* 3) reimbursing HMOs either on a cost basis (thereby removing the financial incentives for HMOs to compete with fee-for-service medicine on the basis of price) or on a fixed-price basis with perverse incentives, e.g., in Oregon an HMO had to absorb all losses, while retaining none of its savings; 4) mandating a very costly benefit package (thereby increasing their premiums relative to the more usual health insurance premiums offered); 5) placing HMOs under permanent regulation by the Secretary of Health, Education and Welfare; 6) requiring open enrollment (persons joining HMOs during the open enrollment periods incur 80 percent greater costs (27); and requiring community rating as the basis for establishing premiums.

Based on their premiums relative to those of traditional insurers, HMOs could compete effectively with the fee-for-service system. However, the requirements necessary to become a federally qualified HMO imposed greater burdens on them than those placed on their competitors. To enable fair competition to exist between HMOs and other delivery systems, they should both face the same rules. Instead, HMOs were forced to compete while carrying a burden of mandated costs higher than that of their competitors.

In more recent years, some of the more stringent requirements imposed on HMOs were loosened. For example, in 1976 Congress relaxed the HMO benefits and eligibility requirements mandated by the 1973 HMO Act. This followed complaints from HMOs that these requirements increased their premiums so they could not be competitive with regular health insurance plans. Also, as part of the 1979 Health Planning Act, large HMOs (enrollment greater than 50,000 persons) were exempted from the CON process. Rather than this being procompetitive legislation for all HMOs, however, the main beneficiaries were the already established traditional HMOs, such as Kaiser, Health Insurance Plan of New York, and Group Health Association of Puget Sound.

EMPIRICAL EVIDENCE ON THE IMPACT OF HMO COMPETITION

Earlier, the theoretical advantages of prepaid health plans were enumerated. Also, comparisons between prepaid plans and fee-for-service coverage showed that the prepaid plans compare favorably with respect to their premiums, total enrollee costs, utilization of their members, and enrollee satisfaction. What has not yet been demonstrated is the competitive effect on fee-for-service providers and insurers. For market competition to have desirable consequences, fee-for-service providers and insurers should respond to HMO competition by attempting to minimize their enrollees' health care costs and to increase consumer satisfaction. Thus, in addition to benefiting their own enrollees, HMOs, through their competition, should benefit all consumers in the area.

---

*According to an interstudy survey conducted in 1973, 48 percent of the responding HMOs said that such CON laws represented moderate or severe barriers to their growth. Richard McNeil and Robert Schlenker, "HMOs, Competition, and Government," *Interstudy*, December 1974, p. 20.

Evidence on competition between prepaid plans and fee-for-service providers and insurers is very limited. However, the available results are consistent with what one would expect under market competition.

Blue Cross and commercial insurance companies compete among themselves and with HMOs on the basis of their premiums, benefit packages, access to consumers, and so forth. Neither the Blues nor the commercials have, until recently, tried to lower their input costs in trying to hold down their premiums. HMOs, however, attempt to decrease their input costs, namely, the hospitalization rates of their enrollees. By reducing hospitalization, HMOs are able to offer a more comprehensive set of benefits at comparable premiums (or similar benefits at a lower premium). Competition between HMOs and Blue Cross would therefore be expected to result in pressure on Blue Cross to also reduce the hospitalization rates of its subscribers. The pressure on Blue Cross to respond to the competitive threat of the HMO is expected to be greater in those situations where the HMO has a larger market share.

Using state data for 1974, Goldberg and Greenberg undertook a multiple regression analysis of Blue Cross's response to HMO competition. Their findings were consistent with the above expectations. In those states where HMO's had high market shares, Blue Cross responded by reducing hospital utilization. The authors concluded that competitive forces work, at least with regard to HMOs and Blue Cross (28).

Another study that provides evidence on the practicality of market competition was the analysis by Christianson and McClure on the competitive response to HMO growth in the Minneapolis–St. Paul area (29). Between 1971 and 1978 HMO enrollment grew at an average annual rate of 27 percent, to where it consisted of 12.4 percent of the population in the Twin Cities metropolitan area. Since overall population growth increased very slowly over this period, the increase in HMO enrollment occurred at the expense of the traditional insurers. What was of particular interest in the Twin Cities area is that there were multiple HMOs competing with the traditional insurers. Often when there is just one HMO in an area, the HMO can increase its enrollment by pegging its premium increases to those of the traditional insurer. With multiple HMOs in an area, however, they were forced into price competition with each other. Also, serving to stimulate competition is the practice of companies in the Twin Cities area of offering their employees a choice of more than one HMO in addition to traditional insurance plans. In addition, the authors report most employers contribute a fixed dollar amount to whichever health plan the employee selects. If the employee selects a plan with a higher premium, the employee must pay the difference.

Two HMOs, both sponsored by different county medical societies, were formed partially in response to the growth of the five existing HMOs. One of these HMOs, an Independent Practice Association (IPA), ran a deficit for its first 2 years of operation. To survive and to be able to offer competitive premiums, tight controls were instituted over its physician members. As a result of such controls on admissions and length of stay, the plan was able to achieve large reductions in its hospitalization rate. The willingness of participating physicians in these plans to accept restrictions on their behavior and to change their style of medical practice was a direct consequence of competitive pressures.

Other health care providers also adapted to the new competitive environment. Hospitals offered discounted prices to HMOs to attract their patients.

Traditional providers and insurers, when faced with a threat to their market shares, responded. They started their own HMOs, reduced hospitalization rates of their subscribers, and, together with the other HMOs, competed on the basis of premiums, access to their facilities, and increased benefit coverage.

In addition to the above two studies, there have been additional examples of the competitive impact of HMOs. California has had substantial HMO growth and, similarly, large declines in hospitalization. In Rochester, New York the local Blue Cross–Blue Shield plan has been engaged in competition with several HMOs. Hospital utilization has also sharply declined. In Hawaii, Kaiser competes with another prepaid plan (an IPA) as well as with traditional insurers. Again, there are low hospital utilization rates (30).

In each of these locations, as well as the earlier study of the Twin Cities, there are unique environmental aspects that may also explain why hospitalization has declined. The statistical analysis by Goldberg and Greenberg can also be faulted (31). Thus until more evidence is available, these findings should be considered preliminary. The responses by traditional insurers to HMO growth, however, are consistent with the predictions of a competitive model. There is increased price (premium) competition, as well as competition along other dimensions: access to facilities, benefit coverage, and consumer satisfaction. Health care providers, when faced with competitive pressures, have shown a willingness to accept restrictions on their behavior and change their style of practice. Hospitals also are willing to compete for HMO business. To stimulate such competition, it appears desirable for the following ingredients to exist: competition among several HMOs in an area; employers who offer multiple choices to their employees; and employees who are required to pay any premium differentials between the health plan they select and their employer's fixed contribution.*

MOVING TOWARD A COMPETITIVE MARKET IN MEDICAL CARE

A number of changes should be made in the legislation affecting HMOs to enable them to compete on an equal basis with the fee-for-service system. HMOs should not have to provide a more extensive benefit package than that being offered by commercial and Blue Cross–Blue Shield insurance companies. In fact, the HMOs should not be subject to regulations any different from those guiding the fee-for-service system and their insurance carriers. HMOs' premiums should not be artificially increased, thereby placing them at a competitive disadvantage. The favorable aspects of the federal HMO legislation should be extended to encompass all HMOs; these beneficial provisions include preempt-

---

*There are two recent publications dealing with competition in the health field the reader should find useful: Kathryn M. Langwell and Sylvia F. Moore, *A Synthesis of Research on Competition in the Financing and Delivery of Health Services*; and Louis F. Rossiter, ed., *Research on Competition in the Financing and Delivery of Health Services: Future Research Needs*, Proceedings of a Conference. Both documents are published by U.S. Department of Health and Human Services, National Center for Health Services Research, Rockville, Md., 1982.

ing state laws that may adversely affect their development, mandating that dual choice be available to all employees, and allowing HMOs to freely advertise. To assure that consumers will be protected from incompetent and unethical providers, a federal quality assurance program should be developed that would monitor the quality of care in all delivery systems, not just that of HMOs. Further, the measures of quality that are developed should emphasize the outcome of treatment, not just the process.

Legislation to control increases in hospital costs is likely to be enacted in the very near future. It is essential that no proposals for reforming hospital reimbursement be adopted that would inhibit innovations in the delivery of medical services. The long-run goal of efficiency in the provision of medical care should not be disregarded in the pursuit of the short-run goal of containing hospital costs. Any rate regulation proposal should allow, and in fact encourage, the development of HMOs. For example, if hospital costs are to be contained by imposing percentage limits on the increase in total hospital revenues from one year to the next, then hospitals that are a part of, or that initiate, HMOs should be excluded from such regulation. (This assumes that HMO involvement consists of a major portion of the hospitals' utilization.) Natural competitive forces should prevent an HMO from raising its premium by too great an amount relative to insurance premiums for fee-for-service medicine.

MAINTAINING A COMPETITIVE FRAMEWORK

The concept of market competition as the basic approach for organizing economic activity in our economy was accepted quite some time ago. This concept, however, has only recently been applied to the health field. Self-regulation by the health professions has, until recently, not only been the norm but also the preferred approach of the professions.

Certain rules of the game must be established and all the participants should abide by these rules if competition is to achieve its desired outcomes. The participants' behavior in the market must be monitored to ensure that they do not violate the rules. Monitoring behavior and intervening when necessary is the role of antitrust activity. Competitors attempt to violate the rules of the marketplace so as to enhance their market position. If health care providers, such as physicians, dentists, and hospitals, or third-party payors can develop a monopoly position through illegal activities, they can increase their revenues. The public is harmed by such activities because they pay higher prices for the services they purchase.

Examples of anticompetitive behavior, all of which have taken place in the health field, are: barriers to entry, economic boycotts, price fixing, and restrictions on truthful advertising and information.* Recent examples of the above

---

*Anticompetitive behavior is illegal on either per se grounds or by virtue of the rule of reason. Per se violations, such as price fixing and economic boycotts, are believed to be obviously anticompetitive and their effects are clearly harmful to consumers. Other forms of competitive behavior are analyzed according to the rule of reason, which attempts to determine the effects of the actions so as to judge whether they are harmful.

types of anticompetitive behavior are: the FTC claimed that the American Medical Association's (AMA) restrictions on advertising and solicitation as stated in its codes of ethics was an unreasonable restraint of trade (32). The U.S. Court of Appeals and the Supreme Court (in 1982) upheld the FTC. The Michigan State Medical Society, which threatened to organize a boycott of Blue Shield if Blue Shield did not change its reimbursement policies, was found to have violated the antitrust laws. The Supreme Court ruled that the setting of maximum prices by the Maricopa Medical Society was illegal. Physicians associated with HMOs were denied hospital appointments by the Forbes Health System Medical Staff as a means of lessening competition.

Not all types of self-regulation by the professions are anticompetitive. Activities by the professional associations that provide increased information on the quality and characteristics of health care providers, such as specialty certification, do not limit either entry or choice of provider. Such actions may improve market performance by providing the consumer with more information. In the past, however, professional regulation resulted in limits on entry and choice of provider, as well as the other forms of anticompetitive behavior listed above.

The application of antitrust laws to the health field is disturbing to many, for reasons of both economic self-interest as well as ideology. Some people have a basic distrust of market forces and of the ability of individuals to cope in such situations. Others fear that their incomes and preferred positions will be competed away. The medical profession has decided not to acquiesce in the Supreme Court's ruling that acknowledged the FTC's jurisdiction over the health professions. As part of its defense in the case brought by the FTC on advertising, the AMA claimed that it is a nonprofit organization and that the FTC only has jurisdiction over organizations and their members that are in business to earn a profit. The FTC Commissioners, U.S. Court of Appeals, and subsequently the Supreme Court upheld the FTC's claim that the AMA, to a significant degree, does operate for the economic benefit of its members. As a result of this ruling, the AMA, the American Dental Association, and other professional associations are lobbying the Congress to pass a law stating that state-regulated professions are exempt from FTC jurisdiction. If successful, the AMA then will attempt to have Congress pass another bill exempting it from the Sherman antitrust laws, which would preclude Justice Department scrutiny of its behavior. Such a legislative success would turn the clock back. No longer would anticompetitive behavior as described above be considered illegal.

Because of their desired outcomes, our society has decided to rely on competitive markets. The maintenance of competitive markets is a proper role of government. In the health field, however, enforcement of the antitrust law is not the only prerequisite for fair competition. As public policy on prepaid health plans is developed, the principles of fair competition should be kept in mind. Particular delivery systems should not be provided with disadvantages or advantages over other health delivery systems. In this regard, the following rules have been suggested to enhance market competition between prepaid plans and traditional insurers and providers.

1. Multiple-choice. Employers should offer their employees a choice of insurance plans. If there are several HMO-type plans in an area then each of those plans, in addition to the traditional health insurers, should have an opportu-

nity to compete for the employee's choice. Restricting the employee's choice to only one plan of each type foregoes the opportunity to have competition between plans of a similar type. To do so would be equivalent to franchising the HMO for the area.

2. Equal employer contributions. It would be desirable if employers contributed equal dollar amounts to whichever plan the employee selects. For price competition to exist between plans, the employee must have an incentive to weigh the benefits of increased coverage against the higher costs of that coverage. If employers merely pay for whichever plan the employee chooses, then the employee's incentive is to select the higher-cost plan. It has been suggested that placing a limit on the amount of the employer contribution that is tax free would provide employees with an incentive to be cost conscious in their choice of health plans. (A tax limit is discussed more completely in Chapter 20 on National Health Insurance.)

3. Design of insurance benefits. If an employee opted for a plan that just offered shallow first-dollar coverage, then a catastrophic illness might exhaust the employee's financial resources and require the state to bear that cost. For this reason, each of the insurance plans should offer, at a minimum, catastrophic coverage. Whether or not the insurance plans should be able to compete on benefit coverage as well as on premiums is controversial. Permitting consumer choice with regard to benefit coverage appears preferable to mandating a single set of benefits for all. Many persons might prefer less comprehensive plans, at lower premiums. For those with lower incomes who are less able to bear out-of-pocket costs, more comprehensive benefits, subsidized by the government, would be desirable.

A MEDICARE VOUCHER

Changes in provider reimbursement under Medicare could provide HMOs with an equal opportunity to serve Medicare patients while also serving as an incentive for HMOs to develop and grow.

An HMO should be permitted to provide services to Medicare patients for a premium that is not based on the HMO's costs. This idea, embodied in several legislative proposals, is referred to as a Medicare voucher. A Medicare voucher would serve two purposes. First, it would limit the federal government's contributions under Medicare to a fixed dollar amount per beneficiary per year, thereby making the government's outlays predictable and controllable. The risk of higher than expected Medicare expenditures would be transferred from the government to private organizations. Second, a voucher system would be a procompetitive strategy in that it would serve to stimulate HMO enrollment. Payment for prepaid health care would become available for a large population group. Currently, Medicare reimburses HMOs on a fee-for-service basis. Therefore an HMO does not share in any savings due to its lower use rate; any savings accrue to Medicare.

Proposals for a voucher system suggest that it should be voluntary for current Medicare enrollees but that it should become compulsory for those newly eligible for Medicare. Once a certain fraction of the Medicare population, such as 50 percent, is part of the voucher system, then the voucher system should become compulsory for all Medicare beneficiaries.

A Medicare voucher would work as follows: the federal government would contribute 95 percent of the value of the voucher, thereby saving 5 percent, by basing the voucher on the average per capita cost for a Medicare beneficiary in a geographic area. This average area per capita cost (AAPC) would be adjusted for age, sex, and health status. The voucher would then be applied toward the purchase of an approved health plan. If the premium is greater than the value of the voucher, then the beneficiary must pay the difference; if it is less, the beneficiary either receives a refund or is provided with additional benefit coverage. The value of the voucher would be increased yearly by an inflation factor.

Some conceptual problems have been raised with the concept of a voluntary or optional voucher (33). The most difficult of these concerns is the issue of adverse selection. It has been estimated that 9 percent of the aged incur 70 percent of the program's expenditures, a large portion of which are spent on services to people who will die within 1 year. Persons who are ill or who have chronic conditions are generally reluctant to leave their physician and switch to an HMO. Under such circumstances the HMO will enroll those aged who are healthier and have lower expenditures. If the HMO receives the average area per capita cost for a Medicare beneficiary, then a voluntary voucher system could end up costing the federal government more money. The government would continue paying for the high-cost aged while HMOs would enroll those with lower average costs. Approaches to resolving this problem, such as adjusting the voucher amount according to health status, are being considered. If the voucher system were mandatory for all aged persons, then this type of adverse selection problem would not cause government outlays to increase. However, a different type of adverse selection problem might still occur. If qualified health plans offered different types of benefit packages to the aged, those who are healthier might choose the less comprehensive plans and thereby receive a large refund. Those expecting to use more services would select the more comprehensive plans. As this phenomenon occurs and as persons switch plans according to their expected use, the premium differential for plans with different degrees of coverage will increase. It is not clear how severe such a problem would be, but again there are methods that could be used to control switching among plans; an extra premium could be charged when a person first enrolls in a comprehensive plan.

Several experiments, using a Medicare voucher, are being undertaken in different parts of the country. As yet, it is too early to judge the receptiveness of the aged and the utilization and cost experience of the participating HMOs.

HOW MUCH SUPPORT IS THERE FOR COMPETITIVE HEALTH PLANS?

It is one thing to propose a market solution; it is another, much more difficult thing to achieve it. There are powerful interest groups that are opposed to organizing the delivery of health services along competitive lines (34). Organized medicine, as discussed previously and more completely in later chapters, believes that its members would be made worse off under competition. HMOs would threaten the practice of fee-for-service physicians, as occurred in the Twin

Cities area. Physicians would have to accept changes in their style of practice and restrictions on their behavior, if they are to survive in such an environment. The growth of prepaid health plans should result in a decreased demand for hospital care—up to 50 percent less. Although some multiinstitutional hospital systems could adapt to a new competitive environment, many hospitals would prefer the security of a regulatory system. Thus another important interest group, hospitals, is unlikely to support such a proposal, if not actually oppose it. Commercial health insurers already believe that there is too much competition among insurers, and have opposed the concept. They are unsure what their future role will be in a system of competing prepaid health plans. The insurance companies would instead prefer some form of hospital rate regulation so that cost shifting and the Blue Cross discount no longer place them at a competitive disadvantage. Hospitals receive greater payments from patients with commercial insurance than from patients with Medicare or Medicaid coverage. In many places, Blue Cross also pays lower prices than the commercial insurers. Tight controls on hospital expenditures and investments, and similar charges regardless of payor class, the commercial insurers believe, would enable them to compete with Blue Cross more fairly on their premiums. So as not to be left behind, however, commercials have started and are experimenting with prepaid health delivery systems.

Blue Cross is another special-interest group that is reluctant to favor changes in the current system of delivery, particularly those Blue Cross plans with high market shares and good provider relations. Although they have also opposed the competition concept, the Blues, like the commercials, have started a number of prepaid health plans.

Business groups, which might be expected to favor competition in general, have been at most lukewarm supporters of competition in health care. Offering multiple choices of health plans to their employees is likely to increase their administrative costs. Many companies believe they currently have preferred-risk groups. Under some competition proposals businesses would have to drop their own self-insurance plans; they fear the premiums they pay on behalf of their employees will increase if their employees join plans that include different risk groups.

Unions are one of the most vocal groups opposing a competitive delivery system. Although unions have been strong supporters of prepaid group practice, those same unions have a basic distrust of competitive markets. They would prefer prepaid health plans to be not-for-profit and that government, rather than markets, be the regulator of provider and insurer performance. There is another important reason why unions oppose a competitive market in health care. Large unions generally have comprehensive health insurance benefits. If a tax limit on health benefits were instituted, the workers in these unions would be worse off. They would no longer receive as much health insurance as they did before; further, their coverage would likely include deductibles and copayments, which have been opposed by unions.

The beneficiaries of a competitive market, as described above, are consumers. Their interests in this legislation are, however, diffuse; they do not see the potential benefits as being great enough to warrant involvement in the political process. The current administration has spoken favorably about introducing competitive market forces into health care. Whether it will do so, and in what manner, remains to be seen. The political future of competitive health proposals is very uncertain.

The market approach to the delivery of medical services has not been tried in recent medical history. The fee-for-service system, which has been the predominant form of delivery of medical services, is not a laissez-faire approach to the market. Fee-for-service practice has been highly regulated by the professions, while market competition was severely restricted. Thus, it cannot be maintained that a system of market competition has been tried and found to be unacceptable. Although there are bound to be problems in the delivery of medical services under any delivery system, people with an anticompetitive bias are too often willing to use their objections to a market system to justify adopting a regulated system. When inequities and inefficiencies are discovered in a regulated system, they are merely used by these same persons to justify even greater regulation. It is very difficult to deregulate an industry. It would, therefore, seem more sensible to attempt a nonregulatory approach before permanently embracing regulation.

This chapter has indicated the benefits of moving toward market competition as a means of improving the allocation of resources in medical care. It should be emphasized again that neither a market approach nor regulation alone will solve all of the concerns that people have with regard to medical care. Redistributing medical services requires government intervention; however, government involvement need not be direct. Government subsidies provided through a market mechanism can more efficiently achieve social objectives concerning redistribution than can a system that relies on regulation and bureaucratic control to make those allocation decisions.

REFERENCES

1. Paul M. Ellwood and Walter McClure, "Health Delivery Reform," *Interstudy* Memorandum dated November 17, 1976.

2. For a more complete discussion of this idea, see: Kenneth Warner, "Health Maintenance Insurance: Toward an Optimal HMO," *Policy Sciences* 10 (December 1978).

3. For a comprehensive review of the advertising literature, see William S. Comanor and Thomas A. Wilson, "Advertising and Competition: A Survey," *Journal of Economic Literature* (June 1979).

4. George Stigler, "The Economics of Information," *Journal of Political Economy* 69 (3) (June 1961).

5. Lee Benham and Alexandra Benham, "Regulating Through the Professions: A Perspective on Information Control," *The Journal of Law and Economics*, October 1975.

6. *Ibid.*, pp. 433, 435.

7. Lee Benham, "The Effects of Advertising on the Price of Eyeglasses," *Journal of Law and Economics* 15 (October 1972).

8. Benham and Benham, "Regulating Through the Professions," p. 438.

9. Statement of the National Retired Teachers' Association and the American Association of Retired Persons on the Economics of the Eyeglasses Industry Before the Monopoly Subcommittee of the Senate Small Business Committee, U.S. Senate, May 24, 1977.

Cited in Lee Benham, "Guilds and the Form of Competition in the Health Care Sector," in Warren Greenberg, ed., *Competition in the Health Care Sector* (Germantown, Md.: Aspen Systems Corp., 1978).

10. Donald Bond, John Kwoka, John Phelan, and Ira Whitten, *Staff Report on Effects of Restrictions on Advertising and Commercial Practice in the Professions: The Case of Optometry* (Washington, D.C.: Federal Trade Commission, Bureau of Economics, 1980). In another study on the effect of advertising restrictions on the price of optometric examinations, the authors found that "price is 16 percent higher in states that ban both optometric and optician price advertising, when examination length, procedures, and office equipment are held consistent." Roger Feldman and James Begun, "The Effects of Advertising: Lessons From Optometry," *The Journal of Human Resources* (Supplement 1978): 247.

11. Various parts of this and the first section were based upon an earlier proposal by the author to permit competition among organizations for the Medicare population based on a capitation payment for their annual medical expenses. See Paul J. Feldstein, "A Proposal for Capitation Reimbursement to Medical Groups for Total Medical Care," in *Reimbursement Incentives for Hospital and Medical Care: Objectives and Alternatives*, U.S. Department of Health, Education and Welfare, Social Security Administration Office of Research and Statistics, Research Report No. 26, 1968.

12. For an excellent conceptualization of the issues as well as a review of the literature on quality, see: Avedis Donabedian, *The Definition of Quality and Approaches to its Assessment*, Vol. I (Ann Arbor, Mich.: Health Administration Press, 1980).

13. M. Roemer and W. Schonick, "HMO Performance: The Recent Evidence," *Milbank Memorial Fund Quarterly* 51 (1973).

14. For a more complete discussion of the idea of institutional licensure, see: N. Hershey, "The Inhibiting Effect Upon Innovation of the Prevailing Licensure System," *Annals of the New York Academy of Sciences* 166 (1969): 951–959.

15. Harold S. Luft, "Assessing the Evidence on HMO Performance," *Milbank Memorial Fund Quarterly* (Fall 1980): 508.

16. *Ibid.*, 511.

17. *Ibid.*, 512.

18. Avedis Donabedian, "An Evaluation of Prepaid Group Practice," *Inquiry* (September 1969): 12.

19. H. Luft, *op. cit.*, p. 519.

20. Similar findings are also reported in a more recent review of HMO performance. See Harold S. Luft, "How Do Health Maintenance Organizations Achieve Their 'Savings'?" *The New England Journal of Medicine*, June 15, 1978, pp. 1336–1343.

21. "Competition Hailed on Health-Care Cost," *New York Times*, August 6, 1977, p. 10.

22. Donabedian, "An Evaluation of Prepaid Group Practice."

23. S.E. Berki and Marie L.F. Ashcraft, "HMO Enrollment: Who Joins What and Why: A Review of the Literature," *Milbank Memorial Fund Quarterly* (Fall 1980).

24. See Reuben Kessel, "Price Discrimination in Medicine," *Journal of Law and Economics*, October 1958. This article is discussed more completely in Chapter 14.

25. The discussion in this section is based on the paper by Richard McNeil and Robert Schlenker, "HMOs, Competition, and Government," *Interstudy*, December 1974. For background on the legislative aspects of the HMO Act and its various amendments, see: The *Congressional Quarterly Almanac*, various years. For a detailed discussion on the early HMO legislation, see: Joseph Falkson, *HMOs and the Politics of Health System Reform* (Chicago: American Hospital Association, 1980).

26. *HMO Industry Report Series*, 4 vols. Vol. 1: Maureen Stadle, *HMO Growth 1980–81* (Excelsior, Minn.: Interstudy, 1982), p. 1.

27. Walter McClure, "A Critique of the Health Maintenance Act of 1973," *Interstudy*, February 1974.

28. Lawrence Goldberg and Warren Greenberg, "The Competitive Response of Blue Cross to the Health Maintenance Organization," *Economic Inquiry* (June 1980).

29. Jon B. Christianson and Walter McClure, "Competition in the Delivery of Medical Care," *New England Journal of Medicine*, October 11, 1979.

30. Jon B. Christianson, *Do HMO's Stimulate Beneficial Competition?* (Excelsior, Minn.: Interstudy, 1978).

31. H. Luft, "Assessing the Evidence on HMO Performance," *op. cit.*, p. 525.

32. For a more complete discussion of these issues see: L. Barry Costilo, "Competition Policy and the Medical Profession," *New England Journal of Medicine*, April 30, 1981; Michael R. Pollard, "The Essential Role of Antitrust in a Competitive Market for Health Services," *Milbank Memorial Fund Quarterly* (Spring 1981); and Clark Havighurst, "Anti Trust Enforcement in the Medical Services Industry—What Does It All Mean," *Milbank Memorial Fund Quarterly* (Winter, 1980).

33. For a more complete discussion of this issue, see: Paul B. Ginsburg, "Medicare Vouchers and the Procompetitive Strategy," *Health Affairs* (Winter, 1981).

34. For a more complete discussion of these issues, see: "Tax Incentives: Competition, Round Two," *Medicine and Health Perspectives*, October 12, 1981; Donald W. Moran, "HMOs, Competition, and the Politics of Minimum Benefits," *Milbank Memorial Fund Quarterly* (Spring 1981); Alain C. Enthoven, "How Interested Groups Have Responded to a Proposal for Economic Competition in Health Services," *American Economic Review* (May 1980); and John K. Iglehart, "Drawing the Lines for the Debate on Competition," *New England Journal of Medicine*, July 30, 1981.

CHAPTER 13

Health Manpower Shortages: Definitions, Measurement, and Policies

Within the context of the overall market for medical care, the various categories of health manpower comprise separate submarkets. The health manpower professions are thus an *input* into the provision of medical services. In Chapter 3, "An Overview of the Medical Care Sector," it was shown that the overall market for medical care consists of a set of institutional markets, a set of health manpower markets, and a set of markets in which the demand and supply of health manpower education occurs. With a change in the demand for medical care, perhaps resulting from an increase in the population with insurance coverage, there will be increases in the demand for the institutional settings in which medical care is provided, and, subsequently, an increase in demand by the different institutional settings for inputs used in the production of their services. The demand for the different health manpower professions is, therefore, a *derived* demand, derived from the demand for medical and institutional services. These demands by the various institutions for different types of health manpower, together with the existing stock of trained health manpower, will determine the wages, the number of persons employed, and their participation rate (what percent of the available stock of each health manpower profession is employed). The health education institutions determine the long-run supply or stock of health manpower in each profession.

How well the different health manpower and education markets perform has an effect not only on the wages and number of health professionals, but also on the price and quantity of medical and institutional services. Since the various submarkets are interrelated and feed into the market for medical services, the efficiency with which the health manpower market performs will affect prices and outputs in each of the other markets; the more efficient a market is, the greater its output will be. Thus an important reason for examining the separate health manpower markets for the different categories of health professionals is to determine how well each market performs. If the markets are determined not to perform well, then we will want to examine alternative approaches for improving their performance, giving due consideration to the reasons for inadequate performance.

The market for health professional *education* will also be examined to determine whether it is performing efficiently—that is, whether the quantity of health professional education is "optimal" for different time periods and whether health education is being produced efficiently. The market for health professional education is important not only because it determines the long-run supply of health manpower, but also because it has been the recipient of a great deal of federal and state funding. Where federal and state health manpower legislation exists in any of the separate health manpower and health education markets, it will be analyzed to determine both its purpose and how effective it has been in achieving its stated goals.

Besides analyzing the efficiency of the separate health manpower markets, the performance of the markets for health professional education, and public policies in these areas, primarily governmental funding policies, we shall examine alternative approaches for forecasting health manpower "requirements." Because forecasts of health manpower have served as the basis for much of the federal and state legislation dealing with health manpower, we shall examine and evaluate the usefulness of different forecasting approaches.

DEFINITIONS OF A HEALTH MANPOWER SHORTAGE

To determine how efficiently a manpower market is performing, we will begin by discussing the concept of health manpower shortages. Shortages of health manpower are often used as an indication of inadequate performance and form the basis for subsequent government intervention.

By a shortage of health manpower different persons mean different things. Often policy prescriptions are proposed to alleviate all shortage situations. Since there are different types of shortages, policy prescriptions vary according to the type of shortage believed to exist. This section therefore will discuss different definitions of shortage, together with the appropriate policy prescription for each. Subsequent sections will discuss the measurement of the various types of shortage situations and then apply the various definitions and their measurement to different health manpower markets.

NORMATIVE JUDGMENT OF A SHORTAGE

There are several *noneconomic* definitions of health manpower shortages. An example is the statement that the demand for physicians "ought" to be greater. It also may be believed that the "need" for physicians is greater than the demand or that the price of physician services is "too high," thereby preventing people from consuming all the physician services they need. These noneconomic definitions of a shortage are based either upon a value judgment of how much care people should receive, or upon a professional determination of how much physician care is appropriate in the population.

Such normative judgments of shortage are based upon a determination of "need" in the population, or upon some professional estimate of health manpower requirements. For example, physician-to-population ratios in high-income states are contrasted with physician-to-population ratios in low-income states. The differences in the ratio are believed to indicate the "need" for physicians in low-income states, which is the number of physicians "required" to achieve a physician-to-population ratio equal to that of the high-income states. The ratio technique will be discussed in more detail in the next section, when the different methods of measuring shortages are discussed. The classic example of professional determination of the number of physicians "needed" was the study by Lee and Jones (1). Lee and Jones based their estimate of the number of physicians required in the population on estimates of the incidence of morbidity and on the number of physician hours required to provide both preventive and therapeutic services to the population. The policy proposals that result from normative definitions of a shortage of health manpower are generally the same: increase the number of trained professionals through increased federal funding. In Figure 13-1 it is assumed that the existing situation is represented by the supply and demand diagrams S_1 and D_1, resulting in the quantity of physician services Q_1. The number of physician services for the population, based on either a need or professional determination, is determined to be Q_2. The usual policy prescription for an increase in the number of physicians is represented by a shift in the supply of physicians to S_2, resulting in an increase to Q_2 in the number of physician services. Q_2 of physician services can also be achieved by shifting the demand schedule to D_2 without shifting the supply or the number of physicians. (A shift in demand can be achieved by a demand subsidy such as insurance coverage for physician services.) Thus, the normative judgment of a shortage of physician services, $Q_1 - Q_2$, can be alleviated either by increasing the number of physicians (shifting S_1 to S_2), or by subsidizing the demand for physician services (shifting D_1 to D_2) along a given supply curve. (A movement along a given supply curve represents increased production by existing physicians.)

Which policy alternative—the demand or the supply shift—is preferable will depend upon the cost of each proposal, which population groups receive the benefits, and the length of time required to achieve the increase in services consumed. Normative judgments of a manpower shortage can be alleviated in various ways; however, these judgments of a shortage say nothing about how well the market for such health professionals is functioning. The market for physicians may be functioning efficiently, though some persons may believe there "should" be more physicians; conversely, the market for physicians may not be producing the number of physicians that would be produced in an efficiently functioning market. However, the basic policy prescription using a normative definition of a shortage is always for federal funding to achieve an increase in the number of physicians. If the market is not functioning well, then there might be alternative ways of achieving an increase in the number of physi-

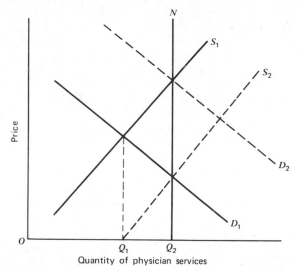

Figure 13-1. Alternative policy prescriptions based upon a normative shortage of health manpower.

cians or physician services *without* resorting to federal funding. Perhaps some legal barriers might be changed to permit an increase in the physician supply without additional federal funds. To determine how well the market for health professionals is functioning, we must establish the economic definitions of a shortage and examine how such shortages may occur. Possible policy prescriptions for correcting these shortages will be an outgrowth of their analysis.

ECONOMIC DEFINITIONS OF SHORTAGES OF HEALTH MANPOWER

In a competitive market, market equilibrium occurs when the value placed on a good or service by its demanders equals the cost of the resources used in its production. When the value placed on that good or service exceeds its cost of production, then too little of that good is produced, creating a shortage.* As the quantity supplied of the good is increased, the costs of its production will rise (which include the higher prices that are necessary to attract the required resources from their other uses) until the cost of production equals the value placed on it by those who demand it. In freely operating markets shortages cannot exist in the long run.

There are two ways of looking at how an economic shortage can occur with respect to health manpower. First, the quantity demanded for a particular health profession (i.e., hospitals' demands for registered nurses) can exceed the quantity supplied at a given market price (wage). The second way in which the value

---

*This situation also occurs when a monopolist establishes a price for its service greater than the marginal cost of producing that service.

placed on a resource can exceed its costs of production is when the income of a health profession exceeds the costs of entering that profession. In this latter instance, the income of a health profession reflects the value of the services that the profession produces. The costs of entering the profession include the out-of-pocket costs of training for that profession, as well as the value of the entrant's time. (Since the time streams at which the income is earned and the costs incurred differ, an appropriate discount rate must be used in equating the two.)

This latter situation may be illustrated by use of Figure 13-2. D_1 is the demand by firms for a particular health manpower occupation. S_L represents the long-run supply curve and is the number of persons willing to enter that occupation at different wage rates. S_1 is the current number of persons in that health profession. (S_1 is unlikely to be vertical, since the supply of work effort from the current stock of trained professionals will depend upon the responsiveness of their hours worked and their participation rate to different wage rates.) The resulting wage rate with S_1 supply will be W_1. If the market were operating freely, then the wage would fall to W_0 as the supply of labor to that occupation increased. If the health manpower profession in question were able to establish entry barriers, S_1 would not shift to the right along S_L. The resulting wage (W_1), which represents the value placed on that labor input by its demanders, would exceed the cost of inducing additions to the supply of that health profession.

Each of the two types of static shortage, the first example where the wage is held below the equilibrium level and the case just considered where the wage exceeds the wage at which persons are willing to enter that occupation, is caused by market power on either the demand or supply side of the health manpower market. When the wage is prevented from rising to its equilibrium level, the demanders of labor are exercising monopoly power; in the latter case it is the suppliers of labor services that are the monopolists. In both of these types of shortage situations, the shortage would disappear with an increase in supply. Supply would increase in the first case if the price of the service were allowed to rise, and in the second case if more persons entered the profession.

These discussions of economic shortage indicate what information should be examined to determine whether or not an economic shortage exists or has occurred. Since each of these approaches will be employed with regard to different health professions, i.e., physicians and registered nurses, these approaches will be discussed in more detail.

When quantity demanded exceeds quantity supplied at a given market price, then, as in Figure 13-3, the price will rise (to P_2), and at the new market price there will be no excess demand. All who are willing to pay price P_2 will be

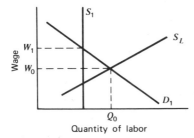

Figure 13-2. A shortage created by a restriction of supply.

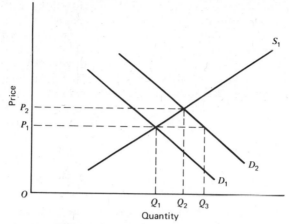

Figure 13-3. An economic shortage.

able to purchase as much as they want of the commodity they are seeking. (There may be persons who cannot afford to buy as much of the commodity as others believe they should purchase at the new, higher price; however, such a normative judgment can still be handled using a market mechanism by providing subsidies directly to such persons.) An economic shortage would occur in the above situation if, with an increase in demand from D_1 to D_2, the price of the service were prevented from rising to its new equilibrium point, P_2. In such a situation, with an increase in demand, at a price of P_1 the demand would be for Q_3 units of service, while at a price of P_1 the supply of that service would be Q_1. The shortage would be the excess of demand over supply at the prevailing price, of $Q_3 - Q_1$.

There can be two types of economic shortage: a temporary (dynamic) shortage or a static (long-run) shortage. Both types of economic shortage are believed to have existed at one time or another in the health professions.

A Dynamic Shortage

A dynamic or temporary shortage will occur when, as in Figure 13-3, there is an increase in demand but the new price has not reached its new equilibrium point of P_2. There will be a greater demand than there is supply at the old price of P_1. Not everyone who is willing to pay P_1 will be able to receive as much as he or she wants. In the long run, however, this form of temporary or dynamic shortage will work itself out: the price will rise to the equilibrium level and there will no longer be a shortage. It is possible that if demand continues to increase, then it will take longer to achieve the equilibrium situation. There will be continued claims of a shortage while the price is rising, although supply will also be increasing. *Increases in quantity supplied, as well as rising prices, distinguish a dynamic shortage from a static shortage,* which will be discussed shortly.

How long will a dynamic shortage persist? In their article on dynamic shortages, Kenneth Arrow and William Capron claim that "the amount of shortage will tend to disappear faster the greater the reaction speed and also the greater the elasticity of supply (or demand)" (2). The reaction speed is the time it takes for price to reach its equilibrium level given the excess of demand over supply. It will take time for firms to realize that there is a shortage at the old price and that they must raise wages to attract more personnel. They must also decide how many more persons they want in the event that they have to pay higher wage rates. It also takes time for employees to react to these higher salaries. If demand and supply are relatively elastic, then it will take smaller price increases to bring about a new equilibrium situation. Thus, in a dynamic situation where demands are increasing, temporary shortages can exist. The magnitude of the dynamic shortage will depend upon how fast demand is increasing, the reaction speed of increased prices to the excess demand, and the elasticities of supply and demand.

The policy prescriptions for a dynamic shortage differ from those prescribed either for a "normative" judgment of a shortage or for a static shortage. Increasing information both to demanders and suppliers in a market where dynamic shortages exist will make the equilibrium situation occur more quickly. Career information given to prospective applicants in professions where demand is increasing, and similar information given to prospective employers regarding the higher wages they will have to pay for such personnel, will bring about a quicker adjustment process. Massive supply subsidies to finance additional applicants entering those professions for which demands are increasing cannot be justified on grounds of economic efficiency. Such subsidies would have to be justified on grounds of a normative shortage, not a dynamic shortage.

Static Economic Shortages

In a static or long-run shortage situation, market equilibrium is not achieved because prices cannot increase. In the typical case of a static shortage, prices are controlled and are thereby prevented from rising to their equilibrium level. If prices cannot be increased, then suppliers cannot pay higher prices to attract personnel away from other occupations. Similarly, a given health professional will not increase the amount of time he or she is willing to work if the wage rate per hour does not increase; at some point the person will prefer leisure to more work. Thus, suppliers will not increase the services they offer unless the prices paid for their services rise. The available supply in such situations is rationed by other methods: there may be long waiting lines to see a physician and only those willing to wait (those with low time costs) will see the physician; there may be a decrease in quality, i.e., physicians may spend less time with each patient; physicians may also refuse to see new patients.

It is possible that a static shortage or a market equilibrium situation could exist in the physician *services* market; in the market for physician *manpower,* there could also be either an equilibrium or a static shortage situation. It is important to keep the analysis of these two markets—the services and manpower markets—separate. For example, in Figure 13-4, the left-hand diagram represents the market for physician services, while the right-hand diagram represents the solo physician as a typical firm in the overall market for physician services. Starting from an equilibrium situation in both markets, with price equal to P_0 and quantity of physician services equal to Q_0, the individual physician as a firm faces a price of P_0 and produces a quantity of services given by Q_0', which is the

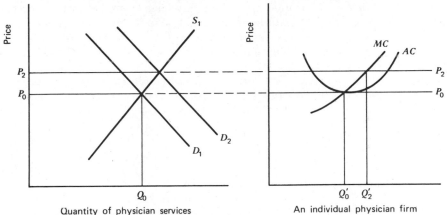

Figure 13-4. The market for physician services and for an individual physician firm.

intersection of the physician firm's marginal-cost curve (MC) and the market price P_0. (For simplicity, we are assuming a competitive market situation in the production and demand for physician services.) The physician firm is in equilibrium (physicians will neither leave the industry nor enter it), since they are earning a normal rate of return, with no excess profits, as shown by the position of the physician firm's average-cost curve (AC) and the market price, P_0.

Given the above initial equilibrium position in both the services and manpower markets, let us assume that there is an increase in demand for physician services, possibly as a result of increased income in the population. The demand for physician services will increase from D_1 to D_2. Given the same number of physicians, physicians will either work longer hours or increase their productivity by hiring auxiliary personnel. This increased output is shown by a movement up the industry's supply curve (S_1), which is the sum of the individual physician firms' marginal-cost curves. The market price will rise to P_2, and each physician will be making excess profits (the distance from P_2 to the firm's average-cost curve at output level Q_2'). The increase in price and output in the market for physician services is the short-run reaction to the increase in demand for physician services.

In this situation there is no shortage in the physicians' services market. If there is an increase in the number of physicians (i.e., firms) in the long run in the manpower market because of excess profits, then the industry supply curve will shift to the right, and each physician firm will be producing at a point where the new price equals average cost and marginal cost. This long-run adjustment of an increase in the number of physicians will also result in an equilibrium situation in the manpower market, and no shortage will exist in either market.

If, however, with an increase in the demand for physician services the price is *prevented* from rising, then a static shortage situation will occur in the services market. Equilibrium could still exist in the physician manpower market, since there will not be an excess of profits (or losses). Alternatively, if the price is allowed to reach its equilibrium level in the services market but new physicians are not permitted to enter the manpower market, then a shortage situation will exist in the physician manpower market. Physicians will be earning excess profits and we would observe little, if any, addition to the number of physicians. *A static shortage in the number of physicians will be represented by high rates of returns (excess profits) to physicians and little or no entry into the physician market.*

The policy implications for a static shortage situation are to allow the price to rise if the shortage is in the services market, or, if the shortage is in the physician manpower market, to relax the entry barriers, which will presumably allow an increase in the number of physicians. With an increase in the number of physicians, the excess profits per physician will theoretically fall until profits are "normal" and there will no longer be an economic shortage of physicians. If a static shortage exists because of barriers to entry, providing subsidies to the new entrants will not resolve the static shortage. The entry barriers are generally not eliminated by such subsidies. Subsidizing the limited number of new entrants will merely increase their return in a profession whose profits are currently considered to be excessive.

In defining and distinguishing between normative, dynamic, and static shortages, we see that the latter two are different types of economic shortages, and that the normative shortage is based upon either a professional determination or on a value judgment of how many of the particular types of manpower are needed. We have also indicated the alternative policy prescriptions for the different types of shortages. In the next section the methods by which each of these types of shortages has been measured will be discussed. The measurement of a shortage is important, since it enables us to distinguish between the different types of shortages.

THE MEASUREMENT OF HEALTH MANPOWER SHORTAGES

In discussing different types of shortages, we have distinguished between economic and noneconomic shortages. Noneconomic shortages have traditionally been measured in one of two ways.

PROFESSIONAL DETERMINATION

The earliest approach, used by Lee and Jones, calculated the number of physicians required in the population based upon an estimate of the number of physician hours needed, as determined by professional judgment, to provide medical care to the population. The authors developed a table of annual expectancy rates for diseases and injuries; they then asked leading physicians to determine the number of services required to diagnose and treat a given illness; the number of physician hours required to provide care for each illness category was then estimated; finally, assuming a 40-hour workweek per physician, the authors translated these hours into a requirement of 165,000 physicians, or a proposed physician-to-population ratio of 135 per 100,000 population. The difference between the current number of physicians and the number of physicians arrived at by the above method is the extent of the "shortage" of physicians.

One of the problems with using such an approach for estimating shortages and for then proposing government intervention to subsidize increases in the number of needed physicians is that the additional physicians do not necessarily go where they are most needed. Further, those persons most in need of physician services may not be able to pay for them even if they are made available. There are additional problems with this approach. What if the current number of physicians exceeds the professionally determined estimate? If such a "surplus" of physicians were to be eliminated, then an *economic* shortage might occur.

Similar in its approach to the Lee and Jones methodology was the recent 1980 Graduate Medical Education National Advisory Committee (GEMENAC) report to the Secretary of Health and Human Services on the future supply and requirements for physicians (3).

Estimates of future supplies of physicians were generated based on estimates of current supplies of medical school graduates, foreign medical graduates, residents, and deaths and retirements. No attempt was made to relate entry into medicine, into different specialties, or entry by foreign medical graduates, to economic factors or to any other causal factors. Instead it was implicitly assumed that such factors would not change over the period studied. Nor did this approach consider changes in physician productivity that might be occurring. It was a mechanical approach to generating future estimates of physicians and their specialty distribution.

The estimates of physician requirements was developed by combining data on current utilization and the "need" for physicians. Within each physician specialty, physicians were asked how many physicians were needed in that specialty. Again such an approach does not explicitly consider patient preferences for care nor economic factors, such as changes in insurance coverage; factors which, in the past, have been important determinants of physician utilization.

The "desired balance" of physician supply and requirements by 1990 does not consider any equilibrating mechanisms such as changes in physician prices or hours worked. The report states that there will be a physician "surplus" of 70,000 physicians by 1990. Although the GEMENAC approach was similar to the Lee and Jones method of 50 years earlier, its conclusions were quite different. Today the concern is with having "too many" physicians.

THE RATIO TECHNIQUE

The second, and major, approach to determining health manpower shortages has been the ratio technique. This method generally uses the existing physician-to-population ratio (or other health-manpower-to-population ratio) and compares it with the physician-to-population ratio that is likely to occur in some future period. To calculate the future ratio, the proponents of this approach estimate the future population and then calculate the likely number of additions of graduates to the stock of physicians, less the expected number of deaths and retirements. The difference between the existing physician-to-population ratio and the future physician-to-population ratio is the difference that must be made up. (In the past the future ratio has always been found to be less than the current ratio.) The policy proposal that always results from a finding that increases in the number of physicians are required is for federal subsidies to health professional educational institutions to produce more graduates. There are some variations on this ratio technique for determining the number of physicians needed. For example, the highest regional or statewide physician-to-population ratio observed might be used as the base ratio to be achieved for the entire country in some future period.

The ratio technique has served as the basis for much of the health manpower legislation in this country. It has been used for physicians, dentists, and registered nurses. Other health professional organizations also make use of this approach in their requests for federal subsidies. Since this approach has had such an important legislative role and has resulted in subsidies of many billions of dollars both by the federal and state governments, it deserves a critical evaluation.

One way of thinking of the physician-to-population ratio is that it is the outcome of an equilibrium situation. At any point in time there is a demand for physicians and a supply of physicians; the intersection of the demand and supply curves results in the physician's income and in a physician-to-population ratio. Attempts to change the physician-to-population ratio generally ignore the fact that this ratio is the result of demand and other supply factors. Any significant change in just the number of physicians should cause changes in the demands for other inputs (substitutes for and complements to physicians), as well as in the demands for physicians themselves, which would mean a movement down the physician demand curve.

Three basic problems are associated with the use of the ratio technique for estimating shortages (or for forecasting manpower requirements). The first problem is that the method does not consider any changes that may occur in the demand for physicians (or other health manpower) services. If demand were to increase, then even maintaining an existing ratio (or striving for a higher ratio as found in other states) might result in an *increase* in the price of physician services, i.e., the shift in demand is greater than the increase in the physician-to-population ratio. Since this approach basically ignores the demand side, differences between the future ratio of physicians to population and the ratio that would be demanded will be resolved through changes in the *price* of physician services. Some persons will be even less likely to be able to afford to buy physician services if the price of those services has increased. Thus, maintaining a given ratio says nothing about whether the future price of physician services will be the same; it may be higher or lower, but it is highly unlikely that it will be the same. Since the future price is likely to be different, and generally will be higher than the current price because of increasing demand, what is the real purpose of maintaining a given ratio? If the objective were to be to provide more services either to certain population groups or to the entire population, then it would be important to lower the price of the service so as to increase its consumption. The ratio technique and its basic policy prescription to change the number of physicians does not even consider price or alternative ways to affect consumption of services.

The second problem with the use of the ratio technique is that it does not consider productivity changes that are likely to occur or possible to achieve. The ratio of farmers to the population has fallen drastically in the last 100 years (from a ratio of 60 farmers to every 100 persons in 1860 to where fewer than 4 in 100 persons are engaged in farming today), yet few people would maintain that there is a shortage of farmers or that it would be desirable to retain the previous farmer-to-population ratio. Because of enormous increases in farm productivity, it takes fewer farmers today to produce more food than their predecessors did. Although productivity gains in medical care appear to be more limited than what has occurred in agriculture, it is still possible to achieve an increase in physician services without increasing the number of physicians. Lesser-trained personnel can be used to relieve physicians of many of the tasks they perform; delegation of tasks would permit an increase in the number of physician visits. If increased productivity is considered, a smaller physician-to-population ratio would be needed in the future. Productivity increases should be considered as an alternative approach to increasing the quantity of physician services in the population; policies to increase productivity require smaller subsidies than policies to increase the number of physicians.

The third problem with the use of the ratio technique is that no indication of the importance of the shortage of physicians is provided. For example, the Bane Report estimated that if the 1959 physician-to-population ratio were maintained (140 per 100,000), then an additional 11,000 physicians would be needed by 1975. These projections assumed that without federal support for medical education there would be 319,000 physicians with a resulting shortage of 11,000 physicians (4). How much is it worth (in terms of governmental subsidies) to reduce this shortage to 7,000 physicians or to no shortage whatsoever? It is difficult, if not impossible, to use the ratio technique to compare the additional cost of decreasing the estimated shortage of physicians with their marginal contribution to medical care or increased health.

A number of technical difficulties are encountered with the use of the ratio technique: omitting research physicians from the physician-to-population ratio, correcting for the age distribution of physicians (since it may affect productivity), and forecasting population in a future period. The three conceptual problems inherent in this approach—no consideration given to demand or productivity changes and no understanding of the importance of the shortage estimate—are, however, more significant shortcomings.

THE RATE-OF-RETURN APPROACH
FOR MEASURING MANPOWER SHORTAGES

We have seen that in the health manpower market three types of market situations can exist: an equilibrium situation, a dynamic shortage, or a static shortage. An equilibrium situation is one in which physicians are earning normal profits. If there were an increase in demand in the physician services market, physicians would, in the short run, experience higher prices leading to excess profits, and in the long run we would expect an increase to occur in the number of physicians, thereby returning their profits to a normal level.

This analogy of the physician as a firm is useful because it helps to delineate what we should expect to observe. Normal profits or excess profits mean that the rate of return to a medical education is either normal or high compared with equivalent investments. Although not all, nor perhaps most, physicians seek a medical education because of its value as a remunerative investment, enough persons do so that if one profession becomes more lucrative than another, some persons will change their preference for the occupation they wish to enter. This is not to say that all persons seeking a professional education do so because it will provide them with a good income. It just means that as some professions and occupations become relatively more rewarding financially, some potential applicants who are relatively indifferent between different professions will switch their preferences to the more rewarding occupation. This switching between occupations and professions will, on the average, equalize returns among the different occupations and professions. (Because there are always large variations in skills, returns *within* an occupation or profession will vary. In the long run, however, the average return should be similar among different occupations.)

When viewing medical education as an investment, one calculates the rate of return by estimating the costs of that investment and the expected higher financial returns. Thus one can compare its profitability with alternative investments, educational and otherwise. The costs of purchasing a medical education are the direct outlays, such as tuition costs and laboratory and book fees, and the income a student foregoes had he or she gone to work immediately upon graduating from college. These opportunity costs of the student's time are the more significant costs of securing a professional education. The high return of an investment in a medical education is the higher income that a physician will earn compared with the income of an alternative occupation. Since these higher incomes occur in the future, they are worth less than if they occurred immediately; the difference in financial returns between being a physician and entering an alternative occupation must be discounted to the present. The comparison between these higher returns and the costs required to receive them is the rate of return to a medical education. (More precisely, the internal rate of return is that discount rate which, when applied to the future earnings stream, will make its present value equal to the cost of entry into that profession, i.e., the present value of the expected outlay or cost stream.)

A normal rate of return might be similar to the rate of return on a college education or on the return the individual could have received had he or she invested a sum of money comparable to what was spent on a medical education. For that reason we are interested in comparing the rate of return with a standard that is based on an alternative rate of return. Returning to our analogy of the physician as a firm, if physicians were receiving "excess" profits, then this would be translated into a high rate of return to a medical education. If there are high rates of return to medicine in comparison with the returns achievable in other occupations, then we expect to observe a greater number of applicants to medical schools until the rate of return again becomes comparable to other occupations or investments.

To distinguish, then, between the two types of economic shortages (a dynamic versus a static shortage), we would want to examine both what happens to the rate of return to a medical education relative to some standard or to other occupations, and the increase in the number of physicians. A dynamic shortage would be characterized by high rates of return in the short run, increases in the number of physicians, and eventually normal rates of return. A static shortage would also be characterized by high rates of return, but they would persist since there would be little or no entry into the profession to drive these rates of return down.* If rates of return remained high and there was a large increase in the supply of physicians, then there might be a persistent dynamic shortage. The key difference between the dynamic and static shortage is whether additions to the stock of physicians occur over time. A dynamic shortage will eventually resolve itself; a static shortage requires intervention, since entry into the profession is prevented.

The main indicators of the performance of the physician market and other health manpower markets are data on relative rates of return and additions to the stock of physicians (or other health manpower). Other indications of a shortage situation, such as greater use of substitute manpower, may be observed; however, such substitution could occur because of changes in the relative wages of different occupations and be unrelated to a shortage situation. For example, if wages and costs of entering a profession increased, the rates of return between occupations could be similar but their relative wages would differ; hence, substitution would occur. Thus, the main method whereby different types of shortages are distinguished is in the use of relative rates of return and entry into the profession.†

The concept of rates of return is also important for public policy. If it is desired to increase the number of persons entering a profession, subsidies can be provided to offset the applicant's training costs. Assuming no excess rate of return, a lower training cost will result in a higher rate of return and consequently an increased demand to that profession. For policy it is important to empirically determine the elasticity of lowering training costs with respect to expected increases in the number of applicants to that profession.

EMPIRICAL ESTIMATES OF HEALTH MANPOWER SHORTAGES

Several studies have attempted to estimate the rate of return to a medical education. The earliest economic study of the physician shortage was by Milton Friedman and Simon Kuznets (5). They studied several professions during the early 1930s and found that for two of the professions, dentistry and medicine, physi-

---

*Similarly, a "surplus" situation will be indicated by a relatively low rate of return. Over time, however, we expect fewer entrants into such a profession, and the rate of return will rise to where it is equal to those in other professions.

†Another approach suggested for measuring whether or not a shortage exists is to examine changes in relative incomes. If one profession's income rises more rapidly than another profession's, then a relative shortage is said to exist. (See, for example, Elton Rayack, "The Supply of Physicians' Services," *Industrial and Labor Relations Review*, January 1964.) The problem with this approach is that it does not consider differences in the relative costs of entering different professions. If training times have increased, or if there is a decrease in the number of working years, we would expect higher relative incomes for this profession in order for the relative rates of return to be similar. Another problem in using the relative-income approach is that the base year for making comparisons among professions is quite important. Depending upon which base year is used, the relative-income approach can show a shortage or a surplus of the manpower in a particular profession. Finally, the relative-income approach cannot distinguish between relative shortages in all professions and a shortage situation in only one profession.

TABLE 13-1. Internal Rates of Return to Male College Graduates, Physicians, and Dentists, and Ratios of Internal Rates of Return of Physicians and Dentists to Male College Graduates, United States, 1939, 1949, and 1956

	1939		1949		1956	
	Rates	Ratios	Rates	Ratios	Rates	Ratios
Male college graduates	13.7	1.00	11.5	1.00	11.6	1.00
Physicians	13.5	.98	13.4	1.16	12.8	1.10
Dentists	12.3	.90	13.4	1.16	12.0	1.04

Source: W. Lee Hansen, " 'Shortages' and Investment in Health Manpower," in *The Economics of Health and Medical Care* (Ann Arbor, Mich.: University of Michigan, 1964), p. 86.

cians earned, on the average, 32 percent per year more than dentists did. (The costs of producing physicians was 17 percent greater than the cost of producing dentists.) Friedman and Kuznets attributed part of the increased income of physicians to greater entry barriers into the profession. This greater return to physicians represented a relative shortage of physicians; that is, their marginal value as represented by their incomes exceeded the costs of producing additional physicians. A later study by W. Lee Hansen found that by 1939 there was a slight *surplus* of physicians and dentists. By 1949 physicians and dentists had a 16 percent greater rate of return than did college graduates, and by 1956 the shortage had decreased slightly: physicians' rates of return were only 10 percent greater than for a college graduate; the comparable figure for dentists was 4 percent. This is shown in Table 13-1, which is reproduced from Hansen's work.

According to more recent studies, the internal rate of return to 4 years of medical school and an internship program were estimated to be (6):

Year	Internal Rate of Return (7)
1956	13.5 percent
1959	14.7 percent
1962	16.6 percent
1963	15.9 percent
1964	16.1 percent
1965	17.5 percent
1966	18.2 percent
1970	22.0 percent
1976	17.5 percent

The 1976 estimate is based on a recent study which estimated the rate of return to a medical education relative to other occupations, each with differing years of education required. It was found that the rate of return (at its midpoint) to a medical degree relative to that of a teacher (i.e., a college graduate) was 17.5 percent in 1976. The rates of return varied greatly depending upon which occupation it was compared to. For example, the rate of return to a medical education was over 100 percent greater than for that of a college professor (8).

What can we conclude based on these data on rates of return? In the pre-World War II period there appeared to be a slight surplus of physicians and dentists. The rate of return to such an education was lower than for comparable investments. After World War II, however, the rate of return to a medical and dental education increased. The rates of return during this period were sufficiently high to indicate a shortage situation. With increasing rates of return, we would expect to observe increased demands for a medical education. If large increases in the stock of physicians were occurring, then we would conclude that a dynamic shortage existed. If, however, the rates of return remained high, and in fact increased, and there were few or no additions to the stock of physicians, then we would have to conclude that a static shortage situation existed and that barriers prevented an adjustment process from occurring. To determine whether a dynamic or a static shortage of physicians existed through the late 1940s, the 1950s, and the 1960s, we turn to an examination of data on changes in the stock of physicians during these periods, as presented in Table 13-2.

In 1950 there were 209,000 active physicians in the United States. By 1965 the number of active physicians reached 277,000, which is a rate of increase of less than 2 percent per year. When the increase in the number of physicians is adjusted for increases in the population, the physician-to-population ratio remained virtually unchanged between 1950 and 1963 (141 physicians per 100,000 population and 140 per 100,000, respectively). After 1963 the total number of active physicians began to increase at a slightly more rapid rate, averaging between 1.5 and 3.7 percent per year until 1975, when the annual increase was 4.5 percent. The physician-to-population ratio also began to show a gradual annual increase during this same period, reaching 167 physicians per 100,000 in 1974. Part of the increase in physicians over this period was a result of increases in foreign medical graduates (FMGs). In 1960, 5.8 percent of the total number of active physicians were FMGs; by 1973, FMGs were 20 percent of the number of active physicians. In 1973 the number of FMGs entering the United States exceeded the number of U.S. medical graduates (USMGs) in that year (12,285 FMGs, 10,391 USMGs). When the physician-to-population ratio is adjusted for the number of FMGs, then between 1960 and 1974 the ratio was virtually unchanged.

The Immigration Act of 1965 facilitated the immigration of foreign-trained physicians (FMGs) into the United States. As a result there was a rapid rise in FMGs between 1966 and 1976. During this period, approximately one-third of the permanent increase in physician supply was attributed to the inflow of FMGs.*

---

*There are two main classifications of FMGs: Those that have permanent immigrant status and those that have exchange visitor status. Exchange visitor FMGs are supposed to return to their own countries after they have received graduate medical training. However, until 1976 many exchange visitor FMGs extended their stays indefinitely, thus clouding the difference between themselves and FMGs permanently immigrating. The annual increase in exchange visitor FMGs exceeded the number of FMGs permanently immigrating up until the mid-1970s. Exchange visitor FMGs were an important component of total FMGs and they were becoming a significant portion of all physicians.

In 1976, as part of the renewal of the Health Professions Educational Assistance Act (HPEA), Congress changed the immigration laws affecting FMGs. Newly entering FMGs were now required to pass more rigorous medical exams as well as exams in written and oral English. The legislation also restricted the number of FMGs who can remain indefinitely by requiring exchange visitor FMGs to return to their own countries after 2 years of U.S. graduate medical education (a 1-year extension is possible). This legislation had its greatest impact on newly entering FMGs with exchange visitor

TABLE 13-2. Number of Physicians and Physician–Population Ratios, United States, 1950–1980

Year	Active Physicians[a]	Annual Percent Change[b]	Physicians Per 100,000 Population[c]	Annual Percent Change[b]	Foreign-Trained Physicians[d]	Foreign-Trained Physicians as a Percentage of All Active Physicians[c]	Physician–Population Ratios Excluding Foreign-Trained Physicians (Physicians Per 100,000 Population)[c]
1950	208,997		141	N.C.			
1955	228,553	1.9	141	N.C.			
1960	247,257	1.6	140	−.1	15,154[e]	5.8	132
1963	261,728	1.9	140	N.C.	30,925	11.3	124
1965	277,575	3.0	145	−1.8			
1967	294,072	3.0	150	1.7	45,816	15.0	127
1969	302,966	1.5	151	.3	53,552	17.0	126
1970	311,203	2.7	158	4.6	54,404	16.8	131
1971	322,228	3.6	161	1.9	59,499	17.8	132
1972	333,259	3.4	165	2.5	64,701	18.7	134
1973	338,111	1.5	166	.6	67,141	19.1	134

1974	350,609	170	3.7	2.4	70,940	19.5	137
1975	366,425	176	4.5	3.5	76,205	20.0	141
1976	378,572	180	3.3	2.3	78,295[f]	20.0	144
1977	381,969	180	.9	N.C.	81,386[f]	20.5	143
1978	401,364	188	5.1	4.4	83,976	20.1	150
1979	417,266	191	4.0	1.6	89,210	20.5	153
1980	435,545	199	4.4	4.2	90,803	20.1	159

Sources: U.S. Department of Health and Human Services, Office of Research, Statistics and Technology, *Health United States 1980*, DHHS Publication No. (PHS) 81-1232 (Hyattsville, Md.: Government Printing Office, 1980), p. 188; Department of Health and Human Services, *Supply and Characteristics of Selected Health Personnel* (HRA 81-20) (1981), p. 36; U.S. Department of Commerce, Bureau of Census, "Estimates of the Population of the U.S. to April 1, 1982," *Population Estimates and Projections*, Series p-25, No. 914 (1982); *Physician Distribution and Medical Licensure in the U.S.*, (1977), Department of Statistical Analysis, Center for Health Policy Research, American Medical Association, Chicago, 1977. *Physician Characteristics and Distribution in the U.S.*, 1981 edition, Division of Survey and Data Resources, American Medical Association, Chicago, 1982; U.S. Department of Health and Human Services, Bureau of Health Professions, *A Report to the President and Congress on the Status of Health Professions Personnel in the United States*, Draft, April 27, 1981; pp. 111–141, Table 7, p. 111–143, Table 9.

[a]MDs only. Excludes inactive and temporary foreign physicians, and those with unknown addresses.

[b]Calculated as an average for each year in a multiyear period (e.g., 9.4 percent increase for 1950–1955 averages to 1.9 percent per year).

[c]Physicians in these columns refers to the sum of MDs and Doctors of Osteopathy (DOs). The number of DOs has fluctuated between 11,000 in 1950 and 17,000 in 1982. Population refers to civilian population.

[d]Includes active physicians and 90 percent of those unclassified. It excludes inactive, temporary foreign physicians, and those with unknown address.

[e]Figure for 1959.

[f]Estimated through interpolation.

TABLE 13-3. Federal and Nonfederal Physicians in the United States and Possessions by Type of Professional Activity, 1963–1980

Year	Total Active Physicians[a]	Physicians Engaged in Patient-Care Activities[b]	Percent Engaged in Patient-Care Activities[c]	Physicians Engaged in Other Professional Activities[d]	Percent Engaged in Other Professional Activities	Physicians with Activities/Specialties Unclassified	Percent Unclassified
1963	261,728	246,951	94.4	14,777	5.6		
1964	269,552	253,543	94.1	16,009	5.9		
1965	277,575	259,418	93.5	18,157	6.5		
1966	285,857	266,766	93.3	19,091	6.7		
1967	294,072	274,190	93.2	19,882	6.8		
1968	296,312	261,722	88.3	34,590	11.7		
1969	302,966	270,737	89.4	32,229	10.6		
1970	311,203	278,535	89.5	32,310	10.4	358	.1
1971	322,228	287,248	89.1	31,451	9.8	3,529	1.0
1972	333,259	292,210	87.7	28,693	8.6	12,356	3.7
1973	338,111	295,257	87.3	29,110	8.6	13,744	4.1
1974	350,609	301,238	85.9	29,028	8.3	20,343	5.8
1975	366,425	311,937	85.1	28,343	7.8	26,145	7.1
1976	378,572	318,412	84.1	30,031	7.9	30,129	8.0
1977	381,969	332,393	87.0	31,226	8.2	18,350	4.8
1978	401,364	342,714	85.4	33,097	8.2	25,553	6.4
1979	417,266	356,783	85.5	36,946	8.9	23,537	5.6
1980	435,545	376,512	87.1	36,404	8.4	20,629	4.8

Sources: *Physician Distribution and Medical Licensure in the U.S.*, (1979), Department of Statistical Analysis, Center for Health Policy Research, American Medical Association, Chicago, 1980. *Physician Characteristics and Distribution in the U.S.*, 1981 edition, Division of Survey and Data Resources, American Medical Association, Chicago, 1982.

[a]MDs only. Excludes inactive physicians and those with unknown addresses.

[b]In office-based practice or in hospital-based practice as interns, residents, and full-time physician staff.

[c]Medical teaching, administration, research and other activity.

[d]The apparent decrease in "physicians engaged in patient-care activities" may in part reflect changes in the activity classification system for physicians made by the AMA in 1968. If "physicians with activities or specialties unclassified" are excluded from "total active physicians," the percentage of physicians engaged in patient-care activities for 1970 through 1980 rises from 89.6 percent in 1970 to 91.4 percent in 1980.

TABLE 13-4. Ratio of Applicants to Acceptances, 1947–1948 to 1980–1981

Year	Applicants Acceptance Ratio	Year	Applicants Acceptance Ratio
1947–1948	2.9	1964–1965	2.1
1948–1949	3.5	1965–1966	2.1
1949–1950	3.4	1966–1967	2.0
1950–1951	3.1	1967–1968	1.9
1951–1952	2.6	1968–1969	2.1
1952–1953	2.2	1969–1970	2.3
1953–1954	1.9	1970–1971	2.2
1954–1955	1.8	1971–1972	2.4
1955–1956	1.9	1972–1973	2.6
1956–1957	1.9	1973–1974	2.8
1957–1958	1.9	1974–1975	2.8
1958–1959	1.8	1975–1976	2.8
1959–1960	1.8	1976–1977	2.7
1960–1961	1.7	1977–1978	2.5
1961–1962	1.7	1978–1979	2.2
1962–1963	1.8	1979–1980	2.1
1963–1964	1.9	1980–1981	2.1

Sources: American Medical Association, "Medical Education in the United States 1971–1972," *Journal of the American Medical Association* 222 (November 20, 1972): 979, Table 12; "Undergraduate Medical Education," *Journal of the American Medical Association* 246 (December 25, 1981): 2917, Table 5. Copyright 1972, 1981, American Medical Association.

Not all active physicians are involved in patient care. When the growth in the number of physicians is examined to determine the total increase in physicians engaged in patient care activities, as shown in Table 13-3, and the number of FMGs is excluded, then the physician-to-population ratio for U.S. physicians engaged in patient care has actually *declined* between 1960 and 1975.

If demand for physicians had been increasing during the period from 1950 to 1965, as indicated earlier by the high rates of return to a medical education, we would expect larger increases in the number of physicians. Increases in the population would also have contributed to an increased demand for physician services and a greater derived demand for physicians. Rather than increasing, the ratio of U.S. physicians in patient care to population was actually decreasing during this 15-year period; the absolute increase in the number of U.S.-trained physicians was extremely small.

The small increase in the number of physicians was not the result of a lack of applicants to medical schools. As shown in Table 13-4, the applicants-to-acceptances ratio during this same period was continually greater than one.

status: their numbers decreased from 2,563 in 1976, to 1,578 in 1977, to finally to 951 in 1978. The number of newly entering permanent immigrants also declined from 4,410 in 1976 to 2,336 in 1978. As a percentage of total new licensees, FMGs decreased from 36.0 percent in 1976 to 23.6 percent in 1978. The data seem to indicate that the annual increase in FMGs has been significantly reduced. U.S. Department of Health and Human Services, Division of Health Professions Analysis, *A Report to the President and Congress on the Status of Health Professions Personnel in the United States* (1981), Washington, D.C.: Government Printing Office, p. III-20; p. III-143.

Congress passed the Health Professions Educational Assistance Act in 1965 in response to claims of a "shortage" of physicians and other health manpower. As a result of this legislation, which provided generous subsidies to health professional educational institutions, medical schools were required to increase their enrollments in order to qualify for federal funds. The effect of this legislation began to be felt in the late 1960s when the number of U.S.-trained physicians began to increase at a more rapid rate.

By 1980, physicians per 100,000 population reached 199. Even when adjusted for the increase in FMGs, the physician-to-population ratio is greater than it has been in recent memory. (The concern currently among a number of persons, and particularly physicians, is with a "surplus" rather than a shortage of physicians.) However, even with the increase in the number of physicians, the ratio of applicants to acceptances is still greater than 1; it reached a high of 2.8 in 1973–1974 and is currently declining—it is now approximately 2.0.

What can we conclude from these data? During the entire post-World War II period, rates of return to medicine were high and rising. Based on these higher returns, we would have expected greater entry into the profession and, consequently, an increase in the number of U.S.-trained physicians providing patient care; however, it appears that there was very little entry into the profession by U.S.-trained physicians. Although there was sufficient number of students demanding a medical education, as indicated by the applicant-to-acceptance ratio, very few additional physicians were produced. Even after the introduction of federal legislation mandating increases in the production of physicians, there was still an excess demand for a medical education. The only possible conclusion, based on the minimal increase in the number of U.S.-trained physicians until the mid-1970s, and the continued high rates of return, is that a static shortage situation existed.

The mechanisms used by the medical profession to create and maintain a static shortage of physicians will be discussed in Chapter 14.

REFERENCES

1. R.I. Lee and L.W. Jones, *The Fundamentals of Good Medical Care* (Chicago: University of Chicago Press, 1933).

2. Kenneth J. Arrow and William M. Capron, "Dynamic Shortages and Price Rises: The Scientist–Engineer Case," *Quarterly Journal of Economics* 73 (1959): 299.

3. *Summary Report of the Graduate Medical Education National Advisory Committee to the Secretary, Department of Health and Human Services,* Vol. I. DHHS Publication No. (HRA) 81-651, (1980), pp. 48–56. Volume II contains a more complete description of the Modeling, Research, and Data Technical Panel.

4. *Physicians for a Growing America,* Report of the Surgeon General's Consultant Group on Medical Education, Public Health Service, U.S. DHEW (Washington, D.C.: U.S. Government Printing Office, 1959).

5. Milton Friedman and Simon Kuznets, *Income from Independent Practice* (New York: National Bureau of Economic Research, 1954).

6. The internal rates of return for the years 1956 to 1966 were estimated by Frank Sloan, *Economic Models of Physician Supply,* unpublished doctoral dissertation, Harvard Uni-

versity, 1968, p. 164. The estimate for 1970, using the same method as Sloan, is in Roger Feldman and Richard M. Scheffler, "The Supply of Medical School Applicants and the Rate of Return to Training," *Quarterly Review of Economics and Business* (Spring 1978): 92, Table 1.

There is a difference in method between Hansen and Sloan. Hansen's income and cost streams begin at the first year of undergraduate college and his foregone earnings are based on those of a high school graduate. Sloan bases his foregone earnings on those of a college graduate and begins his income and cost streams at the first year of medical school.

Sloan calculates two sets of internal rates of return. The first, which is presented above, is for all physicians. The second, published in "Lifetime Earnings and the Physician's Choice of Specialty," *Industry and Labor Relations* (October 1970): 6, is for general practitioners only. His calculated rates of return for general practitioners are: 1955–29.1 percent; 1959–23.7 percent; and 1965–24.1 percent. The rate of return for specialty training is lower than that of a general practitioner.

7. There has been substantial debate about whether the internal rates of return, as calculated above, adequately reflect the true internal rates of return to a medical education. Lindsay claims that a physician, because of his or her training, will receive a relatively high market wage. This high wage will induce the physician to substitute work for leisure; consequently he or she will work more hours than someone with a lower market wage. Lindsay believes that there should be an adjustment for the number of hours worked before the income and cost streams are calculated. When Lindsay adjusts Sloan's data for hours worked (he assumes a 60-hour week for physicians and a 40- to 45-hour week for the alternative occupation) the internal rate of return is reduced.

Sloan's response is twofold; first, he claims that Lindsay overestimated the number of hours that physicians work. Second, Sloan claims that being a physician provides intangible benefits, such as increased status in society, which compensate the physician for any additional hours worked. For this reason Sloan argues, it is not necessary to take into consideration these extra hours when calculating the income and cost streams.

For a more detailed discussion of the Sloan and Lindsay debate see: Cotton M. Lindsay, "Real Returns to Medical Education," *The Journal of Human Resources* 8 (Summer 1973): 331–348; "More Real Returns to Medical Education," *Journal of Human Resources* 11 (Winter 1976): 127–130; and Frank A. Sloan, "Real Returns to Medical Education, A Comment," *Journal of Human Resources* 11 (Winter 1976) 118–126.

8. Stephen Dresch, "Marginal Wage Rates, Hours of Work, and Returns to Physician's Training and Specialization," in *Health Care Financing, Conference Proceedings: Issues in Physician Reimbursement*, Nancy Greenspan, ed. (Washington, D.C.: Department of Health and Human Services, 1981), pp. 199–200. This article also contains estimates of returns to physician specialization, which range from 40.5 percent for internal medicine to −5.0 percent for pediatrics and pediatric surgery. According to Dresch's estimates, unlike those of Sloan, a decision to specialize was profitable for the physician.

CHAPTER 14

The Market for Physician Manpower

In Chapter 13 a dynamic shortage was differentiated from a static shortage according to whether or not there was entry into the market. Persistently high rates of return, it was suggested, could continue only if there were barriers to entry. Based on the small growth in the number of physicians until the mid-1970s, and the continual excess in the ratio of applicants to acceptances to medical schools (as well as the rapid growth in foreign medical graduates entering this country and the increasing number of U.S. students studying medicine overseas), it was concluded that entry barriers must have existed to prevent an equilibrium situation from occurring in the market for physician manpower.

Three entry barriers to the physician's market have been suggested: licensure, graduation from an approved medical school, and continual increases in training, such as the movement to a three-year residency program. There is, however, an alternative hypothesis to explain why barriers in medicine exist: rather than serving to increase the economic returns to physicians, the barriers increase the quality and competence of practicing physicians. It is rationalized that these entry barriers enhance the public interest in a variety of ways. Consumers have very little information on the quality and competence of physicians. Because gathering this information is costly and the consumer may be irreparably injured if the physician is incompetent, licensure provides consumer protection by reducing the uncertainty as to the provider's training. Occupational licensure has also been rationalized on grounds of "neighborhood effects"; preventing an incompetent physician from practicing because he or she may cause an epidemic is an example, because an incompetent physician may harm persons other than the patient being treated. Licensure is thus a means of protecting others from bearing the costs of incompetent practitioners; that is, the social costs exceed the private costs (1).

Given these alternative hypotheses to explain the reasons for entry barriers to becoming a physician—namely, to increase physician incomes or to provide consumer protection from incompetent practitioners—which is the more accurate justification? If the barriers are reduced because they are believed to provide physicians with monopoly incomes, then will the public lose its protection

380

from incompetent providers? Similarly, if it is public policy to maintain such entry restrictions in the belief that they reduce consumer uncertainty and protect society from incompetent providers, but in truth such barriers are meant to provide physicians with monopoly incomes, then is the public really protected from incompetent practitioners? Could the public be better protected using other approaches and at a lower cost?

To determine which hypothesis best describes the reasons for entry restrictions in medicine one must determine how consistent each of these hypotheses is with regard to the assurance of quality or the achievement of monopoly power. If the restrictions that have been developed in medicine are for consumer protection, then the medical profession should also favor other measures that have the effect of improving quality and/or offering consumers protection from incompetent practitioners. If, on the other hand, the entry restrictions are meant to provide a monopoly to physicians and to increase their incomes, then the profession would only favor those quality measures that are in the economic interests of physicians and would oppose quality measures that would adversely affect physicians' incomes.

BARRIERS TO ENTRY IN MEDICINE

The first step in controlling entry into a profession is to establish a licensure requirement. Each state has the authority to license occupations under the power granted to it to protect the public's health. A license to practice medicine, therefore, can be granted only by a state. Beginning in the mid-1800s, when the American Medical Association (AMA) was formed, and extending until 1900, the medical profession sought and received licensure in each state (2). The states, in turn, delegated this licensure authority to medical licensing boards, which have the authority to determine the requirements for licensure. These state licensing boards also have the authority to set the conditions for suspending or revoking a license once it has been granted. The conditions for licensure and for maintaining a license can be set to place the emphasis on the quality of care that the physician provides, or they can be used to impose restrictions on who can practice so as to limit the number of persons entering the profession. The membership of the medical licensing boards in each state is composed of physicians who are either nominated by or representatives of the state and county medical associations. It is in this manner that the county and state medical associations have influenced the conditions for licensure in each state.

The earliest requirement for licensure was an examination. Examination by itself, however, is a weak barrier to entry if a person may try to pass the examination many times and if the number of people who may take the examination is not limited (3). A more effective barrier is one which raises the cost to those wishing to take the examination. Not everyone would be willing to bear this cost, particularly if there was uncertainty as to whether they would pass the licensure exam. The second barrier to entry into the medical profession, therefore, became the imposition of an educational requirement and a limit on the number of institutions that could provide such an education.

This second stage began in 1904 with the AMA's founding of its Council on

Medical Education. This group had the task of upgrading the quality of medical education offered by existing medical schools. Of the 160 medical schools in 1906, the Council on Medical Education found only 82 offering a fully acceptable medical education (4). To achieve greater recognition of its findings, the Council on Medical Education induced the Carnegie Commission to survey the existing medical schools and publish a report. The resulting report, popularly known as the Flexner report, recommended the closing of many medical schools and an upgrading of the educational standards in the other schools. "Flexner forcefully argued that the country was suffering from an overproduction of doctors and that it was in the public interest to have fewer doctors who were better trained" (5).

The result of the Flexner report was that state medical licensing boards instituted an additional requirement for state licensure: before taking an examination for licensure, an applicant had to be a graduate of an approved medical school. The approval of medical schools was conducted by the AMA's own Council on Medical Education. In the years that followed, as expected, the number of medical schools decreased, from 162 in 1906, to 85 in 1920, to 76 in 1930, to 69 in 1944. The graduates of those medical schools that were closed continued to practice. No attempts were made to rectify any supposed inadequacies in their educational backgrounds. Whenever standards are raised, grandfather clauses protect the rights of existing practitioners, regardless of their abilities. The AMA now had control over entry into the profession in two ways: first, through its Council on Medical Education, the AMA was able to limit the number of approved medical schools and, hence, the number of applicants for licensure exams; second, entrants into the profession then had to pass state licensure exams and any other prerequisites promulgated by the individual state medical licensing boards. Thus the AMA, through its Council on Medical Education, was able to determine the "appropriate" number of physicians in the United States.

The third method used by the medical profession to restrict entry, which is also meant to increase the competence of the new physician, is to lengthen the training time required for the student to become a practicing physician. Before entering medical school, a student has to have four years of undergraduate education. The time spent in internship and residency programs after graduation from medical school continually increases; medical school graduates usually take a three-year residency program. For students desiring to enter certain specialties, more than three years is required. The effect of continually increasing the training required before entering a profession is to raise the costs to the entering student. Not only are tuition costs higher the longer are the requirements for undergraduate and medical school education, but more importantly, the income foregone because of the additional years of training is very large. These increased costs reduce the rate of return to someone entering the medical profession. The emphasis in terms of quality is always on the *entering* physician and not on those currently in the profession. It is in the economic interests of current practitioners that the costs of entering the profession continually increase; since their training occurred in the past at a lower cost, they will receive higher prices and higher incomes in the form of economic rent (6).

If the market for physician services were a competitive one, then the more highly trained physicians could advertise their increased training and more recent knowledge and receive a higher price for their services than physicians without this additional training. In such a competitive situation there would be little economic incentive for current physicians to promote higher training requirements for new physicians; therefore, to prevent new physicians from receiving higher returns than current physicians with less training do, it is necessary for the medical profession to maintain the fiction that *all* physicians are of uniform quality. To enforce this impression among patients, the medical profession discourages any intraprofessional criticism and, until recently, prohibits the advertisement of differences in training or any other quality differentials among physicians. Whether or not persons can perform certain medical tasks depends upon whether they are licensed as physicians, thereby being provided with an unlimited scope of practice, rather than whether they have had certain specialized training. Anesthesiologists, for example, can be physicians who are board certified in anesthesiology, or they can be physicians with additional training but who are not board certified, or they can be physicians without any additional training in anesthesia. It appears that merely being licensed is sufficient to allow physicians to undertake most tasks performed by other physicians who may have additional training.

This third barrier to entry, which takes the form of continual increases in the training costs for entering physicians, suggests that measures to increase the quality of physician services are independent of demands by consumers for increased quality and instead are related to the income considerations of the medical profession.

In addition to barriers to entry, another condition is necessary if physicians are to be able to secure monopoly profits. Unless productivity increases among physicians can be controlled, it would be possible for some physicians to greatly increase their output and thereby decrease the price and output and, consequently, the rate of return to competing physicians. Productivity increases are limited in two ways. First, only licensed physicians are allowed to perform certain tasks, thereby severely limiting the ability of physicians to greatly increase their output by delegating tasks to other personnel. Second, when new types of health personnel, such as physician's assistants, are permitted to undertake certain tasks which were formerly the sole prerogative of the physician, the state boards of medical examiners retain the authority to certify their use on an individual physician-by-physician basis. In this manner, a particular physician would not be able to hire a large number of such personnel and greatly increase his or her output. The medical licensing boards' control over physician's assistants can be used to approve their use in situations where demand for physician services has increased, or where no physicians are available, such as in rural areas; their employment can be limited in cases where physician's practices, from the standpoint of the physicians, are underutilized.

The foregoing methods, which have been used successfully by the medical profession to restrict entry into the profession, have been adapted by other health professions as well. The American Dental Association (ADA), after successfully achieving state licensure of dentists, had a study conducted on dental education, which resulted in the Gies report in the early 1920s. As a result of this report, applicants for state dental examinations had to be graduated from approved dental schools, with the accreditation being conducted by the ADA's own Council on Dental Education. The number of dental schools declined as standards, mandated by the ADA and carried out by its Council, were increased.

The length of the training time to become a dentist has also increased; however, the dental profession has not yet instituted any residency requirements such as exist in medicine.

Increased educational requirements increase the investment cost of becoming a physician, thereby decreasing the rate of return to entering physicians. The extent to which the price of physician services and physicians' incomes will rise in response to higher entry costs and fewer physicians will depend upon the elasticities of the demand and supply of physician services. Barriers to entry in the physician market are consistent with a monopoly model which would confer higher incomes on physicians.

We now turn to an examination of these barriers as a means of protecting the consumer from incompetent providers. For this hypothesis to be an accurate description of the justification for such restrictions, the medical profession, through its representatives in county, state, and national organizations, should favor *all* policies, not just entry barriers, to protect the consumer from incompetent practitioners. If the AMA is not consistent in its support of quality measures and only favors those that favorably affect its members' incomes, while opposing those that adversely affect its members' incomes, then we must conclude that the real motivation for such measures is to enhance the monopoly power of its members.

If the AMA were in favor of protecting consumers from incompetent physicians, then one measure the AMA would be expected to favor would be reexamination and relicensure of physicians. One justification given for increased training requirements for new physicians is that there has been an explosion of medical knowledge. Some physicians received their medical education 30–40 years ago; reexamination and relicensure would insure that existing physicians have kept up with this increase in knowledge. Reexamination for relicensure is required in other areas, such as for renewal of driver licenses, or for commercial airline pilot licenses. There can be little justification for favoring increased training for new physicians but not for existing physicians if improving quality is at issue. Yet the AMA is opposed to reexamination and/or relicensure. If reexamination and relicensure were required, then unless the passing level were set so low that everyone always passed, either large number of physicians would fail the reexamination and be unable to practice, or different levels of licensure would be established to recognize what exists in practice.

Not all physicians should be permitted to undertake all tasks even though they are licensed. With the realization that licensure should exist by tasks or levels would come the recognition that it is possible to prepare for different levels by using different educational requirements. It should be possible to have lower training requirements for some tasks; as the complexity of the task to be performed increased, so would the training requirements. One would expect, therefore, that the number of entrants would be greater, the lower the training requirements. If different levels of licensure were to exist, barriers to entry would be lowered and the incomes of practicing physicians would be decreased. Since such an approach to increasing quality among physicians would decrease the monopoly power of physicians, we would therefore expect the AMA to oppose reexamination and licensure by task.

The emphasis on quality control in medicine is on the "process" of becoming a physician and not on the care that is provided ("outcome") once a person has become a physician. Controlling quality and competency of physicians through process measures which require an undergraduate education, four years of education in an approved medical school, a minimum of three years in residency, and, throughout this period, a series of examinations, is consistent with constructing barriers to entry and raising training costs, which thereby lower the entering physician's rate of return. Once the physician has met all of these requirements, then there is no monitoring of the care he or she provides. Physicians may be well trained at at least one point in time, but this does not mean that they will be ethical. A number of studies document the amount of "unnecessary" surgery; other studies show that more than one-half of all surgery is undertaken by unethical or unqualified practitioners. Virtually no quality control programs have been instituted by the medical profession that are directed toward practicing physicians. It was for precisely this reason that Congress passed the Professional Standards Review Organizations (PSROs) legislation in an attempt to develop peer review mechanisms to monitor the quality of care provided by physicians. The AMA opposed this legislation. If the medical profession were concerned primarily with quality rather than with monopoly power, then one would expect that there would be at least some emphasis on the quality of care provided by practicing physicians.

Requiring citizenship for licensure, as a number of states did (it is now unconstitutional), is another example of the use of entry barriers to becoming a physician to achieve monopoly power instead of promoting quality. If a prospective physician has met all the educational and licensure requirements, then a citizenship requirement can *only* be viewed as a means of preventing entry into the profession by foreign-trained physicians. Although the quality of foreign-trained physicians varies greatly, examinations and other procedures, such as monitoring of care, would be more direct and accurate measures of quality than whether or not the individual is a U.S. citizen.

Similar to the citizenship requirement is the requirement by some professional associations (e.g., state dental associations) of residency in a state before the individual is permitted to practice. A year's residency is imposed on dentists who wish to locate in Hawaii. Such a requirement, in forcing the practitioner to be without income for a year, decreases the attractiveness of locating in that particular location. Such a barrier to entry is unrelated to quality, since it does not differentiate among the educational or performance backgrounds of the individuals wishing to locate there. It is solely a device to enhance the monopoly power of the practicing professionals in that location.

It would appear, therefore, that the concern of the medical profession (as well as of other health professions) with quality is selective. Quality measures that might adversely affect the incomes of their members are opposed, such as reexamination, relicensing, continuing education, and any measures that attempt to monitor the quality of care delivered. The hypothesis that quality measures are instituted to raise the rate of return of practicing physicians appears to be consistent with the positions on quality taken by the medical profession.

It has been claimed that the selective approach to quality favored by the medical profession may have served to actually *lower* the quality of care available to the U.S. population (7). Once entry into a profession is restricted, there is an increase in the growth and use of substitutes for that profession. As entry into medicine is restricted, substitutes for medicine such as chiropractic and faith healers are used.

With higher prices for physician services, people also substitute self-diagnosis and treatment for the physician's services. Some of these alternatives may be of lower quality than if the restrictions on medicine were lower. Fewer, more highly trained physicians means that a smaller percentage of the population will have access to medical care. If only physicians are permitted to perform a number of tasks, even though other trained personnel might be equally capable of performing them, this will again mean that a smaller percentage of the population will have access to such services. A relevant measure of the quality of care in society should not be confined to the care received by only those persons receiving physician services; it should also incorporate the size of the population that does not receive any (or much fewer) physician services or use poorer substitutes.*

The current system of medical licensure, with its attendant requirements and emphasis on entry into the profession, imposes certain "costs" on society. The presumed successes of such a system of licensure in protecting consumers against unethical and incompetent practitioners are uncertain. What is desirable is the least costly system for alleviating consumer uncertainty and for meeting society's demand for protection. Several proposals in this regard will be discussed at the conclusion of this chapter.

THE PHYSICIAN AS A PRICE-DISCRIMINATING MONOPOLIST

The establishment of barriers to entry in medicine provides physicians with a greater rate of return than if such barriers did not exist. However large the economic returns are from monopolizing an industry, the monopolist can earn still greater returns if it is possible to become a price-discriminating monopolist. Profit-maximizing monopolists would charge one price to all of their consumers; that price and the resulting output would be determined by the intersection of their marginal-revenue and marginal-cost curves. This situation is shown in Figure 14-1. The profit-maximizing price and output would be P_0 and Q_0, respectively. The amount of "profit" in this situation is the striped area between marginal revenue (MR) and marginal cost (MC). If, however, the above monopolist is now able to become a price-discriminating monopolist (e.g., first degree) and can charge each patient a separate price, then the monopolist's demand curve is also his marginal-revenue curve. A lower price does not have to be charged to *all* patients to sell more services. If the demand curve is now also the marginal-revenue curve, then with the same marginal-cost curve, the monopolist's profit will have increased: instead of being just the striped area, the profit now in-

*Milton Friedman also states that quality has been adversely affected because there is less experimentation in treatment, which tends to reduce the rate of growth in medical knowledge, since a person desiring to experiment in treatment must be a member of the medical profession. The profession also encourages conformity in medical practice. The medical profession has also discouraged malpractice suits against physicians by discouraging physicians from testifying against one another. This action has also limited the consumer's protection against unethical and incompetent practitioners. The possibility of high malpractice awards against them would discourage incompetent practitioners from practicing, thereby providing protection to future patients.

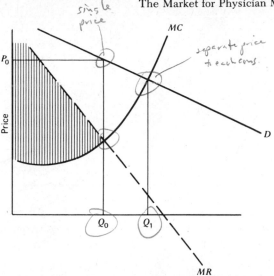

Figure 14-1. Determination of price and output by a profit-maximizing monopolist.

cludes the entire area between the demand and marginal-cost curves. The price-discriminating monopolist's output is also larger (Q_1), since he or she will produce to the point where his or her marginal-cost curve intersects the demand curve, which is equivalent to his or her marginal-revenue curve.

No single price is charged to everyone; the price-discriminating monopolist may charge each patient a different price. Because the profit can be greater if the monopolist can charge different prices to different purchasers for essentially the same service, we would expect monopolists to attempt to become price-discriminating monopolists. Two conditions, however, must be met if price discrimination is to be successfully applied in any market. The first is that the different purchasers of the service must have different elasticities of demand for the same service. Unless the elasticities of demand are different, the profit-maximizing price will be the same for each purchaser. The second condition is that it is necessary to separate the different markets in which the service is sold, so that the purchaser paying a lower price for the service cannot resell it in the higher-priced market. If such markets are not kept separate, then prices will eventually become the same for all purchasers. Figure 14-2 is an illustration of price discrimination. Each diagram represents a different purchaser or market. Assuming a constant and similar marginal-cost curve for serving each market, the profit-maximizing prices would be P_1 and P_2.

In the physician's market we hypothesize that since price discrimination results in greater profits than would result from setting the same price for each purchaser, physicians will attempt to maximize their "profits" by becoming price-discriminating monopolists. The conditions necessary for price discrimination to occur are rather easily met in the physician sector. Patients obviously cannot resell the services they receive, which automatically keeps the markets separate. The elasticities of demand for physician services differ, since persons with higher incomes are willing to pay more than persons with lower incomes for the same services. Ability to pay, however is also affected by the availability of

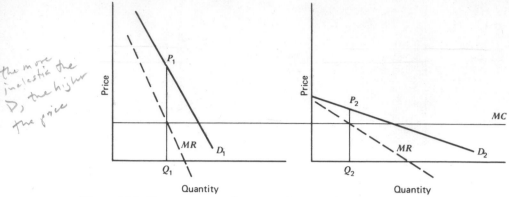

the more the inelastic the D, the higher the price

Figure 14-2. Determination of prices and outputs by a price-discriminating monopolist.

insurance coverage for physician services; thus as insurance coverage for physician services becomes widespread, we expect price discrimination by physicians among their patients to decline.

There is an alternative model to explain physician pricing behavior: differences in prices charged for the same services to different patients means that the physician is acting as a charitable agency. By charging higher prices to those who can afford them, the physician can provide services to persons with lower incomes who cannot afford to pay as much, so the reasoning goes. The physician thus acts as a charitable agency in determining who receives care and how much each is charged. This charity hypothesis has often been used by the medical profession to rationalize the different prices charged for the same services performed. The charity hypothesis would also predict a narrowing over time of the gap in prices charged to different patients. The change will presumably occur when patients with formerly low incomes have increased ability to pay, either as a result of increased income, private insurance coverage, or greater involvement of government in the payment of physician fees.

Each of the two hypotheses—physicians acting either as price-discriminating monopolists or as charitable agencies—suggests that over time there will be a narrowing of fees charged. In one case there will be less of a difference in elasticities of demand as patients' ability to pay increases (hence the profit-maximizing price to both patients is the same).* Under the second hypothesis there is less need to subsidize the lower-income patient by charging a higher

---

*Even with widespread insurance coverage, physicians may still be able to practice price discrimination. When treating a patient, physicians have the option of accepting assignment under Medicare or becoming a participating physician under Blue Shield. Physicians can do so on a case-by-case basis. When the physician either accepts assignment or is a participating physician, he or she agrees to abide by the particular fee schedules. For patients with a greater ability to pay, the physician can decide not to be a participating physician. In this situation the patient pays the physician's fee and applies to either Medicare or Blue Shield for partial reimbursement. The physician receives a greater amount and the patient pays a greater amount out-of-pocket than if the physician accepted assignment or was a participating physician. An illustration of this form of price discrimination was shown earlier in Chapter 9, Figure 9-4.

price to the higher-income patient as lower-income persons' ability to pay increases.

To distinguish between the two hypotheses and test whether physicians have acted as price discriminating monopolists, we would want to examine the past behavior of county and state medical societies. In this way we can determine whether the societies' actions and political positions have consistently been directed toward maintaining a situation which enables individual physicians to price-discriminate. Unless a cartel like organization such as a medical society were able to enforce sanctions against price cutters, price discrimination could not survive in what would otherwise be a competitive market. One might assume that even though entry barriers exist, there is still such a large number of physicians that their market would be a competitive one. If one physician charged a higher price for a given surgical procedure, for example, then other physicians would be able to increase their market share by offering to sell the procedure at a lower price; price discrimination in a competitive situation could not exist. Patients with higher incomes, when charged higher prices, would seek out lower-priced, equally qualified physicians. Prices for medical services would eventually be similar regardless of patient incomes. Differences in price for medical services would be related only to differences in the costs of providing those services and not to differences in the elasticity of demand of the patients. To shed light on the price-discrimination hypothesis of physician pricing, it is necessary to ascertain why, even though there are restrictions on the number of firms (physicians) entering the industry, physician services are not priced as would be expected in a competitive industry. To determine how price discrimination can exist in what could be an essentially competitive industry, we must look for *sanctions* that could be applied to physicians if they were to price their services competitively.

In his classic article entitled "Price Discrimination in Medicine," Reuben Kessel claimed that control over physician pricing behavior was related to the AMA's control over medical education (8). The AMA's control over postgraduate medical training and control over which physicians may take specialty board exams was the source of its control over physicians.

Internship and residency programs are offered only in hospitals approved by the AMA. Physicians want the hospitals they are associated with to be approved for such programs, since interns and residents increase the physician's productivity and income; the availability of interns and residents in a hospital frees up a physician's time both to see more patients and to have more leisure time. Interns and residents are thus demanded by physicians. The hospital pays the salaries of interns and residents, and the physicians receive the benefits of their services as they care for the physicians' patients in the hospital. The Mundt resolution, which was declared unconstitutional in the mid-1960s, required that the entire attending medical staff in the hospital be members in the county medical society if the hospital were to be approved for intern and residency training. Membership in the county medical society thus became important to physicians if they wished to have the hospital privileges which are a necessity for almost all specialties of medicine. Similarly, membership in the county society was a prerequisite for a physician to take examinations for various specialty boards. If a physician engaged in any form of competitive behavior which was branded "unethical," the county medical society, which determines its own rules for membership, could deny such a physician membership in the society and thereby deny hospital privileges.

Those physicians who potentially offer the greatest threat to the existence of price discrimination are new physicians in the community. To establish a market, new firms must advertise their availability, competence, and specialty, and they also must offer lower prices to attract consumers away from established firms. To prevent such competitive behavior from occurring, county medical societies gave new physicians probationary membership. If the new physician engaged in any of the above "unethical" activities to become established in the community, the county medical society would revoke membership and thereby deny hospital privileges to that physician. Probationary status was granted, not just to recent graduates, but also to physicians who had been in practice for a long time in another area (and were members of another county medical society) and had recently moved into the community.

More recently, the sanctions available to the medical societies for use against physicians who wish to compete on price have been state laws which delegate authority to medical licensing boards to determine the conditions for medical licensure. Included in such state laws were severe penalties for advertising and fee splitting. Although the mechanism for inhibiting price competition among physicians has shifted from control over hospital privileges by county medical societies to state laws which prohibit such behavior, the effect has been the same. Strong sanctions and penalties were available to organized medicine (which may be viewed in this instance as a cartel) to inhibit price competition, which would have eroded the physician's ability to price-discriminate.

What is the evidence to support the price-discrimination hypothesis of physician pricing? Does the evidence indicate that the foregoing sanctions were consistently imposed on physicians who attempted to engage in price competition rather than imposed for "quality" reasons? The AMA's position with regard to health insurance is the first evidence Kessel examines in his test of the price-discrimination hypothesis. Insurance coverage to pay for physician services would generally be favored by physicians, since it increased both the demand for physician services and the patient's ability to pay for those services. Health insurance varies with regard to the manner in which the physician is reimbursed. Indemnity plans reimburse the patient a certain dollar amount and allow the physician to charge the patient whatever he or she believes the patient can pay. Such plans are the most conducive to price discrimination by physicians. Health insurance plans that guarantee medical services rather than dollars if the consumer becomes ill would be opposed by the medical profession because they are sold at the same price to consumers regardless of their incomes. Such plans are a form of price competition, since a person with a high income can purchase the same medical services at the same price as could a person with a low income. If the charity hypothesis were the more accurate explanation of physician pricing behavior, then medical societies would not be expected to oppose such plans. The only conceivable reason for the medical profession's opposition to such medical service plans is that they undercut the ability of physicians to price-discriminate in the communities where such plans exist. Examples of such medical service plans are prepaid group practices (PPGPs) where the consumer pays a yearly capitation fee, regardless of family income, and is then entitled both to hospital and medical services when ill. It is interesting, therefore, to examine the sanctions that local medical societies have applied to prevent the development of PPGPs.

The opposition mounted by organized medicine against PPGPs was unaffected by the location of these plans or their sponsorship. The first type of sanction aimed at putting such plans out of business was to deny the physicians associated with them hospital privileges. If the physician was already a member of the county medical society, the medical society would disband and reestablish itself without including the particular physician. New physicians entering the area with the intention of joining a PPGP in the community would not be permitted to join the county medical society. Whether or not a PPGP had its own hospital determined whether it was able to survive. It is for this reason that Kaiser Foundation, a well-known PPGP on the West Coast, operated its own hospitals; otherwise, it could not have offered hospital care to its subscribers and would not have been able to compete. The county medical societies tried other tactics against the Kaiser Foundation. The State Board of Medical Examiners in California tried Dr. Garfield, the medical director of Kaiser, for unprofessional conduct and suspended his license to practice. In subsequent legal rulings the suspension was overruled; the board's action was considered arbitrary in that Dr. Garfield did not have a fair trial.

Another approach used by the medical societies to inhibit the development of PPGPs was to have a higher proportion of physicians who belonged to PPGPs drafted during World War II. (The medical society played a strong role with regard to the drafting of physicians at that time.) A number of physicians serving during World War II were unable to qualify as officers in the Navy and had to serve as enlisted men because they could not obtain a letter from their county medical society stating that they were members in good standing. These physicians believed they were discriminated against because they were associated with PPGPs. In other instances where the local medical societies ousted physicians belonging to PPGPs, successful lawsuits were brought against the medical societies under the Sherman Anti-Trust Act (9).

In addition to attempting to terminate PPGPs through the use of sanctions against physicians associated with them, medical societies attempted to legislate them out of business. State medical societies sponsored legislation in many states, and were successful in more than 20 of them, which placed restrictions on PPGPs, thereby inhibiting their growth. Such restrictive statutes permitted only the medical profession to operate or to control prepaid medical plans. (Federal legislation on health maintenance organizations specifically preempted such restrictive statutes if the HMO qualified under the federal HMO law.)

Another example of the medical profession's interest in maintaining the physician's ability to price-discriminate among patients is the type of medical insurance plan favored by organized medicine. Blue Shield plans, which were developed and controlled by state medical societies, offered physician coverage to consumers under the following terms: if a subscriber's income was less than a certain amount, generally $7,500 a year, then the participating physician would accept the Blue Shield fee as full payment for services provided to the patient; however, if the patient's income was in excess of the stated amount, then the physician could bill the patient an amount in excess of the Blue Shield fee for that service. The medical profession favored Blue Shield because physicians would be assured of payment from low-income subscribers and would still be able to price-discriminate among higher-income subscribers. If the physicians were charitable agencies, then they would not need to charge higher-income patients an additional amount once the lower-income patient was able to pay the full fee for their services. Some medical societies have recently dropped their sponsorship of Blue Shield plans because the plans wished to raise the income limits below which the Blue Shield fee would represent full payment for the patient's use of physician services.

Additional evidence that the charity hypothesis is inapplicable to explain physician pricing behavior is provided in the following statement by Kessel:

> Most of the "free" care that was traditionally provided by the medical profession fell into three categories: (1) work done by neophytes, particularly in the surgical specialties, who wanted to develop their skills and therefore require practice; (2) services of experienced physicians in free clinics who wish to develop new skills or maintain existing skills so they can better serve their private, paying patients; and (3) services to maintain staff and medical appointments which are of great value financially. The advent of Medicare has reduced the availability of "charity" patients used as teaching material, and has led to readjustments in training procedures, particularly for residents. (10)

The sanctions available to the medical profession to prevent price competition have changed over time. Advertising can no longer be prohibited by state practice acts. That the medical profession had been successful in inhibiting price competition is evidenced by the recently successful suit brought by the Federal Trade Commission (FTC) against the AMA and several medical specialty societies. The FTC claimed that the AMA's "Principles of Medical Ethics," which banned advertising, price competition, and other forms of competitive practices, resulted in a situation in which "prices of physician services have been stabilized, fixed, or otherwise interfered with; competition between medical doctors in the provision of such services has been hindered, restrained, foreclosed and frustrated; and consumers have been deprived of information pertinent to the selection of a physician and of the benefits of competition" (11).

The medical profession, then, has been successful in acting in the economic interest of its members. The continually high rates of return to an investment in a medical education and the excess of applicants to acceptances in medical schools are evidence that there has been a static shortage of physicians. To ensure monopoly profits over time, the medical profession has constructed barriers to entry into the profession. Under the guise of controlling quality of care and eliminating unqualified professionals the medical profession emphasized "process" measures of quality control. Quality assurance was present only at the point of entry into the profession by means of requiring attendance at an approved medical school, licensure examinations, and longer minimum times spent in postgraduate training programs; virtually no quality control measures were directed at practicing physicians.

With the authority delegated to it by the state, the medical profession was then able to go beyond establishing a simple monopoly. The medical profession, acting as a cartel to protect the economic interests of its members, was able to establish and enforce the necessary conditions to enable physicians to price-discriminate among their patients. The sanctions used by the medical profession against members who participated in prepaid medical plans were severe enough to retard the development of such organizations for many years. The consequences to society of these actions by organized medicine are that prices of medical services are higher than they would otherwise be, the availability of such services is lower, and, importantly, consumers are not as well protected from unqualified and unethical practitioners as they have been led to believe.

PROPOSED CHANGES IN THE PHYSICIAN MANPOWER MARKET

The objective of proposing changes in the market for physicians is twofold: first, the demand for consumer protection should be achieved in the least costly manner possible, and second, the market for physicians should perform efficiently. The key to improving market performance is to deal first with the concern for consumer protection.

ENTRY INTO THE MEDICAL PROFESSION

If a prospective physician can pass the licensing examination, it is not clear why he or she also has to have attended an approved medical school to be licensed. The only logical reason for also requiring attendance at an approved medical school is that the licensing examination is not a sufficient assurance of the physician's knowledge. If this is the case, then the examination process should be improved and less emphasis placed on the number of years of education required and on attendance at approved schools.

A second approach to lowering the cost of licensure, while also achieving a certain performance level of entering physicians, is to have "task" licensure. Currently physicians are either licensed or they are not, and, once licensed, they are permitted to undertake many tasks, the full scope of medical practice, a number of which they might not be well trained for, such as in the case of the family practitioner who performs general surgery. Instead of such a "zero–one" level of licensure, physicians should be licensed to perform specific tasks. Such task or specific-purpose licenses would recognize what exists in the real world; namely, even though physicians are licensed, the public would be better protected if they performed only those tasks which they are qualified to perform. Task licensure would mean that all physicians would not need to take the same educational training; it might be possible to provide alternative levels of training (or train certain types of physicians) in a much shorter period, which would lower the costs of producing them, since both their educational and opportunity costs would be reduced. If physicians wanted to receive additional specific-purpose licenses, they could return to school to receive additional training before taking the licensure examination for that license. (In this way a career ladder could be developed for medicine.) Under such a proposal, the training requirements to enter the medical profession would not be determined by the medical profession itself but would be related to the *demand* for different types of physicians and the least costly manner of producing them.

CONTINUING ASSURANCE OF THE QUALITY
OF PHYSICIAN SERVICES

As discussed earlier, beyond the licensing of a physician the medical profession undertakes virtually no quality assurance mechanisms. Several proposals to deal with the issue of unethical and unqualified physicians should be considered. First, periodic reexamination and relicensure would require physicians to keep up with their field of practice. Rather than mandating a certain number of hours of continuing education, reexamination would determine the appropriate amount of continuing education on an individual basis. It would also be a more direct measure of whether or not the physician has achieved the objectives of continuing education. Periodic reexamination and relicensure would be consistent with the earlier proposal of task or "specific-purpose" licensure.

If physicians were reexamined and relicensed every few years for specific-purpose licenses, we would have greater assurance that physicians were practicing in the fields of medicine for which they were qualified. There would still be a concern, however, regarding the physician who may be qualified but is unethical in performing services that are not needed and in charging for services not performed. Continual monitoring of the care provided by physicians, with a state agency taking responsibility (with the cooperation of the medical profession), would help to ensure that a minimum of unethical and unqualified actions were undertaken. Penalties assessed by state quality review agencies should be financial and should vary according to the severity of the misbehavior. Penalties that remove or suspend the physician's license are usually considered to be so severe that they are rarely undertaken. Financial penalties would be more likely to be imposed for actions that are not sufficiently flagrant to call for removal of the physician's license but are in need of redress.

Another approach that was developed to safeguard consumers is recourse to the courts, but because malpractice premiums have risen so rapidly recently, proposals have been made to remove the threat of malpractice. Suggestions have been made that the government should pay malpractice premiums for those physicians participating in government programs such as Medicare and Medicaid. The desired effect of such a proposal is to increase physician participation in government medical programs; however, it would negate the relationship between physicians' performance and their malpractice premiums. There are problems associated with the current system of malpractice, such as the uncertainty of future awards, but it would be preferable to improve the current malpractice system rather than do away with it. A well-functioning malpractice system would serve as an incentive to physicians to confine themselves to tasks they are qualified to perform (12).

Now that advertising among physicians and other health professions has been made possible as a result of the FTC action, consumers should begin to have access to greater information on physician qualifications, fees, and availability. One other reform that would improve the performance of the medical profession is to allow productivity increases to occur independent of the permission of the medical profession. Productivity increases through the use of physician's assistants and other paraprofessionals would increase the supply of physician services at a lower cost and in a shorter period than if all tasks had to be performed by highly trained physicians with training requirements in excess of those required for competency. Such productivity increases, occurring at a time of increased supply of physicians, would be strongly resisted by organized medicine. Some physicians will have excess capacity while other physicians will seek to expand their services by employing nonphysician personnel.

Advertising and unlimited productivity increases should create a competitive atmosphere among physicians that should improve the level of consumer protection while increasing the availability of physician services and lowering prices. In conjunction with these proposals, permitting the corporate practice of medicine through HMOs and PPGPs and experimenting with the concept of institutional responsibility for quality of care should result in far-reaching changes leading to improvement in the organization and delivery of medical care.

REFERENCES

1. Thomas G. Moore, "The Purpose of Licensing," *Journal of Law and Economics*, October 1961.

2. Reuben Kessel, "Price Discrimination in Medicine," *Journal of Law and Economics*, October 1958, pp. 25–26.

3. Milton Friedman, *Capitalism and Freedom* (Chicago: The University of Chicago Press, 1962), p. 151.

4. Kessel, "Price Discrimination," p. 27.

5. *Ibid.*

6. This aspect of licensing board behavior is discussed in Simon Rottenberg, "Economics of Occupational Licensing," in *Aspects of Labor Economics,* National Bureau of Economic Research (Princeton, N.J.: Princeton University Press, 1962).

7. Friedman, *Capitalism and Freedom,* pp. 155–158.

8. Kessel, "Price Discrimination," p. 29.

9. This example of Group Health Association in Washington, D.C., and the other examples cited are from Kessel, "Price Discrimination," pp. 30–41.

10. Reuben Kessel, "The AMA and the Supply of Physicians," *Law and Contemporary Problems* (Chapel Hill, N.C.: Duke University Press, 1970), p. 273.

11. United States of America Before Federal Trade Commission in the Matter of the American Medical Association, a corporation, The Connecticut State Medical Society, a corporation, The New Haven County Medical Association, Inc., Docket No. 9064, p. 3, December 1975.

12. For some readings on malpractice, see: Simon Rottenberg, ed., *The Economics of Medical Malpractice* (Washington, D.C.: American Enterprise Institute for Public Policy Research, 1978). Also see: William B. Schwartz and Neil K. Komesar, *Doctors, Damages and Deterrence: An Economic View of Medical Malpractice,* Rand Corporation Publication, R-2340-NIH/RC, June 1978; and Clark C. Havighurst, "Medical Adversity Insurance—Has Its Time Come?," *Duke Law Journal* 6 (1975).

CHAPTER 15

The Market for Medical Education: Equity and Efficiency

In Chapter 14 it was shown that barriers to entry into medicine contribute significantly to the high rate of return from becoming a physician. Perhaps the most important barrier to entry into the health professions is the requirement of having graduated from an approved educational institution. Since such educational institutions determine the number of new graduates, it is important to examine the performance of the medical education sector. Medical schools, dental schools, and other health professional education institutions are the main determinants of the number of health professionals in the United States. They have also been the recipients of large sums of federal and state monies. Because of their combined role as the only approved health professional training institutions, as the determinants of the number of health professionals, and as the recipients of public funds, their performance should be examined in terms of 1) the economic efficiency with which this sector performs and 2) whether there are any redistributive effects (the equity issue) in the manner in which this sector is financed.

THE ECONOMIC EFFICIENCY
OF THE MEDICAL EDUCATION SECTOR

Every market performs certain functions; we are interested in two aspects of efficiency with respect to medical (and other health) education. First, is the industry producing an "optimal" number of health professionals? The appropriate or optimal rate of output in medical (or other health professional) education is concerned with both the number of graduates and their type, i.e., the level of

396

training. Second, is the output (a physician or other health professional) being produced at minimum cost? Efficiency in production is judged on the basis of the extent of economies of scale in medical education (the number of schools) and whether each school is minimizing its costs.

To establish an appropriate yardstick by which to evaluate the performance of the medical education sector, we turn to a model of a purely competitive market. In examining the medical education sector as if it were similar to a competitive market, we look for any divergences between a competitive market and the current system of medical education to determine the reasons (and justification) for such differences. Using the yardstick of a competitive model and any possible economic rationales for differences between the two, we will evaluate the performance of the market for medical education and, if need be, offer proposals for improving its performance.

MEDICAL EDUCATION IN A COMPETITIVE MARKET

Both economic and noneconomic determinants affect the demand for a medical education. The major economic determinant of an investment in a medical education is the expected rate of return. One component of the rate of return is the price, or tuition, of a medical education. If other factors such as physician incomes and the opportunity cost of attending medical school are held constant, a change in the tuition level would cause a movement along the demand curve for a medical education. If physician incomes were to increase, or if the opportunity cost of attending medical school were to decrease, then these changes would cause a shift (to the right) in the demand for a medical education. Tuition, in a competitive market, would be the equilibrating mechanism. In the short run, with a given stock of medical education capacity, changes in demand for a medical education would cause a shift along a given supply curve of medical education; the tuition level would rise, and at the higher levels of tuition all those demanding a medical education would receive it. The level of tuition would serve as a rationing device and there would be no excess demand (applicants over acceptances). The demand and the supply of medical education would jointly determine the number of enrollments and the tuition level.

The supply response in a competitive market would be as follows. In the short run, each medical school facing an increased demand for its spaces would raise its prices (tuition). The higher tuition levels would enable the schools to attract more resources, namely to hire additional faculty by raising salaries. As a response to higher tuition levels, more medical schools might also be started. The long-run effect of the increased tuition would be increased medical school capacity. It would not be necessary for each school to increase its capacity; some schools might prefer to remain small and offer a "higher"-quality product than other schools, such as more inputs per student or longer training times. Tuition levels in such schools would be higher than in those schools that had much larger class sizes and lower training requirements. Whether or not such differences in types of schools could exist would depend upon whether there was a demand on the part of students for such differences in the quality of education. Presumably, just as there are differences in tuition levels and in the perceived quality of undergraduate and graduate schools, there would be a demand for different types of medical education at different levels of tuition. In a competitive system, as in pre-Flexnerian days, the graduates of the diverse educational institutions would have to pass a licensing examination. Some schools would have a much higher passing rate for their graduates than would other schools. Presumably, the schools would advertise such differences as they would their tuition levels and other educational requirements.*

Not all schools under such a competitive situation would be for-profit. Some schools might be nonprofit and have objectives similar to those of medical schools today, such as prestige maximization. As long as entry was permitted into the medical education market, differences in a school's "product"—educational requirements, pass rate on licensing examinations, and the perceived quality of that institution—would have to justify the higher input costs that would in turn be passed on to prospective students in the form of higher tuition levels. Unless students (or their parents) were willing to pay for such differences in quality, these educational institutions would either exit from the industry or, more likely, change their product to conform to what was being demanded.

The supply side of the medical education sector, then, would consist of many firms; economies of scale in medical education such as in library and clinical facilities are not large enough to result in only one school's being sufficiently lower in cost to preclude competition from other firms. Further, it would be expected that the schools would take advantage of any economies of scale that might exist in medical education, since that would improve their competitive position. Each school, in addition to moving to that size of operation that was of lowest per unit cost (for the type of product it was producing), would also attempt to minimize its own costs of operation. Again, the incentives for cost minimization would come either from the school's desire to increase its revenues or from competition from other schools offering prospective students lower tuition levels. Needless to say, schools would be forced to compete among themselves for prospective students.

Thus, a competitive system in medical education, with the only entry barrier into the profession being a licensing examination, would result in a system of medical schools offering a variety of medical education (different training times, different input ratios of faculty to students, and so on) at tuition levels reflecting the minimum costs of producing the different levels of "quality" of education. In a system of education where differences in inputs and outputs were permitted, there would presumably be a higher rate of innovation in teaching methods and curriculum than in a system where inputs and outputs of the educational process were highly structured and little deviation from the norm exists. Such a system should result in efficiency in production, both for the individual school and for the system as a whole.

A competitive system in medical education, as just described, would also result in production of the "optimal" number of medical school graduates. The

---

*Not all professional schools are considered to be similar. Graduates from the Harvard and Stanford business schools are in greater demand than graduates from other business schools. The job opportunities for graduates of law school are also dissimilar. A similar quality spectrum would exist among medical schools. Graduates from higher-quality medical schools would, in addition to having higher pass rates on licensing exams, also find it easier to enter certain residency programs and to gain admission to the staff of certain hospitals.

optimal number of medical school graduates, according to economic criteria, would occur when the benefits of a medical education to the student equaled the costs of that education. The demand for a medical education, at a given level of tuition, would represent the perceived private benefits of that education to the student; tuition would also reflect the costs of producing that education. As the equilibrating mechanism under such a system, tuition would reflect both the costs of producing the education and the benefits received from it. The resulting number of medical school graduates would therefore be optimal, inasmuch as the costs of education would equal the benefits from it.

It may be argued that the private benefits under such a system are less than the social benefits of having a greater number of physicians in society. Under such a circumstance the number of physicians would be too few. If there are external benefits to having a greater number of physicians (this will be discussed shortly), then subsidies can be provided under a competitive system to increase the demand for a medical education. The subsidies can be given directly to students, which, in lowering their tuition, would increase their demand, or they can be provided to the suppliers. If given directly to the students, students would still have an incentive to seek out those medical schools that will provide them with the type of education they desire, at minimum cost.

The foregoing scenario describes how a competitive system for medical education would perform in achieving, at minimum cost, the optimal rate of output of medical school graduates and the different levels of quality in medical education. The crucial role of tuition in this scenario is in equilibrating demand and supply and providing signals to both the demanders and suppliers of medical education.

THE CURRENT MARKET FOR MEDICAL EDUCATION

Tuition, under the current system of medical education, does not serve as an equilibrating mechanism. Medical schools, on the average, receive only 5 percent of their income from tuition payment, as shown in Table 15-1. (For public medical schools tuition is only 2.8 percent of their income while for private schools it is 8.7 percent.) Further, for many medical schools, the amount of funds they receive from the university with which they are associated is unrelated to changes in their enrollment levels. Since medical schools are not very reliant on tuition as a source of revenue, it is not necessary for them to respond to changes in demand for a medical education. They are able to survive and to produce the type of medical education they want to because they receive large, relatively unrestricted, government subsidies. (Revenues from state and local governments represent 34 percent of public medical schools unrestricted support.) The large educational subsidies received by the schools (and research grants and contracts that have also been used to subsidize educational activities) permit the schools to set tuition levels below actual costs of production. According to a study by the Institute of Medicine (IOM) and calculations performed by George Wright, tuition and fees covered less than 10 percent of the cost of education in 1972 (1). When these figures are updated to 1980, tuition and fees consist of approximately 17 percent of the cost of education (2).

TABLE 15-1. Patterns of Support for General Operations of Public and Private Medical Schools, 1968–1969, 1973–1974, and 1979–1980 (Millions of Dollars)

	Years		
	1968–1969	*1973–1974*	*1979–1980*
Public Schools			
Number of medical schools reporting	47	62	73
Total unrestricted support[a]	$305 (48.0)	$732 (55.0)	$2,076 (62.7)
State and local government appropriations and subsidies	171 (26.9)	448 (34.0)	1,078 (33.9)
Professional fee (medical service plan) income	38 (6.0)	121 (9.2)	359 (11.3)
Recovery of indirect cost on contracts and grants	38 (6.0)	61 (4.6)	105 (3.3)
Tuition and fees	16 (2.5)	35 (2.6)	89 (2.8)
Income from college services	3 (0.5)	17 (1.3)	36 (1.1)
Endowment income	1 (0.2)	3 (0.2)	2 (0.1)
Gifts	2 (0.3)	6 (0.5)	31 (1.0)
Hospitals and clinics			191 (6.0)
Other income	36 (5.7)	41 (3.1)	185 (5.8)
Total public schools support	635 (100.0)	1,321 (100.0)	3,178 (100.0)
Private Schools			
Number of medical schools reporting	44	45	46
Total unrestricted support[a]	$272 (37.2)	$473 (39.3)	$1,240 (50.9)
State and local government appropriations and subsidies	17 (2.4)	51 (4.3)	82 (3.3)
Professional fee (medical service plan) income	28 (3.8)	80 (6.6)	311 (12.3)
Recovery of indirect cost on contract and grants	56 (7.7)	100 (8.3)	215 (8.5)
Tuition and fees	36 (4.9)	77 (6.4)	219 (8.7)
Income from college services	19 (2.6)	47 (3.9)	23 (0.9)
Endowment income	31 (4.2)	44 (3.6)	52 (2.1)
Gifts	21 (2.9)	23 (1.9)	49 (1.9)
Hospitals and clinics			189 (9.7)
Other income	64 (8.8)	51 (4.3)	100 (4.0)
Total private school support	731 (100.0)	1,204 (100.0)	2,523 (100.0)
Total medical school support private and public	$1,366	$2,524	$5,701

Source: American Medical Association, *Journal of the American Medical Association*, December 25, 1981: 2929. Copyright 1981, American Medical Association.

[a]The remainder of medical school support is restricted support (this represents funds mandated for specific projects, or purposes). Restricted support was 52 percent in 1968–1969, for public schools, and it declined to 37.3 percent in 1979–1980. For private schools, restricted support was 62.8 percent of total support in 1968–1969. It declined to 49.1 percent of private support in 1979–1980. The sum of restricted and unrestricted support for all schools increased from $1.4 billion to $5.7 billion over the period 1968–1969 to 1979–1980.

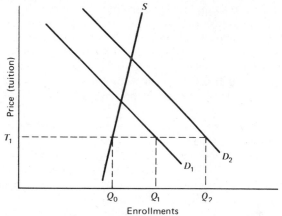

Figure 15-1. The excess demand for a medical education.

The effect of subsidized tuition levels on the demand for a medical education is to cause demand to be greater than it would otherwise be. The increased demand for a medical education resulting from the subsidized tuition is, however, not satisfied. The number of applicants admitted by the medical schools is determined by the number of available spaces. The number of spaces, in turn, is unrelated to the demand for a medical education or to tuition levels; the number is determined by the goals and objectives of the schools themselves. There is thus a continual excess demand for medical education by qualified students, given the increasing rates of return to a career in medicine and subsidized tuition.* This situation is shown schematically in Figure 15-1. With an initial demand for medical education shown by the demand curve D_1, and the supply of spaces shown by S, the amount of excess demand for medical school spaces would be $Q_1 - Q_0$, when the tuition level is T_1, which is below the equilibrium level. As physician incomes increase (or other demand shift variables change), there is an increase in the demand for a medical education to D_2. Again, since tuition does not serve its rationing function, the excess demand for a medical education increases to $Q_2 - Q_0$.

On what basis does the medical school ration its spaces, since it does not rely on tuition to perform this function? It is hypothesized that the medical school will select those students who are most compatible with the goals of the school. Because all approved medical schools are nonprofit, they must have an objective other than trying to make the most money. It is hypothesized that their objective is one of prestige maximization, which is accomplished by retaining a faculty that is interested in research, a low student-faculty ratio that allows more time for research, and training medical students to be teachers and researchers rather than family practitioners. The average medical school is likely to try to emulate Johns Hopkins and Harvard medical schools, with their small class sizes, low

*One study suggests that there are two qualified applicants for each space in medical school. *Report of the National Advisory Commission on Health Manpower*, Vol. I (Washington, D.C.: Government Printing Office, 1967), p. 17.

student-faculty ratios, and emphasis on research. To achieve these goals, medical schools and their faculties want to select students based on high academic qualifications rather than on their future work preferences, such as for working in rural areas. (There is little prestige among medical schools in having the highest percentage of its graduates become primary care practitioners in a rural area.) The excess of applicants resulting from setting tuition levels below the equilibrium level allows the faculty to select those students who most closely correspond to their goals.*

Attaining the goal of prestige maximization requires medical schools to be free from competitive pressures. If a school has to compete, then, as we have seen in the discussion of the competitive model, it will be forced to respond to the demands of the students. Essential to freeing the school from competition are huge outside subsidies that relieve the school of reliance on tuition as a sole source of revenue. Also important are limits on entry into the medical school market by new medical schools that might have different objectives. The manner in which this restriction is achieved is through the accreditation process of new medical schools. It would be very difficult for a new medical school to start if its stated intention was to produce its graduates in a vastly shorter time period, using a different curriculum and different input ratios to train its students. Because it might produce graduates at a much lower cost with the same probability of their passing the licensing examination, such a school would be a potential threat to other schools, and therefore it would be in the other schools' interests to see that such a school was not allowed to start.

What are the consequences of the current system for producing physicians? On the supply side of the market, the educational requirements for producing physicians are determined by the suppliers themselves without regard to demands for such an education. The product is relatively standard and many years of education are required: four years of undergraduate education before admission to a four-year medical school. The product is relatively costly to produce and there are large variations among schools in their costs of production (3). There are strong indications from the wide variations in the cost data that the schools are not minimizing their cost of production, nor do they have any incentive to do so as long as they are the recipients of large government subsidies. It thus appears that efficiency in production is the exception rather than the rule.

It is also highly unlikely that the appropriate number of graduates is produced through the current system of medical education. Since tuition is set way below the actual costs of education, the demand is much greater than it might otherwise be. (Although the price elasticity of demand for a medical education with respect to the tuition rate has been estimated to be approximately $-.4$, i.e., price inelastic, (4) if tuition were to reflect the actual costs of production, demand for such an education would be less than it currently is.) The number of medical

---

*It has also been claimed that the reduction in the number of medical schools as a result of the Flexner report and the consequent excess demand for spaces enabled medical schools to discriminate against certain population groups in society, i.e., Jews, negroes, and women. Reuben Kessel, "The AMA and the Supply of Physicians," *Law and Contemporary Problems*, Duke University, Spring 1970, pp. 270–272. In the *Report of the President's Commission on Higher Education* in 1947 the "Commission concluded that a substantial part of the responsibility for the discriminatory practices of medical schools belongs to the professional associations," Kessel, *ibid.*, p. 274.

school spaces is unrelated to the demand for such spaces. The number of medical school spaces has increased very slowly over time. As shown in Table 15-2, between 1946 and 1947 and 1966 and 1967, the number of medical school enrollments increased by less than 2.0 percent per year. Throughout this period there were continual excess demands for medical school spaces. The number of physicians produced could not have been related to society's demands, or even private demands, for physicians. The number of physicians was determined by the suppliers of education, either in conjunction with other organizations' requirements or solely in response to their own.*

The result of the constraint on the number of medical school spaces was twofold. First, there was a large demand by American students for a foreign medical education. Large numbers of qualified, but rejected, medical school applicants went overseas to study medicine and then reentered the United States to practice. These American students were willing to pay a much higher tuition level in places such as Guadalajara, Mexico, to spend additional years in residence (thereby increasing their opportunity costs), and to receive an education considered inferior to that received in U.S. medical schools. Second, as a result of increased demands for medical care during this period, the rates of return for practicing medicine were much greater in the U.S. than in other countries; consequently there was a large influx of foreign medical graduates (FMGs) into this country. These FMGs came predominately from less-developed countries to work on hospital staffs, and, in many cases, they provided the medical care for the urban poor in the United States.

The U.S. Congress reacted to demands by U.S. citizens for a medical education and also to stem the inflow of foreign-trained physicians by passing the Health Professions Educational Assistance Act (HPEA) in the mid-1960s. The effect of this Act was to increase the supply of medical school spaces. It was, therefore, the perception of Congress that the medical education market was not producing an appropriate number of physicians. To achieve an increase in the supply of physicians, funds were provided for new medical schools and existing medical schools received capitation funds on the condition that they increase their enrollments. Although the AMA and medical schools opposed mandatory enrollment increases, medical schools were in need of additional funds. The Congressional financial incentives to medical schools proved to be effective. As a result of the HPEA legislation, enrollments and graduates began to increase. In 1965–1966 there were 32,835 medical students in 88 medical schools. By 1980–1981, the number of students doubled to 65,497 and the number of schools increased to 126 (see Table 15-2). The consequence of this increase in medical school enrollment was to cause a 50 percent increase in the number of physicians between 1965 and 1980. Between 1980 and 1990 the number of physicians is expected to increase by an additional 36 percent (5).

By the late 1970s, these large projected increases in the supply of physicians led to a concern, particularly among organized medicine and government, that

---

*The goals of the medical schools appear to have been synonymous with the objectives of the American Medical Association. The AMA also prefers small additions to the stock of physicians. It is therefore in the AMA's interest that medical schools be nonprofit. The schools' incentive thereby changes from desiring to increase the number of their graduates to becoming prestigious.

TABLE 15-2. U.S. Medical School Enrollment, First-Year Students and Graduates, 1946–1947 to 1980–1981

| Academic Year | Students[a] | | | Number of Schools |
	Total	First-Year	Graduates	
1946–1947	23,900	6,564	6,389	77
1947–1948	22,739	6,487	5,543	77
1948–1949	23,670	6,688	5,094	78
1949–1950	25,103	7,042	5,553	79
1950–1951	26,186	7,177	6,135	79
1951–1952	27,076	7,436	6,080	79
1952–1953	27,688	7,425	6,668	79
1953–1954	28,227	7,449	6,861	80
1954–1955	28,583	7,576	6,977	81
1955–1956	28,639	7,686	6,845	82
1956–1957	29,130	8,014	6,796	85
1957–1958	29,473	8,030	6,861	85
1958–1959	29,614	8,128	6,860	85
1959–1960	30,084	8,173	7,081	85
1960–1961	30,288	8,298	6,994	86
1961–1962	31,078	8,483	7,168	87
1962–1963	31,491	8,642	7,264	87
1963–1964	32,001	8,772	7,336	87
1964–1965	32,428	8,856	7,409	88
1965–1966	32,835	8,759	7,574	88
1966–1967	33,423	8,964	7,743	89
1967–1968	34,538	9,479	7,973	94
1968–1969	35,833	9,863	8,059	99
1969–1970	37,669	10,401	8,367	101
1970–1971	40,487	11,348	8,974	103
1971–1972	43,650	12,361	9,551	108
1972–1973	47,546	13,726	10,391	112
1973–1974	50,886	14,185	11,613	114
1974–1975	54,074	14,963	12,714	114
1975–1976	56,244	15,351	13,561	114
1976–1977	58,266	15,667	13,607	116
1977–1978	60,456	16,134	14,393	122
1978–1979	62,754	16,620	14,966	125
1979–1980	64,195	17,014	15,135	126
1980–1981	65,497	17,204	15,667	126

Sources: American Medical Association, *Journal of the American Medical Association* 226 (November 19, 1973): 910; and 246 (December 25, 1981): 2917. Copyright 1973, 1981, American Medical Association.

[a]Before 1956–1957, schools in development were not included. For 1973–1974, Harvard University did not provide enrollment data.

"too many" physicians were being produced. As a result, the preferential immigration treatment for FMGs was removed, making it more difficult for FMGs to enter this country, and the HPEA financial assistance to medical schools began to be phased out in the early 1980s.

EFFICIENCY, EXTERNALITIES, AND THE OPTIMAL NUMBER OF PHYSICIANS

The optimal quantity of output in an industry occurs when the cost of producing that last unit equals the additional benefits of consuming it. The price people are willing to pay for that output is an indication of the marginal benefits they hope to receive from consuming it. When price is equal to marginal cost, as would occur in a competitive market, then the marginal private benefits equal the marginal private costs of production, and the optimal quantity of that good or service is produced (assuming no external effects). Those persons receiving the benefits of the good or service are paying the full costs of producing it. When this concept is applied to the number of physicians, the optimal number of physicians' will be produced when the cost of producing physicians is equal to the price (tuition) of a medical education. The price that a student is willing to pay for a medical education reflects the private benefits the student hopes to receive as a result of that education. If the price prospective students are willing to pay for a medical education is greater than the price charged for a medical education, then too few physicians are being produced. More resources should flow into that industry until the cost of producing additional physicians equals the price students are willing to pay for that education.

Under the current system of medical education, however, the costs of producing physicians are greater than they would be in a system where there were fewer artificial educational requirements, such as minimum years required both before entering and during medical school, and where incentives for efficiency were not lacking. Even if the price charged for a medical education were equal to the higher costs of a medical education, too few physicians would be produced under the conditions of the present system. The price students would be willing to pay for a medical education (reflecting their expected marginal private benefits) should be equal to the minimum costs of producing a physician. If the price is not, additional physicians could be produced if the producers were more efficient.

It has been alleged, however, that in addition to the private benefits gained by the student receiving medical education, there are benefits to the public at large from having a greater number of physicians (6). According to this argument, basing the demand for a medical education on just the private benefits to be received by students would result in too low an estimate of the demands for medical education. The existence of additional benefits, to be received by persons other than students, would result in a greater demand for a medical education when added to the private demand by students. For example, as shown in Figure 15-2, *MPB* represents the marginal private benefits received by students from a medical education. *MPC* represents the marginal private costs of producing additional physicians. The intersection of these marginal private benefit and cost curves would result in Q_0 number of physicians. Q_0 physicians is believed

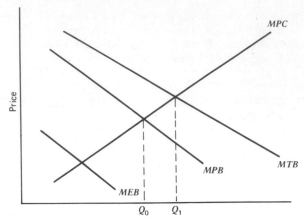

Figure 15-2. An illustration of external benefits in medical education.

by some persons to be a nonoptimal number, i.e., too few, because the external benefits to others from having physicians represented by *MEB* are excluded from this calculation. If these external benefits are included, then the sum of both the private and external benefits, shown by the line *MTB*, would intersect the *MPC* curve at a point to the right of Q_0 physicians, thereby indicating that Q_1 quantity of physicians would be the optimal quantity. The manner in which these external benefits would be included in the foregoing calculation would be to provide a government subsidy, the size of which would reflect the magnitude of the external benefits. This government subsidy could be distributed to prospective medical students, which would lower their tuition costs and increase their demand for a medical education, or else the subsidy could be provided to the medical schools, thereby lowering their cost of producing physicians.

It is important to determine whether or not there are external benefits from having additional physicians. If there are external benefits, then this would warrant government subsidization of medical education for purposes of achieving the optimal number of physicians. (It would still be necessary to calculate the size of the external benefits in order to calculate the number of additional physicians that would have to be produced and the consequent size of the government subsidy.)

Before attempting to answer the question of whether external benefits exist with regard to the number of physicians, it would be best to first discuss what an externality is. When someone undertakes an action, such as purchasing or producing a good or service in the private market, and this action has effects on other individuals or firms, then an externality is said to have occurred. Since the allocation decisions of others are affected by the initial private decisions that created the externality, failure to consider these secondary allocation decisions would result in either too few or too many resources in the market. There are different types of external effects, both positive and negative, as well as externalities in consumption and in production. For public policy purposes it is important to distinguish between technological and pecuniary externalities. The former occur outside the market transaction; as a result of producing a product, a firm pollutes the water, thereby imposing a cost on those using the stream. Pecuniary externalities occur within the market: as a result of an increase in demand by some participants in the market, the price is increased to all other participants in the market. Government intervention is required only in the first case (technological externality) to correct what would otherwise be a misallocation of resources (7). When externalities occur, the government, by calculating the extent of external costs and/or benefits and using a system of taxes and subsidies, should attempt to achieve the optimal allocation of resources. Such a process of nonmarket decisionmaking would involve the use of methodologies such as benefit-cost analysis.

It is not easy to determine the extent of externalities, if any, in medicine. With regard to medical research, traditional public health programs, and water fluoridation, the case for externalities seems clear. Individuals undertaking medical research do not collect from all who benefit from such knowledge. And since all those who benefit do not contribute to the production of that research, too little research would be undertaken if it were based solely on support from those who contribute. The government should, therefore, calculate the size of external benefits, levy the appropriate set of taxes, and subsidize the production of medical research. Only in this manner would the optimal quantity of research be undertaken.

What are the external benefits as a result of having a greater quantity of medical education or a larger number of physicians?* Is it possible to specify the benefits that accrue to others, or to society as a whole, in addition to those who purchase physician services? Without government subsidies to medical education, there would exist a certain stock of physicians. The number of physicians would be determined by the private demand and private costs of producing them. Are there external benefits to having more physicians than would be provided under the private market? (The total contribution of physicians may be large, but their marginal contribution has been estimated to be small.) The case for public subsidies as a result of externalities in education has generally been made with regard to grade-school education: everyone in a democratic society benefits from having a better-educated electorate. The case for public subsidies to higher education is weaker, and for a professional or technical education it is not at all clear that a case can be made for such subsidies (8).

It is not enough to assert that there are external benefits to having a greater number of physicians and then to call for massive government support for our medical schools. Since there is neither clear evidence nor strong argument that external benefits exist in medical, dental, or veterinary education, the case for public subsidies to the health professions educational institutions on grounds of externalities should be reexamined.

There might be other grounds for providing public subsidies to the health professions, such as attracting a certain mix of students, or locating medical graduates in a particular area. Such subsidies are based upon societal value

---

*The situation where an individual includes in his or her utility function the access to medical care by others is an example of external benefits in personal medical care. Government intervention in such a situation should seek to increase the consumption or availability of medical care by low-income persons. This can be more directly achieved through some form of demand-increasing program to such persons rather than by indirectly subsidizing medical schools, which may have little or no effect on increasing the availability of care to such persons.

judgments rather than on externalities. The case for subsidies to medical education on other grounds will be discussed subsequently. These grounds include the improvement of equity in the distribution of medical care to the recipients, or the redress of possible market imperfections if medical education were to be financed through a full-cost tuition program. The equity of the current system of financing education—i.e., who receives the subsidies and who bears the cost—will also be discussed.

SOME PROPOSALS FOR IMPROVING THE EFFICIENCY OF THE CURRENT MARKET FOR MEDICAL EDUCATION

An important defect in the current market for medical education is that there is no linkage between tuition and the role such a price variable should play on both the demand and the supply side. If, as under a competitive system, tuition acted as a price on the demand side, then all who were willing to pay that price would have access to a medical education and there would be no need for 6,000 Americans to be paying higher costs and be studying medicine overseas. If medical schools were not provided with large educational subsidies, then tuition would have to reflect all the costs of a medical education. Allowing tuition to serve as a true price of medical education would encourage the suppliers to be efficient in production. If they were not, and had to charge more than $25,000 a year, which is the educational cost per student per year in some medical schools, they could not fill their spaces. Eliminating or sharply reducing supply subsidies and allowing entry by new suppliers of medical education would enable tuition to become an accurate signal of the number of physicians that would be appropriate (assuming no external benefits). We would then have efficiency in consumption as well as in production.

If, however, tuition reflected all the costs of education and prospective students had to pay all these costs, then low-income students might be precluded from ever becoming physicians. Only students from high-income families would be able to afford what would be very high tuition costs, e.g., possibly in excess of $75,000 for four years of medical school. Full-cost tuition, in a more open and competitive system where the control on quality was based on a number of examinations prior to entering the profession rather than on specific educational requirements for a licensure exam, would probably be much lower than it is under the current system. In addition to lower costs per graduate that might result from a system where greater flexibility would be permitted in curriculum and in teaching methods, the opportunity costs of entering the profession are likely to be greatly lowered. It is not necessary, as in other countries such as Great Britain, to have graduated from a four-year undergraduate school before entering a four-year medical school (9). The training times for entering the profession could be reduced; (10) the opportunity costs associated with these long educational requirements are more costly than increased tuition levels. For example, the average income of a physician starting practice in 1979 was greater than $60,000 (11). In addition to receiving such an income one to two years earlier, the student would save undergraduate tuition and fees if he or she were to enter medical school after two to three years of undergraduate education. Thus medical school tuition could be increased by approximately $15,000 a year to offset the benefit to the student of entering practice one year earlier. If the student entered medical school after two years of undergraduate education, medical school tuition could be increased by much more without adversely affecting the rate of return to a medical education.

An important concern to many persons, however, is that under a system of full-cost tuition the medical profession would still be the province only of children from high-income families. To determine whether such a concern is justifiable and, if so, how to alleviate it, it is necessary to examine the "equity" of the current system of financing medical education.

EQUITY IN THE CURRENT SYSTEM OF FINANCING MEDICAL EDUCATION

In the previous section we were concerned with the economic efficiency of the medical education market. It was determined that, under the current structure of medical education, it was highly unlikely that 1) the optimal number of physicians would be produced, and 2) the production of medical education would be efficient. This section is concerned with the equity—i.e., who receives the benefits and who bears the costs—of the large governmental subsidies that support the current system of medical education.

According to two recent studies, it was estimated that the annual average cost of medical education in 1972 was between $12,650 and $20,370 per enrolled student. During that same period, medical students paid, on the average, approximately $1,200 a year in tuition and fees. Thus, the average medical student received a subsidy of approximately $45,000 from all sources, government and nongovernment, during four years of training (12). The average annual cost of medical education was estimated to be approximately $25,000 per student in 1980. Average tuition and fees were approximately $4,280 (13). Thus the average subsidy for four years of medical school in 1980 was approximately $82,000— about double what it was in 1972. These subsidies are in addition to those received during the student's four years of undergraduate training, since higher education is also subsidized by government funds. The subsidies received by medical students are generally larger than those received by students in higher education or in other professional schools. The reason is that the costs of medical education are greater than the costs in other departments in the university, while tuition rates are generally not much different within the university. With such large subsidies going to each medical student, it is legitimate to question the equitableness of these subsidies. Do such subsidies have desirable redistributive effects, or are they neutral with respect to their effect on incomes in society?

Income redistribution is based upon a societal value judgment that persons with lower incomes should be made better off by being subsidized at the expense of persons with higher incomes. The provision of such subsidies (and the taxes to finance them) may be direct, in the form of cash grants, or indirect, in the form of grants in-kind, such as lower prices for specific goods and services. Education is an in-kind subsidy to all those using it. For an in-kind subsidy to have desirable redistributive effects, low-income persons should receive a proportionately greater share of the subsidy, while the costs of financing it should

TABLE 15-3. Average Family Incomes, Average Higher Education Subsidies Received, and Average State Taxes Paid by Families, by Type of California Higher Education Institution, 1964–1965

	Families Without Children Enrolled in California Higher Education	Families with Children Enrolled in California Public Higher Education	
		University of California	California State College
Average family income	$7,900	$12,000	$10,000
Average higher education subsidy per year	0	1,700	1,400
Average state taxes paid	182	350	260
Net subsidy	− 180	+ 1,350	+ 1,140

Source: Based on data in Table IV-12, p. 76, in W. Lee Hansen and Burton A. Weisbrod, *Benefits, Costs, and Finance of Public Higher Education* (Chicago: Markham Publishing Co., 1969).

come from the predominantly higher-income persons in society. Some redistributive schemes may have perverse effects, as when a greater proportion of the cost is born by the lower-income persons and a greater proportionate share of the benefits is received by the higher-income persons. Such was the case at times with respect to community rating and the manner in which certain services in the hospital were priced. In the typical market situation where a person purchases a good or service, that person receives the benefits from the purchase and pays the cost of producing it. The benefits are fully received and the costs are fully borne by the purchaser, assuming no externalities. With regard to medical education, therefore, are the sizable subsidies that go to each medical student neutral in their redistributive effects, or, if not, which income groups end up subsidizing which other income groups?

There is a growing accumulation of evidence that subsidies to higher education, and particularly to medical education, result in a large redistribution of income; however, the costs are borne by low-income persons and are used to subsidize the highest-income groups in society. Such redistribution, if correct, would be inequitable. First, with regard to higher education, Hansen and Weisbrod, in an examination of the financing of higher education in California and in Wisconsin, have shown that the size of the subsidy received by families that send their children to these state-supported schools is greater than the state taxes they pay for all state-supported services (14). These families have higher incomes, on an average, than families that do not send their children to such schools. As shown in Table 15-3, which is based on the Hansen and Weisbrod study, the average family income of families with children enrolled in the University of California system was $12,000 in 1964–1965. The average family income for families with children enrolled in the California State College system was $10,000. The average for families without children in either system was $7,900. The average amount of state taxes paid by each of these families was $350, $260, and $182, respectively; the *net* subsidy to each of these family groups was + $1,350, + $1,140, and − $180. Because more children from higher-income families attended California's public higher education institutions, these

TABLE 15-4. Family Income of Medical Students, All U.S. Families, by Control of Medical School, 1974–1975

Family Income[a]	Private Schools	Public Schools	All Medical Schools	All U.S. Families[b]
Total	100%	100%	100%	100%
Less than $5,000	5	6	6	13
$5,000–9,999	10	11	11	23
$10,000–14,999	16	19	18	24
$15,000–19,999	14	16	15	18
$20,000–24,999	13	14	13	10
$25,000 or more	42	34	37	12
Estimated median	$21,972	$19,315	$20,249	$12,836

Source: Reproduced from *Descriptive Study of Enrolled Medical Students 1974–75*, DHEW Publication No. (HRA) 76-97, prepared by the Association of American Medical Colleges, p. 26.

[a]Based on students who supplied data.

[b]U.S. Department of Commerce, Bureau of the Census, *Money Income and Poverty Status of Families and Persons in the United States 1974*, Series P-60, No. 99, July 1975.

families were subsidized by the remainder of the families, whose income, on the average, was lower. Hansen and Weisbrod make two additional comments that are relevant to our discussion on financing medical education. First, the additional state taxes paid by the subsidized students, once they begin working and earning higher incomes as a result of their subsidized education, are less than the value of the subsidy they received (on a present-value basis). Second, a number of subsidized students never repay any of their subsidy, since they leave the state. If the evidence in other states is similar to what was demonstrated in California and Wisconsin, then it is clear that prospective medical students (and others) receive substantial subsidies before they even enter medical school.

How are the subsidies in medical education distributed with regard to family income? Table 15-4 presents a comparison of family incomes for medical students with family incomes in the rest of the population. Based on data from this table, it is obvious that the family incomes of medical students were higher than those of all U.S. families. There were three times as many families of medical students with incomes of $25,000 or more than there were in the population at large. Similarly, there were twice as many families in the population with incomes less than $15,000 than among the families of medical students. The estimated median income of families of medical students was almost twice as great as the median family income in the general population. The large subsidies going to medical students, therefore, appear to be going to students whose family incomes are much higher than those in the rest of the population. It is also highly unlikely that the taxes paid to the state by the families of medical students are, on the average, greater than the subsidies received. The redistributive effects of the current method of financing medical education appear to be similar to the earlier examples of higher education in California and Wisconsin. The redistributive effects of the medical school subsidies shown in Table 15-4 are actually an improvement over what they were in the past. In 1967, 20 percent of the medical students came from families with incomes greater than $25,000 a year, incomes that compared with only 2 percent of the families in the general population: a ratio of 10–1. Similarly, 42 percent of the families of medical students had incomes greater than $15,000, whereas only 12 percent of the families in the population had comparable incomes (15).

More recently published data on family incomes of medical students are surprisingly misleading. The highest income level published is "$20,000 or more," which characterizes 46 percent of all medical student families (16). Since inflation has been causing incomes to rise generally, a larger portion of the population also ends up in that highest income category. Thus there is only a 50 percent difference in the proportion of families in that highest-income category. If higher income categories were used, however, the disparities in incomes would become much more obvious. Although it is undoubtedly true that some medical students came from families with low incomes, the major portion of the subsidy going to medical students goes to those with high family incomes.

Another factor bearing on the inequity of the current system of financing medical education is that once medical students graduate, they then enter the top 10 percent of the income distribution in society. It would seem unnecessary to subsidize medical students through their undergraduate and medical education to enable them to enter the highest income distribution, but, on top of that, the students who are being selected to receive the subsidy come from the highest-income families in the first place.

In light of the foregoing discussion, the proposals of the Carnegie Commission Report on Medical Education (1970), suggesting federal subsidies to medical students and medical schools to result in a uniform level of tuition for all schools of $1,000, would worsen rather than improve the performance of the current system of medical education. At such low tuition levels, the excess demand for medical education would become greater than before. Since schools would all charge the same tuition levels, there would be no competition among schools on costs to the students and this would favor the more costly, prestigious schools: if the price is the same, why not go to the "best" school? Such a system would also provide no incentives for schools to be concerned with their costs because they would receive sufficient subsidies to enable each school to charge only $1,000 tuition per year. A more desirable proposal could not have been developed by the deans of the most prestigious, high-cost medical schools themselves.

Are there any justifiable reasons for continuing a method of financing medical education that has the effect of worsening rather than improving the income distribution? Three rationalizations are offered for continuing the present subsidy system. The first states that if it is a societal value judgment to have physicians locate in rural and underserved areas, it is necessary to subsidize medical education (17). Similar to this argument is the one that if a change in the mix of physicians is desired, then subsidies to medical schools are necessary. Compatible with this general line of reasoning is the belief that since medical students leave the state that provided them with a subsidy, to prevent the state that is acquiring them from benefiting, that state should also subsidize its medical students. The common fallacy in each of these arguments is the failure to recognize that subsidies can be provided on a selective basis: for example, only those physicians locating in a rural area would be subsidized by not having to pay all or part of their educational costs. Why should all physicians be subsidized, especially since most of them locate in high-income, urban areas? Similarly, since a small fraction of medical students are classified as minority students, i.e., approximately 10 percent, why should the remaining 90 percent of medical students receive subsidies as well? If the reason a state subsidizes its medical students is that it wants its physicians to locate within its borders, then if medical students were charged full-cost tuition, with those remaining in the state having all or part of their costs forgiven, then those medical students leaving the state would have paid their debt by having paid their full educational costs. This last argument can be applied to any person, including lawyers, accountants, and teachers, who has received subsidized training and then leaves that state to practice elsewhere.

If a state explicitly states the reasons for which it wants to provide a subsidy, it may generate discussion as to whether that is a value judgment that others agree with. Once a policy has been decided upon, it would then be possible to achieve its goal in a much less expensive manner by providing the subsidies directly to persons fulfilling society's needs rather than by providing a generous subsidy to all medical students. Similarly, for a total subsidy expenditure that provides for an equal amount to all medical students, more money would be available to meet society's objectives if the subsidies went only to those participating in a particular agreed-upon program.

A more sophisticated argument favoring subsidies to all students is that the sums of money required to pay for a medical education are so large that very few persons would be able to afford it. Banks would be unwilling to provide loans for tuition and living expenses with no collateral. Further, persons from low-income families have a higher rate of time preference, i.e., income today has a much higher value to the poor than income in the future. As a result, the poor will be less likely to invest in their own human capital, i.e., higher education, than those with higher incomes. Also, undertaking an investment involves some risk that it will not pay off. Medical education is expensive, and future physician incomes may not be as attractive. If physicians have large debts to pay off, so some persons would say, they may select only the most lucrative forms of practice instead of serving certain population groups or perhaps undertaking research.

If all medical students were to be charged full-cost tuition, then such a policy would have to be accompanied by loan programs. A type of loan program that has been advocated by a number of persons is an "income contingent loan repayment plan" (ICLRP). The way in which an ICLRP would work is as follows: students would take out a loan during the period they are in medical school to cover both tuition and living expenses. Once they have graduated and have started to earn an income, they would annually repay a fixed percent of their adjusted gross income. The fixed percent that would be assessed would depend upon how much the student borrowed (18).

By relating the ICLRP to the income of the physician, the program would not distort the preferences of physicians as to the population they serve or the type of practice they enter. A loan repayment plan similar to the one described would also minimize the risk to the student as to the size of the loan that would have to be repaid.* Physicians' incomes have, in any case, been consistently high

---

*A problem with previous student loan programs has been that ex-students have nullified their debts by declaring bankruptcy. In 1977, however, "a new federal law went into effect that binds graduates to their student loan obligations even if they declare bankruptcy." New York Times, November 26, 1977, p. 25.

during the last 30 years. As investments go, an investment in a medical education would carry minimal risk and would be fairly predictable, as attested to by
the continual excess demand for spaces and the willingness of large numbers of
students to pay higher costs to receive such an education overseas.

If, as has been proposed, medical students are charged the full cost of their
education (and medical schools are no longer provided with education subsidies), what will happen to the demand for a medical education? Will the increase in tuition result in a large decrease in the number of medical school
applicants? The rate of return to a medical education was estimated to be approximately 22 percent in 1970 and approximately 17.6 percent in 1976; for many
medical specialties, it was higher than that (19). If full-cost tuition were charged,
it was estimated that the rate of return in 1976 would have declined to 13.5
percent (20). Even at this lower rate of return, an investment in a medical education would still be very worthwhile in that there would still be an excess rate of
return to medicine. In any case, if full-cost tuition were combined with a reduction in the length of the undergraduate program, as discussed earlier, large increases in tuition should be possible to offset the benefit the student would
receive from entering practice one to two years earlier. Thus, there should still
be an excess demand for medical school spaces, at the current level of supply.

A concern that the medical schools would express in the face of a proposal to
eliminate educational subsidies is that they would not be able to finance new
construction. It would be difficult, they would say, for nonprofit educational
institutions to borrow funds. If access to the capital markets were a problem, then
the government could establish mortgage banks or guarantee interest payments.
The current advantage to medical schools of not paying the full cost of medical
school construction is that when there is no cost constraint they can make their
construction programs more elaborate than they would be if the schools had to
repay their costs. Also, there currently may be too much emphasis on medical
school construction just because it is heavily subsidized. Kessel has questioned
both the need to require the medical student to study the first two years of basic
science curriculum in a high-cost medical school, when the same courses are
often taught for much less in other university departments, and the requirement
that the second two years of extensive clinical experience take place within a
medical school and not a community hospital. Innovative experiments along
these lines have begun in a few locations (21).

Perhaps a more important concern for medical schools, if a proposal of full-
cost tuition were implemented, would be that they would have to compete with
one another for students. If students have to pay a substantial cost for their
education, they will be more concerned with the school they select. Even if
subsidies for medical education were provided to some students, the schools
would have to compete for them. Medical and other educational institutions
would much prefer to be subsidized themselves, since the student would have to
go to that institution in order to receive subsidized training. It is for this same
reason that schools prefer to distribute loans and scholarships rather than have
the government or some other central agency distribute them. If the school
distributes the funds, then students can receive them only if they attend the
institution distributing them. If students receive these funds and can then
choose the school they wish to attend, the different schools are forced to compete
for students.

This section has examined the equity of the present system of financing medical education. It was shown that medical students are subsidized through undergraduate education and medical school, and then enter the top 10 percent of the income distribution in society. These same medical students often come from the highest-income groups to start with. Proposals to improve the equity of the current system were suggested, such as having those students who benefit from an investment in a medical education bear the full cost of such an education. Specific value judgments of society, such as having physicians locate in certain areas, should be subsidized directly instead of rewarding all medical students regardless of whether they participate in the particular programs. A method to implement the concept of full-cost tuition, namely, income-contingent loan repayment plans, was suggested.

REFERENCES

1. George Wright, "How Should We Finance Medical Education?" Health Manpower Policy Discussion Paper Series, School of Public Health, University of Michigan, May 1974, p. 1.

2. The earlier IOM estimates were updated by multiplying the 1972 figures by the increase in the Medical Care Price Index between 1972 and 1980. As a rough check on this approach, these results were compared to those arrived at by calculating the ratio of the IOM estimate of educational expenditures per student to total revenue per student (in 1972) based on AMA data and then applying that ratio to 1980 AMA data on revenue per student. Both estimates differed by less than 7 percent with the first method being the lower of the two.

    Data on tuition and fees are from *State Support for Health Professions Education*, Senate Committee on Labor and Human Resources, U.S. Congress (Washington, D.C.: U.S. Government Printing Office, 1981), p. 20.

3. Institute of Medicine, National Academy of Science, *Costs of Education in the Health Professions*, Report of a Study, Parts I and II (Washington, D.C.: 1974). The costs of education vary by approximately 100 percent among schools.

4. Thomas Hall and Cotton Lindsay, "Medical Schools: Producers of What Sellers to Whom," *Journal of Law and Economics* (April 1980). K. Leffler and C. Lindsay, in their article "Student Discount Rates, Consumption Loans, and Subsidies to Professional Training," *The Journal of Human Resources* 16 (Summer 1981): 468–475, argue that subsidies are necessary to compensate for imperfections in the market for human capital. However, they conclude that current subsidies exceed those necessary to alleviate imperfections in this market.

5. John K. Iglehart, "Schrinking Federal Support Brings New Era to Education in the Health Professions," *New England Journal of Medicine* (305) (October 22, 1981): 1027–1032.

6. Rashi Fein and Gerald Weber, *Financing Medical Education*, A General Report Prepared for the Carnegie Commission on Higher Education and The Commonwealth Fund (New York: McGraw-Hill Book Co., 1971), pp. 131–132.

7. For more discussion on this subject, see Neil Singer, *Public Microeconomics: An Introduction to Government Finance*, 2nd ed. (Boston: Little, Brown & Company, 1976), pp. 107–108.

8. See Theodore W. Schultz, "Optimal Investment in College Instruction: Equity and Efficiency," *Journal of Political Economy* (Special Issue: "Investment in Education: The Equity–Efficiency Quandary") 80(3), Part II (May–June 1972).

9. For some suggestions on how educational and opportunity costs might be reduced under a different system for providing medical education, see Reuben Kessel, "The AMA and the Supply of Physicians," *Law and Contemporary Problems*, Health Care Part I, School of Law, Duke University (Spring 1970): 276–278.

10. Robert H. Ebert, "Can The Education Of The Physicians Be Made More Rational?", *New England Journal of Medicine* (305) (November 26, 1981): 1343–1346.

11. *Profile of Medical Practice 1981* (Chicago: American Medical Association, 1981), p. 199, Table 49.

12. George Wright, "Why Should We Subsidize Medical Education," Health Manpower Policy Discussion Paper Series, No. A-6, School of Public Health, University of Michigan, February 1974, p. 32, fn. 6.

13. See ref. 2.

14. W. Lee Hansen and Burton A. Weisbrod, *Benefits, Costs, and Finance of Public Higher Education* (Chicago: Markham Publishing Co., 1969), p. 76.

15. *How Medical Students Finance their Education*, U.S. Department of Health, Education and Welfare (Washington, D.C.: U.S. Government Printing Office, 1970), pp. 8–9.

16. W.F. Dube, *Descriptive Study of Enrolled Medical Students, 1976–1977*, final report from the Division of Student Studies, Association of American Medical Colleges for the Bureau of Health Manpower, Department of Health, Education and Welfare, Washington, D.C.: Government Printing Office, February 1978, p. 55.

17. An important reason why early loan forgiveness programs for physicians locating in rural and underserved areas were ineffective was that it was relatively inexpensive given the heavily subsidized cost of education, for students to buy their way out of their contracted obligations. For a more complete discussion of this topic, see Jack Hadley, "State and Local Financing Options," in Jack Hadley, ed., *Medical Education Financing: Policy Analysis and Options for the 1980s* (New York: PRODIST, 1980). Also see: *State Support for Health Professions Education, op. cit.*, pp. 42–54.

18. The idea of an ICLRP is not new. It was proposed over 20 years ago as a means of financing higher education. Yale and Duke Universities have experimented with such plans. A good theoretical discussion of the ICLRP is presented in Marc Nerlove, "Some Problems in the Use of Income-Contingent Loans for the Finance of Higher Education," *Journal of Political Economy* 83 (February 1975): 157–183. The author also discusses the Yale Plan. A proposal to use such a plan for medical students has been proposed by Bernard Nelson, Richard Bird, and Gilbert Rogers, "An Analysis of the Educational Opportunity Bank for Medical Student Financing," *Journal of Medical Education* (August 1972). A computer simulation of such repayment plans to indicate their feasibility is performed in William C. Weiler, "Loans for Medical Students: The Issues of Manageability," *Journal of Medical Education* (June 1976).

19. Stephen P. Dresch, "Marginal Wage Rates, Hours of Work, and Returns to Physician Training and Specialization," in Nancy Greenspan, ed., *Health Care Financing Conference Proceedings: Issues in Physicians Reimbursement* (Washington, D.C.: Department of Health and Human Services, 1981), p. 199.

20. *Ibid.*

21. George Wright, "Why Should We Subsidize Medical Education," p. 13.

CHAPTER 16

The Market for Registered Nurses

In the past years there have been numerous claims of a shortage of nurses in the United States. The evidence used to support such claims has been data which establish the ratio of registered nurses to the population and vacancy statistics of unfilled nursing positions in hospitals. For example, in 1956 it was estimated that there was a shortage of 70,000 nurses in the United States. By 1966 that estimate had increased to 125,000, and it was estimated (in 1963) that by 1970 the magnitude of the shortage would reach 200,000 nurses (1). Vacancy rates (as a percent of total positions) were increasing from between 13 and 16 percent in the mid-1950s to 23 percent by 1962 (see Table 16-1). As a result of these claims of nurse shortages, the U.S. Congress in 1964 passed the Nurse Training Act (NTA), which provided $300 million over a five-year period to alleviate the alleged shortage. The NTA was subsequently renewed and amended in 1966, 1968, 1971, 1975, and 1979. In all, more than $2 billion has been authorized by the U.S. government to alleviate the nurse shortage.

Since there has been such a large federal commitment to nursing education, it is important to understand the bases for public policy in this area. The first step toward understanding the various claims of shortages and the subsequent massive support for nursing education is to investigate the performance of the registered nurses market. If this market had been functioning well, then there would be no reason for any government intervention, let alone the large federal support which has been devoted to increasing the supply of nurses. If such federal support occurred when the market for nurses was performing efficiently, then we must look for other reasons to understand the demand for subsidies to nursing education. One example of such an alternative explanation would be a value judgment that medical care should be more readily available to the population and that one way to achieve this increase in availability is to subsidize one input (nurses) to the supply of medical care. If such a value judgment is the basis for federal support to this area, then it should be evaluated by comparing this supply subsidy to alternative supply subsidies to determine which subsidy program achieves the largest increase in supply of medical care per dollar spent. Alternatively, such supply subsidies should be compared to demand subsidy programs

417

TABLE 16-1. Vacancy Rates in Hospitals
for General-Duty Nurses

Year	Vacancy Rate
1953	14.6
1954	13.0
1956	16.8
1958	13.0
1961	23.2
1962	23.0
1967	18.1
1968	15.0
1969	11.2
1971	9.3
1980	10.6

Source: Reprinted by permission of the publisher, from Donald E. Yett, *An Economic Analysis of the Nurse Shortage* (Lexington, Mass.: Lexington Books, D.C. Heath Co., Copyright 1975, D.C. Heath Co.), p. 138, Table 3-13. The 1980 vacancy rate came from unpublished data provided by American Hospital Association from its annual hospital survey.

which would also achieve an increase in quantity of medical care consumed for a particular beneficiary group.

If, on the other hand, it is found that the market for registered nurses has not been functioning well, then certain policy prescriptions might be called for. Depending upon the particular reasons for its poor performance, federal subsidies might be one policy alternative; other forms of government intervention, not requiring the use of federal subsidies, might also be appropriate. Only after examining the performance of the market for nurses can it be determined whether there was or is any justification for federal subsidies to nursing education and, if not, what possible explanations might be offered for the use of such subsidies. Also, by examining the effect of the federal subsidies we might gain some insight into their intended as opposed to their stated purpose.

MEASURING THE PERFORMANCE OF THE MARKET FOR REGISTERED NURSES

If the market for nurses were performing relatively efficiently, then we would expect it to operate as is shown in Figure 16-1. Starting from an initial equilibrium point, with the demand for registered nurses (RNs) represented by D_1 and supply by S_1, the equilibrium wage would be W_1 and the number of RNs employed, Q_1. The assumption that the demand for RNs has been increasing over time would be represented by a shift in the demand curve to D_2. With a higher demand for RNs, we would expect wages to increase to W_2 and the quantity of

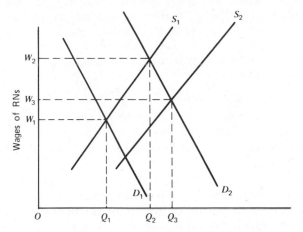

Figure 16-1. The market for registered nurses.

RNs employed to increase to Q_2. The increase in RNs employed would come from the existing stock of RNs, i.e., the total number of trained nurses. A measure of the increase in number of those RNs in the existing stock of RNs who are working is the "participation rate," i.e., the percent of the stock of RNs that are active (employed).* Thus the short-run effects of an increase in demand on the market for nurses is an increase in their wages, from W_1 to W_2; an increase in their employment, from Q_1 to Q_2; and an increase in their participation rate (not shown in Figure 16-1). The long-run effect of the increase in demand, from D_1 to D_2, is an increase in the supply of nurses, which is shown in Figure 16-1 by a shift in the supply curve to the right, to S_2. The reason for the shift in the supply curve is that as the wage of RNs is increased, from W_1 to W_2, nursing becomes a relatively more attractive profession when compared with, for example, teaching. Assuming that all the factors that affect the demand for a nurse's and a teacher's education do not change, with the exception of the increase in nurses' wages relative to the wage of teachers, some prospective applicants for a teacher's education may decide to enter nursing. This change in career patterns does not mean that all candidates will switch their educational choices, nor does it mean that the persons who do change are motivated solely by financial return. What it means is that for *some* people, the choice of one profession over another is a matter of indifference; a change in the relative incomes of the professions will mean that more of these people select the profession with the highest income. How many people switch depends upon the difference in relative incomes and how many people are relatively close to the margin in their choices.

---

*For the majority of trained nurses who are women, a number of factors influence whether or not she will seek employment. Her wage is only one such factor. Whether or not she has young children and what her husband's income is are additional factors. However, if nurses' wages increase, while all other factors remain unchanged, then some inactive nurses will decide to become active. The elasticity of the participation rate with respect to nurses' wages will indicate the percent increase in employment for a given percent increase in nurses' wages. This will be discussed in more detail later.

Thus, the long-run effect of the increase in demand is that we would expect to find an increase in the wages of RNs, relative to other occupations with similar training costs, and an increase in the number of persons entering nursing. The performance measures of an efficiently operating market that we would look for with an increase in demand are:

- an increase in the wages of RNs;
- an increase in the rate of return to one who becomes an RN, both in absolute terms and relative to other occupations;
- an increase in the number of registered nurses employed and in their participation rate; and
- an increase in the use of substitutes. As RNs' wages increase, RNs become relatively more expensive to use. We would expect to observe their employers substituting *away* from the use of RNs to the use of other nursing personnel whose wages haven't increased as rapidly.

If we wanted to test whether the market for RNs is adjusting to changes in the demand for RNs, then we would collect data on each of these measures. Before turning to an examination of the data, however, we should discuss the indications that a market is not performing efficiently. In this way we will be able to determine the efficiency with which this market is operating and also the possible reasons for inadequate performance, if that should be the case.

As we observed in Figure 16-1, with an increase in demand from D_1 to D_2, we would expect the wage to rise, and this would bring about an increase in the number of nurses employed—in the short run through an increase in their participation rate, and in the long run through an increase in the number of persons becoming nurses (a shift to the right in the supply curve). One possible market imperfection, therefore, would be that nurses wages do not increase, or do not increase sufficiently to reach a new equilibrium level. Such a situation could be the result of a dynamic shortage. With an increase in the demand for nurses, the major employers of nurses may not know how much they have to increase nurses' wages to bring about an increase in their employment; similarly, it takes time for working nurses to learn which hospitals are paying higher wages and for inactive nurses both to learn of the increase in wages and to decide to become active again. A dynamic shortage for RNs is illustrated in Figure 16-2. With the increase in demand from D_1 to D_2, the demand for RNs will initially be Q_2, which is W_1 at a point on the new demand curve D_2. Thus, in a dynamic shortage, until information becomes available to nurse employers that they have to raise wages if they are to hire more nurses, and the information becomes available to nurses that they could receive higher wages if they were to become active, there will be a shortage of magnitude $Q_1 - Q_2$. As the wages of RNs increase, the shortage will begin to decrease, which means that those employers who are willing to pay the higher price will be able to employ more nurses. The existence of a dynamic shortage is a temporary phenomenon and should slowly disappear with time. Unless demand for RNs continually increases faster than the increase in the supply of RNs, which would allow the dynamic shortage to persist, equilibrium will eventually occur in the market. The only indication that a dynamic shortage existed (or continues to exist) would be that together with continued vacancies for RNs (budgeted but unfilled positions) there would also

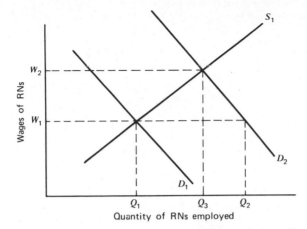

Figure 16-2. A dynamic shortage in the market for registered nurses.

be observed in the market for nurses higher wages, increased rates of return, and increases in employment, in participation rates, and in use of substitutes.

Another possible imperfection that might occur in the market for nurses (and which is more serious than a dynamic shortage) is a static shortage. In a situation of a static shortage, the nurses' wages are prevented from increasing to an equilibrium level. Because the wages are below the market-clearing wage, there will be a continual shortage that, unlike the situation of a dynamic shortage, will not be temporary and work itself out. A static shortage can also be illustrated with use of Figure 16-2. With an increase in demand from D_1 to D_2, the quantity of nurses demanded at the old wage would be Q_2. If the wage is prevented from rising, then the shortage, $Q_1 - Q_2$, will not disappear. In distinguishing between whether there has been (or is) a static shortage or a dynamic shortage, we would expect to observe measures of shortages, e.g., vacancy rates for nurses, in both cases, but in a static shortage we would *not* expect to observe large increases in nurses' wages, in their participation rates, or in their rates of return. In both cases we would expect substitution away from the use of RNs to occur, since it is more difficult to employ as many RNs as the employers would like, in one case because nurses' wages have gone up and they have become relatively more expensive to employ, in the other because employers cannot hire all the nurses they would like to at the old wage.

Having specified the measures of performance to be used in determining which of the foregoing market descriptions best characterizes how the market for nurses has operated in the past, we now turn to an examination of the data; we now know which data to look for and how to interpret them.

THE PERFORMANCE OF THE MARKET
FOR REGISTERED NURSES

Nurses are predominantly employed in hospitals. As shown in Table 16-2, of the 1,272,851 registered nurses employed in 1980, 65.6 percent were working in

TABLE 16-2. Number and Distribution of Active Registered Nurses by Place of Employment, 1980

Place of Employment	Number of Active RNs	Percentage of RNs
Hospitals	835,647	65.6
Nursing homes	101,209	8.0
Schools of nursing	46,504	3.7
Private duty	20,240	1.6
Community health	83,440	6.6
School nurses	44,906	3.5
Occupational health	29,164	2.3
Offices	71,974	5.7
Other and not reporting	39,498	3.0
Total	1,272,851	100.00

Source: U.S. Department of Health and Human Services, Division of Health Professions Analysis, *The Registered Nurse Population, An Overview from National Sample Survey of Registered Nurses, November 1980* (Revised June 1982), Rockville, Md.: U.S. Department of Health and Human Services, 1982, Report No. 82-5, p. 13.

hospitals. The remaining places of employment and their respective percentages were: nursing homes (8.0 percent), occupational health (2.3 percent), nursing education (3.7 percent), private duty and office (7.3 percent), and public health and schools (10.1 percent).(3.0 percent were employed in other nursing fields or did not report.) Thus, what happens in the hospital sector has the largest effect on the employment of registered nurses. When we examine the way in which the demand for hospital care (hence the demand for RNs) has been changing over time, we have seen in Chapter 10 that both admissions and patient days in short-term general and other special hospitals (which have approximately 80 percent of all hospital admissions) have been increasing since the end of World War II. The demand for hospital care has been increasing over time as a result of a number of factors: the age distribution of the population has been changing, income and health insurance coverage has increased, and there were large government programs in the mid-1960s which began to lower the cost of hospital care to the poor and aged. Medical advances, which changed the hospital from an institution providing chronic care to one that provides acute care, and modern medical technology have resulted in increased demands for RNs per patient day—for example, in intensive care units. There has thus been an increase in use of medical care, and more of this care has been provided in hospitals. Because fewer nursing students have been providing care in hospitals, there has also been a greater demand for nurses as a result of a shift to more care by RNs. An increase in the responsibilities delegated to RNs for tasks that were formerly performed by physicians in hospitals has added additional burdens. These factors have resulted in a 65 percent increase in the use of general-duty nurses per patient (in nonfederal hospitals) between 1949 and 1966 (2)*.

---

*A demand function for RNs in short-term hospitals was estimated by Donald E. Yett et al., and it was determined that the effect of a 1 percent increase in patient days would result in a .86 increase in RNs, in hospitals of 200 or more beds. The effect of a 1 percent increase in RN wages would lead to a -1.75 decrease in number of RNs employed, and the cross-elasticity of demand for RNs with respect to the wages of aides was 1.43. D. Yett, L. Drabek, L. Kimball, and M. Intriligator, *A Forecasting and Policy Simulation Model of the Health Care Sector* (Lexington, Mass.: Lexington Books, 1979), p. 95.

As a result of such forces, which would tend to increase the demand for RNs, unless the supply of RNs increased faster, we would expect to observe increases in nurses' salaries and in rates of return to a nursing education, substitution toward the use of nonregistered nurses, and increases in the nurse participation rate. According to Table 16-3, between 1946 and 1980 average annual salaries of "all active nurses" increased 649 percent, from $2,136 per year in 1946 to $15,992 per year in 1980. Salaries, however, also increased in other occupations in which women were predominately employed over that same time period. When we examine the increase in salaries both before and after the introduction of Medicare and Medicaid in 1966, we see that nurses' salaries increases by 154 percent between 1946 and 1966. However, teachers' salaries increased 233 percent and salaries of "female professional technical and kindred workers" increased 187 percent over the 1946–1966 period. After 1966, nurses' salaries had the largest percentage increase: 194 percent between 1966–1980, compared with only 131 percent for teachers and 171 percent for "female professional technical and kindred workers." Thus when we examine nurses' wages relative to the wages in comparable professions, it appears that the overall percent increase has been similar for the entire 1946–1978 period; however, nurses' wages increased less rapidly before Medicare and more rapidly afterward. The ratio of nurses' salaries to those of teachers was 1.03 in 1946, declining to a low of .75 in 1963, and thereafter increasing to 1.00 in 1980. (See Table 16-4.) Nurses' wages were 1.05 to those of "Female Professional Technical and Kindred Workers" in 1946, declining to .86 in 1961, rising to 1.10 in 1972 and then declining to 1.02 in 1980. (It is also of interest to note that the ratios of "All RNs" and "Hospital RNs" have become more similar in the last decade.)

Based on these data on relative wages, it would appear that since the wages of other female workers increased more rapidly during the period before 1966, there was a relative *surplus* rather than a relative shortage of nurses during this period! This same observation is supported by the data on relative rates of return to a nursing education when they are compared with "females with one to three years of college training." In 1946 there appears to have been a sizeable shortage of nurses; i.e., the rate of return was higher for nurses than for the comparison group. By 1959, however, the relative rate of return to nursing declined, thereby indicating a *surplus* of nurses; i.e., women could receive a higher rate of return by entering an occupation other than nursing. By 1966, however, the relative rate of return to nursing had increased, indicating a shortage situation again (3).

What is of interest in the 1946–1966 time period is that wage increases to nurses have not been uniform according to place of nurse employment. Wages (nominal) increased much more rapidly between 1946 and 1966 for nurse education (224 percent) and school nurses (215 percent) than for hospital-employed nurses (157 percent). After 1966 the opposite occurred, as hospital nurses experienced the largest percent increase in their wages.

When we examine the increase in supply of nurses over this same time period, we observe that there has been an increase in the number of nurses employed in nonfederal hospitals, an increase of 109 percent between 1949 and 1966. However, as we would expect, the increase in the number of nurses employed in nurse education positions, and in other areas which have had larger percent increases in their wages, was much greater, 254 percent, over the same time period (4).

It thus appears that within nursing there have been increases in wages but

TABLE 16-3. Percentage Increase in Nominal Incomes of Registered Nurses, Teachers, Female Professional, Technical, and Kindred Workers, and Licensed Practical Nurses[a]

Year	Female Professional, Technical, and Kindred (%) (1)	Teachers (%) (2)	LPNs (%) (3)	RNs (%) (4)	Hospital RNs General-Duty Position (%) (5)	Nurse Educators (%) (6)	School Nurses (%) (7)
1946–1980	187	671		649	736	804	567
1946–1966	171	233		154	157	244	215
1966–1980		131		194	225	163	112
1966–1972	52	44	85	77	88	63	39
1972–1975	22	22	27	21	22	21	17
1975–1978	24	20	23	22	23	18	17
1978–1980	18	9		12	16	13	11

Sources: Columns 1, 2, 4, 5, 6, 7, rows 1, 2, 3, 4: Donald E. Yett, *An Economic Analysis of the Nurse Shortage* (Lexington, Mass.: Lexington Books, 1975), pp. 154–57, 184–186, 188–189; Column 1, rows 5, 6, 7: Department of Commerce, Bureau of the Census, *Current Population Reports*, Series P-60, Nos.: 90, p. 138; 103, p. 23; 123, p. 255; 132, p. 199; Column 2, rows 5, 6, 7: W. Vance Grant and Leo J. Eiden, eds., *Digest of Education Statistics, 1981* (National Center for Educational Statistics), p. 60; Column 3, rows 2, 3, 4, 5, 6, 7; and column 5, rows 5, 6, 7: U.S. Department of Health and Human Services, Public Health Service, Health Resources Administration, *The Recurrent Shortage of Registered Nurses: A New Look at the Issues*, DHHS Publication No. (HRA) 81-23 (Washington, D.C.: U.S. Government Printing Office, 1980), p. 3; Columns 6, 7, rows 5, 6, 7: American Nurses Association, *Facts About Nursing, 1972–1973* ed., pp. 10, 34, 145, 152; 1974–1975 ed., pp. 124, 137; 1976–1977 ed., pp. 40, 165, 179, 186; 1980–1981 ed., pp. 14, 197, 203, 230; Columns 5, 6, 7, row 7: U.S. Department of Health and Human Services, Public Health Services, Health Resources Administration, Bureau of Health Professions, Division of Health Professions Analysis, *The Registered Nurse Population, An Overview from National Sample Survey of Registered Nurses, November, 1980* (Revised June 1982), Report No. 82-5, p. 21.

Note: The percentage changes in income do not include changes in benefits. According to the Department of Health and Human Services, *The Recurrent Shortages of Registered Nurses: A New Look at the Issues*, pp. 5–8, nurses' benefits were comparable to those in similar occupations by 1978, whereas in 1960 they were considered to be inferior.

[a]The values in rows 1–6 were determined by taking a weighted average of the salaries of nurses in various nursing fields.

TABLE 16-4. The Ratio of All Registered Nurses' and Hospital General-Duty Registered Nurses' Salaries to Those of Teachers and Female Professional, Technical, and Kindred Workers

Year	Female Professional, Technical, and Kindred Workers		Teachers	
	All RNs	Hospital RNs	All RNs	Hospital RNs
1946	1.05	.97	1.03	.95
1948	1.00	.95	.92	.87
1951	.97	.92	.86	.82
1954	.89	.82	.82	.76
1957	.91	.85	.79	.74
1961	.86	.79	.77	.70
1963	.90	.87	.75	.73
1966	.93	.87	.79	.73
1969	1.02	.95	.87	.81
1972	1.10	1.08	.97	.96
1975	1.08	1.08	.96	.96
1978	1.07	1.06	.98	.97
1980	1.02	1.04	1.00	1.03

Sources: Donald E. Yett, *An Economic Analysis of the Nurse Shortage* (Lexington, Mass.: D.C. Heath Co., 1975), pp. 154, 160, 188. Department of Commerce, Bureau of the Census, *Current Population Reports*, Series P-60, Nos. :90, p. 138; 103, p. 23; 123, p. 255; 132, p. 199. W. Vance Grant and Leo J. Eiden, eds., *Digest of Education Statistics, 1981,* National Center for Educational Statistics, p. 60. U.S. Department of Health and Human Services, Health Resource Administration, *The Recurrent Shortage of Registered Nurses: A New Look at the Issues,* Department of Health and Human Services, Publication No. (HRA) 81-23 (Washington, D.C.: U.S. Government Printing Office, 1980), p. 3. U.S. Department of Health and Human Services, Division of Health Professions Analysis, *The Registered Nurse Population, An Overview from National Sample Survey of Registered Nurses,* November 1980 (revised June, 1982), Report No. 82-5, p. 21.

that these wage increases have been more rapid for nonhospital-based nurses. Similarly, the percent increase in nurse employment has been greater in the nonhospital sector, which employs only about 23 percent of all nurses. It appears that particular submarkets within nursing are adjusting—there are relatively larger increases in the nurses' wages in those markets. It is perplexing that nurses in the nonhospital sector should experience higher increases in their wages. If there are no barriers to movement between the two sectors and if the training costs are similar, then we would expect wage increases to be similar in both the hospital and nonhospital sectors (or if training costs differ, then the relative rates of return to be similar in the two different sectors).

With regard to substitution of other nurses (e.g., aides and licensed practical nurses) for registered nurses, we observe (according to Table 16-5) that although the relative salary differential of registered nurses to practical nurses has changed very little in the 1949–1978 period, a great deal of substitution within nursing has been occurring. From 1949 to 1966 the ratio of licensed practical nurses (LPNs) to registered nurses increased by 181 percent, from .16 in 1949 to .45 in 1966. Substitution would be expected if salary differentials increased or if

TABLE 16-5. The Ratio of LPNs' to RNs' and the Ratio of LPNs' to RNs' Salaries in Nonfederal Short-term General and Other Special Hospitals

Year	Employment LPNs/RNs	Income LPNs/RNs
1949	.16	
1955	.29	
1959	.37	
1960		76.6
1962	.40	
1963		74.6
1966	.45	72.1
1968	.50	
1969		70.2
1970	.51	
1972	.50	73.3
1973	.49	
1974	.48	
1975	.46	76.1
1976	.45	
1977	.43	
1978	.41	76.2
1979	.39	
1980	.37	
1981		74.1

Source: The employment and income ratios for the years 1949–1978 came from the U.S. Department of Health and Human Services, Public Health Service, Health Resources Administration, *The Recurrent Shortage of Registered Nurses: A New Look at the Issues*, DHHS Publication No. (HRS) 81-23—data on relative employment rates are on p. 6, and data on relative wage rates are on p. 5. The employment ratios for 1979 and 1980 were derived with permission from data in: American Hospital Association, *Hospital Statistics* (Chicago: AHA), © 1980, p. 21. The income ratio for 1981 was derived from preliminary reports of the Department of Labor, Bureau of Labor Statistics, *Industry Wage Survey: Hospitals* (1981).

there was a change in relative productivity (however, if their productivity changed, then this should have been reflected in a change in relative salaries). However, the increase in RNs relative incomes over this same period was slight. The upward trend in the use of LPNs relative to RNs began to reverse itself beginning in the early1970s, with the use of LPNs relative to RNs decreasing from .51 in 1970 to .37 in 1980. There was, however, virtually no change in their relative salaries over this same period.

What can we conclude about the market for nurses based upon the foregoing data? Starting from the late 1940s, the base period for comparison with changes over time and other occupations, nursing appeared to be a relatively attractive profession from a financial standpoint. Its rate of return was relatively higher than in comparable professions; one might even say that there was a slight shortage of nurses at that time. However, from that base period to the mid-1960s the attractiveness of nursing as a profession declined relative to comparable professions. This could be interpreted in the following way: although there was an increase in demand for nurses, it was smaller than the increase in demand for comparable occupations, and therefore wages rose faster in other professions. With a smaller increase in wages, and a decline in relative rates of return, fewer persons would be expected to enter nursing. Such a model would not explain a shortage situation but instead one characterized by a relative surplus of nurses.

This characterization of a surplus situation (i.e., demand increasing less rapidly than supply so that there is a decline in the relative wages of nurses) does not coincide with what a great many people believed was occurring during this time period. The common belief was that there was a shortage rather than a surplus of nurses. The indications of a shortage were the substitution of practical nurses for RNs and the increasing vacancy rates of RNs in hospitals. If the market were characterized by a dynamic shortage, then as demand increased faster than supply, we would expect an increase in vacancies as hospitals found they could not hire as many nurses as they would like at the prevailing wage, and the substituting toward less expensive personnel would begin. However, a dynamic shortage would also be characterized by rising wages of RNs and higher wages for RNs relative to practical nurses. Thus the data would be most characteristic of a dynamic shortage situation except for the fact that hospital nurses' wages (and their rates of return) were not rising more rapidly.

The only type of market situation which logically incorporates these contradictory data is one characterized by a static shortage. In a static shortage we might start from a point of equilibrium (1946–1949), represented by the intersection of the demand and supply curves, D_1 and S_1, in Figure 16-2. As the demand for hospital and medical care rises, bringing with it an increased demand for RNs, the demand curve shifts to D_2. If nurses' wages, instead of rising to the new equilibrium point, were kept below it in some way, then Q_1 Q_2 would represent the shortage, i.e., vacancies in hospitals; hospitals would have to substitute toward greater use of practical nurses because they could not employ all the RNs they would want to at the RNs' previous wage. Similarly, hospital RNs' wages, relative to those of RNs in other nursing employment, would increase less rapidly if they were held down in the hospital sector but not in other nurse employment sectors. As RN wages were prevented from increasing, they would begin to fall behind those in comparable occupations and the RNs' relative rate of return would similarly decline.

A static shortage situation, where RNs' wages show some increase but less than was necessary to clear the market and less than what was occurring in other areas of nursing or comparable occupations, would also explain why hospital nurse employment has also gone up less than in the nonhospital sector; with a rising supply curve for RNs, a small increase in hospital wages would result in only a small increase in the number employed in hospitals.

The data then appear consistent with a somewhat static shortage in the hospital market for RNs in the period during the late 1950s and early 1960s. Given this explanation or hypothesis of what has occurred, it is necessary to explain how such a static shortage could have persisted, i.e., what mechanism would have prevented nurses' wages from reaching the equilibrium level, and, second, why the static shortage disappeared in the period after 1966.

IMPERFECTIONS IN THE MARKET FOR RN SERVICES

The explanation for a possible static shortage of nurses in the hospital sector prior to 1966 is that hospitals have acted as a cartel in setting nurses' wages and are monopsonists or oligopsonists with respect to the employment of registered nurses. Ten percent of all hospitals are the only hospital in an area, 30 percent of hospitals are located in areas where there are only one or two hospitals, and 45 percent of hospitals are in areas where there are less than four hospitals; more than 60 percent of hospitals are in areas where there are fewer than six hospitals (5). As purchasers of nurses' services, therefore, hospitals have a great deal of market power; they employ 75 percent of all nurses (both hospital-based and private duty nurses), and since there are few hospitals in any one area it is relatively easy for them to collude in setting nurses' wages. In most sectors where a firm is only one of many other firms hiring people in a certain occupational category, it is difficult for the firms to collude to begin with or to ensure later that each firm does not violate the collective agreement. When there are many firms, it is in the interests of any one firm to raise the wage slightly and attract people from other firms. Hospitals, however, can quickly find out whether or not another hospital in the area has changed its wage policy. Also, since they employ almost all of the active nurses, it is difficult to attract nurses from other firms. The hospitals, in facing an increase in the demand for their services and believing that the short-run supply of nurses is relatively inelastic (i.e., increasing the wage would result in only a small increase in the number of nurses seeking work, either through a change in their status from inactive to active or from immigration from other areas), will decide to hold down nurses' wages. RNs' wages represent a significant portion of a hospital's budget (25 percent); increasing the wage rate to attract new nurses would require an increase in the wage to all existing RNs as well.

RNs employed in nonhospital settings would receive higher wages because these other employment settings would be more willing to pay higher RN salaries to enable hiring as many RNs as needed. RNs represent a small portion of the cost of operation in these other employment sectors. Further, in some employment situations, e.g., government, the RN's wage would be related to the wages of other occupational groups and would, therefore, increase at the same rate as these other personnel categories.

To test this hypothesis of hospital collusion in the setting of nurses' wages, Donald Yett conducted a survey of the 31 largest hospital associations to determine whether or not they had wage stabilization programs. Fourteen of the 15 hospital associations that responded reported that they did have wage stabilization programs (6). [The one hospital association that did not have one asked how it could start one (7).] Additional evidence of the attempt by hospitals to fix nurses' wages in their area is the following statement that appeared in the *Los Angeles Times*: "The majority of hospitals fix wages for nurses on recommendations from the Hospital Council of Southern California. The Council's recommendations have always been accepted and are based on recommendations from the management consulting firm of Guffenhagen-Kroeger Inc." (8).

As hospitals found it difficult to hire more nurses during the period of continued shortage, they intensified their efforts along two other lines to increase the number of nurses. Hospitals began recruiting foreign-trained nurses and they lobbied for legislation to provide subsidies to increase the number of registered nurses.

Before evaluating how effective the subsequent nurse training legislation was, it is interesting to examine what happened to the market for nurses in the post-1966 period. After 1966 two events occurred which substantially changed the market for nurses. The first, and perhaps most important, was the passage of Medicare and Medicaid. The second was the increase of collective bargaining among hospital nurses.

When Medicare and Medicaid were passed, the demand for hospital care increased because the aged population was provided with hospital coverage. At the same time, hospitals were reimbursed on a "cost-plus" basis. The effect was to increase the demand for RNs and, at the same time, to make the demand more inelastic with respect to their wages. If hospitals hired more nurses and increased their wages, these costs could then be passed on to the government (on a proportional basis according to the ratio of charges to charges to cost of aged patients). Depending upon what portion of their hospitalized population was covered under some form of cost reimbursement, e.g., government, Blue Cross, or other third-party reimbursement, hospitals were relieved from pressures to contain their costs. Wage increases to hospital-employed nurses increased rapidly in the post-Medicare period, more rapidly than wage increases to nonhospital-employed nurses and to persons working in nonhealth-field occupations with comparable training. Nurses' wages, which were artificially held down for a number of years, were allowed to rise. Thus, by 1969 rates of return to hospital-employed nurses were comparable to other occupations.

Registered nurses employed in nonprofit hospitals were expressly exempt from the legal provisions of the National Labor Relations Act between 1947 and 1974, and did not, therefore, have legal protection of their rights to organize or support a union. (In 1974, an amendment to the Taft-Hartley Act repealed the provisions that excluded hospitals from its jurisdiction.) Collective bargaining on behalf of hospital nurses, therefore, started slowly. In addition to the impediments to collective bargaining contracts which legally permitted hospitals to refuse to bargain with unions representing hospital employees, the American Nurses' Association (ANA) had not been a strong proponent of unionization. In 1970 approximately 38,000 RNs were included under collective bargaining agreements (9), which represented only about 5 percent of employed RNs. By 1977 200,000 RN's, more than 20 percent of employed nurses, were included under collective bargaining agreements, a substantial increase over 1970 (10). The effects of collective bargaining agreements, however, are felt beyond the numbers of nurses covered. To forestall such agreements, hospitals may offer higher wages to RNs.

The effects of unionization in a market dominated by monopsonists will be to increase wages and possibly employment; whether or not increased employment will occur will depend on how much the wage is increased. Such a situation is described in an appendix to this chapter.* This monopsonistic hospital

---

*Several studies have been conducted to determine the effect of a monopsonistic market on nurses' wages and then the effect on wages in these markets of collective bargaining. In one study, using 1973 data, it was found that, "Unionization of at least 75 percent of the nursing workforce is associated with

control over nurses' wages was weakened by the growth (both actual and expected) of nurses' unions.

To sum up, then, the effects of Medicare and Medicaid and the increase (also the threat) of nurse collective bargaining after 1966 resulted in an increase in wages for nurses at a rate that was more rapid than had been the case both in the past and for nurses not employed in hospitals. The effect of those wage increases was to decrease the reported vacancies in hospitals (refer back to Table 16-1) so that by 1971 the vacancy rate dropped to 9.3 percent from its high of 23.2 percent in 1961.† From 1969 on, the various market indicators no longer suggest a static shortage, but rather a situation characterized more by a market adjusting toward an equilibrium situation. It appears, therefore, that in the past there was probably a static shortage of registered nurses, created by the collusion of hospitals to keep nurses' wages from rising. Such a situation no longer exists. The appropriate public policy in the past would have been to allow nurses' wages to rise, which would have resulted in increased hospital costs—normal occurrence in an industry experiencing a rising demand for its services and facing a rising supply curve for its factor inputs.‡ Allowing nurses' wages to rise would have brought forth an increase both in the stock of nurses and in their employment (participation rates). Federal legislation to increase the supply of nurses would not have been necessary.

Since there no longer appears to be any shortage of nurses (11), it would also appear to be unnecessary to continue federal assistance to increase the supply of nurses. Yet new federal funding for support of nurse training was renewed in late 1975 (Congress overrode President Ford's veto of that legislation in order for it to become law) and again in 1979. To better understand the probable intent of the federal legislation to support nurse training and how effective it has been in achieving its stated goals of increasing the supply of nurses, it is worthwhile to examine the Nurse Training Act in some depth.

FEDERAL SUPPORT FOR NURSE TRAINING

The stimulus for the Nurse Training Act of 1964 was the estimate of the impending shortage of nurses that would occur without federal legislation. The Surgeon

---

an addition to yearly starting salaries of $803. The size of the negative monopsony effect remains statistically significant but is again reduced to $383." Charles Link and John Landon, "Monopsony and Union Power in the Market for Nurses," *Southern Economic Journal* 41(4) (April 1975): 655. See also Richard W. Hurd, "Equilibrium Vacancies in a Labor Market Dominated by Non-Profit Firms: The 'Shortage' of Nurses," *Review of Economics and Statistics*, May 1973.

† There is some evidence to suggest that vacancy statistics are overstated. One independent survey of nurse vacancy rates made by the U.S. Employment Service (USES) in April 1966 found a 5 percent vacancy rate, as contrasted to the American Nurses' Association estimate for that same period of 13.5 percent. If the ANA statistics are roughly twice as great as the USES vacancy statistics, then this would suggest that in 1971, when the American Hospital Association (AHA) reported a vacancy rate of 9.3 percent, a more realistic vacancy rate was half that amount, approximately 4.5 percent. Such a low vacancy rate suggests that there is no shortage of registered nurses. John Edgren, "The Federal Nurse Training Acts," *Health Manpower Policy Studies Group Discussion Paper Series*, School of Public Health, University of Michigan, 1977, pp. 6–7.

‡ Claims of a "shortage" in this type of situation are merely a matter of employers' not wishing to pay higher prices for their inputs. Government intervention in such situations is not economically justified.

General's Consultant Group on Nursing, appointed in 1961 to study the problem, concluded in its report in 1963 that indeed there was a serious shortage. The shortage forecast was made using the ratio technique and was thus unrelated to any economic criterion of shortage. The forecast was also not based on any conclusion regarding the performance of the market for nurses.

Support for federal legislation on nurse training came from several groups: Congress recognized the potential political rewards of backing health legislation; the federal bureaucracy—specifically, the Division of Nursing in the U.S. Public Health Service—helped to justify the need for the legislation with an eye toward an expanded role in administering it; hospitals believed they would gain from such legislation because it would increase the supply of nurses, thereby slowing down the rate of increase in nurses' wages; and support came also from the American Nurses' Association, which must have perceived the effects of the federal legislation to be different from the effects perceived by hospitals, if we are to interpret nurse training as being consistent with the goals of the ANA membership. Among other things, the ANA seeks to increase its members' incomes. If the legislation were to have the effect desired by hospitals, namely, an increase in the supply of nurses, then it would inhibit the rise in nurses' wages, which would be the opposite of the ANA's objective. It must, therefore, be assumed that the ANA saw the legislation as an opportunity to change the role of registered nurses. If the educational subsidies provided under this legislation could be redirected toward producing fewer, more highly trained nurses who could undertake more responsibilities, then the effect of these fewer nurses, each with more training, would be a greater increase in nurses' wages.

Thus, the reasons for federal subsidies for nurse education varied. Such legislation would not have improved the functioning of the market for nurses; in an economic sense there was no justification for federal legislation. The true intent of the legislation was to benefit either hospitals (by providing them with cheaper inputs) or nurses (by changing educational requirements and graduating fewer nurses capable of performing more tasks). By analyzing how the legislation was implemented and what its effects were we can determine who actually benefited from the legislation.

Two broad purposes were stated in the Nurse Training Act (NTA) of 1964: to increase the quantity of nurses and to improve their quality. These two goals matched the separate interests of the ANA and AHA. The goals and programs enacted in the NTA of 1964 were those recommended in the Surgeon General's report of 1963. To achieve both an increase in the quality and quantity of nurses, there were four broad areas of federal support in the NTA of 1964, which were continued in subsequent renewals and amendments to that act. The two most important areas, comprising 93 percent of the total funds expended on nursing training between 1964 and 1981, were, first, a program of grants to schools of nursing for distribution in the form of scholarships and loans to students (40 percent of total funds were for this purpose). The second area of federal support was for grants to the nursing schools for construction, planning or initiating programs of nursing education, or for general financial support (53 percent of the funds went for this purpose).

With regard to the quantity objective of the nurse training legislation, i.e., an increase in the number of nurses, the 1963 Surgeon General's report stated that with the federal support requested, 680,000 nurses would be a "feasible" goal by 1970. In updated estimates made in 1967, it was predicted that 1,000,000 RNs would be needed in 1975. To achieve these increases in the number of nurses, it was proposed that schools of nursing increase the number of their graduates to 53,000 a year by 1969, which represented a 75 percent increase over 1961 (12).

The goal of 680,000 RNs by 1970 was surpassed; it was achieved a year earlier than expected. The number of nurses in 1975 was also very close to what was desired. Though it would appear that the nurse training legislation achieved its goals, upon closer examination it is doubtful whether these achievements were a result of the federal support for nurse training. The number of graduates being produced by schools of nursing in 1969 was 42,196, not the 53,000 per year that was supposed to occur as a result of the federal program. In fact, the number of graduates was only 1,196 more than what the Surgeon General's report estimated would have been the case *without* any federal legislation (13). Although the quantitative goals underlying the NTA were achieved, the funding of nursing schools and students did not achieve the increase in graduates believed necessary to achieve these goals. How then were the desired goals met?

An increase in the number of RNs employed can occur in one of two ways: 1) an increase in the number of nursing graduates, or 2) an increase in the number of trained nurses (the stock of RNs) who are employed, i.e., the participation rate.* The federal program was directed exclusively at increasing the number of nursing graduates and thus probably had no effect on the nurse participation rate.†

The number of nurse graduates could have been increased under the federal programs as a result of 1) funding for new construction to result in an increase in the number of spaces in nursing schools, 2) the loans and scholarships programs to induce people to enter nursing who would otherwise not, and 3) financial assistance to the nursing schools, which could have resulted in either more attractive facilities or lower tuition rates to attract potential students. Several economists have estimated the increase in the number of nursing graduates as a result of the federal support for nursing education. Donald Yett estimated that "the increase in enrollment of marginal entrants resulted in approximately 2,660 graduates over the years 1968 to 1970" (14). John Edgren estimated a total increase of 6,813 additional graduates between 1966 and 1972 as a result of the federal subsidy program.‡ It would appear that the federal subsidies led to an increase of less than 1,500 new graduates a year.

Why was the increase in nurse graduates so small, given the large federal subsidy program? Nursing education is typically provided in one of three types of settings; diploma schools, community colleges offering a two-year associate degree, and four-year colleges offering a baccalaureate degree. Diploma schools, generally located in or associated with hospitals, have in the past provided the

---

*An increase in nurse employment can also occur if there is a change in the rate at which nurses retire or die and also if there is a change in the immigration of foreign-trained nurses.

† It might be argued that the loan forgiveness portions of the loans and scholarship program might have increased the participation rate of new graduates; however the majority of nurses are active anyway immediately upon graduation.

‡ The 6,813 additional graduates between 1966 and 1972 were out of a total 247,753 graduates over that same period. Edgren, "The Federal Nurse Training Acts," p. 26.

majority of nurse graduates.* While attending classes, students in diploma schools work in hospitals and receive a stipend. Hospitals subsidize the cost of their diploma schools to assure themselves a supply of nurses upon graduation. However, as the mobility of nurses has increased, hospital diploma schools have become a diminishing source of nurses for the particular hospitals subsidizing them. Hospitals could no longer be assured that their subsidies to such schools would be repaid when the nurses left to work elsewhere. As tuition costs to the students in diploma schools rose, enrollments declined (15). After World War II diploma schools of nursing rapidly declined, from 1,118 in 1950 to 344 in 1978. Hospitals hoped that the federal subsidies under the NTA would be used to increase the number of nurses graduating from diploma schools of nursing. There was sufficient capacity in those schools to accommodate increases in enrollment. However, the American Nurses' Association stated in 1965 that they wanted nursing education to occur in institutions of higher learning. The National League for Nursing (NLN) was designated as the accrediting agency for dispensing federal support to schools of nursing; its goals were, of course, similar to those of the ANA. Until 1968, payments to diploma and associate degree schools under the NTA fell short of what Congress authorized (50 percent), while payments to baccalaureate programs were approximately equal to what was authorized (16).

Although the number of diploma school programs declined, graduates from these programs still made the largest contribution to the number of new active nurses during the period from 1950 to 1972. The number of baccalaureate degree programs increased from 195 to 293 over that same period, yet the number of new active nurses they contributed was only twice as great as the number of graduates from associate degree programs, which grew in numbers from one program in 1950 to 541 in 1972. The large growth in associate degree programs began before the funds for the NTA became available. (The number of graduates from each of these programs is shown in Table 16-6).

It appears that in administering the NTA, no attempt was made to maximize the number of nurse graduates. If that had been the goal, the funds would have been allocated differently according to the different types of nursing schools.

---

*Of the approximately 1,272,851 employed RNs in 1980, 70.9 percent or 876,000 graduated from diploma nursing schools and associate degree programs; 20.6 percent or 255,000 graduated from 4-year baccalaureate degree programs; and 5.3 percent or 65,000 graduated from masters and doctorate programs.

As of 1950, there were 1,314 state-approved schools of nursing. Of these, 1,118 were diploma schools, 195 were BA programs, and 1 was an associate program. By 1965 there were 1,193 programs; of these, 821 were diploma schools, 198 were BA schools, and 174 were associate degree schools. By 1978, there were a total of 1,374 programs; of these, 344 were diploma schools, 353 were BA schools, and 677 were associate degree schools. *Source Book of Nursing Personnel,* U.S. Department of Health, Education and Welfare, Division of Nursing, Bethesda, Md., DHEW Publication No. (HRA) 75-43, December 1974. American Nurses Association, *Facts About Nursing,* 1980–1981 ed., p. 152; U.S. Department of Health and Human Services, Bureau of Nursing, *Report of the Secretary of Health and Human Services on The Supply and Distribution of and Requirements for Nurses as Required by Section 951, Nurse Training Act of 1975, April 27, 1981,* p. 156. U.S. Department of Health and Human Services, Division of Health Professions Analysis, *The Registered Nurse Population, An Overview: From National Sample Survey of Registered Nurses, November 1980,* Report No. 82-5, p. 11.

TABLE 16-6. Nursing Graduates by Type of Nursing School Program

Academic Year	Total		Diploma		Associate Degree		Baccalaureate	
	Number	Annual (% Change)	Number	% of Total Graduates	Number	% of Total Graduates	Number	% of Total Graduates
1952[a]	29,016		26,720	92.1	298	1.0	1,998	6.9
1955[a]	28,729	−.3	25,826	89.9	199	.7	2,704	9.4
1960–1961	30,019	.9	25,071	83.5	917	3.1	4,031	13.4
1965–1966	34,909	3.1	26,072	74.7	3,349	9.6	5,488	15.7
1970–1971	46,455	5.9	22,065	47.5	14,534	31.3	9,856	21.2
1975–1976	77,065	10.7	19,861	25.8	34,625	44.9	22,579	29.3
1976–1977	77,755	.9	18,014	23.2	36,289	46.7	23,452	30.1
1977–1978	77,874	.2	17,131	22.0	36,556	46.9	24,187	31.1
1978–1979	77,132	−1.0	15,820	20.5	36,264	47.0	25,048	32.5
1979–1980	75,523	−2.1	14,495	19.2	36,034	47.7	24,994	33.1

Sources: For 1952 and 1955: U.S. Department of Health, Education and Welfare, Division of Nursing, *Source Book of Nursing*, DHEW Publication No. (HRA) 75-43 (Washington, D.C.: Government Printing Office, 1974), p. 98. For 1960–1980, National League of Nursing, *Nursing Data Book, 1981* (New York: National League of Nursing, 1982), p. 39, Table 36. Used with permission.

[a]These represent calendar years.

Instead, there appears to have been a conscious decision to favor growth in the number of nursing graduates from baccalaureate degree programs. From the ANA's point of view, such graduates would be more likely to take on additional responsibilities. Shifting away from diploma schools to baccalaureate schools would also coincide with the ANA's goals, since a likely result would be a smaller increase in the number of nurse graduates, thereby resulting in an eventual increase in their wages. The starting salaries of nursing graduates are similar regardless of the type of school from which they are graduated. A graduate from a baccalaureate school spends more time in school compared with graduates from associate degree or diploma schools, yet the wage differential does not compensate baccalaureate graduates for the additional training time or foregone income.

The growth in demand for associate degree education was related to its relatively high rate of return when compared with comparable occupations (17). It is thus likely that associate degree programs would have grown without federal NTA support (18). The diploma-school enrollments probably declined because the higher rates of return in these programs, relative to BA and AA degrees, were not high enough to offset "certain non-financial disadvantages (e.g., apprenticeship-type work requirements, restrictions on social life, little or no access to job opportunities other than in nursing, etc.)" (19). The rate of return to a BA degree program was lower than the diploma or associate degree programs. In order to compensate for this lower rate of return, the ANA has attempted to provide such students with greater direct financial support and indirect support through payments to the collegiate schools for construction and operating expenses, to eventually result in lower tuition levels. The reasons, therefore, for the small increase in nurse graduates as a result of the federal legislation is the change in educational emphasis in nursing toward baccalaureate degrees and the allocation of the federal funds to promote this change in the type of nursing graduate. Whether or not this is a desirable federal objective is another question.

If the federal subsidies for nurse education produced few additional nurses, then how were the quantitative goals for the number of nurses achieved? Based upon an econometric model of the nursing sector, which was used to stimulate changes that have occurred in nurse employment over time, one author concluded:

> The predicted nurse graduations, which by 1969 are equal to 39,250, are not even close to the 53,000 set as the 1969 goals by the Surgeon General's Consultant Group on Nursing, necessary to achieve the 680,000 employment figure. In fact, the model's predictions of nursing school graduations are considerably below this level throughout the forecast period. Therefore, the achievement of the 1969 level of nursing is to be attributed to the increases in participation rates and the change in the age distribution of the stock of nurses, as well as increased graduations, and none of these events are even remotely influenced by the existence of the subsidy programs in question. (20)

Labor force participation rates for nurses increased from 48.8 percent in 1950, to 55.3 percent in 1960 (21), to 65.2 percent in 1966, to 70.5 percent in 1972, and to 76 percent in 1980 (22). There was a net increase of 414,815 employed RNs from 1966 to 1977. It has been estimated that the sources of this net increase in employed RNs were: a change in the participation rate and in reinstatements (RNs who have renewed their lapsed licenses), 33.9 percent; foreign-trained

RNs, 9.1 percent; and new graduates, 57.1 percent (23). Graduates from associate degree programs represented 3 percent of graduates in 1960–1961, 31.4 percent by 1970–1971, and 47.1 percent by 1977–1978. The higher nurse participation rates were in large part due to the increase in nurses' wages. During the time period that the federal subsidy program to nurse education was in effect, there were large increases in the wages of nurses as a result of the Medicare and Medicaid programs. It is believed that these wage increases resulted in a higher nurse participation rate, which was a major contributing factor in the increase in nurse employment. It appears, therefore, that the achievement of the employment goals underlying the NTA of 1964 were the result of other factors (e.g., increased nurse participation rate), rather than the federal subsidy program itself.

It is possible to compare the costs of increasing nurse employment through subsidizing nursing education, as under the nurse training legislation, with an approach which would subsidize nurses' wages directly. The cost (in terms of federal subsidy dollars required) for increases in the number of employed nurses is several times lower if direct wage subsidies are provided to nurses instead of providing federal subsidies to nursing schools to increase the number of their nursing graduates. For example, earlier it was estimated that the number of additional nurses employed as a result of the federal support to nursing schools was approximately 1,500 nurses per year or 24,000 for the 16-year period 1965–1981.* The estimated federal expenditures under nurse training legislation during that time period was $1.57 billion. This comes to $65,000 per employed nurse as a result of the federal subsidy program. If an alternative federal program for increasing the supply of active nurses were implemented, namely, to simply provide a wage subsidy to all employed nurses, how much would this cost? Several studies have attempted to estimate the elasticity of the participation rate with respect to nurses' wages, holding other factors constant. These studies have derived elasticity estimates ranging from a negative elasticity to an elasticity of 2.8 (24). In our example we will use an elasticity estimate of 1.0; i.e., a 1 percent increase in nurses' wages leads to a 1 percent increase in the number of active nurses.

If the wage elasticity with respect to the nurse participation rate were 1.0, then it would require a 1 percent increase in nurses' wages, multiplied by all employed nurses, to achieve a 1 percent increase in the number of employed RNs. In 1963 there were approximately 550,000 active RNs receiving an annual wage of $4,714. A 1 percent subsidy to increase their wage would be $47 per nurse multiplied by 550,000 active nurses, for a total subsidy cost of $25 million. This would result in a 1 percent increase in the number of active RNs, or 5,500 additional nurses. The federal subsidy per additional nurse employed under this program comes to $4,545. Table 16-7 shows the federal subsidy per active nurse under this type of a program for different time periods. As the number of active

---

*The number of nurses produced as a result of the NTA would be lower than this estimate, since there is a long lead time necessary before the federal funds have their effect. Legislation enacted in 1964 contained authorizations for 1965 and began to affect nursing schools in 1966. First graduates from associate degree programs would appear in 1967, and graduates from baccalaureate programs, which were the recipients of a large part of the funds, would not appear until 1969.

TABLE 16-7. Cost of an Alternative Federal Subsidy Program to Increase the Number of Active RNs

Year	Annual Wage	1 Percent Increase in Wage	Number of Active RNs	Total Cost of 1 Percent Increase Col. 3 × Col. 4	1 Percent Increase in Employed RNs	Cost per Additional RN Col. 5 ÷ Col. 6
1963	$4,714	$47	550,000	$25,000,000	5,500	$4,545
1966	5,763	57	600,000	34,000,000	6,000	5,666
1969	7,815	78	630,000	50,000,000	6,300	7,936

RNs increases, so does the annual number of subsidy dollars required to produce an additional active RN under this approach—from $4,545 per active RN in 1963 to $7,936 per active RN in 1969. To produce an equivalent 24,000 nurses through a wage subsidy program would have taken approximately 4 years at a total subsidy cost of $120 million, for an average cost of $5,000 per additional nurse. When compared with the cost of $65,000 per active RN produced under the actual nurse training legislation, the cost per active RN under this alternative subsidy program is approximately 10 times less expensive. Even if one were to vastly change the assumptions used in these calculations, i.e., the elasticity of the nurse participation rates or the number of nursing school graduates produced under the NTA, this alternative subsidy program is still less expensive.* (The attractiveness of this program would be increased further if the subsidies *were discounted*.) Other advantages of the alternative subsidy program are that the administrative costs of this subsidy program are lower and that the increase in active nurses will occur much more quickly than it would as a result of a subsidy program which relies on increased nursing graduates. Also, under the alternative subsidy program, the federal government does not make a *continuing* commitment of financial support to schools of nursing. Once federal funds have subsidized these institutions, a new constituency for federal support has been created, and it is difficult to reduce support even if it is no longer believed that there is a nursing shortage.

An important difference between the nurse training legislation and the alternative subsidy program is that the more successful the federal government is in increasing the number of nursing graduates, the lower the increases in nurses' wages will be. The increased supply of new nurses will hold down potential increases in nurses' wages; this dampening effect will have an adverse impact upon the participation rate. Thus, the subsidy to nursing schools may be self-defeating!

CONCLUDING COMMENTS

An analysis of the market for registered nurses appears to indicate that it is currently performing well. That is, as demand for nurses increases, the wage of registered nurses rises so that there is no economic shortage or surplus of nurses. The measures used to evaluate the performance of the nursing market were the rise in the number of hospital-employed nurses, their rate of return compared with other nurses and other occupations with comparable training, the increase in the number of nurses entering nursing, and the participation rate of nurses. As would be expected in an efficiently operating market, as the demand for nurses increased, so would their wages, their relative rate of return, the number of students entering nursing, and the percentage of trained nurses who are active. From the late 1940s to the current time, the nursing market appears to have achieved a new equilibrium point; rates of return to nurses are again comparable

---

*If a .25 elasticity estimate were assumed, then a wage subsidy program would have taken 14 years at a total subsidy cost of $888 million to produce 24,000 nurses—almost half the cost of the program adapted by the government.

to other occupations. (The rates of return, however, vary, depending upon the type of nursing school that the nurse has graduated from.) However, the adjustment process that has occurred during this 20- to 25-year period has not always worked well. During the period between the late 1950s and the mid-1960s, there appeared to have been a shortage situation; there was a greater demand by hospitals for nurses than was being supplied at the going wage. From an analysis of the percent increase in wages of hospital employed nurses relative to other nurses, it appeared that the shortage situation was not a dynamic one but rather was the result of hospital collusion to prevent nurses' wages from rising. This collusion, which was an attempt by hospitals to keep their costs from increasing, led to intensified recruiting of foreign-trained nurses and to greater substitution of practical nurses and nurses aides for registered nurses by hospitals. Hospitals also lobbied for federal subsidies to increase the supply of nurses so as to be provided with cheaper inputs. The "shortage" situation began to disappear when Medicare and Medicaid were passed. As the demand for hospital care (and the consequent demand for nurses) increased as a result of this legislation, the hospitals were able to pass on to the government the increased costs of higher nurses' wages and the increase in number of nurses employed. Collective bargaining agreements between hospitals and nurses began at this time. These two factors resulted in a large increase in nurses' wages in the post-Medicare period and in nurse participation rates; they also led to increased enrollments in associate degree programs.

It thus appears that the market for nurses began to correct itself. The federal legislation to support nurse training had been passed by this time (1964), and the increased federal support coincided with the increased demand by prospective nurses for associate degree programs. The American Nurses' Association and the accrediting agency for disbursing the federal funds, the National League for Nursing, saw the federal training subsidies as a chance to change the educational requirements and eventually the roles and responsibilities of nurses. Greater emphasis was placed on baccalaureate programs by these organizations.

The original manpower goals underlying the 1964 Nurse Training Act were achieved, although it appears that they would have been achieved without the federal subsidy program. Regardless of the accuracy of the original rationale for the federal subsidy to nursing education, since the quantitative goals have now been achieved, what further justification is there for continued federal subsidies to nursing schools? If continued increases in the number of active nurses are desired, then it would be many times less expensive to achieve these increased numbers through a different subsidy program. If the objective of continued subsidies is to raise the educational level to prepare nurses to undertake additional responsibilities, then it is questionable whether this is a sufficient criterion for federal intervention in the nursing market and for use of public funds for this purpose. If there is a greater demand for such personnel, and state practice acts permit nurses to undertake additional responsibilities, then the increased return for doing these tasks would justify increased investment by nurses for this training. It is not clear why federal subsidies are required. The goals used by the nursing profession to justify continued subsidies to nursing education should be made explicit so it can be determined whether it is a goal agreed to by the rest of society and whether the proposed approach is the least expensive way to achieve it.

A recent proposal by the American Nurses' Association, if implemented, should have an important effect on the supply of nurses. The ANA has proposed that beginning in 1985 all nursing graduates should receive a BA degree. If the ANA is successful in raising nurse educational requirements in this manner, there should be a sharp reduction in the number of new graduates each year. Currently, graduates with a BA degree represent only 31 percent of new nurse graduates. If implemented today, this policy would result in a loss of 54,000 graduates per year. The impact of this policy over time should be an increase in salaries of nurses, with a consequent rise in hospital costs. These higher costs would, in part, be shifted to patients, government, and other third-party payors.

APPENDIX: THE EFFECTS ON WAGES AND EMPLOYMENT OF REGISTERED NURSES OF UNIONIZATION IN A MONOPSONY MARKET

A monopsonist, with a demand curve D_1, will face a rising supply curve for nurses described by S_1 in Figure 16-3. Since the monopsonist must pay a higher wage to all currently employed nurses each time it pays a higher wage for an additional nurse, it faces a marginal factor cost (MFC) curve which lies above the supply curve. The MFC curve represents the cost to the monopsonist of hiring an additional nurse. At each point on the supply curve, the MFC curve indicates the additional cost in terms of higher wages that must be paid to all previously hired nurses. Thus the equilibrium quantity of nurses the firm will hire and the wage it will pay under such circumstances is given by the intersection of the demand curve and the MFC curve. Drawing a line down to the supply curve will indicate the wage it would pay and the quantity of RNs employed. At the equilibrium

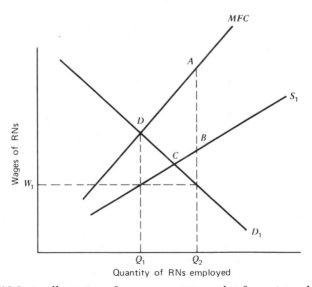

Figure 16-3. An illustration of a monopsonistic market for registered nurses.

wage of the firm, W_1, the monopsonist would be willing to hire Q_2 quantity of nurses, which is the point on the firm's demand curve at a wage of W_1. However, if the firm were to actually hire Q_2 number of RNs, it would have to pay a wage much higher than W_1. The new wage would be at that point on the supply curve above Q_2 shown by B. The cost to the firm of that wage and Q_2 number of nurses would be point A *on the MFC curve. Since point A* on the MFC curve would be greater than the firm's demand curve, the firm would not want to hire Q_2 nurses at a wage represented by point B on the supply curve. Thus W_1 and Q_1 are equilibrium points for the monopsonist. However, at that wage, W_1, the firm will report $Q_1 - Q_2$ vacancies for nurses. These are the number of nurses it would be willing to hire at wage W_1. Vacancies are thus expected and quite normal in a monopsony situation.

In this situation, if a union were started and set a minimum wage for its employees, then the supply curve for nurses would change. It would become horizontal up to the point of the minimum wage on the original supply curve. This would indicate that under the collective bargaining agreement, nurses cannot be paid below a certain minimum union wage. The hospital can hire all the nurses it wants at that wage. The MFC curve would also change. It would become equal to the new minimum wage, since there is no additional cost to the hospital as it hires an additional nurse; i.e., it does not have to increase the wages of those nurses currently employed. Up to the point where the negotiated wage intersects the original supply curve the hospital can hire all the nurses it wants at the negotiated wage. Beyond that point the hospital will have to increase its wages and also pay higher wages to its existing nurses. Thus at that point the hospital will again face a rising supply curve and a rising MFC curve. In situations involving a monopsony purchaser and a union representing the employees, it is possible for the union to set a wage that is higher than the previous wage and also increase employment. This is illustrated in Figure 16-4. If the union sets a

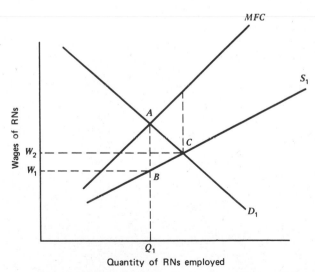

Figure 16-4. Collective bargaining and a monopsony market for registered nurses.

wage rate anywhere between A and B, it will raise the wage (since the current wage is W_1) and it will increase the number of nurses hired. Any wage between A and B will make the supply curve and the MFC curve horizontal up to that point. For example, a wage rate of W_2 is the point where employment of RNs is greatest. The new wage rate intersects the demand curve at the same point that the supply curve does. Therefore the wage rate (W_2) is the new MFC and supply curve up to the point where it intersects the original supply curve. To hire more nurses after that point, the firm will have to pay a higher wage and thus face a rising MFC and rising supply curve. Above point A on the demand curve, a union wage will decrease employment of RNs, unless the demand curve shifts to the right.

REFERENCES

1. Donald E. Yett, *An Economic Analysis of the Nurse Shortage* (Lexington, Mass.: D.C. Heath Co., 1975), p. 19.

2. *Ibid.*, p. 110.

3. *Ibid.*, p. 182.

4. *Ibid.*, p. 199.

5. *Ibid.*, p. 221.

6. F. Sloan and R. Elnicki construct a model to test the monopsony hypothesis and several other hypotheses about nurses' wages for the year 1972. Their model and conclusions may be found in Frank Sloan and Richard Elnicki, "Determinants of Professional Nurses' Wages," in Richard Scheffler, ed., *Research in Health Economics,* Vol. 1 (Greenwich, Conn.: JAI Press, 1979), pp. 217–254.

7. Yett, *op. cit.*, p. 221.

8. *Ibid.*, p. 221.

9. Stuart Altman, *Present and Future Supply of Registered Nurses,* U.S. Department of Health, Education and Welfare Publication No. (NIH) 72-134, Division of Nursing, Washington, D.C.: Government Printing Office, November 1971, p. 15.

10. Myrtle K. Aydelotte, "Trends in Staffing of Hospitals: Implications for Nursing Resources Policy," in Michael L. Millman, ed., *Nursing Personnel and the Changing Health Care System* (Cambridge, Mass.: Ballinger, 1978), p. 132.

11. A recent government study has also concluded that there is no economic shortage of nurses. See: Jesse S. Hixson, Jack Reid, Jack Rodgers, and Stephen Boehlert, "The Shortage of Nursing Personnel—A New Look at the Issues," Division of Health Professions Analysis, Bureau of Health Professions, Health Resources Administration, February 26, 1981 (mimeographed).

12. Yett, *op. cit.*, p. 246.

13. *Ibid.*, p. 247.

14. *Ibid.*, p. 248.

15. *Ibid.*, p. 29.

16. *Ibid.*, pp. 32–33.

17. *Ibid.*, p. 251.

18. *Ibid.*, p. 249.

19. *Ibid.*, p. 249.

20. Robert T. Deane, "Simulating an Econometric Model of the Market for Nurses," unpublished doctoral dissertation, Department of Economics, University of California at Los Angeles, 1971, p. 218. A further discussion of the ineffectiveness of the Nurse Training Act (NTA) may be found in Robert Deane and Donald Yett, "Nurse Market Policy Simulations Using an Econometric Model," in Richard Scheffler, ed., *Research in Health Economics* (Greenwich, Conn.: JAI Press, 1979).

21. Altman, *Present and Future Supply of Registered Nurses*, p. 102.

22. *The Registered Nurse Population: An Overview*, from a national sample of registered nurses, November 1980, U.S. Department of Health and Human Services, Bureau of Health Professions, Division of Health Professions Analysis, Report No. 82-5, Rockville, Md.: U.S. Dept. of Health and Human Services, December 1981.

23. John Edgren, "The Federal Nurse Training Acts," *Health Manpower Policy Studies Group Discussion Paper Series*, School of Public Health, University of Michigan, 1977, p. 39.

24. The reasons for the differences in the estimates relate to the types of data used, aggregate versus micro, characteristics of the nurses, and the econometric methods employed. For a further discussion of these estimates see: Frank A. Sloan, *Equalizing Access to Nursing Services: The Geographic Discussion*, Department of Health, Education and Welfare Publication No. (HRA) 78-51, Washington, D.C.: Government Printing Office, March 1978; and Charles R. Link and Russell F. Settle, "Wage Incentives and Married Professional Nurses: A Case of Backward-Bending Supply?," *Economic Inquiry* 19 (January 1981): 144–156.

CHAPTER 17

The Pharmaceutical Industry

INTRODUCTION

Drugs provide society with enormous benefits. They reduce mortality and morbidity, relieve pain and suffering, are less expensive forms of treatment than surgery and hospitalization, are more readily accessible to a larger portion of the population than more expensive technologies, and have enabled physicians to see more patients with improved treatment outcomes.

Many serious diseases have had their incidence and severity greatly reduced by modern drugs. For example, penicillin and the antibiotics have caused a large decline in the mortality and morbidity associated with infectious diseases such as pneumonia, meningitis, and tuberculosis. Pneumonia used to be a widespread, greatly feared, and often fatal disease. Tranquilizers and chemotherapy of mental patients have resulted in changes in the treatment of mental illness and large reductions in use of mental institutions, enabling many who would have been incapable of functioning adequately to actually work and live at home. Antihypertensive drugs reduced the death rate from hypertensive heart disease from 44 per 100,000 in 1960 to 11 per 100,000 in 1970. Synthetic hormones and birth control pills have had a worldwide impact. People have been able to plan their families conveniently. Many childhood diseases, such as measles, diphtheria, and polio, that are potentially fatal or crippling have been virtually eliminated by the use of vaccinations.

Drugs also reduce the direct and indirect costs of illness. They reduce the need for hospitalization and the length of time needed as an inpatient when it is required, a very large savings of the direct cost of illness. By reducing both the length and severity of illness, drugs enable the patient to return to work sooner, thereby lowering the indirect costs of sickness. Drugs are an integral part of medical treatment, whose benefits in medical, social, and economic terms would be incalculable should their availability be withdrawn.

For all of its enormous impact on health status and in the alleviation of pain, personal expenditures on drugs have been rising less rapidly than personal medical care expenditures over the past 30 years. Drug (and medical sundry) expenditures were $3.7 billion in 1960, increasing to $8.0 billion in 1970 and to $21.4 billion in 1981, for an average annual rate of increase of 8.7 percent per year (1). This is in contrast to the increase in total personal health care expenditures, which rose from $23.6 billion in 1960 to $255.0 billion in 1981, for an average annual rate of increase of 12 percent per year. As a percentage of total personal health care expenditures, drugs have fallen from 15 percent in 1960 to 9 percent in 1980. This is shown in Table 17-1.

Drug prices have also been subject to less price inflation than have medical care prices. According to the Bureau of Labor Statistics, the drug price index has increased from 115.3 in 1960 to 154.8 in 1980. Over this same period of time, the Medical Care Price Index has risen from 79.1 in 1960 to 265.9 in 1980, while some components of this index, such as hospital services have increased from 57.3 to 418.9 over this same period of time. These data are shown in Table 17-2.

Given the impact that drugs have had, their relatively small proportion of total health expenditures, and their small annual rates of increase in prices, why has so much attention been given to the ethical drug industry, which consists of drugs promoted and distributed primarily to health professionals and which are available to consumers by prescription only? There are two reasons for such

TABLE 17-1. Personal Expenditures on Drugs and Personal Health Care Expenditures, 1950–1981

Year	Personal Health Care Expenditures (Billions of Dollars)	Drug and Medical Sundries[a]	Drug Expenditures as a Percentage of Personal Health Care Expenditures (%)
1950	$10.9	$1.7	15.9
1960	23.7	3.7	15.4
1965	35.8	5.2	14.5
1970	65.1	8.0	12.6
1975	116.8	11.9	10.1
1980	217.9	19.2	8.8
1981	255.0	21.4	8.4

Source: Robert Gibson and Daniel Waldo, "National Health Care Expenditures, *Health Care Financing Review*, vol. 3, 1980" (September 1981): 20–31; and *Health and Human Service News*, July 26, 1982.

[a]Note: The category "Drug and Medical Sundries" includes spending for prescription drugs, over-the-counter drugs, and medical sundries dispensed through retail channels. Expenditures for drugs purchased or dispensed by hospitals, nursing homes, other institutions, physicians, and dentists are excluded. About 57 percent of all dollars for drugs and medical sundries are spent for prescription drugs alone, and another 31 percent are spent for over-the-counter drugs. Whether prescription expenditures as a percentage of personal health care expenditures parallel the trend exhibited by drug and medical sundries as a percentage of personal health care expenditures was examined by studying the annual survey of prescription sales published by the *American Druggist*. The *American Druggist* estimates for dollar volume of retail prescription sales should approximate the total consumer expenditures for prescriptions. The *American Druggist* estimates show that the dollar volume of prescription sales is a declining percentage of personal health care expenditures, over the period 1955–1979. It declines from 8.21 percent in 1955 to 7.74 percent in 1965, to 5.22 percent in 1975, to finally 4.75 percent in 1979. It appears then that, in relation to personal health care expenditures, drug and medical sundries and prescription expenditures do behave similarly.

TABLE 17-2. Selected Average Consumer Price Indices, Calendar Years 1950–1980

Year	Medical Care	Prescription Drugs	Hospital (Semiprivate Room)	Physicians' Services
1950	53.7	92.6	30.3	55.2
1955	64.8	101.6	42.3	65.4
1960	79.1	115.3	57.3	77.0
1965	89.5	102.0	75.9	88.3
1970	120.6	101.2	145.4	121.4
1975	168.6	109.3	236.1	169.4
1980	265.9	154.8	418.9	269.3

Sources: Two sources were used. Data for 1950–1970 came from U.S. Department of Labor, Bureau of Labor Statistics, *Handbook of Labor Statistics, 1975—Reference Edition* (Washington, D.C.: Government Printing Office, 1975), pp. 326–336; data for 1970–1980 came from U.S. Department of Labor, Bureau of Labor Statistics, *Consumer Price Index Detailed Report*, various years.

attention. First, there has been concern that selling costs and profits in this industry are too high and that this is indicative of monopoly power among pharmaceutical companies. Second, that the drugs manufactured and marketed by this for-profit industry should be safe.

The issue of drug safety and efficacy have been dealt with in the Food, Drug and Cosmetic Act of 1938 and in the 1962 Kefauver–Harris amendments to that act. In the second half of this chapter, the federal regulations to improve drug safety and efficacy and their effect on the industry's rate of drug innovation are analyzed. The first part of this chapter is devoted to an analysis of the economic performance of the industry. Public policies that have been proposed to improve the industry's performance will also be evaluated. Policies to change the economic performance of the industry, such as curtailing promotional expenditures, reducing prices, and lowering the rate of profits, also affect the industry's rate of drug innovation. For purposes of analysis, however, each of these effects on drug innovation will be discussed separately.

THE ECONOMIC PERFORMANCE OF THE PHARMACEUTICAL INDUSTRY

Critics of the pharmaceutical industry have been concerned by what they perceive as monopoly power and its attendant abuses. They cite many examples of these abuses: the continuous high rates of profit, the extraordinary large and wasteful amounts that are spent on detailing and other promotional expenses, the high prices at which drugs are sold in relation to their costs of production, and the existence of price discrimination, as evidenced by the fact that the same drugs are sold for less to large purchasers, such as hospitals, than they are to retailers, and that brand name drugs sell for so much more than generic drugs. These measures of inadequate industry performance are believed to be a result of a highly concentrated industry, caused by high entry barriers, and consequently little competition among its members.

If an industry were competitive, then profits would be normal, similar to what is earned in other industries, and there would be a greater degree of price competition; price discrimination would also therefore be less likely. High promotion expenditures would not be necessary as firms competed more on price.

Thus critics of the pharmaceutical industry and earlier economic studies have viewed the industry from a traditional perspective. They concluded that high profits, prices, and promotion expenditures could only exist in an industry characterized by monopoly power. With an emphasis on these aspects of monopoly power, they proposed policies that would change both the structure of the industry and the behavior of firms in the industry. For example, decreasing the effective life of patents would lessen one source of monopoly power. Having the federal government reimburse for drug prescriptions according to the price of generic drugs only (the maximum allowable cost regulations), would result in a lowering of drug prices. Contrasting the performance of the pharmaceutical industry to that of a theoretical competitive industry, led the critics of this industry to propose wide-ranging policies to change what they perceived as an inadequate performance.

This traditional or static view of the pharmaceutical industry has recently come under sharp attack for two reasons. First, emphasizing the more visible monopoly abuses neglects the tremendous beneficial impact that product innovation has had, not only on society, but also on industry competition. A more dynamic analysis of the drug industry, based on the competitive effects of product innovation, suggests an entirely different picture of the industry's performance. Second, economists have recently begun to question whether the indicators of monopoly power are in fact accurate. It has been suggested that industry profits are greatly overstated using traditional accounting methods, that there is in fact a great deal of price competition, and that high promotion and selling expenses serve important economic functions, such as providing physicians with information and as an important means by which firms enter new markets, rather than being a barrier to entry.

The "dynamic competition" view of the pharmaceutical industry reaches quite opposite conclusions on the industry's performance. Further, when the policy prescriptions of the traditionalists are examined in this new light, the impacts of their proposals are seen to be quite harmful in terms of their effects on product innovation and competition.

In analyzing the drug industry, the structure of the industry is examined first. Examples of structure are the conditions of entry into the various therapeutic markets and the importance of economies of scale in determining firm size. Structural characteristics determine the number of competing firms, given the size of the market. This information is usually summed up in the measure referred to as the *concentration ratio*, which is the percentage of the industry's sales accounted for by the four (or eight) largest firms.

After industry structure, the pharmaceutical firm's behavior is examined. Examples of firm behavior are the degree of price competition, product promotion, and product competition. Last, we attempt to evaluate the industry's performance.

While viewing the drug industry within this traditional framework, the importance of dynamic competition, as manifested through product competition, will be examined in terms of how it influences the industry's structure, conduct, and performance. Within this context, the accuracy of profitability, which has been the basis of much of the criticism of the pharmaceutical industry, will also be discussed.

CHARACTERISTICS OF THE DRUG INDUSTRY

When economists examine the structure of an industry, the concentration ratio is used as an indication of monopoly power. The concentration ratio is the percentage of total industry sales provided by a small number of firms. Thus a four firm concentration ratio indicates the percentage of total sales supplied by the four largest firms. If this concentration ratio is high, then it is often assumed that these firms have monopoly power; that is, the fewer the number of firms there are, the easier is it for these firms to collude in the setting of prices. A low concentration ratio suggests that the market shares of firms are generally small and that there is more competition among firms. Scherer claims that "when the leading four firms control 40 percent or more of the total market, it is fair to assume that oligopoly is beginning to rear its head" (2).

The determinants of the concentration ratio depend on how easy it is to enter that industry. The greater the barriers to entry, the higher the concentration ratio. Entry barriers may differ by industry; some may involve control over the resources used in production, such as was the case with bauxite which was used in the production of aluminum. The more typical entry barrier is economies of scale in production. In the drug industry it has been suggested that patents are the prime barrier to entering a therapeutic market. Other barriers that have been mentioned are economies of scale in research and development and high promotion expenditures, which are used to differentiate a brand name drug in the minds of physicians.

There are approximately 600 drug firms in this country. The four firm concentration ratio in the pharmaceutical industry (as of 1973) was 27.8 percent (3). This is certainly lower than for automobiles, which is 99 percent; cigarettes, 84 percent; and soaps and detergents, 62 percent (4). However, it is not appropriate to look at the concentration ratio with respect to total drug sales because there are many separate markets within the overall drug industry in which firms either cannot or do not compete. The question then is what is the relevant market over which concentration ratios should be calculated? One analyst has observed that one should not

> ignore the fact that the overall drug market is fragmented into a number of separate, noncompeting therapeutic markets: antibiotics are not substitutes for antidiabetic drugs, and tranquilizers are not substitutes for vitamins. Manufacturers do not compete on an industrywide basis, and hence concentration must be evaluated within the various therapeutic groups of drugs in which competition does occur. (5)

A more general definition of markets has been proposed by Stigler:

> An industry should embrace the maximum geographical area and the maximum variety of productive activities in which there is a strong long-run substitution. If buyers can shift on a large scale from product or area B to A, then the two should

be combined. If producers can shift on a large scale from B to A, again they should be combined.

Economists usually state this in an alternative form: All products or enterprises with large long-run cross-elasticities of either supply or demand should be combined into a single industry. (6)

Thus even though therapeutic markets appear to be a more relevant definition than overall industry sales, there is still the problem of which are the relevant therapeutic markets. For example, one investigator, Vernon, classified drugs into 19 therapeutic markets after consulting with various marketing people in the drug industry (7). The criteria used for categorizing drugs was the degree of demand side substitutability between different drugs. In another study, Hornbrook classified drugs into 69 therapeutic markets. The criteria used by Hornbrook was whether the drugs produced essentially the same therapeutic effects; if so they were then classified into the same therapeutic market (8). In still another study the investigators developed their definition of therapeutic markets by evaluating physicians' prescribing habits (9). This study resulted in only 10 economic markets.

Each of the above studies is based on demand side substitutability. None fulfill the supply side criterion suggested by Stigler, namely, if a producer in market A can shift on a large scale to producing product B, then both should be combined into a single market. Thus if a firm is currently producing antibiotics and it can quickly shift and produce antiarthritics, they should then be included in a single market definition. Supply side substitution is more difficult for researchers to determine than demand side substitution. The supply side definition would be likely to result in lower concentration ratios than a market definition based on demand side substitution alone.

Using Vernon's classification of therapeutic markets, as shown in Table 17-3, the four firm concentration ratio is quite high. The lowest four firm concentration ratio in a therapeutic market was 46 percent. There are several in the 90 percent range, and the unweighted average was 68 percent. These concentration ratios indicate a high degree of market concentration by a few firms.

If we were to rely on the traditional method of analyzing monopoly power in an industry, namely high concentration ratios, we would conclude that drug firms possess a high degree of monopoly power in various therapeutic markets. This conclusion, however, has been disputed by a number of economists. Concentration ratios are a "static" measure of market power. While particular therapeutic markets may have high concentration ratios at a given point in time, there is a high rate of turnover in market shares. Instability in market shares is a result of intense competition among firms through new product innovation and is indicative of "dynamic" competition. Unless this dynamic aspect of competition among drug firms is analyzed, the use of static concentration ratios provide a misleading impression of monopoly power over time.

An investigation of the instability of market shares among 20 different industries was undertaken using an index of market instability (10). Of the 20 different industries, only the petroleum industry had a higher index of market instability than the drug industry. See Table 17-4.

Another indication of the degree of product competition in the drug industry and its effects on market shares was a study of entry and exit in different thera-

TABLE 17-3. Concentration of Sales in the U.S. Ethical Drug Industry, by Therapeutic Markets, 1968

Therapeutic Market	Four-Firm Ratio
Anesthetics	69
Antiarthritics	95
Antibiotics–penicillin	55
Antispasmodics	59
Ataractics	79
Bronchial dilators	61
Cardiovascular hypotensives	79
Coronary–peripheral vasodilators	70
Diabetic therapy	93
Diuretics	64
Enzymes–digestants	46
Hematinic preparations	52
Sex hormones	67
Corticoids	55
Muscle relaxants	59
Psychostimulants	78
Sulfonamides	79
Thyroid therapy	69
Unweighted average	68

Source: John M. Vernon, "Concentration, Promotion and Market Share Stability in Pharmaceutical Industry," *Journal of Industrial Economics* 19 (July 1971): 246–266. Reprinted with permission by Basil Blackwell Publisher, Ltd.

peutic markets. Seventeen therapeutic markets were studied over the period 1963–1972. In 15 of the 17 markets there were more than five new entrants. The market shares of new entrants exceeded 10 percent and in some cases went as high as 33 and 43 percent. Exit from the industry also occurred in 16 of the 17 therapeutic markets (11).

Although concentration ratios in the various therapeutic markets are high, it is necessary to examine changes in market shares over time to better understand the degree of competition in the drug industry. As evidenced by the turnover of leading firms and the instability of market shares, these findings suggest that monopoly power is eroded over time. It is through new product development that firms compete in various therapeutic markets.

NEW PRODUCT COMPETITION

Patents provide a firm with protection against competitive suppliers providing the identical compound. Since a large proportion of prescription drugs, more than two-thirds, have patent protection, entry into specific therapeutic markets requires some kind of chemical product differentiation (12). However, the importance of patent protection for achieving monopoly power in a therapeutic market can be overstated. The various therapeutic markets are not monopolized

TABLE 17-4. Indices of Market Share Instability

Industry	Instability Index[a]	Number of Firms
Food	10.83	119
Tobacco	9.06	12
Textile mill products	9.30	61
Apparel	1.48	7
Lumber and wood products	4.45	16
Furniture and fixtures	3.86	8
Paper	9.63	49
Printing	14.82	25
Chemicals	17.42	74
Petroleum	24.38	35
Rubber	9.16	14
Leather	5.69	8
Stone, clay, and glass	13.25	31
Primary metals	14.25	76
Fabricated metals	8.70	51
Machinery (except electrical)	12.71	NA
Electrical machinery	17.24	46
Transportation	19.92	70
Professional and scientific	17.19	19
Drug industry	22.80[b]	21

Source: Douglas L. Cocks, "Product Innovation and Dynamic Elements of Competition in the Ethical Drug Industry," in Robert B. Helms, ed., *Drug Development and Marketing* (Washington, D.C.: American Enterprise Institute, 1975). Reprinted with permission.

NA, not applicable.

[a] All indices are computed with mergers excluded. Hymer and Pashigian calculated their indices on the basis of shares of assets: the calculation for the drug industry is based on shares of hospital and drugstore sales.

[b] Calculated by Cocks (see text).

by single drugs. It is through the development of both major and minor chemical modifications and new dosage forms that firms enter markets and compete.

Critics of the drug industry claim that much of the product differentiation are for minor modifications that provide little social value and that large promotional expenditures are used to establish brand name loyalty amongst physicians. Further, most of the product innovations were derived from discoveries at universities and in nonindustrial settings. The drug industry, of course, disputes these criticisms. How important are the products produced by the drug industry?

Several studies have attempted to assess the relative importance of the drug industry to other institutions and organizations in their contribution to new drug discoveries. In one study, Schnee determined which drugs were important drug discoveries over different periods by using data on significant drug discoveries prior to 1963 from a study conducted by the Commission on Cost of Medical Care of the American Medical Association. The commission determined significant drug discoveries by asking "400 physicians and pharmacologists to select the most important advances from a preselected list of eighty-nine drugs introduced after 1934. His selection of important drug introductions in the 1963–

TABLE 17-5. Schnee's Distribution of Drug Discoveries, 1935–1970

Source	1935–1949	1950–1962	1963–1970
Industry	52	69	82
Universities, hospitals, or research institutions	34	16	9
Other	14	15	9
Total	100	100	100

Source: Based on Jerome Schnee, "The Changing Pattern of Pharmaceutical Innovation and Discovery," mimeographed (New York: Columbia University, Graduate School of Business, 1973). This table was reprinted with permission from David Schwartzman, *Innovation in the Pharmaceutical Industry* (Baltimore, Md.: The Johns Hopkins University Press, 1976), p. 77.

1970 period was largely based on a survey by *The Medical Letter* of 170 physicians at medical schools" (13). Schnee found that the share of important drugs discovered by the drug industry has been increasing over time. As shown in Table 17-5 the drug industry's share has increased from more than 50 percent in the period 1935–1949, to 69 percent between 1950 and 1962, and to 82 percent between 1963 and 1970. The drug industry, according to Schnee, had always been an important source of drug discoveries and is now the prime source in the development of significant new chemical entities.

Another study, with similar results, was undertaken by the Food and Drug Administration (FDA) in 1974. The FDA determined those drugs introduced in the periods 1950–1962 and 1963–1970 that in its opinion represented important gains in medicine. As shown in Table 17-6, the distribution of those new drugs attributed to development by the drug industry was 69 percent and 82 percent, respectively, for the two periods studied (14).

All product innovation and competition is not the result of significant medical discoveries. However, as a source of new drug discoveries, the drug industry has played a leading role in the past, and in recent years it has increased in importance to where it is the major source for such drug discoveries. Different studies, using different definitions of major drug discoveries, reach similar conclusions. In addition to major drug discoveries, minor modifications and different dosage forms can have important social and economic advantages. For example, "The modification of an injectible drug to permit oral self-administration is an economic advance, if not a major medical advance" (15).

EXPENDITURES ON RESEARCH AND DEVELOPMENT

An indication of the importance of product competition to the drug industry are their expenditures on research and development. The drug industry spends approximately 11.5 percent of its sales on research and development. This percentage has varied between 10.5 and 12.1 percent since 1965 (16). These expenditures were approximately 1.5 billion dollars in 1979. When compared to other industries, the drug industry has the second highest research and development expenditures as a percent of sales. The communications industry has the highest

TABLE 17-6. Percentage Distribution of Discoveries of Important New Drugs Introduced in 1950–1962 and 1963–1970, Selected by FDA

Source	1950–1962	1963–1970
Industry	69	82
Other	31	18
Total	100	100

Source: Commissioner Schmidt's statement to the Subcommittee on Health of the Senate Committee on Labor and Public Welfare, August 16, 1974, appearing in August 26, 1974, FDC Reports. Discoveries assigned by Paul de Haen, *Nonproprietary Name Index,* and the *Merck Index.* This table was reprinted with permission from David Schwartzman, *Innovation in the Pharmaceutical Industry* (Baltimore, Md.: The Johns Hopkins University Press, 1976), p. 79.

ratio. However, government funding finances 43 percent of that industry's research and development, whereas the government finances less than one percent of the drug industry's research and development expenditures (17).

It has been suggested that research and development expenditures serve as a barrier to entry into various therapeutic markets. If there are large economies of scale in research and development, then product competition will only occur between the largest drug firms. Market instability and turnover will be traded off among the same large firms. However, several studies have concluded that research and development as a percent of sales was similar for different-sized firms in the period before 1962. With respect to the output of research and development expenditures, product innovation, it was also determined that small firms were not at a disadvantage. In fact, the "firms that contributed the most innovations, relative to their size, were not the largest firms but somewhat smaller ones" (18).

These findings with respect to expenditures on research and development and product innovation changed when data from the post-1962 period was examined. Schwartzman found that in the period 1965–1970 larger firms spent a larger portion of their sales on research and development than did smaller firms. Similarly, larger firms had an advantage over smaller firms in terms of the number of product innovations produced (19). These findings are reinforced by another study.

Grabowski and Vernon examined production of innovations in three different periods, 1957–1961, 1962–1966, and 1967–1971. The number of firms having a new chemical entity declined in each of these three periods from 51, 34, and 23 firms, respectively. Also the four largest firms in terms of sales have increased their output of new chemical entities, from 24 and 25 percent in the first two periods to 48.7 percent of innovational output in the 1967–1971 period. It would thus appear that innovational output is becoming more concentrated in the largest drug firms (20).

These findings, which indicate economies of scale in the post-1962 period, suggest that the 1962 FDA Amendments (which will be discussed more fully later) may have provided an advantage to larger firms. The time and resources required for developing and testing new products as a result of the FDA Amendments have been increased (21).

PROMOTIONAL EXPENDITURES

The role of promotional expenditures is controversial. Its critics believe it to be wasteful, and as a means of providing physicians with information, a relatively inefficient mechanism with its reliance on detail men and heavy journal advertising. Many people oppose large advertising expenditures, not only in the drug industry but also for automobiles, breakfast cereals, and other products. It is also believed that advertising is misleading and that it attempts to manipulate consumers into choosing products they do not need.

In perfectly competitive markets advertising is viewed as unnecessary, since buyers have perfect information and products are homogeneous. When advertising is viewed with respect to oligopolistic markets, such expenditures are viewed as a means of avoiding price competition by attempting to differentiate their products. Again, advertising is considered wasteful, if not misleading. Traditionally, advertising within the drug industry has been analyzed within a similar context. Within therapeutic markets, products have been considered to be relatively homogeneous, and the large promotional expenditures are seen as an attempt to create product differentiation and brand loyalties in the minds of physicians.

In recent years, drug industry promotional expenditures have undergone a reevaluation. Promotion expenditures are seen as serving two important purposes: information and as a means of achieving entry for new product innovations (22).

When prescribing, physicians should be aware of which drugs are most appropriate for treatment, the correct dosages, the appropriate dosage form, the effects of patient characteristics, such as weight, age, other drugs being taken, the patient's health condition and the price to the patient of the drug. Learning about all the possible drugs that might be used for all the physicians' patients is a formidable task. There are many thousands of drugs available to choose from. New drugs, modifications, and changes in dosage forms are constantly coming on the market. There are a number of ways physicians may stay informed: medical journals, *The Medical Letter*, and books such as the *Physician's Desk Reference*. To stay abreast of the literature is very time consuming for a physician.

Based on several studies, it appears that marketing efforts by drug firms play an important role in keeping physicians informed. One study, based on a survey of physicians, found that physicians regarded detailmen as either a very good or fairly good source of information (23).

Further, that 60 percent of the reporting physicians believed the information provided by the detailmen was sufficiently valuable so as to warrant seeing all the detailmen who tried to make appointments with them.

Promotion by itself does not guarantee success for a new drug. Physicians are apparently able to distinguish among claims for various drugs. Schwartzman cites the case when a number of drugs were heavily promoted and yet their sales turned out to be less than their promotion costs. These were new drugs that were ranked by the FDA as having little or no therapeutic gain over existing drugs

(24). Similarly, drugs that were rapidly accepted as a result of strong promotion efforts were of significant benefit compared to alternatives available. In fact, it has been estimated that at times too little has been spent on promotional activities. Peltzman examined the consequences of failure by physicians to adopt drugs due to a lack of information. When certain innovations in drug therapies occur, there is a benefit to society if physicians are sufficiently knowledgeable to prescribe such drugs as soon as possible. He cites the case of tuberculosis (TB), estimating that if the use of TB drugs had spread as rapidly as the Salk vaccine, 80,600 lives would have been saved. Similarly, if major tranquilizers had been more heavily promoted, this might have resulted in a savings of 645 million patient days in the hospital (25).

Drug industry promotion may not be the ideal way of disseminating information to physicians. Physicians differ on what sources they rely on for information. Patients who go to physicians who keep up with developments in drug therapies through the medical literature bear the cost of heavy drug promotion that attempts to reach other physicians who rely on the drug companies for their information. There is, unfortunately, no way of lowering the price of drugs to the patients of physicians who do not rely on drug company promotion (26). If drug promotion expenditures are to be reduced in the future, there must be changes in the incentives and/or costs to physicians for relying on other sources for information on drugs.

In addition to providing information, promotional expenditures enable firms to enter new markets. Contrary to the previous belief that promotional expenditures served as a barrier to entry, more recent studies have concluded the opposite. Telser studied drug entry in 17 therapeutic markets over the period 1962–1972 in order to determine whether promotional expenditures deter or facilitate entry into the market for new drugs. Entry in a market was measured by the percentage of sales in a market as of 1972 for a drug which did not have any sales in that market previously. Using a multivariate analysis, Telser found a positive relationship between promotional expenditures and entry. He therefore concluded that promotional expenditures facilitate entry, without which new products would be unable to compete with existing drugs (27). In another study, Hornbrook found similar results and concluded that "promotion has a procompetitive effect, other things being the same, in that it acts as a means of entry—a market penetration tool—more effectively, on balance, than as a barrier to entry" (28).

What would be the possible savings to consumers if all promotional expenditures were eliminated? Schwartzman estimates that if all promotional expenditures were eliminated, the amount of the savings that would eventually be passed on to consumers would represent approximately 5 percent of their drug bill (29). This potential savings, however, must be offset by a cost to physicians (and most likely shifted to their patients) of the costs to replace the information previously provided by the drug companies. Another cost would be a delay in introducing new products into highly concentrated markets. Product competition would undoubtedly decline as the marketing of new products becomes more difficult without promotional expenditures. Both nominal and quality-adjusted prices would remain high with less product competition. The slower dissemination of new drug innovations also results in a cost to patients; the foregone benefits they may have received had they had earlier access to a newer, more beneficial drug.

PRICE COMPETITION

It has been commonly believed that there is no price competition among drug companies. The reasons for this belief are, first, that patents provide a firm with monopoly power, hence protection against close substitutes. Second, physicians do not pay for the drug and are therefore less sensitive to drug prices. Physicians also prescribe by brand name thereby limiting the patient's choice. Further, there are legal restrictions, i.e., antisubstitution laws that limit competition in those cases when close substitutes may exist. And lastly, given the high degree of concentration in therapeutic markets, it is easier for drug firms to collude on pricing policies. Their desire for wanting to maintain high drug prices is that the price elasticity of demand for drugs is low. Thus if a firm were to engage in price competition and the other firms were to follow, total sales revenue in that market would fall.

The evidence offered in support of this lack of price competition is that drugs are sold at prices much higher than their marginal costs of production. Second, based on a study over the period 1949–1959, Markham observed a great deal of price inflexibility. Of the 308 drugs examined, more than 50 percent did not change their price over this period (30). If prices were competitively set, they would change in response to changing demand and cost conditions. And last, price discrimination appears to exist in the pricing of drugs; prices are higher in retail markets than for hospitals, and prices differ in domestic and international markets.

To understand the degree of price competition in the drug industry, it is again necessary to view it within a dynamic framework. At a given point in time, prices are "high" in relation to their marginal costs. However, over time different forms of price competition emerge. Close substitutes enter markets, not protected by patents, and prices begin to decline. In other cases, improvements occur in competing drugs that sell for similar prices as existing drugs; hence their quality-adjusted prices decline. Over time both the number and closeness of substitutes within a therapeutic market increase. As this occurs, the price elasticity of demand for each of the drugs increases, and prices begin to decline. There is thus a life cycle to therapeutic markets.

Drugs that are considered to be major innovations, i.e., to have large therapeutic gains, and not having any close substitutes, can obtain a high market share despite a high relative price. However, drugs that are considered to be minor innovations are more likely to be introduced at low prices relative to other drugs in that market. Such pricing strategies are consistent with pricing according to the perceived elasticity of demand for that drug. The closer the substitutes (the case of a minor innovation) the greater the price elasticity of demand, hence the lower the price to obtain a share of the market.

Multiple-source drugs, which are generic type drugs supplied by several manufacturers under their own brand names, comprise more than 44 percent of total prescriptions (31). Once a patent has expired, entry into that market is relatively easy. FDA approval is required before a new drug can be marketed. But if the drug is a duplicate of an existing drug then FDA approval is more easily acquired. For a new entrant to gain a share of a market, with a similar type of product, it usually lowers price. Even though price cutting will have an adverse impact on profits, it may be the only way for a new multiple source drug to gain a share of the market. Given the low price elasticity of demand for drugs, the total number of drugs sold in the market is unlikely to change as a result of lower prices. Changes in market sales will be at the expense of existing firms. The pattern appears to be that as more duplicate drugs are offered in a market, the later entrants reduce their prices much more than the earlier entrants; eventually the original drug manufacturer and others must match these price reductions at least in part.

Demand elasticity also increases over time. In markets where price exceeds marginal cost, there is an incentive for firms to enter. As more and closer substitutes enter a market, the price elasticity of demand of the original firms increases and prices are eventually reduced. For example, with respect to tetracycline, there were five major manufacturers. Lederle, which had an 85 percent share of the market in 1962, declined to 72 percent in 1964 at which time Squibb started sharply reducing its prices, from $15.60 to $3.98. Squibb's market share increased over the next several years. One of the major losers was Lederle, which did not respond to price cutting; its market share declined from 72 percent to 33 percent before it finally started to compete on price (32).

Evidence of greater price elasticity over time is also provided by data on overall drug price trends. Drug prices have declined even though there has been inflation in the general economy as measured by the rise in the Consumer Price Index. Thus the "real" price of drugs has declined even faster than their nominal prices.

Still another approach that has been used to indicate price competition in different therapeutic markets is to adjust drug prices by a quality measure. When the prices of different drugs are compared, it is usually assumed that the brands are of equal quality. If the newer drug is improved compared to existing drugs, and it is sold for a similar price, then the actual price, i.e., the nominal price divided by quality, has actually declined. Just looking at nominal prices therefore can be misleading.

To understand the reason behind drug manufacturer's willingness to engage in price competition it becomes necessary to reexamine our beliefs as to the prescribing habits of physicians and the role of pharmacists. Apparently drug manufacturers assume that at least some physicians are price conscious when they prescribe for their patients and that some pharmacists are willing to act as the patient's agent. This behavior among physicians and pharmacists will serve to increase price competition among drug firms.

> Pharmacists will use a low-priced drug rather than the original brand to fill a generic prescription. This is not universally true, but the proportion of generic prescriptions filled with low-priced drugs is much higher than the proportion of prescriptions that specify a brand accounted for by the low-priced brands. Substitution occurs. The pharmacist, in effect, acts as a price agent for the consumer. (33)

Also, antisubstitution laws are not as great an inhibiter of price competition as is believed.

> Before it was legal to do so, pharmacists did substitute; and frequently they did so without asking permission from the prescriber. For example, there was brand substitution in 33 percent of all ampicillin prescriptions, and the pharmacists did

not obtain permission to make such substitutions in 82 percent of these cases; so they were doing so illegally. When they substituted, they tended to substitute a low-priced brand for the prescribed brand. Again they were acting as a price agent. (34)

These findings suggest much more price flexibility and competition than previously believed (35). Patented drugs and major innovations provide greater monopoly power in pricing a drug. Uniqueness in the short run, however, gives way to imitations and a greater number of substitutes over time. As price elasticity increases, there is greater price competition. "Historically, no leading product has maintained its market share position for more than a limited number of years. Preeminence is temporary" (36).

PROFITABILITY IN THE PHARMACEUTICAL INDUSTRY

One of the criticisms of the drug industry is the high rate of profits that are made as a result of other people's illnesses, many of whom are of low incomes. Most critics will acknowledge that a normal rate of return is appropriate so as to enable the industry to continue to supply drugs and to provide for an incentive for research. However, published data on profitability of the drug industry, compared to other industries, show that drug companies receive an "excessive" rate of return. The average rate of return on equity for all manufacturing companies over the period 1958–1975 was 11.1 percent. For drug companies it was 18.1 percent (37). Since these "excessive" profits have continued over a large number of years, it is used as evidence of the drug companies' monopoly power.

Recently, economists have reexamined the rate of profit received by drug companies. The conclusion of many of these studies is that published profit data are seriously in error and that they *overstate* the true rate of profit earned by drug companies. When corrections are made to the published data, the rate of return earned by drug companies are approximately comparable to rates of return earned in other industries. It has been further said that since the passage of the 1962 FDA Amendments the true rate of return to drug firms has been falling.

To the extent that these new findings on drug industry profitability are correct, there are important public policy implications: Previous estimates of the relatively high rate of return to drug firms have been the impetus for policies to lower prices, require the cross-licensing of patents, and to reduce the patent life of new drugs. If implemented, each of these policies would decrease drug industry profitability. If drug firm profitability has not been excessive, then policies to further decrease profitability in this industry would cause the rate of return to be below that earned in other industries; with a lower return on investment, there would be a consequent decline in research and development, hence drug innovation would fall.

The finding that drug industry profitability is relatively normal also suggests that there are no strong barriers to entry into various drug markets; while firms might have temporary monopoly power, it is eroded over time.

To understand this change in perception of drug industry profitability, it is necessary to examine how profits are calculated and to discuss some of the determinants of industry profitability.

The manner in which accountants calculate profitability (R_{acc}) is to subtract all expenses (E) from sales revenue (S) and divide this by the firm's capital or the stockholders' equity (C).

$$R_{acc} = \frac{(S - E)}{C}$$

Net income ($S - E$) is the income remaining after all expenses and taxes have been paid. This accountant's definition of profitability is the method used to compare profitability between different industries. According to the above definition, advertising, research and development, and promotional expenses are all treated as current expenses; they are deducted from sales revenue in the year they are incurred. Economists have argued that these expenditures are more than current expenses. They are, in fact, intangible capital, since their effect continues beyond the year in which they are incurred. For example, research and development expenditures might not yield any benefit in the current year; but if a successful drug is developed, benefits will accrue in future years. It takes a number of years before a successful drug is finally marketed. The testing process to receive FDA approval alone may take a few years. These expenditures are incurred so as to receive future benefits. A similar case can be made for advertising and promotional expenditures; their effects are longer lasting than for the year in which they were made. Because the above types of expenditures provide future benefits, their economic life is greater than one year. They are a form of intangible capital of the firm and should therefore be depreciated rather than expensed all at once.

In accordance with conservative accounting principles, such expenditures are expensed since there is uncertainty as to the future benefits they may provide and over how many years such future revenues may accrue. Therefore the most conservative approach is to assume that there are no benefits in future periods from these expenditures.

If the economists' definition of profitability (R_{econ}) were to be used, and these expenditures were treated as intangible assets (A), then a certain portion of these assets should be depreciated (D) each year, i.e., treated as an expense. The remainder, that is, the undepreciated portion of the asset, should then be added to the firm's capital investment. Thus the economists' definition of profitability would be stated as follows:

$$R_{econ} = \frac{(S - E - D)}{C + (A - D)}$$

The effect of this change in the treatment of advertising, research and development, and promotional expenditures is to cause net income to be greater than it would otherwise be, since only a part of the expenditure is deducted from sales revenue rather than the entire amount. However, the capital base of the firm is increased by the amount of the undepreciated asset.

Each year new expenditures are incurred for research and development, advertising, and promotion. At the same time, previous year's expenditures are being depreciated. To see why failure to capitalize these expenditures leads to an overstatement of profitability, one has merely to think of a situation when the absolute profit in a given year is equal, i.e., the amount being depreciated is equal to the current year's expenditures on intangible capital. Under the accountants' definition of profitability (R_{acc}) the capital base is smaller than under the economists' definition of profitability (R_{econ}); the economist includes the undepreciated asset as part of capital while the accountant does not. Therefore the accountants' definition will show a higher rate of profitability than would the economists'.

In accordance with generally accepted accounting principles, the accountants' definition of profitability is used by all industries. The pharmaceutical industry, however, is more affected by this definition of profit than any other industry. As a percentage of sales, expenditures for advertising, promotion, and research and development are greater in the drug industry than for any other industry. For example, the pharmaceutical industry spent 5.3 percent of its sales for research and development during the period 1961–1971. For other industries such as food, the comparable percentage was .4 percent. The highest percentage for other industries was in the electrical machinery and aerospace industries where it was 3.6 and 3.5 percent, respectively. With respect to advertising, no other industry had as high a percent of sales as did the drug firms, which was 3.7 percent over the period 1949–1971. Companies that were relatively high on research and development (as a percentage of sales) were generally low on advertising expenditures (as a percentage of sales), although the pharmaceutical industry was highest in both categories (38).

How large an overstatement of accounting profitability is caused by a failure to include these expenditures as intangible capital depends upon several factors: which expenditures should be considered as current versus capital outlays, the depreciation schedule for each category of expenditure, and how rapidly the capital base of the firm is growing over time. As the economic life of intangible capital increases, the effect is a decrease in the rate of return to the industry (39).

Several studies have estimated "corrected" rates of return to the drug industry using the economists' definition of profitability. The differences between the corrected and uncorrected rates of return are striking. The accounting rate of return for the drug industry in the late 1960s was estimated at greater than 18 percent a year. The economic rates of return for those same years was less than 12 percent. Over the 10-year period, 1965–1974, the average rate of return, using the accounting definition, was 17.3 percent; the estimated economic rate of return for that same period was 11.1 percent (40).

When similar corrections for intangible capital are made to rates of return in other industries, it can be observed that while the rate of return is still higher for the drug industry, they are much closer to those in other industries. These data are shown in Table 17-7.

There are a number of other factors which have been suggested as the reasons for the remaining differences in the rates of return between the drug industry and other industries. One reason to expect higher rates of return in the drug industry is that they have faced a continual rising demand for their products. Drug sales have risen at a faster rate than many other industries. Since the 1950s, drug sales have increased more than twice as fast as the Gross National Product. Growth in overseas sales has also been increasing at more than twice the rate of sales in this country (41). Some of the reasons for the high rate of growth in sales, in addition to the therapeutic benefits of new drugs, has been changes in payment mechanisms, such as Medicare, Medicaid, and the growth of

TABLE 17-7. Average Accounting and Corrected Rates of Return on Net Worth, 1959–1973 (Percentages)

Industry	Accounting Rates of Return	Corrected Rates of Return	Difference
Pharmaceuticals	18.3	12.9	−5.4
Electrical machinery	13.3	10.1	−3.2
Foods	11.8	10.6	−1.2
Petroleum	11.2	10.8	−0.4
Chemicals	10.6	9.1	−1.5
Paper	10.5	10.1	−0.4
Office machinery	10.5	9.9	−0.6
Motor vehicles	10.5	9.2	−1.3
Rubber products	10.1	8.7	−1.4
Aerospace	9.2	7.4	−1.8
Ferrous metals	7.6	7.3	−0.3
Average	11.2	9.6	−1.6
Variance	7.5	2.5	

Source: Kenneth W. Clarkson, *Intangible Capital and Rates of Return* (Washington, D.C.: American Enterprise Institute, 1977), p. 64. Reprinted by permission from *Issues in Pharmaceutical Economics*, edited by Robert I. Chien. Lexington, Mass.: Lexington Books, D.C. Heath and Company, Copyright 1979, D.C. Heath and Company.

health insurance. Changes in the demographic composition of the population, such as the increasing portion that is aged, has led to increased demands for medical care and consequently an increase in the demand for drugs.

Another reason for increased returns in the drug industry is the greater risks in returns. In competitive markets the rate of return would move toward the opportunity cost of capital adjusted for risk. Those industries with less predictable returns on their investment would require a greater risk premium to attract investors. The uncertainty from return to research and development expenditures contains an element of risk that is perhaps greater than in other industries.

Several studies have attempted to empirically estimate the effect on drug industry profitability as a result of higher than average growth in sales and a premium for greater risk. These studies suggest that drug industry rates of return are several percentage points higher than in other industries because of these two factors (42).

After the effects of these factors, i.e., growth in demand and higher risks, on rates of return in the drug industry are allowed for, Schwartzman concludes that the effects of patents as a means of providing monopoly profits are surprisingly small. He estimates that they provide only a normal rate of return on investment, contrary to what is commonly believed.

> The average realized rate of profit of pharmaceutical manufacturers has not exceeded the average realized rate of all manufacturing after adjustment for expensing research and development, riskiness of investment, and the growth of sales, despite the importance of patents for this industry. The patent protection has resulted in a large investment in research and development rather than a high expected rate of profit. The public policy of granting patents has had the intended effect of increasing investment in research which has reduced the profit rate to the same level as in other industries where patent protection is unimportant. (43)

An important implication of capitalizing intangible capital has occurred since the passage of the 1962 FDA Amendments. The effect of these Amendments has been to increase the time and resources required to develop and test a new drug before it can be marketed. This is to increase the probability that there are no harmful side effects and that the proposed drug is effective in treatment. The effect of the increased time and resources required to bring a new drug to market is an increase in the capital (undepreciated assets) of the drug firm (the ratio of research and development capital to other capital increases) with a consequent decrease in the economic rate of return to the firm. (The accounting rate of return may be unchanged.) One study has estimated that an increase of two additional years for development time would decrease the economic rate of return by 2 percent while leaving unchanged the accounting rate of return. Another study estimated that the 1962 FDA Amendments will cause a 50 percent decrease in the economic rate of return (44). If investment in research and development is related to the expected economic rate of return to be earned by the firm, then the effect of the 1962 Amendments will be a decrease in investment in research and development.

One other unintended consequence of the 1962 Amendments with respect to profitability is that entry barriers have been increased. It now costs more and takes longer for drug firms with competitive products to enter a given therapeutic market. Drug firms with established products will be able to earn larger profits for a longer period of time until competitive products are introduced.

Published data on drug industry profits, based on the accounting rate of return, showing continual high rates of profitability, have been one of the reasons for proposals to change the structure of the industry. It would be unfortunate, not only for the drug firms but for consumers of drugs as well, if public policies to reduce industry profitability were based on misleading profitability data rather than on the more accurate economic rate of return measures.

FEDERAL REGULATION OF DRUGS

HISTORY OF FEDERAL DRUG LEGISLATION

The passage of the Pure Food and Drugs Act of 1906 was the beginning of federal regulation over drugs. The major emphasis of this legislation was not on drugs but was instead concerned with abuses in food adulteration and with patent (secret) medicines. Under this law the government had control only over the labeling of drugs; it was not concerned with advertising, testing, or even the content of the drug. The government sought to protect the public from medical quacks and the false claims made for patent medicines (45).

It was not until the 1930s that the modern drug era began. As new drugs were introduced in this period, a tragedy occurred and was the impetus for new drug legislation. A company seeking to make a liquid form of sulfanilamide for children, the first therapeutic discovery of the modern era, dissolved it in ethylene glycol (antifreeze). The company was unaware of its toxic effects and did not test it on animals. This resulted in the death of more than 100 children (46).

The passage in 1938 of the Food, Drug and Cosmetic Act (FDC) not only increased the government's control over the advertising and labeling of foods, drugs, and cosmetics, but also, for the first time, said a drug had to be considered safe. The Food and Drug Administration was given the authority for judging safety. The 1938 law was intended to protect the public from unsafe, potentially harmful drugs. Before the FDA gave a company approval for a new drug, the New Drug Application (NDA) had to indicate that the drug was safe for the use suggested on the label. Drug companies instituted premarket testing to prove the safety of the drug. (Drug testing was also in the companies' interest since it would limit their potential liability by excluding potentially hazardous drugs from the market; thus it is likely they would have instituted such safety procedures in the absence of any legislation.) It was left up to the drug companies to decide the amount of clinical research necessary to prove a drug was safe. The FDA did not specify the procedures for premarket testing.

The next step in the federal regulation of drugs, and the most controversial, was the 1962 Amendments to the FDC Act. Starting in 1959, Senator Kefauver held hearings on the drug industry. Pervasive throughout these hearings was the belief that existing regulations permitted new drugs to be sold, at high prices, that were of questionable efficacy. Senator Kefauver apparently believed that it was possible to sell drugs at high prices, of dubious quality, because of patent protection, heavy promotion by the drug companies, consumer and physician ignorance, and minimal incentives for physicians to be concerned with their patients' drug costs. Heavy promotion and extravagant claims for their effectiveness, it was believed, misled physicians and patients into purchasing their drugs. Underlying this attitude of drug company behavior was the belief that much of their research was for minor innovations. Senator Kefauver believed that only if the federal government regulated drug company claims about their effectiveness would the public receive accurate information (47).

A number of people believed that the 1962 Amendments would not have passed had it not been for another drug tragedy, this time thalidomide. Thalidomide was first distributed in Europe. An American drug company began to distribute it in this country to some physicians on an experimental basis. The 1938 legislation permitted such limited distribution to qualified experts as long as the drug was labeled as being under investigation. The American drug company withdrew the drug from use after reports from Europe that deformed babies were born to mothers who had taken the drug during their pregnancy. Thalidomide was effectively kept off the U.S. market by the 1938 legislation. However, there was great concern that there was insufficient testing of new drugs. These concerns, in addition to the earlier concerns arising from the Kefauver hearings, led to the 1962 Amendments (48). In response to these concerns, the Amendments made two major changes in the 1938 legislation. There was now greater specificity over the premarket testing of new drugs and, second, the criteria for introducing new drugs was changed.

The 1962 Amendments enabled the FDA to specify the testing procedures a drug manufacturer must use to produce acceptable information for evaluating the drug company's NDA. Extensive data on animal tests were now required before the FDA would permit testing on human subjects. With respect to the new criterion for introducing new drugs, a proof of efficacy was added to the proof of safety that was required under the 1938 legislation. Previously, under the 1938 law, the FDA had to determine that it was safe to market a new drug (the proof being left to the drug company), but now under the 1962 Amendments, the FDA also had to find that the drug was effective in its intended use. Effective was interpreted as achieving the claims made for it by the drug company. To prove efficacy, drug companies were required by the FDA to conduct double-blind "experiments," i.e., neither the patient nor physician was aware of the drug therapy being administered.

Numerous other changes were made with regard to regulation of drugs in the 1962 Amendments such as those with respect to advertising and promotion. Generic names were required on drug labels and advertised claims were restricted to those approved by the FDA. However, the increased emphasis on premarket testing (and its specificity) and the proof of efficacy were the two most important changes. It was toward these two aspects that much criticism has been directed.

A FRAMEWORK FOR ANALYZING THE 1962 AMENDMENTS

How can anyone oppose increased testing requirements for new drugs and proof that the claims made by the drug companies are in fact accurate? Any additional benefits accruing to the public as a result of the 1962 legislation, however, are not without additional costs. Public policy that attempts to increase benefits without regard to their costs may in fact make the public worse off than they were before. Increasingly, researchers, including economists, pharmacologists, and others, are suggesting that this is what has occurred as a result of the 1962 Amendments. To understand how increased testing of drugs and proof of efficacy can result in a greater harm to society, it is necessary to have a framework within which the 1962 Amendments can be evaluated.

As a result of increased federal regulation over drugs, there has been an increase in both the benefits and costs to the public. First the presumed benefits will be discussed and then the costs.

The positive aspects of the legislation were expected to be threefold: Ineffective drugs will no longer be marketed, thereby saving consumers money. Second, because of the more stringent testing procedures and the requirements for animal testing, it was expected that drug safety would be enhanced. And third, greater control over the accuracy of drug claims and the dissemination of information on their benefits and risks was expected to stimulate price competition among drug companies. Drug companies would be less able to "artificially" differentiate their products, thereby decreasing promotional expenditures and consequently drug costs. If these lower prices are passed on, then consumers should benefit through lower drug prices.

In a classic study, Peltzman has attempted to quantify the value of these benefits to consumers (49). To estimate the savings due to keeping ineffective drugs off the market, Peltzman attempted to compare the change in demand curves of new drugs both before and after the 1962 Amendments. If ineffective drugs were introduced before 1962, then their demand curves should decline over time as physicians discover that they are ineffective drugs. Demand curves in the post-1962 period should not decline but should instead increase since they are "effective" drugs. Other factors also affect the demand for drugs. However, once these other factors are controlled for, we would expect the pre-1962 demand curves growing less than post-1962 demand curves. Peltzman found that there was no substantial difference between pre- and post-1962 Amendment new drugs with respect to their market shares or prices. "If pre-amendment efficacy claims were substantially exaggerated, it would be expected that pre-1962 new drugs would not hold their market share as well as post-1962 new drugs, or that they would do so only if their prices were reduced once the exaggeration was revealed by experience in use. But . . . [the data] . . . suggests the experience with them did not generally cause doctors and consumers to regard their initial evaluations as exaggerated" (50). Peltzman claims the reasons for such a small regulatory effect on ineffective drugs is that, "The penalties imposed by the marketplace on sellers of ineffective drugs before 1962 seems to have been sufficient to have left little room for improvement by a regulatory agency" (51).

The issue of efficacy from the perspective of patient treatment was addressed by Professor Wardell as follows:

> Failure to show a difference in efficacy between a new drug and an older one should not be taken to mean that the new drug cannot be a worthwhile advance. . . . First, each drug's efficacy may be exerted on a different segment of the population; if both drugs were available, the proportion of patients treatable might be much higher than if either drug were available alone. By the same argument, a drug that is "on average" less effective and more toxic than existing therapy may still be highly desirable for some segments of the population. Our current simplistic statistical concepts of efficacy and safety usually fail to take this into account. Second, it is common to find that the spectrum of side effects differs for each drug, or that the pharmacokinetics are different enough to confer different dosage regimens upon each drug. Third, in the actual treatment of many types of conditions, a patient should receive several drugs in turn on a trial-and-error basis until the one that is best for his needs is determined empirically. These realities of therapeutics for individual patients are generally ignored in the current requirements for evidence of drug efficacy. All these factors can be crucial for tailoring therapy to an individual patient to achieve maximal efficacy, safety, comfort, convenience, and compliance with the therapeutic regimen. To achieve these goals it is desirable to have a number of alternative therapies from which to choose. (52)

With respect to the benefits from increased testing requirements, Peltzman expected to observe fewer health risks (reduction in loss of life and morbidity) and a consequent reduction in medical expenditures as a result of safer drugs. To calculate the expected value of increased safety requirements, Peltzman estimated the losses that would have been prevented if the 1962 Amendments had been in effect earlier. He examined those cases where drugs were implicated in either fatal or harmful effects to patients. "Thalidomide-type products do not appear to have been introduced frequently in the years before 1962" (53). In estimating the consequences of a thalidomide disaster in this country Peltzman assumed it would have been on a scale that occurred in West Germany, even though thalidomide was kept off the U.S. market by the 1938 FDC Act in 1961. (He further assumed that such drug tragedies occurred once every decade.)

The yearly savings due to all of the above benefits was estimated by Peltzman to be less than $100 million (54).

Turning to the cost side, Peltzman lists a number of negative consequences as a result of the 1962 Amendments. These are:

1. Since fewer new drugs are introduced and the time required to do so increases, older drugs can command higher prices for a longer period of time than previously. Barriers to entry increased and fewer new drugs led to a decline in price competition.
2. As a result of the increased testing requirement, there is now a greater delay in the introduction of new drugs. Because of an increased delay, physicians have had to use older drugs that were less safe than newer ones to which they did not yet have access.
3. The cost of developing a new drug has now increased because of the more stringent testing requirements. This has led to a permanent decrease in the number of new drugs.

Peltzman estimates the cost to consumers of higher prices as a result of the decline in price competition at $50 million. A much larger cost, estimated at $300–400 million, results from the reduced flow of new drugs. The net cost of the drug amendments from these "measurable effects add up to a net loss of $250–350 million, or about 6 percent of total drug sales" (55).

Each of the above "costs" is discussed in more detail.

Effects on Price Competition

It was believed by its proponents that the 1962 Amendments, with its proof of efficacy and controls over drug advertising, that price competition would be increased. Drug companies would be less able to differentiate their products; drugs would be seen as having closer substitutes. In setting their prices, drug companies would be more sensitive to the prices of close competitors. However, if there are fewer new drugs entering a market and there is a longer time period before drugs can enter, then a barrier to entry has been created. Rather than increase price competition, a barrier would serve to *decrease* it. In support of the view that there is price competition between new and old drugs, Peltzman finds that prescription drug prices have risen slightly faster than they would have in the absence of the amendments. He estimates the cost to consumers of this anticompetitive effect to be approximately $50 million a year (56).

Drug Lag

Drug controls over drug safety are almost completely based on premarket testing. Once a new drug has been approved by the FDA, there is relatively little postmarketing surveillance. In the premarket phase animal testing is required before the drug can be tested in human trials. This increase in premarket testing has led to a delay in the introduction of new drugs. Peltzman suggests that this delay is, at a minimum, two years (57).

The necessity of animal testing has been questioned by some experts. It has been criticized because of the limited relationship between the results of animal tests and subsequent results on humans. The effects of some drugs are observable only in humans (58). And some important drugs, such as penicillin, are lethal in animals.

Sir Alexander Fleming once remarked that the success of the penicillin project depended on the fact that, since he was not a pharmacologist, he had not tested the drug in animals at all and that, knowing in retrospect its animal toxicity, he would never have had the courage to try it on man! If even one new drug of the stature of penicillin or digitalis has been unjustifiably banished to a company's back shelf because of excessively stringent animal requirements, that event will have harmed more people than have been affected by all the toxicity that has occurred in the history of modern drug development. It is entirely conceivable that the losses from excessively conservative interpretation of animal toxicity tests are more harmful than the toxicity that would be experienced if drugs were tested in man, with appropriate safeguards, at an earlier stage. (59)

A related but no less important problem of the emphasis on premarket testing is that given the limited number of persons that can be tested in the premarket phase, only the most frequent harmful effects can be detected. Once a drug is marketed and used in a larger population, the less frequent adverse drug reactions begin to show up. It is in the postmarketing phase that drug tragedies can occur. Thus postmarketing surveillance should be an important concern of those empowered to protect the public safety. Unfortunately, while pre- and postmarket testing may be viewed as substitutes, the emphasis is placed on the premarket phase.

Peltzman has attempted to estimate the cost to the public of the drug lag. He does this by examining past drug innovations in drug therapy and calculates what the loss in benefits from these innovations would have been had they been introduced two years later than they had. It turns out that the losses would have been substantial and several times greater than the estimated value of the benefits of the legislation (60). While such an exercise is conjectural, it does serve to indicate the immense importance in lives saved, decreased morbidity, and lower use of medical treatment from a more rapid introduction of important drug discoveries. When estimates are made to indicate the potential savings of drugs that would decrease heart disease and cancer by a small percentage, it is clear from Peltzman's calculations that the loss in potential payoffs are so great as to outweigh any possible benefits due to fewer ineffective drugs and decreased drug toxicity as a result of the new amendments.

One means of documenting the drug lag is to compare how long important new drugs were available in England before they became available in this country. Wardell, a noted pharmacologist, claims that "in many therapeutic areas, useful and even uniquely effective or safe drugs have been introduced in Britain substantially earlier than in the United States, and at any given time the United States lacks a number of such drugs" (61). He concludes his cross-country comparison by saying, "In view of the clear benefits demonstrable from some of the drugs introduced in Britain, it appears that the United States has lost more than it has gained from adopting a more conservative approach than did Britain in the post-thalidomide era" (62).

As a specific example of the harmful effects of the drug lag Wardell cites the case of the beta-blocking agent propranolol:

[It was] available in Britain in 1965 but was not available at all in the United States until 1968, and then it was approved only for relatively minor uses. It took another five years for the same drug to be approved for its first major use, angina, and still another three years (until 1976) before it was approved for its other major use, hypertension. This, and the lack of availability of certain other beta blockers in the United States, resulted in a marked backwardness in American sophistication in the treatment of hypertension over much of the past ten years.

Other beta blockers, such as practolol and alprenolol, have been shown abroad to produce a 40 percent reduction in the incidence of myocardial reinfarction and cardiac death in postcoronary patients. Although this effect could result in saving several thousand lives annually in the United States, these beta blockers are no longer available in this country even for investigational purposes. *As a result of these interminable delays, American textbooks of pharmacology and medicine are in some fields so hopelessly out of date that when used abroad they are often irrelevant.* (63)

Rate of Drug Innovation

The most controversial aspect of the 1962 Amendments has been its effect on the rate of drug innovation. Economists have suggested that the production of innovation can be explained within a traditional demand and supply framework. If drug companies anticipate a rising demand for drugs, the companies will respond with an increase in their supply of new products. Similarly, if the costs of innovation are increased, this should result in a decrease in the supply of new drugs. Within this framework, therefore, we would have expected to observe a decrease in the rate of drug innovation as a result of the 1962 Amendments.

In the post-1962 period the cost of developing a new drug was greatly increased. These higher costs of development occurred for three reasons. There were more stringent testing procedures before a drug company could apply for a new drug approval from the FDA. Second, there was an increase in the number of years between the time the development of a new drug was initiated and its approval by the FDA. One economist has estimated that costs must be incurred for 10 years instead of five years before a company can begin to receive revenues from a new drug (64). A third reason is the greater risk and uncertainty of innovation. One such measure of risk is the attrition rate of new drugs. In the 1950s it was estimated that the attrition rate of new drugs was two out of three. Now less than one new drug out of ten undergoing chemical testing is marketed (65).

It has been estimated by one analyst that the cost of developing a new drug has increased tenfold by 1971 compared to the pre-1962 period. (After allowing for inflation the cost was still more than five times greater.) Another economist estimated the costs in 1974 to be more than 10 times greater than they were in 1960 (66). Hansen (cited earlier) concluded that the cost (in 1976 dollars) of each new chemical entity that is marketed represents a cost of approximately $61 million. (It is not surprising that new drugs that would serve potentially small markets are less likely to be developed. Even though such drugs may be badly needed, the increased costs of developing such drugs, given the size of the market, make such investments unprofitable.)

The increased development time, higher cost, and greater uncertainty of success resulted in a sharp decline in profitability of new drugs in the 1962–1972 period (67). We would therefore expect to observe a decline in the number of new drugs introduced in the post-1962 period. As anticipated, during the period

1957–1961 there were 233 new chemical entities. This declined to 93 during 1962–1966 and further to 76 in 1967–1971 (68). Peltzman attributes most of the reasons for this decline to the 1962 Amendments.

The FDA does not, of course, agree with this assessment. They have responded that the reasons for this decline are twofold. Ineffective new drugs were eliminated from the market and, second, there has been a natural decline in drug innovation worldwide. It has become more difficult to develop new innovations as the opportunities for new research has declined. This latter reason is unrelated to the 1962 Amendments.

With respect to the FDA reply that the decline is a result of keeping ineffective drugs off the market, Peltzman refers to several studies to demonstrate that, at most, 10 percent of pre-1962 drugs were ineffective. Further, even though there is not agreement on what constitutes a significant new chemical entity, Peltzman used data from an unpublished FDA study to show that there was an annual average of 12.3 "important therapeutic advances" between 1950 and 1962 and only 9.1 per year between 1963 and 1970 (69). Thus the decline in the rate of innovation since 1962 is real.

In a recent study, Grabowski, Vernon, and Thomas examine the reasons for the serious decline in drug innovation since 1962. To determine whether the 1962 Amendments contributed to this decline, they undertook a comparative study of the rate of innovation in this country and in the United Kingdom (UK). Until 1971, drug regulation in the UK was similar to regulation in this country in the period prior to 1962. If the reason for the decline in the rate of drug innovation was the worldwide phenomenon of a lack of research opportunities then the UK should have been similarly affected. Since the regulatory environment differs between the two countries, this comparison should help to isolate these separate effects. The authors state, "The data . . . clearly show that there has been a significant decline in the R&D productivities for the two countries over the post-amendment period. However, perhaps the most interesting result is the much stronger *relative* decline in R&D productivity that the United States experienced in the decade after 1962. . . . Hence, over this period in which the United States shifted to a much more stringent regulatory environment than the United Kingdom, it also experienced a much more rapid decline in R&D productivity" (70).

It is difficult to determine whether the downward trend in innovation due to the nonregulatory effect in both countries is an adequate test of the depletion of research opportunities or whether it is due to other reasons. Another possible explanation is the thalidomide tragedy and scientific advances in the pharmacological sciences, both of which resulted in greater amounts being spent on research and development, and consequently resulted in fewer drug innovations. Under this explanation, the drug companies have been willing to incur higher development costs so as to preserve their reputations and to minimize their legal liabilities by forestalling any drug tragedies.

Thus the cross-country comparisons demonstrate that there has been an effect on new drug introductions as a result of the 1962 Amendments. The general downward trend in drug innovations in both countries, however, may be due to several reasons and to date it has not been possible to determine the exact reasons for the decline.

CONCLUDING COMMENTS

All policies have trade-offs. It is not possible to receive benefits without also incurring costs. Policymakers should consider both aspects, the costs as well as the benefits of their decisions. Drug safety can be increased, that is, the risks of harmful side effects of a new drug can be lowered, by requiring still further testing and delaying for a greater number of years the marketing of new drugs. The cost of that policy, however, is to deny new drugs to people in need of them. Wardell cites the case of benzodiazepine hypnotic (nitrazepam) which was available in Europe five years before it was approved for marketing in this country in 1971. An advantage of this drug over other hypnotics is its safety in overdosage. Based on data in foreign markets and U.S. deaths due to overdosage of hypnotics, Wardell concluded that the five-year delay in availability in U.S. markets resulted in more than 1,200 deaths in this country (71). If a drug marketed in this country caused these many deaths, it would be considered a major drug disaster. But the fact that these were deaths that could have been prevented by earlier introduction of a new drug went unnoticed.

The difference between preventable deaths and deaths caused by drug toxicity are that the latter are visible; the victims have names and families, and their pictures may be in the paper. They are identifiable. Preventable deaths are statistical, as such they are anonymous. An agency such as the FDA is likely to place a greater emphasis on minimizing visible deaths rather than being as concerned with anonymous beneficiaries. In so doing, the FDA limits criticisms of its actions by the press and the public. Comprehensive premarket testing can also be viewed as a means by which the FDA protects itself.

From a societal perspective, however, criteria different from those used by the FDA should be considered. Given the enormous benefits from the early introduction of new drugs, greater emphasis should be given to the earlier introduction of new drugs rather than seeking to minimize the risks of drug toxicity through extensive premarket testing. Perhaps appropriate policy would be to encourage greater risk taking when introducing new drugs with a consequent strengthening of postmarketing surveillance to minimize the risk of drug toxicity.

PUBLIC POLICY TOWARD THE PHARMACEUTICAL INDUSTRY

ECONOMIC PERFORMANCE OF THE INDUSTRY

The concern that critics of the pharmaceutical industry have had with respect to its economic performance have resulted in several proposals, each of which would result in lower drug prices and drug profits. Several of these proposals, together with their effects, both direct and indirect, will be discussed.

Compulsory Licensing of Patented Drugs

An important source of monopoly power in the drug industry is patent protection. Critics believe that the length of time over which a patent protects a manufacturer is too long. If the patent were for a shorter period of time (it is currently for 17 years), the manufacturer would still be able to earn sufficient profits to provide incentives for research, without resulting in excessive profits. To lessen this source of monopoly power, it has been proposed (by Senator Kefauver and subsequently by Senator Nelson), that after several years of exclusive patent rights, the manufacturer be required to license other drug firms to manufacture and market the patented drug, while paying the original manufacturer a "fair" royalty rate.

Cross-licensing proposals have varied in their definition of how long the original patent holder is to have exclusive rights and on what royalty rate should be paid to the original patent holder. Under the Kefauver proposal, exclusive patent rights to new drugs would start at the date of filing the new drug application. Given the long period of time before a new drug is marketed, for many drugs the exclusive period would be over before the commercial life of a drug started (72). Other proposals suggest three to four years of commercial life, sales of a certain magnitude, and perhaps a return of five to one over the cost of the drug.

Cross-licensing would increase price competition among the various manufacturers and distributors of the drug. Drug prices would be reduced as would profits to the original patent holder.

An important consequence of cross-licensing is that while it will not affect the supply of the patented drug, it would result in a decrease in the supplies of yet undiscovered drugs. Not all research and development results in patented and profitable drugs. Only a small number of drugs eventually become profitable. Proposals that limit the profit on those that become successful will decrease the overall rate of return to research and development and consequently lead to a decrease in drug innovation.

Recently, legislation has been introduced that would lengthen the effective life of a drug patent. With the longer development time before a new drug can be marketed, it is estimated that the effective life of a drug patent is now about 9 years. This is a decline from almost 14 years in 1966. The proposed legislation would increase the patent life, up to a maximum of 7 years, due to time lost as a result of the testing and regulatory process (73).

Generic Versus Brand Name Prescribing

Another means of lowering drug prices is to encourage the substitution of generic drugs for those prescribed by brand name. Generic drugs are less expensive than brand name drugs and they are believed by many to be equally safe, since the FDA is responsible for monitoring their quality. The issue of generic versus brand name prescribing has been manifested in two types of policies: repeal of antisubstitution laws in a state and the federal maximum allowable cost regulations.

Antisubstitution Laws.   Pharmacists and a number of consumer groups have favored repeal of state laws that prohibit the pharmacist from substituting a generic drug for a brand name drug specified in a prescription without the prescribing physician's permission. The pharmacists claim that they are able to judge the quality of substitute drugs and that by substituting to generic drugs they can save the consumer money. According to one survey many pharmacists make such substitutions in states where it is illegal to do so (74).

Repeal of antisubstitution laws is opposed by the pharmaceutical industry and by many physicians. Their argument goes as follows: If a physician believed it was acceptable to substitute a generic type drug for the brand name one prescribed, then this could be indicated on the prescription form. To substitute without the physician's permission is to diminish the physician's role in caring for the patient. When prescribing for a patient, the physician should consider the patient's health history, whether the patient has any allergies, how the prescribed drug acts with other medications the patient may be taking, the price of that drug relative to others, and the quality of the drug, as indicated by the physician's confidence in certain manufacturer's products. Price is clearly a secondary consideration. It is generally difficult to monitor the drug response by an ambulatory patient, and this difficulty is increased when the drug taken by the patient is not the one prescribed by the physician.

Federal Maximum Allowable Cost Regulations. Through the Medicaid program, the federal government has adopted regulations to encourage generic substitution. Under the maximum allowable cost (MAC) regulations, pharmacists are to substitute the chemically equivalent drug which is generally available at the lowest cost for any prescribed brand name drug. Pharmacists participating in the MAC program would, among multiple source drugs (comprising approximately 40 percent of ethical drugs), receive a dispensing fee plus the lowest cost of generic drugs that are "generally available." By use of the term "generally available," the drug manufacturer must reduce the price of their generic drugs to all buyers and not just to those on Medicaid. Thus, to be able to compete for Medicaid patients, drug manufacturers cannot maintain differential prices to Medicaid patients and private pay patients.

The effect of the MAC regulation is to lower the price of drugs for patients under the government-reimbursed program as well as to all other patients. The marginal cost of a drug is a small fraction of both the price and the average cost of a brand name drug. Thus intensive price competition of generic drugs among drug manufacturers should result in large reductions in both prices and profits.

Two objections have been raised with the MAC regulation, which would also be applicable to repeal of antisubstitution laws. The first is with respect to the quality of generic drugs. It is assumed by many that the quality of all generic drugs is equal. Schwartzman, however, claims that with so many drug manufacturers [there were 757 drug manufacturing facilities in 1977 (75)] the FDA has, in the past, not been able to adequately monitor the quality of drugs produced by all manufacturers (76). Since the emphasis of the MAC regulation is on price competition according to chemically equivalent drugs, Schwartzman claims that the incentives for manufacturers to be concerned with quality is less than if they were producing drugs under their own brand name.

A second concern with the MAC regulation (and with other proposals that attempt to lower drug prices) is that it results in a decrease in drug industry profitability. A lower rate of return on drug firm research and development will result in a smaller output of product innovation. These long-run consequences of decreased profitability are less obvious to the public than the immediate savings to the government of lower drug prices. Less drug innovation is an important cost to society which the government gives less weight to when considering its own immediate needs for reduced expenditures.

FEDERAL REGULATION OF DRUG SAFETY

Public policy should attempt to achieve an appropriate balance between minimizing the risk from early introduction of potentially hazardous drugs and providing ready access to therapeutically important drugs to patients who need them. It appears that the FDA has overemphasized the former while neglecting the latter. To achieve a more optimal mix between these two concerns, several policies have been suggested.

Postmarketing Surveillance

One way of permitting consumers to benefit from the early introduction of new drugs while helping to ensure that the public is adequately protected is to place a greater reliance on postmarketing surveillance. Present policy virtually neglects postmarketing surveillance and relies too heavily on premarket testing. Usually it is not possible to detect widespread drug toxicity in the early stages of a drug's development. In that phase, its use is limited to a small number of people and it is prescribed under close supervision. Widespread toxicity can occur when a drug is used by a much larger number of people, over a long period of time, and in an unsupervised manner.* Thus surveillance is particularly necessary once a drug is widely marketed.

This country has one of the lowest voluntary reporting rates of drug toxicity of all countries reporting to the World Health Organization's International Drug Monitoring Program. On a per capita basis, Britain's voluntary reporting rate was 10 times that of the United States. The lack of an effective postmarketing surveillance system has also been criticized by the Government Accounting Office (77).

Restricted Use of Drugs

It has been suggested that the restrictive regulations on use of drugs should not apply equally to all physicians. Currently, medical specialists in university hospitals are treated the same as general practitioners with respect to their access to

---

*Proposals to speed up the approval process for new drugs are likely to be rejected as a result of the recent problems with the drug Oraflex. An antiarthritic drug, Oraflex was separately tested in both Britain and the United States. After the drug was marketed, there were allegations that the drug was implicated in 60 deaths in Britain and 12 in the United States. The drug company voluntarily withdrew the drug before the FDA took any action. Even though the drug had been tested, it is not possible to judge all the potential side effects of a drug until it is placed in wider use than when it is studied in clinical trials. There may have been a combined effect between Oraflex and other drugs. Sick elderly patients may have been taking several drugs simultaneously.

Speeding up the approval process by relying more on drug companies for information does not absolve the drug company from the economic liabilities of a drug tragedy. These economic consequences are likely to be the main determinant of how much information is necessary before a drug company is willing to market a new drug.

drugs. In order to make certain drugs available that have not yet undergone their complete premarket testing, their distribution could be restricted to certain types of patients for whom the benefits of the drug would be particularly great. Earlier drug usage could be made available to those physicians that are expert in particular areas or that have undergone special training in their use.

These are just several of the ways in which patients can benefit from early availability of new drugs without permitting the widespread early release of powerful new drugs whose complete uses and effects are not yet fully known (78). Rather than placing stringent restrictions on the introduction of new drugs, a more flexible and responsive policy to patients' needs should be encouraged. In fact, the 1962 Amendments and their enforcement by the FDA should be held to the same standards that they would apply to new drugs.

> Indeed, if judged by the same standards they themselves set for drugs, the 1962 laws could not be approved because no evidence of their safety or efficacy exists: They were implemented in a scientifically uncontrolled manner, and no measures of their effects were even sought. We are only now beginning to evaluate in retrospect the effects of the changes that began in 1962, and it is doubtful whether their full impact can ever be known. (79)

Additional Reforms

Other countries with less restrictive drug regulations are able to introduce new drugs more quickly than in this country. When these drugs are shown to be important therapeutic discoveries, the FDA should be willing to accept data based on foreign use of the drug. Prior to 1975 the FDA did not accept any foreign data for a new drug. The FDA has recently begun accepting such data; however, additional studies in this country must still be conducted. The drug lag could be greatly reduced if, for some drugs, greater reliance were placed on the experience of other countries with the drug.

Other countries place a greater reliance than the United States on expert advisory committees for decisions on approval of new drugs. If the FDA were required to act similarly, then these advisory committees would not have the same reluctance as the FDA to delay approval of new drugs. The committees would, as in other countries, balance both the hidden as well as the visible costs and benefits of new drugs. The FDA would not bear the onus of visible deaths due to early introduction of new drugs.

The 1962 Amendments have resulted in such bizarre situations that drugs (such as benzodiazepine hypnotic) were kept off the market when they were safer than the drugs they were meant to replace.

In 1974 Congressional hearings were held on the FDA's performance with respect to the drug lag. In response to this criticism, the FDA gave greater priority to significant new drugs. This "fast track" clearance was supposed to permit significant new drugs to be introduced sooner than they would otherwise have been. While this has been a move in the right direction, there is great concern that drug approval times are still too long.

In 1978 the Carter Administration introduced drug legislation that would have, among other things, speeded up the approval of new drugs. Though an amended bill passed the Senate, it did not pass the House before the 96th Congress adjourned.

The policy of the Reagan Administration is to seek administrative reform of the FDA's drug approval process rather than achieve these goals through new legislation.

Unfortunately, there is still a significant lag in the introduction of new drugs. A recent Government Accounting Office (GAO) study on FDA procedures found that the FDA policy of giving priority to important new drugs has produced some progress. The GAO found that while approval times for new drug applications lengthened in four of the FDA's six reviewing divisions they were reduced in the remaining two (80). Unless public and Congressional pressures on the FDA for more rapid introduction of drugs persist, the main losers would once again be the anonymous beneficiaries; that large number of people who could benefit and yet are denied access to beneficial drugs.

CONCLUDING COMMENTS

An important imperfection in the pharmaceutical market is that while the physician prescribes drugs, he or she is not responsible for the cost of the prescription; it is paid for by the patient or a third-party payor. It is time consuming, hence costly, for the physician who desires to be well informed on the latest in drug therapy, new minor chemical modifications, side effects of various drugs, alternative dosage forms, and prices. Faced with high informational needs and an incentive system whereby someone else pays for the drug, it is not surprising that the current system of drug marketing is what it is.

The physician's role in the pharmaceutical market, however, is no different than the physician's role in the broader medical care delivery system. To change physician behavior, it is necessary to change the incentives facing the physician. If there were competition among prepaid health plans, based on a capitation payment, both the incentives and information requirements facing physicians would change. Assuming drugs were included as a benefit in a prepaid health plan, then there would be a change in the financial incentive facing the participating physician. Drug costs become one more component of care whose costs are to be minimized. Prepaid health plans would be likely to purchase drugs at lower prices than they are sold on the retail market. They would purchase larger quantities and, being more informed buyers, would be better equipped to shop around. The informational needs of physicians in such a setting might also be lessened. The physician might develop sufficient confidence in the organizations' pharmacists to be willing to delegate some of the decisionmaking on drugs to them. In several health maintenance organizations (HMOs) today physicians are able to indicate on their prescription form whether it is permissible for the pharmacist to substitute.

The pharmaceutical industry does not perform as well as many would prefer; it devotes more resources to promotion than its critics believe is necessary; the prices of drugs are higher than its costs of production; and low-income persons have difficulty paying for needed drugs. It is important, however, to retain a proper perspective on this industry. Many proposed policies to decrease promotion expenditures, prices, and profitability may result in greater long-term harm than their immediate benefits.

Drug costs represent a small percent of the costs of medical care and have been rising at a less rapid rate than medical care prices. The benefits of drug therapy are enormous. Drugs prolong life, alleviate pain, and are a very low-cost substitute for more expensive medical treatment; for example, Tagamet, an anti-ulcer drug, saves millions of dollars in hospital and surgical costs each year (81). A new class of heart drugs might eliminate coronary bypass surgery. Drugs are very cost effective. The main emphasis of public policy toward the pharmaceutical industry therefore should be to *increase* drug innovation. Too great an emphasis on correcting perceived monopoly abuses, such as through requiring cross-licensing, and policies to decrease drug prices and profits, will result in a lower rate of return on research and development and, hence, on product innovation. Further, the monopoly abuses may be more perceived than real. Profitability estimates are not as high as originally believed and promotional expenditures serve an important information function as well as being a means of entering new markets. There is also a greater degree of price competition than formerly believed. It would therefore be unfortunate if policies were instituted, based on incorrect perceptions, the net effect of which was to decrease drug innovation. Policies should instead be developed to provide greater incentives for research and development and to decrease the time required to bring new drugs to market. The benefits to society from increased drug innovation will far outweigh the immediate savings of lower drug prices. In this regard the FDA Amendments should be reevaluated with these objectives in mind.

REFERENCES

1. Drug and medical sundry expenditures include expenditures for both prescription and nonprescription drugs. Approximately 56 percent of drug and medical sundry expenditures are for prescription drugs. See the footnote to Table 17-1.
2. F.M. Scherer, *Industrial Market Structure and Economic Performance* (Chicago: Rand McNally and Co., 1970), p. 60.
3. Henry G. Grabowski and John M. Vernon, "New Studies on Market Concentration, Theory of Supply, Entry, and Promotion," in Robert I. Chien, ed., *Issues in Pharmaceutical Economics* (Lexington, Mass.: Lexington Books, 1979), p. 32.
4. *Ibid.*, p. 31.
5. Walter S. Measday, "The Pharmaceutical Industry," in Walter Adams, ed., *The Structure of American Industry*, 4th ed. (New York: Macmillan Company, 1971), p. 167.
6. George J. Stigler, "Introduction," in *Business Concentration and Price Policy*, National Bureau of Economic Research (Princeton, NJ: Princeton University Press, 1955), p. 4.
7. Henry G. Grabowski and John M. Vernon, *op. cit.*, p. 32.
8. *Ibid.*, pp. 33–35.
9. *Ibid.*, pp. 35–36.
10. The study by Douglas Cocks, "Product Innovation and the Dynamic Elements of Competition in the Ethical Pharmaceutical Industry," in Robert B. Helms, ed., *Drug Development and Marketing* (Washington, D.C.: American Enterprise Institute, 1975) used the Hymer–Pashigian instability index, which is calculated as follows:

$$I = \sum_{i=1}^{n} \left(\frac{S_{t,i}}{S_t} - \frac{S_{t-1,\,i}}{S_{t-1}} \right)$$

where I = index of instability
$S_{t,i}$ = sales of the ith firm at time t
S_t = total industry sales at time t

11. A.T. Kearney, *Study of Economics of Entry and Exit in the Pharmaceutical Industry*, Pharmaceutical Manufacturers Association, April 30, 1974.

12. Henry Grabowski and John M. Vernon, *op. cit.*, p. 39.

13. As reported in David Schwartzman, *Innovation in the Pharmaceutical Industry* (Baltimore, Md.: The Johns Hopkins University Press, 1976), p. 76.

14. As reported in David Schwartzman, *ibid.*, p. 79.

15. *Ibid.*, p. 18.

16. *Fact Book*, Pharmaceutical Manufacturers Association, 1980, p. 22.

17. *Ibid.*, p. 26.

18. Jerome E. Schnee and Erol Caglarcan, "Economic Structure and Performance of the Ethical Pharmaceutical Industry," in Cotton M. Lindsay, ed., *The Pharmaceutical Industry* (New York: John Wiley & Sons, Inc., 1978), p. 32.

19. *Ibid.*, pp. 32–33.

20. Grabowski and Vernon, *op. cit.*, p. 48.

21. Hansen estimates that when expenditures are capitalized to the date of marketing approval at a 10 percent interest rate, the estimated cost per marketed new chemical entity is 61.6 million dollars (in 1976 dollars). Ronald W. Hansen, "The Pharmaceutical Development Process: Estimates of Development Costs and Times and the Effects of Proposed Regulatory Changes," in Robert I. Chien, ed., *op. cit.*, p. 168.

22. A recent article discussing these two aspects of promotional expenditures is Keith B. Leffler, "Persuasion or Information? The Economics of Prescription Drug Advertising," *The Journal of Law and Economics* (April 1981).

23. This was a survey conducted in 1966 of British physicians and reported in David Schwartzman, *op. cit.*, pp. 188–189.

24. *Ibid.*, p. 194.

25. Sam Peltzman, *Regulation of Pharmaceutical Innovation* (Washington, D.C.: American Enterprise Institute, 1974).

26. For a more extensive discussion of promotion expenses, its magnitude, and components, see Chapter 9 in David Schwartzman, *op. cit.*

27. Henry G. Grabowski and John M. Vernon, *op. cit.*, p. 44.

28. *Ibid.*, p. 45.

29. David Schwartzman, *op. cit.*, p. 202.

30. J. Fred Weston, "Pricing in the Pharmaceutical Industry," in Robert I. Chien, ed., *op. cit.*, p. 77.

31. David Schwartzman, "Pricing of Multiple Source Drugs," in Robert I. Chien, ed., *op. cit.*, p. 97.

32. David Schwartzman, "Pricing of Multiple Source Drugs," *op. cit.*, pp. 99–100.

33. *Ibid.*, p. 99.

34. *Ibid.*, p. 99.

35. It is possible to reconcile the above evidence on price competition with the earlier evidence on price inflexibility cited by Markham through the findings that there is a

difference in the manufacturer's posted prices and the price at which transactions occur. Apparently Markham was observing posted prices rather than "real" prices.

36. J. Fred Weston, *op. cit.*, p. 94.

37. Walter J. Campbell and Rodney F. Smith, "Profitability and the Pharmaceutical Industry," in Cotton M. Lindsay, ed., *The Pharmaceutical Industry* (New York: John Wiley & Sons, Inc., 1978), p. 114.

38. Kenneth W. Clarkson, "The Use of Pharmaceutical Profitability Measures for Public Policy Actions," in Robert I. Chien, ed., *Issues in Pharmaceutical Economics* (Lexington, Mass.: D.C. Heath Co., 1979), p. 117.

39. As additional proof that corrected rates of return are a more accurate measure of profitability in the pharmaceutical industry, Clarkson finds that corrected rather than accounting rates of return are a more useful explanatory variable for explaining variations in stock prices of drug firms. *Ibid.*, p. 118.

40. *Ibid.*, p. 113. In another part of his article, Clarkson presents a sensitivity analysis of the rate of return to different economic lives of various expenditure categories.

41. David Schwartzman, *op. cit.*, p. 156.

42. These studies are discussed in David Schwartzman, *op. cit.*, pp. 156–158; and in Campbell and Smith, *op. cit.*, pp. 113–115.

43. Schwartzman, *op. cit.*, p. 159.

44. These studies are reported in Oswald H. Brownlee, "Rates of Return to Investment in the Pharmaceutical Industry: A Survey and Critical Appraisal," in Robert I. Chien, ed., *op. cit.*, p. 139.

45. A brief history of federal regulation over drugs appears in Jerome E. Schnee, "Government Control of Therapeutic Drugs: Intent, Impact, and Issues," in Cotton M. Lindsay, ed., *op. cit.* For more detailed information, see the references in that chapter. A recently published history of drug regulations is: Peter Temin, *Taking Your Medicine: Drug Regulation in the United States* (Cambridge, Mass.: Harvard University Press, 1981).

46. William M. Wardell, "The History of Drug Discovery, Development, and Regulation," in Robert I. Chien, ed., *op. cit.*, p. 8.

47. A discussion of the Kefauver hearings and the congressional debate which preceded the 1962 Amendments was written by Richard Harris, *The Real Voice* (New York: Macmillan Company, 1964).

48. Wardell states, "The fact that thalidomide had not been approved for U.S. marketing was somehow irrelevant, as was the fact that the new requirements in the amendments, had they been in effect, would not have prevented a thalidomide-type tragedy." William M. Wardell and Louis Lasagna, *Regulation and Drug Development* (Washington, D.C.: American Enterprise Institute, 1975), p. 1.

49. Sam Peltzman, *op. cit.*

50. *Ibid.*, pp. 37–38.

51. *Ibid.*, p. 45.

52. William M. Wardell, "Therapeutic Implications of the Drug Lag," *Clinical Pharmacology and Therapeutics* 15(1) (January 1974): 76.

53. *Ibid.*, p. 52.

54. The exact method by which Peltzman calculates the value of each of these benefits is described in the Appendix of his book.

55. Peltzman, *op. cit.*, p. 81.

56. *Ibid.*, pp. 47–48. This estimate is based on 1970 drug sales. It would be higher in current prices.

57. *Ibid.*, p. 57.
58. Wardell and Lasagna, *op. cit.*, p. 138.
59. *Ibid.*, pp. 138–139.
60. Peltzman, *op. cit.*, pp. 72–73.
61. Wardell and Lasagna, *op. cit.*, p. 97.
62. *Ibid.*, p. 105.
63. William M. Wardell, "The Impact of Regulation on New Drug Development," in Robert I. Chien, ed., *op. cit.*, p. 147. (Italics in original quote.)
64. Oswald H. Brownlee, "The Economic Consequences of Regulating Without Regard to Economic Consequences," in Robert I. Chien, ed., *op. cit.*, p. 216.
65. Henry G. Grabowski, John M. Vernon, and Lacy G. Thomas, "Estimating the Effects of Regulation on Innovation: An International Comparative Analysis of the Pharmaceutical Industry," *Journal of Law and Economics* (April 1978): 136.
66. Brownlee, *op. cit.*, p. 216. Additional cost estimates are cited in Wardell and Lasagna, *op. cit.*, p. 46.
67. Grabowski, Vernon, and Thomas, *op. cit.*, p. 158.
68. Grabowski and Vernon, *op. cit.*, in Robert I. Chien, ed., p. 47.
69. Peltzman, *op. cit.*, pp. 86–87.
70. Grabowski, Vernon, and Thomas, *op. cit.*, p. 151.
71. As reported in Peltzman, *op. cit.*, p. 89.
72. David Schwartzman, *op. cit.*, p. 332.
73. Henry G. Grabowski and John M. Vernon, "FDA Regulation of Pharmaceuticals," *Working Paper No. 15* (Washington, D.C.: American Enterprise Institute, November 1981), p. 70.
74. David Schwartzman, *op. cit.*, p. 271.
75. A company may have more than one discrete manufacturing facility. *Fact Book* (Washington, D.C.: Pharmaceutical Manufacturers Association, 1980), p. 14. The government's General Accounting Office has estimated that the FDA must inspect 5,400 plants manufacturing drugs. David Schwartzman, *op. cit.*, p. 24.
76. David Schwartzman, *op. cit.*, p. 328.
77. Wardell and Lasagna, *op. cit.*, p. 99.
78. For a more complete set of suggestions for public policy in this area, see Wardell and Lasagna, Chapter 13.
79. Wardell and Lasagna, *op. cit.*, p. 164.
80. "FDA Approval of New Drugs is Speedier, But More Progress is Needed, GAO Says," *Wall Street Journal*, September 16, 1981.
81. John F. Geweke and Burton A. Weisbrod, "Some Economic Consequences of Technological Advance in Medical Care: The Case of the New Drug," in Robert B. Helms, ed., *Drugs and Health* (Washington, D.C.: American Enterprise Institute, 1981).

CHAPTER 18

The Political Economy of Health Care

INTRODUCTION (1)

A number of studies have been conducted to evaluate the effectiveness of federal subsidy programs in the medical care sector. In examination of federal manpower subsidies to increase the number of dentists it was found that an equivalent number of dental visits could have been produced, at less than one-tenth the cost, if the federal subsidies had been provided in a different manner, namely, if the wages of dental auxiliaries had been subsidized (2). Evaluations of the federal Nurse Training Act revealed that an increase in the number of employed registered nurses could have been achieved at between one-fifth and one-tenth the cost had an alternative approach been used; namely, if the wages of registered nurses had been stabilized, thereby increasing their participation rate in the market (3). These analyses of the federal manpower subsidy programs have questioned the justification offered for such programs, based, as it was, on the use of health-manpower-to-population ratios to indicate a "need" or "shortage." The method used to distribute the subsidy funds is also open to question. A possible conclusion is that further economic analysis is needed if governmental programs are to be cost-effective. The assumption is that with additional information, policymakers would generate better legislation. However, another interpretation of the type of health legislation that results from the legislative process is that the resulting legislation is actually what is intended. Under this hypothesis the participants in the legislative process are assumed to have rational goals and to be aware of the effects of the legislation that is proposed. If the resulting legislation is not cost effective, it is because it was not meant to be cost effective.

An examination of the beneficiaries of such legislation lends support to this hypothesis. The major beneficiaries of health manpower legislation were the health professional schools, because they were the recipients of the vast majority of funds distributed, and the health professionals themselves since their educational costs were subsidized.

If the outcome of legislation is the result intended, then the prospects for improving the cost-effectiveness of future health legislation by merely providing additional economic analyses of its intended effects is uncertain. To predict legislative outcomes it becomes necessary to develop a model, not of the most cost-effective approach to achieving the stated objectives of the legislation, but rather of the supply and demand for legislation (4). In other words, a model of the political economy of health care is required. A theoretical framework to explain the outcome of the legislation would include the following participants in the legislative process: legislatures and/or the particular legislative committee with jurisdiction over the proposed legislation; the health interest groups affected by the legislation, such as the American Hospital Association (AHA) and the American Medical Association; the bureaucracy that will administer the legislation; the executive branch of the federal government; and other interest groups, such as industry and unions. Those who may be affected by the proposed legislation undoubtedly would like to influence it so that it coincides with their particular interests.

For example, legislators favor (or propose) particular legislative actions because they improve their chances of being reelected: if the legislation is viewed favorably by their constituents or other proponents, support will be forthcoming to the legislators, either in the form of campaign funds, volunteers for helping in the election campaign, or simply votes. The health interest organizations have a demand for legislation because it benefits their members. The demand for legislation by these interest groups, which is an indication of how much a group would be willing to "pay" for those legislative benefits (in terms of campaign funds and so on), depends upon what benefits the legislation provides beyond the legislative benefits the members of the group already possess. The cost of obtaining these legislative benefits, as determined by the direct monetary and nonmonetary outlays necessary to achieve them, depends, among other things, on the action of other interested parties to that legislation. The greater the adverse effect of the legislation upon other interest groups, the greater will be their willingness to "pay" to forestall or defeat the proposed legislation, which in turn increases the cost of having such legislation passed. The cost of obtaining the legislation may well exceed the positive benefits to members of a group favoring the legislation, in which case they will be unsuccessful in achieving their legislative program.

Another interested participant in the legislative process is the bureaucracy which is to administer the legislation. Bureaucrats wish to see their own bureaucracies survive and grow, thereby justifying their larger salaries as the size of their agencies and responsibilities increase. The particular bureaucracy administering the legislation can promise benefits to legislators or particular interest groups if the legislation increases the agency's budget. The executive branch of government, which has overall responsibility for the government budget, may have an interest in the legislation because it would affect total government expenditures. The executive branch of government would like to start new programs so as to increase its own reelection chances. To do so, it may be interested in constraining expenditures on old programs, since new legislation would require additional dollars, which could come either from politically unpopular higher taxes or from underfunding current programs.

These are some of the participants in the legislative process. Other possible participants are industry and labor unions, who would be affected in their costs of production, and in number of workers employed or wages, respectively. A complete model to explain the actual outcome of legislation would have to quantify the perceived benefits and the costs of the proposed legislation to all of these participants.

This chapter examines the legislative behavior of only one of the participants in the legislative process: the health interest groups. The reason for selecting them is that in the past much of the health legislation at both state and federal levels has been strongly influenced by these groups. In fact, the structure of our health care system is, in many respects, the result of legislative activity by these health associations. Health interest groups often provide the only testimony on legislation; their positions are well publicized and are presented as being synonymous with that of the public interest. All legislation is complex and requires knowledgeable persons to understand it. In the past the public has been inclined to believe that health legislation is best understood by health professionals and therefore has been willing to accept the politics of health as espoused by health professionals. A simple example of this point is President Ford's veto of the Nurse Training Act, which was overridden by Congress. Health professionals decried President Ford's action. Given the limited analysis in the media of the reasons for that veto, Congress believed it was on safe political grounds in overriding it.

The potential impact of health interest groups is enormous. From 1965 to 1981 state and federal expenditures on health care increased from $8 billion to $103 billion. Total expenditures on health care increased during this same period from $36 to $255 billion. Had the health legislation which was passed during this period been written in a different fashion—less to the liking of the health interest groups—health expenditures would undoubtedly have risen at a slower pace. This massive redistribution of income from patients and taxpayers to health professionals during this same period is an indication of the legislative success of health professionals. Yet few persons would maintain that the level of health in this country has risen primarily as a result of these massive increases in health expenditures.

The belief that legislation can confer large monetary benefits to interest groups is not new. Nearly two hundred years ago, in *The Federalist,* James Madison expressed this idea (5). The reason special-interest legislation is enacted is that the economic interests of producers are concentrated while the economic interests of consumers are diffused over many areas of economic activity. The benefits to special-interest groups from legislation are potentially so large as to provide them with ample incentive to secure legislation on their behalf. The cost to each consumer from special-interest-group legislation is relatively small, since the costs are spread over a great many consumers. The proponents of such legislation are rarely so bold as to admit that their incomes will be increased by imposing what is the equivalent of a tax on all consumers of their products. Instead, such legislation is presented as being in the public's or country's interests.

While producers often receive their entire incomes from the products they produce, consumers rarely spend more than a small portion of their income on any one product; thus, their economic interests are considered diffuse. Further, for consumers to learn of the special-interest legislation that is being proposed, to ascertain the effects of such legislation on the prices they must pay for the affected products, and to inform other consumers and mobilize them against such legislation is clearly more costly to the consumer than any monetary benefits that would be derived from having the legislation defeated.

The beneficiaries of special-interest-group legislation have been documented in a number of studies; milk producers benefit from milk marketing boards, domestic producers benefit from tariffs on imported goods, maritime workers benefit from maritime subsidies, and northern industrial workers benefit from federal minimum wage legislation. A less obvious, but no less important interest group that has benefited from legislation is health professionals. The activities of health associations and their success in the legislative marketplace have been virtually unnoticed.

In the health services industry, as with other industries, consumers on the average spend a small portion of their incomes on medical care, approximately 10 percent. Because expenditures for medical care are a relatively small percentage of consumers' incomes, it is to their advantage to allocate their time and efforts to other activities that have a greater impact on their budgets and incomes. For health professionals, however, health legislation determines almost all of their income. Therefore, it is in their interests to be involved in the legislative process; they are willing to contribute money and time to political campaigns, testify at legislative hearings, and provide information to legislators and the public on their positions.

Most health legislation that is of importance to health associations has been at a state level. This is to the advantage of the health associations, since it increases the costs to consumers and others who may wish to oppose them. Opponents would have to organize and bear the necessary costs of becoming involved in the legislative process 50 times rather than once. What makes it even more difficult for the consumer to become involved in health legislation at a state level is that such legislation does not outwardly appear to affect the consumer's dollars. State practice acts, which define the tasks to be performed by different health professionals and set the requirements for licensure and state appropriations for medical, dental, and other health professional educational institutions are policy decisions that appear to be too remote to affect the consumer's pocketbook.

THE DEMAND FOR LEGISLATION BY HEALTH ASSOCIATIONS

To gain a better understanding of the type of health legislation that exists in this country it is necessary to develop a model of the demand for legislation by health interest groups. Such a framework should indicate the type of legislation that different health associations would favor or oppose. If the framework presented is a fairly accurate predictor of the political behavior of different health associations, then it should also be possible to anticipate future legislative changes and the form that such legislation might take. The political behavior of two types of health associations will be examined: first, those health associations that represent the interests of health manpower professions, namely, the American Medical Association, the American Dental Association, and the American Nurses' Association, and second, those associations that represent nonprofit providers, namely, the American Hospital Association, the Blue Cross Association, the Association of American Medical Colleges, and the American Association of Dental Schools.

A framework of the demand for legislation will be presented to describe the specific types of health legislation that the various health associations desire. The necessity for having a framework is twofold: 1) it is not possible to merely state that health associations act in their own interests without first defining their interests, and 2) a model is required to indicate how particular legislation works to achieve those interests. Without such a framework it is not always obvious how legislation promotes the interests of the health associations. The test of the validity of the proposed approach is how accurately the proposed framework predicts the political positions of the health associations. Finally, the implications of such a framework for explaining the political behavior of health associations with regard to the structure, organization, and financing of medical care will be presented.

SEVERAL CAVEATS

Before discussing the economic model of political behavior, however, it is important to clarify certain situations where the model would predict that an association would take a certain political position on legislation but we observe the association clearly taking a different position. One such situation sometimes occurs when we observe the current political position of an association. If the preferred position of the association is no longer politically possible, and other persons and organizations are proposing positions that are much more to the disadvantage of the association's members, then the current position taken by the association will be better than the alternatives being proposed by others. An example of a preferred and a current position is the American Hospital Association's position on cost containment for hospitals. As will be shown, hospitals do not want constraints on what they can charge or on how fast their costs can rise. The American Hospital Association's favorable attitude toward prospective reimbursement might be considered a rejection of the proposed framework; however, when one analyzes the current political climate of the government and the attitudes of others toward hospital cost control, it can be seen that more severe approaches are being suggested and are even being proposed in the form of legislation to place tighter constraints on hospitals. Thus, the American Hospital Association's willingness to accept some cost constraints is perfectly consistent with what the model would predict.

Another instance where the model would appear to be inaccurate, when in fact it is not, is when there has been a change in the perceived self-interest of the association's members. Such a change in self-interest would occur when the organization's very survival is threatened. An example of such a situation is Blue Cross's relationship to hospitals. Hospitals started Blue Cross to ensure payment for their services. In many cases hospitals provided initial capital for Blue Cross, controlled the board of directors, and until recently, owned the Blue Cross emblem. One would therefore expect Blue Cross's self-interest to be synonymous with that of hospitals. However, in the last several years Blue Cross has come under attack for not performing its intermediary function adequately. Blue Cross had not monitored hospital costs nor had it been an innovator in containing the rapid rise in hospital costs. Such behavior is not unexpected because hospitals controlled Blue Cross. But if Blue Cross is to survive in an increasingly competitive environment, it must be able to do more than merely reimburse hospitals. In order to create a new image for itself, and survive, Blue Cross has begun, at least in its public statements, to become an adversary of hospitals. Blue Cross's political positions have shifted in the last several years as it has had to redefine its self-interest in order to convince a skeptical group of government officials, legislators, unions, and industry that it can perform and should not be replaced either by a state rate review commission or by another insurance company. A similar situation has occurred with Blue Shield and its relationship to organized medicine.

There are two other minor instances where it may appear that the political positions of a health association diverge from the self-interest of its members. The first is when an association is fearful that its continually negative position on legislation may be of greater cost to its members than any possible benefits to be derived from opposing it. An example of such a situation is the American Hospital Association's position on applying the minimum wage law to hospital employees. For many years the AHA was successful in exempting hospitals from such legislation. More recently, however, it did not take a position when such legislation was once again being proposed to include hospital workers. One reason is that hospital workers were now being paid in excess of the minimum wage and so its effect would have been small. More importantly, however, the AHA could see that this time such legislation was going to pass and therefore it would be a needless loss of political capital to oppose the legislation.

The second example of an association not opposing legislation that is inimical to the interests of its members occurs when it decides to go along with the desires of other health associations in hopes of receiving their support for legislation which is of greater importance to its members' interests. Such trade-offs would not be a refutation of the model's prediction that health associations act in their members' interests regardless of the effect on the "public" interest.

DEFINITION OF HEALTH ASSOCIATION MEMBERS' SELF-INTEREST

Since the predictions made by the economic framework are based on the premise that the health association will demand legislation according to the self-interest of its members, it is necessary to more precisely define the self-interest of the different health associations to be analyzed. Whether legislation has a positive, negative, or a neutral effect on the association members' self-interest depends upon what the members perceive their interests to be.

When defining self-interest for a large number of health professionals such as physicians, dentists, and nurses, or for organizations that may be quite diverse even though they are considered to be one type of institution, such as hospitals, there is a natural tendency to make the definition complex so that it encompasses the diversity. If, however, the self interest goals are complex, or if new goals are specified for each separate piece of legislation, then it is not possible to develop a good predictive model. However satisfying a complex goal statement may be, it is easier to evaluate the effect of legislation using a relatively simply defined goal. Besides, unless the goal that the association is pursuing is easy for its membership to understand, the members may be distressed over the activities on which the association is spending their dues. The true test of whether the specified goal of the association is an accurate measure of the self-interest of its membership is how well the model is able to predict the legislative behavior of the association.

For each of the associations that have health professionals as members (AMA, ADA, and ANA), the legislative goals of the association are assumed to be to *maximize the incomes of its current members.* Health professionals have many goals, of which income is only one; however, income is the only goal that all the health professionals in an association have in common with one another. (Increased autonomy and control may be another goal, but they are highly correlated with increased incomes. Income is thus a more general goal.)

The goals or "self-interest" of the associations representing the nonprofit institutions (AHA, BCA, AAMC, and AADS) must differ from those of the health professional associations, since such organizations cannot retain any "profits." Hospitals and medical and dental schools are assumed to be interested in *maximizing their "prestige."* Prestige for hospitals is seen in terms of their size and the numbers and types of facilities and services. The availability of a full range of facilities and services also makes it easier for a hospital to attract physicians to its staff. Administrators of large prestigious hospitals are held in esteem by their peers and earn high incomes. Prestige for a medical school is usually defined as having students who wish to enter one of the specialties, most probably to become teachers and researchers themselves, a faculty that is primarily interested in research, and a low student-faculty ratio. Little prestige accrues to a medical school that trains students to enter general practice or practice in a rural area.

Blue Cross plans have a goal other than that of profit or prestige: it is assumed that Blue Cross seeks to *maximize its growth in enrollment and revenues.* A larger organization provides management with greater responsibility, which justifies greater management incomes. It is further assumed that prestigious hospitals and medical schools and large Blue Cross plans also have some form of satisficing behavior as a goal. For example, a Blue Cross plan with a high percent of the health insurance market in its area can afford to be less concerned with efficiency. In prestigious hospitals and medical schools, the return to efficiency similarly falls as the organization approximates its prestige goals.

Although there are differences in the objectives of the health associations, the members of these associations all try to make as much money as possible, either to retain it themselves, as in the case of health professionals, or to expend it to achieve either prestige or growth goals. Thus, the model of demand for legislation is the same for all health associations. Basically, each health association attempts to achieve for its members through legislation what cannot be achieved through a competitive market, namely, a monopoly position. Increased monopoly power and the ability to price as would a monopolist seller of services is the best way for them to achieve their goals.

Specifically, there are five types of legislation a health association will demand. Four of these legislative actions have the effect of increasing the association members' revenues, while the fifth should decrease the member's costs of operation. Legislation to increase revenues is legislation that 1) increases the demand for the members' services, 2) causes an increase in the price of services which substitute for those produced by the members, 3) limits entry into the industry, and 4) enables the providers to charge the highest possible price for their services, such as by preventing competition based on prices and by charging different prices according to the willingness to pay of different purchasers (i.e., price discrimination). Legislative policies which lower the provider's cost of operation are 1) subsidies to the inputs used in the production of the provider's services and 2) changes in the state practice acts which allow for greater productivity of the inputs used in production. Each of these legislative policies will be discussed in more detail, with illustrative examples of legislative behavior of the various health associations.

DEMAND-INCREASING LEGISLATION

An increase in demand along a given supply curve will result in an increase in price, an increase in total revenue, and, consequently, an increase in income or net revenue. The most obvious way of increasing the demand for the services of an association's members is to have the government subsidize the purchase of insurance for the provider's services. No health provider, however, wishes the government to insure all persons in the population, such as is done by the British National Health Service. Instead, the demand for insurance subsidies is always discussed in relation to specific population groups in society, namely, those persons with low incomes. The reason for selective government subsidies is twofold: first, those persons with higher incomes presumably have private insurance coverage or can afford to purchase the provider's services. The greatest increase in demand would result from extending coverage to those currently unable to pay for those services. Second, extending government subsidies to those currently able to pay for these services would greatly increase the cost of the program to the government. Greater commitment of government expenditures would result in greater government control over the provider's prices and utilization. Thus, for the purpose of increasing the demand for the provider's services, government subsidies are always requested in relation to specific population groups rather than for the population at large.* A related point is that

---

*Even when demand subsidies are requested for a particular population group, it is proposed that such demand subsidies be phased in gradually. If the increase in demand is too large, this might create dissatisfaction among the patients because of the limited supply; prices and waiting times would tend to increase rapidly, possibly resulting in pressure on the government to enter the market. If the increase in demand is large, it may result in pressure to cause a greater increase in the number of providers than the association believes is in the best economic interests of its members.

health associations always want an intermediary between the government and the provider of services. The reason is the fear that the government would otherwise interfere in the setting of prices.

Examples of such demand-increasing policies are the AMA's program for national health insurance, which proposes demand subsidies for low-income groups, and the ADA's program for national health insurance, which is also related to the incomes of the recipients. A further example of what is preferred by the health professional associations was the AMA's Blue Shield plan. The AMA initially started and controlled Blue Shield. Blue Shield provided coverage for physician services only and covered the patient's entire bill only if the patient's income was below a certain level. The physician was able to charge patients with higher incomes an amount above the Blue Shield fee. In this way the physician was able to price-discriminate, a factor which will be discussed in the following section.

The American Nurses' Association, whose members work for other providers, has favored demand-increasing proposals that increase the demand for those institutions in which registered nurses work. Increased demand for hospital care will result in increased demand for registered nurses (RNs). The ANA has also favored policies which would increase the demand for RNs directly, such as requiring increases in the use of RNs in hospitals and nursing homes. Another demand proposal favored by nurses is one which increases their role, i.e., increases the number of tasks that nurses are permitted to perform. If they are successful at this strategy, the demand for nurses will increase because their value has increased in that they can do more remunerative tasks. Nurses that can be used more flexibly than before can perform the tasks that might have required the hiring of two different types of health professionals. As nurses and other health professionals try to increase their roles, they also wage a struggle in the legislative marketplace to prevent other health professionals from competing with the nurse. Other examples are the attempts by optometrists to increase their role at the expense of ophthalmologists, podiatrists and orthopedic surgeons, and psychologists and psychiatrists. The health professional association that is successful in enabling its members to increase their role while preventing other health professionals from encroaching upon that role will assure an increased demand for its members' services and, consequently, higher incomes.

The major attempt made by the American Hospital Association to increase demand has been the establishment and control of the Blue Cross Association. In its establishment it was intended to pay for the costs of hospital care only, thereby lowering the costs of hospital care to consumers and increasing their demand for services. Blue Cross also assured that the hospitals would be paid for their services. The American Hospital Association also favored government subsidies for the aged under Medicare, which would have increased the demand for hospital care by a high user population with generally low incomes. The AHA also sought government payment for such services through an intermediary (their own Blue Cross Association) rather than directly from the government, which would have gotten the government more directly involved with the hospitals' charges for Medicare patients.

Blue Cross's legislative strategy with regard to demand-increasing proposals is to remain an intermediary under any national health insurance plan that may be passed. Therefore, its legislative proposal for national health insurance had been one which ensured a place for Blue Cross, and was not particularly concerned with any other specifics of the plan.

The Association of American Medical Colleges (AAMC)'s tactic to increase the demand for medical schools has been to demand legislation, at both a state and federal level, that would provide schools with unrestricted operating subsidies. Such subsidies would enable the schools to set tuition levels that are greatly below the actual costs of education. With artificially low tuition levels, the schools would experience an excess demand for their spaces by prospective applicants for a medical education. (The same is true for a dental education.) As long as there is an excess demand for a medical education—and the schools do not willingly expand their spaces to satisfy this excess demand—then the schools can determine the type of educational curriculum that comes closest to meeting their (and the AMA's or ADA's) preferences. If there were no excess demand for a medical education, then the schools would have to respond, as would any other supplier, by providing the type of product the demanders were willing to pay for. Under a demand-oriented system, the schools (and the health professional associations that originally controlled the schools) would not be able to determine the type of educational system in the United States. By retaining a monopoly over the provision of medical and dental education, and by charging tuition levels that are so low as to encourage excess demand for such an education, the schools can select the type of students they prefer from the excess of applicants and establish the training times and educational requirements for entering the profession.

SECURING THE METHOD OF HIGHEST REIMBURSEMENT

Whether the association members' goal is income, prestige, or growth, the method by which the provider is reimbursed is crucial to its attainment. High prices, netting larger revenues, increase incomes and facilitate the achievement of institutional objectives through the expenditure of those revenues. There are two basic approaches to being able to secure the highest possible reimbursement for services. The first is to charge different patients or payors different prices according to their ability to pay. This method of pricing (price discrimination) will result in greater revenues than will a system of charging all patients the same price. The second approach is to preclude price competition among competing providers. Essential to price competition is the provider's ability to advertise differences in prices and any other differences in service, such as availability and competency measures. Price competition is most important for the new practitioner or firm entering an area, who must let potential patients know they are available and be able to attract them away from established providers. To prevent such competition from occurring, health professional associations have included advertising and other forms of competition in their practice acts as reasons for suspending practitioners' licenses and for assessing penalties for "unethical behavior." Since such competitive behavior was not necessarily related to low quality, its inclusion as part of the unethical practices for which a practitioner can be penalized can only be interpreted as a means of preventing price competition among providers.

Physicians and dentists have a strong preference for "usual, customary and reasonable" (UCR) fees. Such a method of pricing essentially lets the providers charge what the market will bear. Patients with higher incomes (who would be willing to pay more) can thus be charged higher fees than those with lower incomes, as has been the case with the use of Blue Shield income limits. In his classic article, "Price Discrimination in Medicine" (6), Kessel describes how county and state medical societies attempted to forestall the development of prepaid group practices, which are a form of massive price cutting since they offer to provide medical services at the same price to all persons regardless of their income. More recently, Blue Shield in Spokane, Washington, boycotted physicians if they offered their services through a health maintenance organization. It ended its boycott only when ordered to do so by the Federal Trade Commission, acting on its belief that it was an anticompetitive tactic. Physicians want to be free to either accept or reject assignment on a case by case basis under Medicare and Blue Shield payment. By doing so, the physician is assured of payment from low-income persons while still able to charge a higher price to the higher-income patient. It is interesting to note that the method that is proposed for payment of providers under proposed legislation is often crucial to its acceptance by the provider association.

The fee-for-service approach, based on UCR fees, and used so successfully by the AMA, is being imitated by other health professional associations. Registered nurses are striving to become nurse practitioners who will be able to bill the patient directly under fee-for-service. The ANA has attempted to secure such an amendment to the Medicare law. Other health professionals have also tried to gain the authority to bill under fee-for-services. Fee-for-service, using UCR fees, which in most cases are reimbursed by the government or other third-party payor, is the most direct route for a health profession to increase its income.

The methods of reimbursement favored by the American Hospital Association for its members are ones which either discourage or do not provide consumers with any incentive to compare prices among different hospitals, and methods which enable the hospitals to charge different payors different prices for their services. When hospitals started the Blue Cross Association, Blue Cross plans were required to offer consumers a service benefit plan. A service benefit provides the hospitalized patient with services rather than dollars. In so doing, it actually provides the consumer with an incentive to enter the most expensive hospital, since the services at such a hospital, which are presumably of higher quality, will not cost the consumer anything extra. Thus, under a service benefit policy, hospitals cannot compete for patients on the basis of prices.

If hospitals are to be able to generate sufficient funds to expand their facilities and services, then they must be able to set prices in excess of their costs. The manner in which this is done is to charge different prices to different payors and to set prices for different services according to what the market will bear, i.e., according to price elasticity of demand. Hospitals thus prefer multiple sources of payment, rather than one major purchaser of their services, so that they can charge some payors higher prices for the same services. An example of this pricing behavior is to charge commercial insurers and patients responsible for their own bills higher rates than those charged to Blue Cross (which receives a discount) or to Medicare (which pays on the basis of ratio of charges to charges to cost). Another method by which the hospital is able to use price discrimination in its rate setting is to set higher price-cost ratios for those services where the demand is believed to be more price inelastic, such as ancillary services, than for services which are price elastic, such as obstetrics. That hospitals have used their pricing strategy to their benefit can be seen by the large increase in net revenues after Medicare was instituted. This resulted both from the favorable payment terms and from the inclusion in their reimbursement structure of previously unreimbursable expenses such as unfunded depreciation.

The use of community rating, which was originally used by Blue Cross as a means of setting premiums, may also be viewed as a method of price discrimination. Under community rating all groups are charged the same premium regardless of their utilization experience. High-user groups are thus subsidized by low-user groups. High-user groups were also, in many cases, groups of people with low incomes who could not afford to pay the higher premiums. This method of pricing resulted in the largest enrollment for Blue Cross.

Medical and dental schools, as stated earlier, would rather be reimbursed by the federal and state governments for their costs than charge the students the full costs. The government, for one reason, has a much greater ability to pay than does the individual student. Further, unrestricted operating subsidies allow the school to produce the type of education the faculty prefers without having to respond to the demands of students. That the schools have been relatively successful in charging the government a monopoly price for their services is an observation supported by data which indicate that public medical schools receiving state support have higher per student costs than private schools. Medical and dental schools are opposed to the government's providing those same subsidies directly to the student. If government subsidies went directly to the student, then the student would be able to select the school, and the schools would have to compete for students.

Under the current system of providing subsidies, the student can receive a subsidy only by attending a subsidized school. The current system guarantees the survival of the schools and requires the students, not the schools, to compete. Similar to their preference for receiving operating subsidies, the schools prefer to distribute loans and scholarships themselves rather than having the students apply directly to the government for such financial assistance.

When one observes the method of pricing used by health professionals and health institutions and the success those providers have had in increasing their revenues through those pricing methods, it is difficult to believe that the distinction between profit and nonprofit has any meaning with regard to which group can provide services at a lower price.

LEGISLATION TO REDUCE THE PRICE AND/OR INCREASE THE QUANTITY OF COMPLEMENTS

It is difficult in medical care to know when an input, such as a nurse, is a complement or a substitute based just on the task to be performed. A nurse may be as competent as a physician to perform certain tasks; if the nurse works for the physician, however, and the physician receives the fee for the performance of the task, then the nurse is a complement and will increase the physician's productivity. If, however, the nurse performs the same task and is a nurse practitioner operating and billing independently of the physician, then the nurse is a substitute for the physician in providing that service. The essential element in determining whether an input is a complement or a substitute is who controls the use of that input and who receives reimbursement for the services provided by that input.

The legal authority for the different tasks each health profession can perform and the source of stipulations defining under whose direction health professionals must work are the state practice acts. A major legislative activity for each health association is to seek changes in the state practice acts; health associations representing complements attempt to have their members become substitutes, while other health associations whose members currently control complements seek to retain the status quo. For the physician, almost all of the health professions and health institutions are complements; nurses and optometrists are examples of professionals who desire to expand their scope of practice and practice independently of physicians.

With an increase in the demand for health services, providers can increase their incomes if that increased demand is met through greater productivity on their part rather than through an increase in the number of competing providers. The provider's incomes can be increased still further if their productivity increases are subsidized and if they do not have to pay the full cost of increasing their productivity. Examples of legislation that would have the effect of subsidizing increased productivity are educational subsidies, capital subsidies, and changes in the state practice acts to permit greater delegation of tasks. The American Hospital Association, for example, favored the Nurse Training Act, in their belief that subsidizing the training of registered nurses would increase the supply of nurses. With a greater number of nurses, nurses' wages would be lower than they would otherwise have been. The AHA has favored both the Hill-Burton program, which provided capital subsidies to modernize hospitals, and educational subsidies to increase the supply of allied health professionals. The AHA has opposed legislative actions which would have increased the hospitals' costs of inputs. It opposed the extension of minimum wage legislation to hospital employees and has called for a moratorium on the separate licensing of each health professional. (Separate licensing of each health profession would limit the hospital's ability to substitute persons and to use such persons in a more flexible manner.)

The AMA has similarly favored both subsidies to hospitals, because hospitals are inputs to physicians, and increases in the supply of registered nurses under the Nurse Training Act. However, the AMA has opposed the increased educational standards that the ANA wanted to impose on nursing institutions as a condition for receiving funds under the Nurse Training Act. Higher educational standards for nurses do not necessarily increase the productivity of nurses, but they limit the supply of nurses and increase the nurse's qualifications as a substitute for the physician. The AMA has also favored internship and residency programs. Interns and residents are excellent complements to physicians, since they can take care of the physicians' hospitalized patients and also relieve the physician of serving in the hospital's emergency room or having to be on call at the hospital. For this reason the AMA has favored the use of foreign medical graduates to serve as interns and residents. Because interns and residents, once they have graduated, become substitutes for existing practitioners, the AMA has favored the return of foreign medical graduates to their home countries once their residencies are completed. To forestall competition from U.S. medical graduates, the AMA has always favored increased training times so that prospective physicians would serve a longer time as complements to practicing physicians.

An interesting example of the AMA's attitude toward a new complement is its position on the physician's assistant (PA). Physician's assistants are potential substitutes for the physician if they practice independently. Thus, the AMA wants to ensure that the fee from services rendered by the PA always goes to the physician. In fact, whether there is direct or indirect supervision of the PA is less important to the AMA in determining its political position toward this new category of health professionals than is who gets the fee. Another important characteristic of the AMA's attitude toward the use of PAs is whether or not the introduction of such personnel in an area will create excess capacity among physicians in the community, resulting in greater competition among them for patients. If the physician did not have sufficient demand to keep as busy as he would like, then the introduction of inputs that would increase the physician's productive capacity would be against the interest of those physicians who would like to be busier. However, as demand for physician (and dental) services increases, there will be a greater tendency to allow productivity increases to occur. Thus, physicians had to secure the permission of their local medical society on an individual basis whenever physician's assistants were to be used in an area. Regardless of the training of such personnel, if there was insufficient demand per physician in an area, it was unlikely that permission to use PAs would be granted.

Similarly, state practice acts were changed to permit greater delegation of tasks as demand for physicians or dentists increased. We would expect to find those state practice acts with the least delegatory authority in those states where there is the lowest level of demand per practitioner. The introduction of new types of health professionals and methods to increase productivity is more related to local demand conditions than to the competence of such personnel to perform the tasks for which they were trained.

The AAMC has been relatively successful in its demands for input subsidies. Medical schools have received subsidies for construction, for research (which has been used to subsidize teaching programs), for teaching hospitals, and for the cost of education. After years of receiving unrestricted subsidies, the schools had to provide for small enrollment increases to receive federal capitation grants. These programs have been phased out. The schools had, of course, opposed all conditions attached to receiving government subsidies. The subsidies received from the states, however, are unrestricted. It is not surprising that the schools have been more successful in their legislative efforts at a state level than at a federal level, where it is relatively easier for opponents to lobby against the schools with Congress.

Blue Cross's main political activity directed toward lowering the price of its inputs has been to favor the development and strengthening of hospital planning agencies. Because Blue Cross reimbursed hospitals according to their costs, hospitals had an incentive to add facilities and services and pass the costs of these additional services on to Blue Cross and its subscribers, who must then pay higher health insurance premiums. In a number of instances the addition of facilities and services, and even additional bed capacity, was duplicative in the community in which they were built. Hospitals compete among themselves for physicians and patients. (And since the hospitals were reimbursed on an individual cost basis and the patient had no incentive under a service benefit policy to select the lowest-cost hospitals, the process of adding duplicative beds and facilities could continue.) Blue Cross's premium consists almost entirely of the costs of hospital care. To remain competitive against commercial insurance companies whose premiums are comprised of a smaller portion of hospital care and whose policies may reimburse patients a fixed dollar amount rather than the complete costs of their hospitalization, it is in Blue Cross's interests to keep the cost of hospital care (both hospital use and the cost per unit) from rising.

Because of Blue Cross's traditional relationship with hospitals, it was difficult for Blue Cross to directly monitor hospital costs. An alternative, indirect approach to restraining the cost of the Blue Cross premium, and one which was *not* opposed by the major hospitals in Blue Cross's area, was to prevent the development of new hospitals and the expansion of beds and facilities in smaller existing hospitals. The existing large hospitals either had the latest facilities and services or were the likely candidates to receive the approval of the planning agency to add such facilities. As a means of restraining competition, these large hospitals favored the strengthening of planning agencies. Limiting the increase in hospital beds and the addition of services, whose costs Blue Cross had to pay even if they were duplicative, were expected to hold down both hospital utilization and Blue Cross's premiums. Although Blue Cross has been a strong advocate of limiting hospital utilization and duplicative facilities and services, its efforts to date have not been successful in limiting the rise in hospital costs. Although Blue Cross's competitive position has been eroding (the market share of non-Blue Cross carriers has been rising both in the Medicare and non-Medicare markets), Blue Cross has still been reluctant to directly approach the problem of rising hospital costs by aggressively monitoring utilization and to change the basis of hospital reimbursement.

LEGISLATION TO DECREASE THE AVAILABILITY AND/OR INCREASE THE PRICE OF SUBSTITUTES

Any health association will attempt to have the price of a service increased (or its availability decreased) that is considered to be a substitute for the services delivered by its members. If it is successful in doing so, then the demand for services provided by its members will be increased. Three general approaches are used in the legislative arena to accomplish these goals. The first is to have the substitute service declared illegal. If substitute health professionals are not permitted to practice, or if substitutes are severely restricted in the tasks they are legally permitted to perform, then there will be a shift in demand away from the substitute service. The second approach, usually employed when the first approach is unsuccessful, is to exclude the substitute service from coverage for payment by a third party, including any government health programs. This latter policy raises the price of the substitute to a person who is eligible to purchase that service under the third-party coverage. The last approach is to try to raise the costs of the substitute, thereby necessitating a higher price for the services if the substitute is to remain in business. Examples to illustrate the political behavior of health associations in each of these areas will be provided.

For many years the AMA regarded osteopaths as "cultists." It was considered "unethical" for physicians to teach in schools of osteopathy. Unable to prevent their licensure at a state level, however, the AMA attempted to deny osteopaths hospital privileges. A physician substitute is less than adequate if that substitute cannot provide a complete range of treatment. As osteopaths developed their own hospitals and educational institutions, the medical societies decided that the best approach to controlling this potential increase in the supply of physician substitutes was to merge with the osteopaths, make them physicians, and then eliminate any future increases in their supply. An example of this approach, which was used in California until it was overturned by the Supreme Court of the State of California, was to allow osteopaths to convert their D.O. degree to an M.D. degree on the basis of 12 Saturday refresher courses. (By 1966, 15 states had similar merger agreements between the medical and osteopathic societies.) After the merger between the two societies occurred in California, the Osteopathic Board of Examiners was no longer permitted to license osteopaths.

Optometrists and chiropractors are potential substitutes for ophthalmologists and family practitioners. One approach used by the AMA toward such substitutes has been to attempt to raise their price relative to that of physicians. Medicare, which reduces the price of physician services to the aged under Part B, has been the vehicle for much legislative competition. The AMA has opposed both optometrists and chiropractors from qualifying as providers under Part B, thereby effectively raising their price to the aged relative to that of physicians, whose services are reimbursable.

An example of the legislative behavior of dental societies toward substitute providers is illustrated by dentistry's actions toward denturists. Denturism is the term applied to the fitting and dispensing of dentures directly to patients by persons who are not licensed as dentists. Independently practicing denturists are a threat to dentists' incomes, since they offer to provide dentures at lower prices than do dentists. Dentists have, however, been successful in having denturism declared illegal. (Denturists are legal in seven out of Canada's 10 provinces. As a result of their success in Canada, denturists in the U.S. have become bolder by attempting to have certain state practice acts changed to permit them to practice.) Occasionally, denturists illegally sell dentures to patients. To combat this potential competition, local dental societies, such as in Texas, have responded in two ways: first, they offered to provide low-cost dentures to low-income persons; second, they pressured state officials to enforce the state laws against the illegal denturists.

A special ADA commission set up to study the threat of denturists reported that the number of persons who are edentulous is much greater in the lower income levels, and it is among these persons that the denturists have met with great success in selling low-cost dentures. An editorial commenting on this special study commission's report proposed that:

> Organized dentistry should set up some system for supplying low-cost dentures to the indigent or the near indigent all over the country, but especially in those states where the legislatures are considering bills that would allow dental mechanics to construct dentures and deliver them directly to the patient . . . this is the type of program that would have a favorable impact on the public—not to mention legislators . . . .The supplying of dentures to low income patients by qualified dentists at a modest fee (or even at no fee in special cases) and in quantities meeting the public demands would go a long way toward heading off the movement for legalized denturists. (7)

It is only the threat of competition that results in the dental profession's offer to provide low-cost dentures to the indigent or near-indigent. If this competitive threat by denturists is eliminated through dentistry's successful use of the state's legal authority, the net effect will be to cause the public to pay higher prices for dentures.

One of the most important substitutes for registered nurses training in this country is the foreign-trained RN. Because nursing salaries are considerably higher in the United States than in many other countries, there is a financial incentive for foreign nurses to come to the United States. The manner in which the American Nurses' Association has tried to decrease the availability of a low-cost substitute for nurses trained in the United States has been to make it more difficult for the foreign nurse to enter the United States. The ANA has attempted to have the Department of Labor remove the preferential status of foreign nurses from the immigration regulations. The ANA has also proposed that foreign nurses who wish to enter the United States be screened by examination in their home country before being allowed to enter. The ANA's advocacy of screening prior to admittance to the United States, where they would be screened again by having to pass state board exams, is consistent with a policy of reducing the inflow of foreign nurses. If the screening exam were administered in the United States, then foreign nurses could still work in some nursing capacity even if they did not pass the exam, and then retake it in the future. Establishing an additional screening mechanism before nurses emigrate erects another barrier to nurses' entering the United States; if they do not pass the exam, they are unlikely to emigrate.

There are two additional legislative approaches that the ANA has used to raise the cost of substitutes for RNs. The first is to favor increases in the wages of other health professionals. A great deal of substitution of licensed practical nurses for RNs has occurred. The greater the wage increases of RN substitutes, the less likely it is that there will be substitution away from the RN because of increasing disparity between the wages of RNs and other health personnel. The second legislative tactic used by the ANA is to prevent other personnel from undertaking nursing tasks performed by RNs. The ANA has opposed policies which would have permitted physicians to have greater delegatory authority over which personnel can perform nursing tasks; the ANA has opposed permitting licensed practical nurses to be in charge of skilled nursing homes, since this would cause substitution away from RNs who currently perform such functions; the California Nurses' Association opposed a bill that would have authorized firemen with paramedic training to give medical and nursing care in hospital emergency departments; and the ANA, as a means of preventing physician's assistants from moving into a role which the ANA would like to see reserved for RNs, has favored a licensing moratorium. Such a moratorium would prevent any new health personnel from being licensed to undertake tasks that RNs perform or would like to be permitted to perform.

Two examples of the approach used by the AHA to raise the price of substitutes has been to oppose free-standing surgicenters and to attempt to raise the relative price of for-profit hospitals to patients. Surgicenters are outpatient surgical facilities and therefore low-cost substitutes for hospitals. Any increase in the use of surgicenters will decrease the demand for inpatient care. In order to limit the availability of such low-cost substitutes, hospitals have argued that surgicenters should be permitted only when they are developed *in association* with hospitals. In this manner hospitals would be able to control the growth of a competitive source of care, and they would be able to benefit (since presumably they would operate the substitute service) as such surgicenters develop. Hospitals have also favored including surgicenters under certificate-of-need legislation. If such substitutes were subject to the approval of planning agencies, which are heavily influenced by the hospitals in the community, then it is unlikely that a low-cost substitute would be permitted to develop. The existing hospitals would claim that the growth of these institutions would leave them with excess inpatient surgical facilities, which, under cost-based reimbursement, the community (through Blue Cross) would have to pay for anyway.

Methods used by nonprofit hospitals to raise the cost of a substitute are to oppose the granting of tax-exempt status to for-profit hospitals, thereby raising their costs, and to oppose granting Blue Cross eligibility to for-profit hospitals, or even to new nonprofit hospitals, when the existing nonprofit hospitals claim that there are sufficient beds in an area. Denying third-party reimbursement to potential or actual competitors in effect precludes the use of the facilities by patients whose costs of hospitalization would be reimbursed if they entered a hospital that was eligible for Blue Cross reimbursement.

The political position of Blue Cross with respect to substitutes is similar. Blue Cross would favor having the Social Security Administration excluded, by law, from being able to compete with the Blues as an intermediary under any government payment program. Further, Blue Cross opposes granting to commercial insurers the same tax-exempt status that Blue Cross plans enjoy, which causes their competitors' costs to be increased.

The substitute sources for the American medical and dental educational system are foreign schools whose graduates then immigrate to the United States. To reduce the likelihood of foreign medical schools' substituting for U.S. medical schools, the AAMC has favored strong restrictions on the number of foreign medical graduates who can enter the United States, thereby reducing the attractiveness of a foreign medical education. The ADA and the AADS have similarly attempted to reduce the attractiveness of foreign dental education as a substitute for U.S. dental schools by increasing the requirements of a dentist who has received a foreign dental education. Not only are the time requirements of foreign-trained dentists increased, but additional requirements are then imposed upon these same persons once they enter the United States. To date, such restrictive practices in dentistry have been successful: as of 1973 less than 1,000 foreign-trained dentists (less than 1 percent of all practicing dentists) were estimated to be practicing in the United States.

LEGISLATION TO LIMIT INCREASES IN SUPPLY

Essential to the establishment of a monopoly position are limits on the number of providers of a service. The justification given by health associations for supply-control policies is that they ensure high-quality care to patients. At the same time, however, these same health associations oppose quality measures that would have an adverse economic effect upon existing providers. This apparent anomaly—stringent entry requirements and then virtually no quality-assurance programs directed at existing providers—can be consistent only with a policy that seeks to establish a monopoly position for existing providers. If the health associations were consistent in their desire to improve and maintain high quality standards, then they should favor all policies which ensure quality. Quality control measures directed at existing providers, such as reexamination, relicensure, and monitoring of the care actually provided, would adversely affect the incomes of some providers; more importantly, such "outcome" measures of quality assurance would make the entry or "process" measures unnecessary, and thereby permit larger numbers of providers into the industry.

A test of the hypothesis that entry barriers are primarily directed toward developing a monopoly position rather than improving quality of care would be to determine the position of the particular health association on any quality measure that would have an adverse effect on its members' incomes. If the health association were truly interested in quality, it should favor all quality measures, even those that would have an adverse effect on some of its members. It is virtually impossible to find instances where a health association has favored such measures. On the other hand, if the health association only favors those quality measures that have a favorable impact on its members' economic position, then it can be concluded that the real intent of those quality measures is the improvement of the competitive position of its members rather than the assurance of quality of care in the most efficient manner.

The following examples illustrate measures to assure quality that are in the interests of the members of health association and those that are not and are therefore opposed by the association.

The health professions are always in favor of licensing. The profession ends up controlling the licensure process by setting the necessary requirements for licensure and having members of the profession itself comprise the licensing board. Once licensing requirements have been legislated at a state level, the profession, through its representatives on the licensing board, imposes additional requirements. The major requirement is that before any person can take a licensing examination, he or she must have had a specified education, usually of a minimum number of years (which keeps increasing), and this education must have taken place in an educational institution approved by the profession or its representatives. The number of educational institutions is always limited so that, as in medicine and dentistry, there is continually an excess demand by applicants for admission. Limiting the number of educational spaces, and specifying an educational curriculum that imposes training requirements in excess of the skills required to practice in the profession, reduces the number of persons who can take the licensing examination. If the licensure requirement just specified passing an examination, then potential practitioners could secure the necessary knowledge in a number of different ways, in different lengths of time, and in different institutions. In such a situation, the number of persons who could potentially take the exam and pass it would be much greater than if the number of those applying to take the exam were limited by the number of approved educational spaces.

The foregoing policies have been successfully developed in medicine and dentistry. Nursing is also moving in this direction through attempts to require that nursing education take place only in colleges that offer a baccalaureate degree. Previously, the predominant place of education for a nursing degree was in a diploma school, generally operated in conjunction with a hospital. By proposing that the educational requirement for nursing be increased, the ANA must be well aware that fewer nurses will be trained, since the costs of training have increased (and persons trained for a baccalaureate degree might decide to receive training for a profession other than nursing). The ANA also must be aware that with the additional training it would presumably be easier to justify having nurses perform additional tasks, thereby increasing nurses' incomes.

It is interesting to note that no health profession favors methods that would reduce the time required to prepare a person to enter the profession. Further, no health profession favors establishing additional training requirements for its existing members, even though additional requirements are continuously being imposed on new entrants to the profession. No health profession favors relicensure or reexamination requirements for its current membership. The reason for opposing them is that it would lower the incomes of their membership if they had to take additional training or if they could not pass reexamination. Favoring additional requirements just for new members, without permitting those new members to advertise their increased competence, provides a windfall to the current membership. The public is led to believe that all persons in a profession are equally (or at least minimally) qualified when this may no longer be the case, particularly for those practitioners who were trained 30 years ago and have not maintained their knowledge. If the members of a profession are concerned with quality, then they should favor the maintenance of quality among themselves, yet they have opposed any attempt to review their performance. Health professional associations that have proposed continuing education for their members have done so in response to demands by those *outside* the profession for stronger continuing education requirements. The continuing education requirements are always relatively easy to achieve, at low cost to the members of the profession. Also, the profession never proposes using continuing education as a prerequisite for reexamination.

At times the profession imposes requirements on new entrants into the profession that are blatantly barriers to entry. Examples of such requirements are U.S. citizenship for foreign medical and dental graduates in order to practice in some states and a one-year residency requirement if a duly trained and licensed professional, such as a dentist, wishes to practice in another state, such as Hawaii. Such requirements cannot be remotely related to a concern for quality. The current method of quality assurance for health professionals is aimed solely at entry into the profession rather than at monitoring the quality of care practiced by the professionals. The inadequate performance of state licensing boards in disciplining their members is evidence of this practice. The public is less protected against unethical and incompetent practitioners than it has been led to believe.

Hospitals, medical and dental schools, and Blue Cross plans are also advocates of supply-control policies, since they provide these institutions with a monopoly position in their market. Since such institutions cannot achieve a monopoly position through the normal competition of the marketplace, they seek to achieve it through legislation. Large hospitals favor certificate-of-need (CON) legislation. CON agencies, which are likely to be controlled by the administration of the large existing hospitals, will use legislative authority to limit the growth of potential competitors in their areas. With fewer providers in a community, patients will have less choice among providers, and the existing providers will more easily be able to increase their costs and prices. The survival of existing hospitals will also be assured, since competing hospitals will have been excluded. Larger hospitals are likely to be favored over smaller hospitals in their requests for the addition of new specialized facilities. Because many specialized facilities are useful to a limited number of patients in the community, it is likely that the larger hospital will be able to justify having the facility more easily than a smaller institution; also, larger hospitals are more likely to have complementary facilities that may be required for new specialized services. CON legislation does not control the increase in hospital costs; it merely restricts expansion and additions to capacity and facilities. If another mechanism to control the large annual increases in hospital costs must be found, why not use this mechanism to determine which hospital is more efficient and has the demand that would warrant adding beds and new facilities?

The supply-restriction policies favored by medical and dental schools have specified uniformly high educational standards for a professional education and eliminated any incentives for such schools to compete among themselves for students. Eliminating for-profit medical and dental schools emphasizes prestige as the basis for competition. As a result of the Flexner Report (Gies report for dental education in 1926), beginning in 1910 the number of medical (and dental) schools was drastically reduced, curriculums standardized, and educational requirements lengthened. The number of schools was reduced, as was the incentive to compete for students on the basis of costs. More recently there have been pressures for expansion in medical and dental education. In order to continue receiving large government subsidies, the schools have been required to increase their enrollments. As a means of forestalling the growth of new, competing schools, the AAMC has proposed that new schools be located in areas that did not always have a medical or dental school to supply their needs. If schools were established in areas that already had schools, competition would develop to attract students from within the area and for receiving funds from the legislature.

Blue Cross plans do not compete with one another. The manner in which Blue Cross plans are set up in an area (they must sign up 75 percent of the hospitals and beds) generally precludes more than one plan from being established. Since no other health insurance plan offered a service benefit policy for hospitalization, each Blue Cross plan in an area had a virtual monopoly over the type of product it was selling. Even though the criteria for awarding the Blue

Cross emblem enabled each plan to be a monopolist, the plans were not able to preclude the development of close substitutes such as commercial insurance companies.

CONCLUDING COMMENTS

Because the separate members of each of the health associations cannot achieve a monopoly position through the normal competitive process, they seek to achieve it through legislation. They then attempt to improve their monopoly position by further demanding legislation that will increase the demand for their services, permit them to price as would a price-discriminating monopolist, lower their costs of doing business, and disadvantage their competitors either by causing them to become illegal providers or by raising their prices. Health associations have been relatively successful in the legislative arena, as is indicated by the large sums of money being spent on their services and by their members' position in society's income distribution. What are the "costs" or implications to the rest of society of the success of these interest groups in the legislative marketplace?

IMPLICATIONS OF THE POLITICAL ECONOMY MODEL

The more successful health associations are in enabling their members to achieve their goals, the higher will be the price of their members' services. The greater the price competition between members of different health associations, the lower the prices of both groups will be. State dental societies' establishment of low-cost denture clinics to compete with denturists is an example. When the competition is reduced, as is the case when the state dental societies apply pressure to have the laws against denturists enforced, the price of dentures will once again increase. Allowing surgicenters to compete with hospitals will lower the cost to the patient for minor surgical procedures, but once hospitals are able to control the number of such centers and require them to be associated with hospitals, the competition will decline and the price will likely increase. Other successful tactics used by health associations to prevent price competition among their members have included prohibiting advertising, limiting productivity increases, and establishing relative value scales (which the Federal Trade Commission believes has enabled the profession to engage in price fixing). The beneficiaries of policies to increase prices are, of course, the health professionals themselves. These higher prices are borne by patients and taxpayers who finance government health programs.

The second implication of successful legislative behavior by health associations is that the public is provided with a false assurance with respect to the quality of the medical care it receives. The state has delegated its responsibility for protecting the public to the individual licensing boards which are controlled and operated in the interests of the providers themselves. The approach toward quality assurance is not necessarily the least costly or most efficient, nor is it concerned with unethical or incompetent providers. That state licensing boards rarely take disciplinary action against their members has resulted in pressure by outsiders to establish Professional Standard Review Organizations (PSROs) to improve the quality of care being delivered. The effect of granting control over quality to providers has increased the costs of their services and has still not resolved the original problem of protecting the populace from incompetent or unethical providers, e.g., those who perform unnecessary surgery. The patients are not as well protected as they have been led to believe.

Finally, the creation of legislative monopolies has inhibited innovation in the delivery of medical care. Innovation provides greater choice to consumers, higher quality, and lower costs. Innovation, however, threatens the monopoly position of the separate provider groups. In protecting fee-for-service health care delivery, the AMA has retarded the development of prepaid group practices and health maintenance organizations. The AMA and ADA have inhibited the development of new types of health personnel, such as physician's assistants and expanded-function auxiliaries, because they might become potential substitutes. The AHA has sought, through certificate-of-need legislation, to stifle the growth of free-standing surgicenters. It was only through the competition of commercial insurance companies that major medical insurance was developed.

THE OUTLOOK FOR LEGISLATIVE CHANGE IN MEDICAL CARE

The incentive and reason for the legislative success of health associations is that the benefits to their members are greater than the costs imposed on individual consumers. Proposed legislative changes that would remove the monopoly protection that members of health associations currently enjoy would be difficult to achieve. Because the members of the health associations have more to lose than the individual has to gain from such legislative changes, they will be more involved in trying to prevent such legislative changes.

Are there alternative approaches to structural change in the delivery system that will achieve the twin goals of quality assurance and minimum cost? One proposal that has been suggested is to place consumers on the boards of health institutions and on licensing boards. I believe this to be a false panacea. Even assuming that consumer representatives would know the most efficient manner of structuring the delivery system (which is unlikely), it is improbable that they would be effective. Consumers are currently represented on all the boards mentioned. To date the consumers have not been able to make Blue Cross plans more aggressive in their monitoring of hospital costs, they have not been able to deter their hospitals from establishing duplicative facilities and services, nor have they moved licensing boards to become more active in disciplining their errant members. Consumers are usually nominated by the professions or administrators of the institutions themselves, and it is far easier to remove a particular board member than for a particular board member to change the performance of the profession. Consumers also do not have all the necessary information; they must rely on the professionals and administrators themselves for the appropriate information. Thus it is difficult to conclude that improved performance of an institution or of a profession will be in proportion to the number of consumers on their boards.

Another approach that has been suggested to improve the performance of the delivery system is to have greater government intervention and regulation of the industry or profession. When one examines the performance of regulatory agencies in other fields, it can be observed that these agencies rarely perform in the consumer's interests. Such agencies either are captured by the industries they are meant to regulate or they respond in a manner that seeks to minimize outside conflict. There is no reason to believe that health care regulatory agencies would perform any differently. A growing body of evidence with regard to CON agencies and state agencies responsible for regulating nursing homes has not produced the hoped-for accomplishments. It is unlikely that additional government regulation would succeed any better.

Certain other developments may have some beneficial effects in the legislative marketplace. The first of these is the involvement of a greater number of interest groups in the legislative process. The success of the AMA and the ADA has not gone unnoticed by other health professional associations. Greater competition among health associations in the legislative process is occurring. As more health associations attempt to increase the benefits to their members through changes in the various state practice acts, the cost to the AMA and ADA of preventing such changes increases. The possible gains to these other health associations from becoming substitutes for, rather than complements to, the physician and dentist are very large. They are becoming more willing to assess their members the necessary costs to compete for legislative changes.

Other interest groups that are becoming more active are industry, unions, and the states themselves. As the costs of health care continue to rise at a rapid rate, such costs, when embodied in wage agreements as fringe benefits, are passed on to the worker in terms of lower wages (since the cost of his fringes have increased), and in terms of higher prices to the consumer for manufactured goods (as the wage costs of producing these goods and services have increased). Unions, to receive higher wages for their members, and industry, so as not to have to raise the prices of its products, have become more concerned with the rise in costs of medical services. In the past, certain large unions attempted to resolve this problem by proposing to shift the costs of medical care to the federal government through national health insurance. It is increasingly being recognized, however, that the costs of health care cannot be completely shifted to other taxpayers and that a significant part of that cost will be borne by industry and labor (ultimately, by consumers) through various payroll taxes. Because both industry and labor are affected by the rise in medical costs, and because the costs to each of them of gathering the necessary information and participating in the legislative process are much less than the possible benefits if they are successful in reducing the rise in medical costs, we would expect them to become more active participants in the legislative process.

A number of large states have been greatly affected by their share of the cost of administering the Medicaid program. The annual cost to certain states for Medicaid is in excess of one billion dollars. These funds are no longer available to meet the demands of other interest groups within a state, and to continue paying such large amounts of money each year may necessitate increases in the state income tax. If these states cannot shift this burden to the federal government, they will become very interested in making legislative changes that will ease their burden.

It is possible that because of the rise of new health interest groups, industry, unions, and the states themselves, there will be greatly increased competition in the legislative process. As a result of this competition, more information will be provided by the different interest groups regarding the cost, quality, and efficiency of different systems of delivery for medical services. It is thus more likely that changes in the state practice acts and in the delivery system will be possible in the future.

A second development related to the foregoing is the role of the government in quality assurance. As more information has become available on the poor performance of health associations in monitoring (through their licensing boards) the quality of care practiced by their members, the government has become more involved. An example of this involvement is PSRO legislation. At a state level it is likely that there will be changes in the state's role in assurance of quality of care. As different health associations seek to become licensed and establish their own licensing boards, there is an awakening interest in preventing this proliferation, which would create an inflexible system to decide which persons can perform specific tasks. Some states are moving in the direction of *combining* licensing boards, with a number of different provider groups having representation on those boards. It is possible that such licensing boards would allow greater delegation of tasks and would also become more flexible in the prerequisites for licensure. It is hoped that such boards would begin to monitor the quality of care practiced.

In the past the states have delegated their responsibility for protecting the public from unqualified practitioners to the separate health professions. The states should not be allowed to abrogate their responsibilities in this manner. The state agency responsible for this function should be required to develop performance measures to determine how well it performs its monitoring function. Further, the legislature should hold annual oversight hearings on the performance of the responsible state agency. If this were to occur, interested persons, as well as organized interest groups, would be able to participate (at a low cost) in the process of structuring the delivery system and in quality assurance. To further ensure that the responsible state agencies perform their tasks of quality assurance, patients and consumers should have recourse to the courts. Greater publicity and accountability in the area of quality assurance should permit changes and innovations in the delivery system which have in the past been inhibited by health associations whose members' monopoly position would have been adversely affected.

REFERENCES

1. This chapter is based upon Paul J. Feldstein, *Health Associations and the Demand for Legislation: The Political Economy of Health* (Lexington, Mass.: Ballinger Publishing Co., 1977). Included in the book are additional examples, references, and more extensive discussion of the topics covered in this chapter. In 1975, the Federal Trade Commission (FTC) charged that the American Medical Association (AMA), the Connecticut State Medical Society, and the New Haven County Medical Association restricted the

ability of their members to advertise. The AMA claimed that since they were a not-for-profit organization, the FTC did not have jurisdiction over them. The approach used in this chapter and in the above book, with its applications to the AMA, was the basis for testimony by the author to demonstrate that the AMA acted in the economic interests of its members. The administrative law judge found in favor of the FTC on both the advertising and jurisdictional issues. These decisions were upheld on appeal and in 1982 the Supreme Court, by a tie vote, upheld the lower court rulings.

2. Paul J. Feldstein, "A Preliminary Evaluation of Federal Dental Manpower Subsidy Programs," *Inquiry*.

3. See Chapter 16, "The Market for Registered Nurses."

4. See the references in Chapter 11, this volume, on the economic theory of regulation.

5. James Madison, *Federalist No. 10*, 1787.

6. Reuben Kessel, "Price Discrimination in Medicine," *Journal of Law and Economics,* October 1958.

7. "Action Urgently Needed on 'Denturist' Movement," editorial, *JADA* 92 (1976):665.

CHAPTER 19

The Role of Government in Health and Medical Care

The involvement of government in the health and medical sector in the United States has been increasing very rapidly. Federal government expenditures for personal medical services have risen sharply since the passage of Medicare and Medicaid in the mid-1960s. Various levels of government are also suppliers of medical services: the Veterans Administration's system of hospitals, and medical services supplied to military dependents in military facilities under the auspices of the Department of Defense. Different levels of government also provide indirect subsidies for medical services in the form of subsidies for medical research, for hospital construction (under the Hill-Burton Act), and for health manpower under federally supported programs, and subsidies by states for health professional education. At least as important as this financial involvement of government in medical services is the less obvious role of government in setting the rules under which medical services are paid for, organized, and provided, and the protection it provides to patients through mechanisms such as licensing. Although government has long been involved in establishing the rules of the game for medical care, it is its relatively recent and more obvious role in financing medical care that has generated more debate, particularly with regard to financing national health insurance.

Some people view this increasing involvement of government in the medical sector as inevitable and beneficial; to others it is improper and the cause of inefficiencies. To clarify the debate over the increasing involvement of government in medical care, it is useful to review the traditional criteria for the role of government in a market system and to apply these criteria to medical care. Differences in opinion over the role of government in medical care can then be separated into differences regarding 1) whether the traditional criteria for government involvement are appropriate, and 2) given the appropriateness of the criteria, whether such criteria warrant government involvement in medical care. The first set of differences involve value judgments over the role of government. The sooner these differences are recognized as such, the sooner the participants will be able to focus the debate on whether there are more appropriate alternatives to the traditional criteria for government involvement. Given a set of criteria for government involvement, whether or not government involvement is warranted is more easily resolved because the existence of certain situations in medical care can be empirically determined. The evaluation of government programs in medical care, therefore, depends both upon appropriate criteria for government involvement and upon the applicability of such criteria to medical care.

There are two traditional areas where government is acknowledged to have a role in a market-oriented system. Each of these areas will be briefly discussed.

MARKET IMPERFECTIONS

In a competitive market system, economic efficiency on the demand and on the supply side typically cannot be achieved when the assumptions underlying competitive markets are violated. The most important assumptions that are not fulfilled in medical care are that consumers have perfect information, that there is complete mobility of resources,* and that patients and providers have an incentive to minimize their costs of purchasing and providing medical treatment. Although advertising has recently been permitted, consumers still lack information concerning their medical diagnosis, treatment needs, the quality of different providers, and the prices charged by different providers. Barriers to mobility of resources exist in restrictions placed on the tasks that various personnel are permitted to perform, entry into health manpower professions, and entry by institutions into various institutional markets. The incentives of patients and providers to be concerned with the costs of medical care have been reduced by the purchase of excess insurance coverage resulting from the tax deductibility of health insurance premiums, the purchase of insurance by employers as a nontaxable fringe benefit to their employees, and the reliance on cost-based reimbursement to providers by third-party payors, including government.

The effect of a lack of price information is empirically evidenced by the wide dispersion of prices for a given service and the significantly lower prices in states which permit advertising. The patients' ignorance as to their medical need, diagnosis, treatment requirements, and the quality of the provider gives rise to a situation where physicians, it is generally believed, can create their own demand; studies show different surgery rates for similar patient populations depending upon the method of physician reimbursement. Attempts to provide

---

*Another imperfection would be with respect to the capital markets. If full-cost tuition were charged to medical students, then students would not be able to borrow from banks based just upon their prospective earnings and without collateral. This type of market imperfection exists for all forms of higher education and is not peculiar to just medical or dental education. At present, however, other market imperfections in the health education market, such as barriers to entry, are of greater overriding concern, since they prevent full-cost tuition from being instituted.

more information to the patient in this regard have been made by having patients receive second opinions before undergoing surgery.

Examples of the widespread existence of barriers in medical delivery are the continual excess of demands by applicants for a medical (and dental) education, continually high rates of return to the medical profession with relatively little entry into the profession, and the willingness of prospective students to bear higher costs and study for a longer period of time overseas in order to practice as physicians in the United States. In the institutional sector, lack of consumer information and barriers to entry result in prices' exceeding average costs. For example, Blue Cross was able to use a community rating scheme for many years to price its hospital coverage; currently, a number of plans still use a modified form of that method, called merit rating. Hospitals are able to price their services so as to cross-subsidize different services and patients. Their ability to price according to the patient's elasticity of demand (as does the physician) is indicative of a lack of price competition. Excess insurance for patients and cost-based reimbursement to providers have resulted in inappropriate utilization and a concern for efficiency, excessive duplication of facilities, and rapidly rising medical costs.

The effect of barriers to entry and the lack of price competition is that the price patients pay for medical care does not reflect their marginal valuation of using those services. Utilization of medical services by patients when insurance is subsidized (either by the government or through tax deductions) exceeds what they would be willing to pay for that care if they had to pay the full price. Similarly, the price that is paid for medical care by third-party payors, the government, and patients (both through their out-of-pocket expenditures and through their taxes) exceeds the minimum costs of providing that care (and it is believed that the level of quality is greater than what patients would be willing to pay for if they were required to pay the full costs of that care).

Thus, it is apparent that there are imperfections in the market for medical services. Many have been created by the government. To discuss the appropriate role of government in the face of these imperfections, it is first necessary to explain why these imperfections were originally instituted. The *ostensible* reason for placing restrictions on entry, information, and price competition was to provide consumer protection. Given the technical nature of medical services and the potential harm that may be inflicted upon an uninformed patient by an incompetent provider, the government, working through the health professions and health institutions, placed its emphasis for consumer protection on nonprofit providers. Training requirements in nonprofit institutions were specified; licensure, which was to be carried out by the health professions, placed strong restrictions on who was permitted to practice and was responsible for performing medical services; information on prices, quality, and accessibility was prohibited to prevent unethical providers from misleading the sick. Thus, the very imperfections that prevent the medical sector from performing more efficiently were instituted under government auspices.

How can the demand for consumer protection* be satisfied while eliminat-

*A demand for consumer protection might be considered an externality; namely, if the government or some agency were to insure that all providers are competent, then all consumers would benefit from the lower risks and lower search costs when seeking a provider. The reason for including a discussion of consumer protection in this section rather than in the following one, which discusses externalities, is

ing those imperfections that result in inefficiencies in the medical sector? There are several possible policy prescriptions that would remove the imperfections and improve the efficiency of the medical sector. On one hand, the government could eliminate the barriers that limit entry into the health profession. This approach would rely on the development of private mechanisms, such as malpractice and improved consumer choice, to insure that the goals of consumer protection are achieved. Alternatively, the government could retain the responsibility for consumer protection, not delegate it to professional associations, and eliminate the market imperfections that would no longer occur once competence and quality were monitored directly by the government. An example of this latter approach would be for the government to annually license institutions rather than individuals for delivery of medical services. The cost of monitoring quality of care would be lower when institutions rather than individual practitioners were periodically examined.

If, in fact, the above barriers were meant to insure quality of care, then this goal could be achieved more directly and more efficiently by an approach that actually monitored the quality of care provided. It would no longer be necessary to rely solely on the proxy methods to accomplish this goal.

Eliminating the foregoing imperfections would enable the market mechanism to allocate medical resources efficiently. Providing government subsidies to alleviate the consequences of such imperfections, rather than eliminating the imperfections themselves, cannot be justified on theoretical grounds. If entry and practice barriers limit the availability of medical care by increasing its price, then a system of government construction or manpower subsidies, which have as their stated goal an increase in availability of medical resources, cannot be justified on grounds of economic efficiency. Such subsidies merely mask the effects of the market imperfections. These subsidies would have to be justified on grounds other than as a means of improving market efficiency. The appropriate role of government when faced with imperfections in the marketplace should be to eliminate restrictive practices and directly address the need the restrictions were ostensibly imposed to meet (i.e., consumer protection). Government subsidies cannot be justified as a means of improving market efficiency when there are imperfections of the type discussed.

Many people, however, oppose the elimination of restrictions on information and on medical practice. The elimination of market imperfections would not be, in their opinion, an improvement over the current system. Such persons oppose a market approach for determining the quantity and quality of medical care to be provided and the most efficient method for delivery of such care. Their opposition to competition under a market approach is not based on grounds of greater economic efficiency, but instead is a result of a value judgment that such criteria are inappropriate in medical care. Patients, in their opinion, do not have sufficient information, nor are they rational enough to competently choose the appropriate providers and the correct amount of medical care when they are ill. Indeed, they feel, such a decision should not involve the consumer at all but

---

that whether or not externalities are in fact the real reason for the market imperfections mentioned, the proposed policy prescriptions are similar to what would be the situation if such imperfections were simply a result of monopoly behavior on the part of the providers.

should be professionally determined; the professional determination, or allocation, of medical care should be based on medical need and not on consumer choice.

One of the criteria for economic efficiency in the demand for a service is that consumers will use a service until the price they pay for the last unit purchased equals the additional value they receive from it. When the marginal utility of the last unit consumed equals the price paid, the consumers are maximizing their utility. Since the price they must pay represents foregone utility that could be received from other goods and services, consumers adjust their utilization when prices change so that the marginal value of their last unit equals the new price. Consumers use different quantities of services, even though they face the same prices, because the marginal utilities to them of additional units differ. Each consumer, however, is matching the marginal utility of that last unit to the foregone utility of other goods and services. Further, when the consumer is the sole beneficiary of his or her purchases, then it is said that his or her marginal private benefit is equivalent to marginal social benefit.

If consumers are not assumed to be rational, or if persons do not believe that consumer choice should prevail, then the traditional demand curve does not represent marginal social utility. Under such circumstances, traditional economic policy, which favors removing imperfections in order to satisfy consumer wants, will not achieve the goals of those persons who do not believe in consumer choice and sovereignty in determining the amount of medical care to be provided.

What criteria do those who oppose consumer sovereignty in medical care suggest for determining the quantity of medical care in society? Determination of need or establishment of health priorities for consumers, which they favor, is difficult to operationalize. Government bureaus would presumably be required to establish resource levels. The criteria such agencies would use for the marginal value placed on allocating more resources to permit greater utilization, or for reducing need by a given percentage, have not been developed. Nor would everyone agree that a person should not be allowed to consume something that he or she is willing to pay for (as long as it does not have any negative effects on other persons). Based on their valuation of their own time, some people may prefer to pay a higher price rather than wait longer for the receipt of a service. Substituting collective judgment for an individual judgment to determine how much medical care is to be available represents a difference in values and is unrelated to whether a market system will be more efficient than an alternative system for achieving the same set of values.

This difference in values regarding whose satisfaction is to be achieved is also often reflected in the opposition by these same persons to use of competition on the supply side. Competition in supply among provider groups is based upon the assumption that to survive and grow, suppliers will compete for consumers, and in so doing, they will minimize their costs (enabling them to sell their service at a lower price) and attempt to provide those services that consumers desire. Persons who do not believe that consumers should determine what providers should produce often express similar disbelief in the ability of suppliers to compete with one another without harming patients. We often find that such persons want to substitute regulation and monopolies for competition on the supply side. Regardless of differences in values regarding who should determine the quantity and quality of medical services, it should be possible to allow different delivery systems to compete on the supply side. Although there may be a distrust of competition to achieve efficiency, allowing such competition to exist and to be an alternative to a more controlled delivery system, e.g., a system of VA hospitals, would provide a fairer test of which approach is more efficient at achieving the level of output established by government agencies.

This somewhat extended discussion of differences in values that exist in medical care was undertaken because the appropriate role of government is being assessed with regard to the values and criteria that underlie a market system. Much of the criticism of a market approach is not based upon the market system's ability to achieve the specified economic criteria. Because much of the disagreement is a result of differences in values and unspecified criteria, the discussion on the role of government and public policy alternatives would be sharpened if these distinctions were more apparent.

MARKET FAILURE

There are certain situations where markets, with no imperfections, will still not produce the optimal amount of output, which is defined as price equaling marginal cost. One such situation would be a "natural" monopoly in the provision of a particular service. In a natural monopoly the economies of scale are so large that, given the size of the market, it would be less expensive to have one firm produce that service. If competition prevailed, one of the firms would be able to lower its costs by increasing its scale of production, thereby driving other firms out of business. In a situation of natural monopoly, competition cannot exist; because of the monopolists' pricing strategy, the output is likely to be less than optimal. The situations in which natural monopolies exist in the health field are rare. Relatively good substitutes exist for most medical services at a local level. Economies of scale in hospitals are slight; individual hospital services such as cobalt therapy units may be subject to relatively large economies. Such services, however, serve a much larger market than is served by the hospital in which they are located. Thus, the market served by such specialized facilities and services is large enough for competition to exist between several of them. Because few services in medical care appear to have the characteristics of a natural monopoly, the natural-monopoly argument has not been an important justification for government intervention or subsidies in medical care.

Another possible reason for market failure in medical care is the existence of externalities. Externalities occur when an action undertaken by an individual (or firm) has secondary effects on others, which may be favorable or unfavorable. Externalities result in a nonoptimal amount of output being produced, because an individual or firm considers their benefits and costs only when making a production or consumption decision. If costs or benefits are received by others as a result of someone's private decision, the level of output produced in the market will be based upon either too small a level of benefits (i.e., positive external benefits), or too small a level of costs of production (i.e., positive external costs). For example, as shown in Figure 19-1, when there are external benefits (MEB), the result of an individual's considering only the (marginal private) benefits

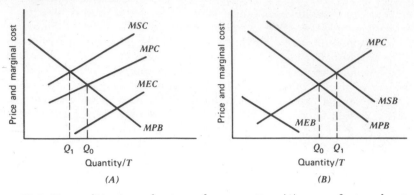

Figure 19-1. Externalities in production and consumption: (A) a case of external costs, (B) a case of external benefits.

(MPB) he or she expects to derive from that purchase would be a level of output determined by the intersection of the marginal-private-benefit (MPB) schedule and the marginal private costs (MPC) of producing that service. The resulting level of output, Q_0, would be smaller than if the external benefits to others (MEB) were also included. If the marginal private benefits and the marginal external benefits were added together [to result in the marginal-social-benefits (MSB) curve], then the resulting level of output would be Q_1, which is greater than Q_0.

A situation where external costs are imposed on others would be similar in approach, though opposite in effect, for purposes of determining the optimal level of output. A firm deciding how much output to produce would consider only the marginal private benefits and marginal private costs; it would not take into account any costs imposed on others, such as through air pollution. If the marginal costs imposed on others (MEC) were added to the firm's costs of production, then the resulting costs of producing that output, the marginal-social-cost curve (MSC), would represent the full costs of production. The level of output that would be produced in this latter case would be smaller, Q_1, than when the external costs were not considered, Q_0.

Individual consumers and producers in a competitive market do not normally take into consideration the external benefits or costs imposed on others as a result of their decisions. When such external costs and benefits are not incorporated into the private decisionmaking process, then the resultant output level is not optimal. Some persons receive benefits for which they would be willing to pay but do not, while others bear additional costs for which they did not receive any benefits. (In the latter case, the persons purchasing the good or service that results in an external cost are paying a price that is less than the full costs of producing that service.) Externalities therefore have two effects. The first is the effect on economic efficiency: it is only when all the marginal benefits (MSB) equal all the marginal costs (MSC) that the optimal level of output is determined. The second effect is redistribution: some persons receive an external benefit for which they do not compensate those providing it, or a cost is imposed on them for which they are not reimbursed.

To incorporate external costs and benefits into the private decisionmaking calculus when large numbers of individuals are involved requires some form of collective, nonmarket decisionmaking.* When large numbers of persons are involved, it becomes difficult to make voluntary arrangements that are satisfactory to all concerned. Group or collective decisionmaking, in which all persons must abide by the decision, is required to determine both the optimal level of output and to whom the compensation is to be paid (and on whom the taxes should be assessed). It is a legitimate role for government to serve as the group's agent in a nonmarket situation (1).

The existence of externalities legitimizes a role for government in health care, but what should that role consist of? It is not sufficient merely to claim that externalities exist and then justify all types of government intervention and financing of health and medical care. The proper role of government is twofold. First, it must determine the exact nature and size of external benefits and costs, if externalities are believed to exist. The measurement of externalities is a difficult task, both conceptually and empirically, as will be discussed below. Nonmarket studies, referred to as benefit/cost analyses, are important for determining the optimal level of output in situations where externalities exist. A problem with benefit/cost studies that have been undertaken in the health field is that they suggest it is appropriate for the government to undertake *any* program that has "favorable" benefit/cost ratios. It is important to determine whether such programs have any external effects; if there are no external effects, then the role of government if any, must be justified on other grounds. An example of inappropriate benefit/cost analysis is its application to personal health programs that have no external effects. The analyst may propose a system of government subsidies based solely on a finding of a favorable benefit/cost ratio. If there are no external effects and the individuals involved do not wish to spend their own funds on the program, then it would not be appropriate to have the government intervene, unless one is willing to declare that the individuals making the decision are not rational or, as is more likely, that the individuals do not share the same values as the analyst.

The second proper role of government when externalities exist is to determine how the externalities shall be financed—who shall be compensated and who shall be taxed. To use the previously mentioned example of air pollution as an example of a situation where external costs are imposed on others, the government should determine the magnitude of the external costs and then place a unit tax (equivalent to the size of the external costs) on those who are producing the particular product that is causing the pollution. The per unit tax will cause an increase in the polluters' costs of production and a consequent decrease in production and pollution (as shown in Figure 19-1A). The proceeds of the tax can then be used to reimburse those who bear these external costs. Similarly, when there are external benefits, as in the case of medical research, then those receiving the external benefits should be similarly taxed and the proceeds used to subsidize an increase in medical research. The financing principle should attempt to affix the taxes and subsidies to those who generate the external costs and

---

*When few individuals are involved, it is possible that they will reach agreement among themselves as to the proper levels of compensation, and the resulting level of output will be optimal.

benefits. A system of financing based on ability to pay would be inappropriate unless such a system reflected the extent of the external benefits and costs (2). Not all nonmarket decisionmaking should be based at a federal level, however. For some health programs, the benefits and costs are purely local in character, e.g., water fluoridation; the appropriate level of financing, therefore, is local in that case.

Situations involving externalities do not necessarily require government production or provision of particular services. If a particular service does not have the characteristics of a natural monopoly, then there is no reason why there could not be competition in the provision of that service. Medical schools and other research institutions could compete for research grants. Research is not necessarily produced more efficiently if undertaken solely by federally employed researchers. The criterion for whether the service should be governmentally or privately provided should be efficiency; there is nothing inherent in the nature of externalities that suggests services should be publicly provided.*

Several types of situations in the health and medical fields give rise to externalities. The first type may be referred to as the "consumer protection" argument, which was discussed previously. Given the technical nature of medical care, the usual lack in a patient's knowledge regarding diagnosis, treatment needs, and the provider's competence, consumers might benefit from the establishment of certain minimum standards and the provision of information. If the private market did not provide minimum standards (possibly through malpractice actions) or the necessary information required by consumers, or if all consumers desired the government to insure some minimum standards, then consumer protection would become an externality and hence a legitimate role for the government. The methods by which the government could fulfill this public demand for protection would be similar to those discussed previously.

Another externality with regard to personal medical services is what may be referred to as "externalities in consumption." If healthier and wealthier individuals do not want to see persons less fortunate than themselves go without necessary medical care and are willing to contribute to their medical care, then an externality in consumption is said to exist. This is because the utility of individuals depends not only upon the quantity of goods and services they themselves purchase, but also upon the amount of certain goods and services (such as medical care) purchased by others. Under such circumstances, if some persons contribute to the medical services of the less fortunate, then other persons, who similarly would have been willing to contribute, receive an external benefit;

---

*Using the criterion of efficiency, is there any reason for allowing the federal government to have a monopoly on the provision of medical care for veterans? Presumably, the government could determine how much it was willing to spend on medical care for a specific class of veterans (those with a service-connected disability) and then allow them a choice as to whether they wished to purchase care in the private medical sector or in the government's Veterans Administration hospitals. Such potential competition would be threatening to the Veterans Administration bureaucracy. Prohibiting competition for the provision of governmentally financed services often has less to do with efficiency and choice considerations than with the survival of an entrenched government bureaucracy. It would also reduce the size of the VA organization, since 85 percent of its beds are filled with veterans who do not have a service-connected disability. (Instead of reducing the size of its bureaucracy and budget as the number of veterans of the type for whom it was originally established to provide medical care decreases, the VA would prefer to maintain its institutions and budget by expanding the eligible class of veterans.)

everybody receives the benefit of seeing the less fortunate receive medical care, even though everybody did not necessarily contribute. Theoretically, each person who receives an external benefit should contribute according to the size of the external benefit. Unless there is some form of nonmarket decisionmaking, it will not be possible to collect from all the persons who receive an external benefit.

The implications from the preceding discussion are twofold. First, government, acting as the agent for the collective desires of those wishing to contribute, should tax those persons (assuming the government knows the utility functions of each individual exactly) the amount they would be willing to contribute and should provide a subsidy to the desired recipients equivalent to the magnitude of the collected tax. Second, the form of that subsidy (e.g., medical services) and the determination of its method of distribution (possibly an income-related determination of recipients), should represent the desires of the *donors*, not the recipients (3). This is because some donors may be willing to contribute, and thereby receive an external benefit, only if their contributions go to a particular income group, for a particular type of service, and are distributed in a certain manner. There are a number of ways in which subsidies could be provided to help those who are ill or who have low incomes. These persons could be given an income supplement rather than just an increase in their medical services; with an increase in their incomes, they could spend those funds on housing, nutritional foods, or medical services. If it is a lack of access to medical services that the more fortunate wish to redress, then it would be inappropriate, from the donor's perspective, to allow those funds to be spent on goods and services other than medical care. Under circumstances of externalities in consumption, in-kind subsidies are efficient.

The justification for national health insurance and other forms of in-kind subsidies (to be discussed more completely in subsequent sections) is presumably based on the assumption that there are externalities in consumption; otherwise, proposed in-kind subsidies would not be efficient. If the objective of the subsidies were the redistribution of income, then direct cash supplements would be a more efficient means to this end. The recipients of the subsidy would always prefer cash, which can be used to satisfy their most important needs, rather than a subsidy that can be used for only one of their needs, a need which may not represent their highest priority (4). For in-kind subsidies to be efficient, therefore, the intent must be to satisfy the preferences of the *donors* rather than the recipients. When an in-kind subsidy is called for, as in the case of externalities in consumption, then the type of person the donors are willing to subsidize and the amount of subsidy to be provided to each person are probably inversely related to the recipient's income: the lower the recipient's income, the greater the donor's willingness to provide a subsidy will be. It is unlikely that a person will receive an external benefit from seeing a person with a possibly higher income than his own receive a subsidy. These aspects of in-kind subsidies should be kept in mind when national health insurance and other in-kind subsidies are discussed subsequently.

Requiring everyone to purchase minimum health insurance that includes catastrophic coverage might also be justified on grounds of externalities. If a person decides to self-insure, then other persons are bearing part of the cost of that decision. If the person who self-insures is unfortunate enough to incur a catastrophic medical expense that he or she is unable to pay, then the community (through welfare payments) will have to reimburse the medical providers for that person's medical services. The rest of the community will have to bear part of the cost (in terms of higher taxes) of that individual's decision to self-insure (or purchase less than catastrophic insurance). It would be more equitable, therefore, if these costs were borne in full by individuals at risk, similar to an uninsured motorists fund.

The third type of externality that occurs in the health field is usually associated with public health programs rather than with personal medical services. Vaccination programs, clean water supplies, air pollution abatement, and medical research are examples of goods that result in large external benefits. It has generally been with respect to these types of programs that a great many benefit/cost studies have been undertaken.

REDISTRIBUTION USING IN-KIND SUBSIDIES

There are many types of in-kind subsidies in medical care. Some of these are demand subsidies, others are supply subsidies; some are indirect with regard to the beneficiary groups they hope to affect, others are direct. National health insurance would be classified as a direct demand subsidy. Before discussing national health insurance, it would be instructive to first discuss the different types of in-kind subsidies in medical care, their magnitude, their probable effects, and their probable beneficiaries. When we develop a better understanding of in-kind subsidies, their actual as compared with their stated purposes becomes clearer, and a context within which national health insurance can be analyzed is provided. If national health insurance is enacted, it is then questionable whether current in-kind subsidies should be continued. If national health insurance is a more efficient in-kind subsidy, then perhaps current in-kind subsidies should be used to help fund a national health insurance program.*

The major in-kind subsidies on the demand side are Medicare and Medicaid. Expenditures under these programs (and other direct subsidies on the demand side such as maternal and child health care) were $73.0 billion in 1981 (5). The other demand-side subsidies are indirect: there is the tax deductibility of one-half of health insurance premiums (up to a $150 maximum), the tax de-

---

*Regardless of their stated intent, in-kind medical care subsidies do not have as their actual objective an increase in health status. Instead, their goal appears to be an increase in use of medical services. For example, the Medicare program, which is a direct demand subsidy to the aged, provided, on average, a subsidy of $1,279.55 per aged person in 1978, as opposed to government medical expenditures of $218.13 per person aged 19–64 and $81.99 per person under 19 years of age. If the actual purpose of government medical care expenditures were to achieve an increase in health levels, then these expenditures might well have been allocated to different population groups, disease categories, and to non-medical-care programs. Even if it were agreed that the in-kind subsidy was to be provided to the aged alone, a different allocation of funds for non-medical-care services would be called for. An equivalent cash supplement to the aged to enable them to increase their consumption of food, housing, and heating would probably contribute more to their health than a subsidy restricted to medical services alone. Charles R. Fisher, "Differences by Age Groups in Health Care Spending," *Health Care Financing Review* (Spring 1980): 81, Table A.

ductibility of medical expenses in excess of 3 percent of adjusted gross income, and the provision of employer-paid health insurance premiums as a fringe benefit, which are excluded from the employee's taxable income. These indirect subsidies are estimated to cost approximately $20 billion a year (6).

On the supply side there are subsidy programs for health manpower education, at both federal and state levels, federal subsidies for hospital construction, and federal and state provision of medical services through the Veterans Administration and state and local government hospitals. There are also numerous indirect supply subsidy programs, for example, which grant tax-exempt status to nonprofit providers such as nonprofit hospitals and Blue Cross plans, and state assistance in financing hospital bond issues.

The size of these demand and supply subsidies, both direct and indirect, is very large: roughly $128 billion in 1981 (7). Since expenditures for personal medical care totaled approximately $255 billion in 1981, it is clear that the role of government in the financing and provision of personal medical services is large and increasing.

Given the significant role of government in personal medical services, it is important to determine who the beneficiaries of these subsidies are and how efficiently these subsidies are being distributed. These two issues are interrelated; as previously discussed, the argument for in-kind subsidies is based upon externalities in consumption. As such, the primary beneficiaries should be those persons with low incomes and/or poor health (plus indirectly those who favor such programs). If the subsidies are distributed in such a way as to benefit higher-income groups or provide them with a greater proportionate share of the subsidy, then the distribution of the subsidy is inefficient; i.e., the desired beneficiary group (low-income persons) could receive a greater amount of the subsidy if it were provided in a different, presumably more direct, manner.*

It is generally easier to calculate the beneficiary groups under demand rather than supply subsidies. Under the Medicaid program, for example, the designated beneficiaries are the medically indigent. Since Medicaid is a federal-state matching program, the definition of medical indigency and the benefits provided under the program vary by state. However, as shown in Table 19-1, expenditures under Medicaid go predominately to the poor and near-poor. This relationship between income level and Medicaid expenditure holds for both per capita as well as total Medicaid expenditures. When one examines indirect demand subsidy programs, it becomes even less obvious that the subsidies are going to those persons with the lowest incomes and/or greatest medical needs. Under Medicare, because the beneficiary group is defined by age rather than income level, the effect of the subsidy by income level is more even than for Medicaid. Not all aged persons have lower incomes or are of poorer health than nonaged persons. Although per capita Medicare expenditure decreases with higher income levels, the percent of Medicare expenditures going to each income level is more evenly distributed. The poor and near-poor received 28 percent of total Medicare expenditures as compared to the high-income group, which received 21 percent.

---

*This assumes that the method of distribution is not prescribed by the same externalities argument that gave rise to the subsidy in the first place.

TABLE 19-1. Major Federal Government Expenditures on Health Services, 1977

All Persons	Income Tax Savings	Medicare[a]	Medicaid	Total Federal[b]
Per Capita Government Expenditures				
Poor and near-poor	$ 2	$141	$184	$327
Other low-income	16	99	63	178
Middle-income	43	57	16	116
High-income	90	48	4	142

Total Government Expenditures (Billions of Dollars)

	$	%	$	%	$	%	$	%
Poor and near-poor	0.1	1	4.3	28	5.6	62	10.0	29
Other low-income	0.5	5	3.1	20	2.0	22	5.6	16
Middle-income	3.5	34	4.7	31	1.3	14	9.5	27
High-income	6.2	60	3.3	21	0.2	2	9.7	28
Total expenditures	10.3	100	15.4	100	9.1	100	34.8	100

Sources: This table is from Gail R. Wilensky, "Government and the Financing of Health Care," *American Economic Review* (May 1982): 205, Table 2.

[a] Less Part B premiums.

[b] Excludes expenditures from veterans programs and small federal programs. The definition of income groups are as follows: The "poor" include those whose family income was less than or equal to the 1977 poverty level as well as those whose income was between 101 and 125 percent of that level. "Other low income" includes those whose income is 1.26 to two times the poverty level, "middle income" is 2.01 to four times the poverty level, and "high income" is 4.01 times the poverty level or more. For a family of four in 1977, these four groups distribute as follows: less than $8,000 to $9,999, $10,000 to $15,999, $16,000 to $31,999, and greater than $32,000. The percent of the population in each group is 14, 15, 39, and 32 percent, respectively.

When tax subsidy programs, such as the exclusion of employer-provided health insurance premiums from taxable income and the deduction of medical expenses in excess of 3 percent of adjusted gross income are examined, the benefits are received by the higher-income groups. Middle-income and high-income groups together receive 94 percent of those subsidy dollars.

When government expenditures for all three programs are combined, the total benefits are very evenly divided among the different income groups; the biggest losers, however, appear to be the other-low-income group, with 16 percent of total government expenditures. The poor and near-poor, middle-income, and high-income groups received 29, 27, and 28 percent, respectively. Medicaid expenditures, which heavily favor the low-income groups, are offset by the tax subsidy programs. The redistributional effects of Medicare are small.

The government is attempting to reduce its expenditures on Medicare and Medicaid. As it does so, the redistributional effects of government health expenditures will go more to the higher income groups, unless changes are also made in the tax subsidy programs.

It would thus appear that the more directly the demand subsidy is aimed at a designated population group, the more likely it is to provide the intended recipients with a larger proportion of that subsidy. Direct subsidy programs of this sort would be more in accordance with legislative intent. Indirect demand subsidy programs would be a less efficient way of subsidizing a particular beneficiary group. An increase in taxes to provide subsidies to higher-income persons would be approved by legislators only if it were uncertain that the subsidies would go to higher-income persons or if it were not obvious to the voters. If in-kind medical subsidies are to be justified, then the beneficiaries should presumably be those with lower incomes and/or greater needs for medical care than the persons favoring such subsidies. Direct demand subsidies would be both a more obvious and a more direct means of assuring that this objective is achieved.

Demand subsidies impose costs on those persons not receiving them in two ways. First, there is an increase in taxes to pay for the subsidy program. Second, an increase in demand by the recipients of the subsidies leads to an increase in the prices of medical services. These higher prices for medical services will both increase the price and decrease the use (depending upon the price elasticity of demand) of those persons not being subsidized. After Medicare and Medicaid were introduced, prices in the medical sector more than doubled as shown in Table 19-2.

The demand subsidy will have secondary effects throughout the entire medical care sector. A demand subsidy will cause an increase in demand in the different institutional markets: hospitals, physician services, and so on. How large the increase in demand will be in each of the separate institutional markets will depend, in part, upon the type of demand subsidy—i.e., how much price is reduced to the beneficiaries—in each of the institutional settings and the elasticity of supply in that market. A more inelastic supply will result in greater price increases, which will tend to reduce demand in both the beneficiary and nonbeneficiary groups. As demand increases in each of the institutional settings, there will be an increase in the derived demand for the inputs (different types of health manpower and nonlabor inputs) used in that setting. With increased demands for health manpower, wages and incomes in the manpower markets will increase, together with participation rates. In the long run, an increase in the incomes of health personnel will result in increased demands for a health professional education, and if the health education market responds, there will be an increase in the stock of trained health manpower. How much of the demand subsidy will end up in higher prices rather than increased services will depend upon the elasticity of supply in the various medical markets. The greater the number of restrictions on entry into the health professions, on the tasks that different health personnel can perform, and on the methods of reimbursement used, the greater the inelasticity of supply and the higher the increases in medical prices will be.

Supply subsidies may also be classified according to whether they are directly targeted to a beneficiary group or whether their benefits are diffused among a number of population groups. An example of a supply subsidy that is directed at a designated beneficiary group is the provision of funds to establish a clinic in a low-income neighborhood. Even if there is no corresponding demand subsidy, the new clinic will result in an increased use of medical services because it will decrease the patients' cost of travel to the facility. Most direct supply subsidies are not of this type; the major direct supply subsidies are the Veterans Administration hospitals and the hospital services provided by state and local governments.

The Veterans Administration medical system is fairly extensive, consisting

TABLE 19-2. Average Annual Percent Changes in Consumer Prices and Selected Medical Care Prices, 1961–1981

Years	CPI All Items	CPI All Services Less Medical Care Services	Medical Care Services	Semi-private Room Charge	Physician Fee
1961–1966	1.1	1.8	2.9	5.3	2.8
1967–1970	3.8	5.0	5.6	9.8	5.0
ESP[a]	6.1	5.0	6.0	4.9	3.2
1975	9.1	9.1	12.5	17.2	12.3
1976–1981	9.9	11.3	10.0	12.3	10.0

Source: The data for the years 1961–1976 are from Congress of the United States, Congressional Budget Office *Expenditures for Health Care: Federal Programs and Their Effects* (Washington, D.C.: U.S. Government Printing Office, August 1977). The data for 1977–1981 are from Bureau of Labor Statistics, *CPI Detailed Report* (various issues), Tables 1A and 5A.

[a] Economic Stabilization Period (August 1971–April 1974).

of 120 general hospitals, 50 mental hospitals, and numerous clinics and rehabilitation centers. Although the major stated role of the VA is to provide medical care to veterans with a service-connected disability, only 15 percent of the veterans in VA hospitals are there for that purpose. The remaining 85 percent have low incomes and receive care for illnesses unrelated to their military service (8).

State and local government hospitals account for approximately 20 percent of all admissions to short-term general hospitals and approximately 25 percent of all hospital outpatient visits. These hospitals have served as important sources of medical care for the indigent and have relieved the private hospitals and physicians of the financial risk of caring for these patients.

In view of the increase in Medicare and Medicaid, and the possibility of enacting national health insurance, all of which are targeted to the same population groups served by the VA and other government hospital systems, what is the likely and proper role for these providers? If the medically indigent were to receive a demand subsidy with benefits at least as complete as those presently available to them in the VA and other government hospitals, then the demand for care in these institutions is likely to decline sharply. State and local government hospitals have had a reputation for providing care of lower quality or of less satisfaction to patients than is provided by community nonprofit hospitals. VA hospitals are inconveniently located in relation to their beneficiary population (there are only 120 VA hospitals as opposed to more than 3,500 community hospitals), and it is unlikely that the advantages of being in a VA hospital are sufficient to offset the patient's considerable travel costs. If the benefits (i.e., price) under national health insurance for the 85 percent of the VA patient population who are medically indigent were the same as the benefits for the community's medically indigent, it is likely that the VA patient population would choose care in a community hospital.

If the current medical care system, the VA and the other government hospitals all had to compete for patients under a demand subsidy arrangement, the VA and governmental hospitals would either have to change or they would not be able to survive in a competitive environment. For the VA system to compete for the 85 percent of its population who use the VA because they are medically indigent, it would have to provide ambulatory services, change its organizational and reimbursement arrangements with its physicians, increase its relative efficiency by lowering length of stay and using less costly substitutes for inpatient care, and compete on a more local basis for patients, since patient travel costs and time are likely to be significant determinants in choosing medical delivery systems.

The VA hospital system has been able to survive since the passage of Medicare and Medicaid because the VA was able to fill the gaps in that coverage for the medically indigent veteran. Will there be a role for the VA if the benefits under national health insurance are more complete for the medically indigent? It is unlikely that a bureaucracy as large as the VA will accept the market's judgment of an 80 percent reduction in its budget, but it is equally unlikely that such a large, centrally controlled bureaucracy will be able to undertake the drastic changes in its role, organization, and delivery system that are necessary to compete on an equal basis with the private medical system. If the VA cannot survive under these conditions, what economic justification is there for providing additional large subsidies to enable the VA to maintain its current expanded role?

The role of state and local governmental hospitals under national health insurance is also uncertain. With the passage of Medicare and Medicaid, these hospitals were able to bill for their services and increase their source of revenues. Patients also came to these hospitals because there were gaps in their Medicare coverage. The hospitals became less dependent upon local governments for financial support. With additional funds, these hospitals were able to increase their staffing (from 234 employees per 100 patients in 1965 to 387 in 1977; this compared with 252 and 369, respectively, in community hospitals) and improve their plant and equipment. It has been hypothesized that because these governmental hospitals were controlled on a local basis and operated with more decentralized management than the VA hospital system, it was easier for them to adapt and to compete with community hospitals (9). If the medically indigent served by these hospitals were to be provided with more comprehensive benefits under national health insurance, then it is possible that these hospitals would be able to adapt and survive without additional subsidies. It would be questionable that direct supply subsidies would still be necessary if the population group originally served by these institutions were provided with a direct demand subsidy and chose to exercise those benefits in a different medical care delivery system.

Indirect supply subsidies, the other major type of in-kind supply subsidies, are exemplified by funds for training additional health manpower and capital grants to hospitals. These indirect supply subsidies have their initial effects on a particular medical market. For the subsidy to result in increased medical services, its effects must eventually be transmitted through several medical markets. For example, when a subsidy is given to medical schools to increase the number of physicians, several years pass before there is an increase in the number of additional graduates. These graduates will then work in a number of settings, ranging from hospitals to physicians' offices. The increase in the amount of services eventually received by the members of a particular beneficiary group will depend upon their elasticity of demand for those services. (The increased supply of services is a downward shift along a patient's demand curve for that service.) If demand by members of the beneficiary group is relatively inelastic, i.e., not very responsive to changes in the price of the service, then there will be relatively little increase in their use of medical services. Since indirect supply subsidies are not generally targeted to particular beneficiary groups, the beneficiaries will be all those persons using the service; they will be paying a lower price than before the subsidy. Because low-income persons do not use medical services as much, they may receive less benefit from such subsidies than high users do; the high users may also have relatively higher incomes.

In addition to their being inefficient, in that the highest proportion of the subsidy does not go to low-income persons, general supply subsidies present further problems. When only one input into the process of producing medical care is subsidized, a manager who is attempting to use the lowest-cost combination of inputs will tend to use more of the subsidized input because its cost has been artificially reduced. For example, a subsidy to train additional registered nurses will, if it is successful, result in a greater increase in the supply of nurses and a relatively lower wage for them. Because the wage of nurses is lowered with the subsidy, hospitals will substitute away from other nursing personnel toward more registered nurses in providing patient care. This is a more costly approach to providing patient care than if the hospital were merely awarded an equivalent unrestricted subsidy. In the latter case, the hospital would use a combination of registered and nonregistered nurses and other inputs based on their relative prices and productivities. The hospital consequently would use fewer registered nurses than if only wages were artificially reduced through a subsidy. Subsidies that increase the supply of a particular input are therefore less efficient (more costly) than an equivalent dollar subsidy.

It is also often difficult to determine what additional services have been produced as a result of a supply subsidy. Although one might be able to count the number of additional persons trained as a result of the subsidy (which is not as easy as it might appear), it is more difficult to calculate the net increase in services resulting from the additional health manpower. Without additional nurses, the wage rate of existing nurses would have risen more rapidly, which in turn would have caused a greater increase in the participation rate of trained nurses not currently employed. In the long run, with higher wages in the profession, there would be an increase in the number of persons seeking a career in nursing. Similarly, without a subsidy to increase the number of physicians, the productivity of existing physicians might be greater. Thus, to assume that the additional services provided by the subsidized manpower are the net benefits of the supply subsidy program is to greatly overstate its benefits.

To understand exactly what impact supply subsidies have on increased utilization of services, and for which beneficiary groups, it is necessary to use a complex econometric model of the medical sector. For example, a subsidy to increase the number of registered nurses will have its initial impact on the nursing education market. How many additional nurses will be graduated as a result of that subsidy will depend, in part, on the objectives of the different types of nursing schools and on which schools receive the subsidies. The number of nurses will also depend upon the elasticity of demand for a nursing education by prospective nurses, since the subsidy will reduce their educational costs. The impact of additional nurses on the market for nurses will affect nurses' wages, participation rates, and nurse employment. How many additional nurses will be employed in the various institutional settings will depend upon the elasticity of demand for nurses in each of the different settings and the new wage for nurses. (The determination of wages and employment will, of course, be a simultaneous process.) The greater the substitutability of registered nurses for other types of nursing personnel, the higher the elasticity of demand will be and the greater the decrease in demand for nonregistered nurses will be. Each of the institutional settings that employ registered nurses will have a slightly lower cost for its nursing personnel; the cost of care in each institutional setting will also be lower. How much lower it will be will depend upon how many registered nurses are employed and the elasticity of the demand for nurses (i.e., whether many more nurses are hired as a result of their relatively lower wage). The effect of the nurse subsidy on cost of care will vary for each institutional setting; hospitals, which hire the majority of nurses, would receive the largest cost reduction. Since the relative cost of the different institutional settings has changed, how much the price of care will be reduced in each of the institutional settings as a result of a lowering of costs will depend upon the elasticity of demand for services and the environment in which an institution competes. If there are no competitive pressures on the institution, if the institution attempts to maximize its prestige, and if the institution is reimbursed on a cost basis, it is less likely that the cost savings will be passed on to patients and other third-party payors. Thus, the final impact of supply subsidies on supply of medical services as compared with the impact of demand subsidies is much more difficult to determine. It is equally difficult to determine which consumer or payor group receives the major benefit of the subsidy, if any of them receives any benefit at all.

Supply subsidies in medical care have generally been direct in their impact on low-income persons when the government itself has served as the supplier. When supply subsidies have been indirect, in-kind subsidies have provided benefits to all those persons who use medical services; but, as with the Hill-Burton program for hospital construction, nothing was done to help those who could not afford to use the hospital. A demand subsidy was still required for the medically indigent. In-kind supply subsidies take longer than direct demand subsidies do to provide greater access to medical services to a beneficiary group. They are also economically inefficient, either because patients have no choice as to which provider they must go to, as under the VA system, or because the relative cost of inputs is distorted. Finally, the benefits of indirect supply subsidies are overstated, since employee participation rates and productivity increases are, in fact, likely to be lower than what they would otherwise have been.

Although direct demand subsidies would appear to be a more efficient method of providing an in-kind subsidy, supply subsidies are legislatively popular. The probable reason is not that legislators are necessarily unaware of which is the more efficient subsidy method, but rather that the providers of medical care and manpower education are important beneficiaries of such proposals. Legislators are likely to be receptive to the lobbying efforts of these groups because supply subsidies are obvious to their constituents and are favorably received, such as when there is an increase in the number of physicians and nurses or a new hospital building appears in a community.

The intent of the preceding discussion on existing in-kind subsidies in medical care was to provide both an indication of the current magnitude of their support and some criteria by which to judge the efficiency of alternative types of in-kind subsidies. If national health insurance is to be undertaken, then one should specifically determine which of the many demand and supply (direct and indirect) subsidies should remain; any funds saved might be used to bear part of the cost of national health insurance.

REFERENCES

1. For a lengthier exposition of this point, see, for example, Neil M. Singer, *Public Microeconomics: An Introduction to Government Finance* (Boston: Little, Brown & Company, 1976).

2. For a complete explication of the issues involved in financing government activities such as this, see Richard Musgrave, *A Theory of Public Finance* (New York: McGraw-Hill, 1959).

3. For a more extended discussion of this proposition see Paul Feldman, "Efficiency, Distribution, and the Role of Government in a Market Economy," *Journal of Political Economy* 79(3) (May–June 1971): 508–526.

4. A proof of this statement may be found in a number of texts on microeconomics. See, for example, Donald S. Watson and Malcom Getz, *Price Theory and Its Uses* (Boston: Houghton Mifflin Company, 1981), p. 119.

5. Robert M. Gibson and Daniel R. Waldo, "National Health Expenditures, 1981," *Health Care Financing Review*, vol. 4 (Baltimore, Md.: Health Care Financing Administration, September 1982), p. 1.

6. Charles E. Phelps, "Public Sector Medicine: History and Analysis," in *New Directions in Public Health Care* (San Francisco: Institute for Contemporary Studies, 1980), pp. 130–131.

7. Phelps's fraction of government expenditures as a percent of total health spending, which was 51 percent, was applied to total health spending in 1981.

8. *Ibid.*, p. 153.

9. *Ibid.*, p. 162.

CHAPTER 20

National Health Insurance: An Approach to the Redistribution of Medical Care

This discussion on national health insurance (NHI) begins with a theoretical framework that can be used to analyze various proposals in terms of the efficiency with which they achieve the different values that underlie proposals for NHI. No attempt will be made to select one set of values over another; instead, the analysis will be concerned with the most efficient means for achieving a given set of values. Some empirical evidence based on Medicare will be used to support the theoretical conclusions. This theoretical discussion will then be used as a basis for developing a set of criteria for evaluating alternative health insurance proposals. The current system of financing medical care and several suggested proposals for NHI will then be discussed according to the criteria developed. No attempt will be made to provide a detailed discussion of current legislative proposals, inasmuch as a number of other publications have provided such detailed analyses (1). Also, since new legislative proposals are constantly being made, a basic understanding of the concepts underlying such proposals should be more useful for understanding both current and future proposals.

ACHIEVING EFFICIENCY FOR DIFFERENT VALUES UNDERLYING NATIONAL HEALTH INSURANCE

A THEORETICAL DISCUSSION

National health insurance (NHI) may be viewed as an in-kind demand subsidy based on the argument that there are externalities in consumption. If the nonpoor wish to subsidize the poor, this will result in a demand for government subsidies. The degree of subsidization will differ depending upon the values held by the nonpoor with respect to redistribution of medical care services. One set of values may be termed minimum provision, meaning that no person in society should receive less than a certain quantity of medical care in case of illness. A second set of values might be called equal financial access to medical care. If these values were the basis for the externalities in consumption, then they would suggest an NHI plan that would equalize the financial barriers to all persons; in other words, the price of medical services would be the same for everyone. The third set of values that people may share with respect to redistribution of medical care services goes beyond equal financial access to require equal treatment for equal needs—in other words, equal consumption of medical services regardless of economic or other factors affecting utilization. The different demands for government subsidies reflect varying sets of values that are believed to exist in the population. The first set of values would require the smallest level of subsidization; the third set of values would be the most expensive to achieve.

It is not possible to state which set of values is the most appropriate one; whichever set of values the population selects would be the proper basis for the level of government subsidies under NHI. Although it is not possible to determine a priori the set of values that is likely to be chosen by the population, it is possible to determine the most efficient approach for achieving each of the three sets of values. It should be possible to state which types of national health insurance are likely to be more efficient than others, regardless of the set of values that one holds.

Minimum provision may be achieved in one of two ways: those persons whose consumption of medical care is below the minimum may be subsidized to bring their consumption up to the minimum, or, alternatively, a subsidy can be provided to *everyone* so that at the resulting new, lower price, no one person's consumption would be below the minimum specified by society. These two alternatives are shown in Figure 20-1. Assuming that there are three different income groups—high incomes (HY), middle incomes (MY), and low incomes (LY)—their demands for medical care would be shown by the three demand curves, *HY, MY,* and *LY*, respectively. The aggregate demand curve of all three income groups is shown by *HYMYLY*. The reason the three demand curves do not result in the same consumption of medical care at zero price is that there are factors, other than financial ones, that result in differences in demand between different income groups. For example, low-income groups may incur greater costs in traveling to providers than do higher-income groups; differences in attitudes may also affect their utilization. Provider preferences in dealing with different income groups may also play a role. If the current price of medical care is P_{MC}, then the utilization of the three income groups would be Q_1, Q_2, and Q_3, and their aggregate utilization would be Q_0, which is the intersection of the aggregate demand curve and the supply of medical care (assuming, for simplicity, perfect elasticity). If society wanted to assure that no one received less than a minimum amount of medical care, Q_m, then a system of national health insurance that reduced the price of medical care to everyone, or that sets the price at zero for everyone, would achieve this goal. A system of subsidies that lowers the price of medical care for just those whose consumption is less than the minimum

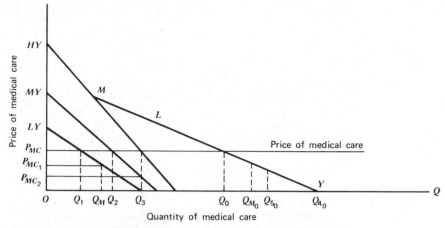

Figure 20-1. Demand curves of different income groups.

would also achieve this goal. If medical care were free, then everyone's consumption would increase, with the total going from Q_0 to Q_{4_0}. If, instead, a subsidy were provided to just those persons whose consumption was below the minimum (i.e., by lowering the price to lower-income persons to P_{mc_1}) then the aggregate increase in use of medical care would be less, from Q_0 to Q_{m_0}. The cost to society of this approach to achieving minimum provision would be the subsidy required to increase the low-income group's utilization, which is $P_{mc} - P_{mc_1}$, multiplied by that group's utilization, Q_m. The cost of making medical care free to all persons would be the price of medical care multiplied by the new and greater quantity that would result when the price was reduced for everyone, which is P_{mc} multiplied by Q_{4_0}. Since both approaches would achieve the goal of minimum provision, the approach that provided a subsidy to the lower income group only would be less costly, hence more efficient, than a scheme that reduced the price to everyone.*

If society's values with respect to redistribution of medical care were that all persons should have equal financial access to medical care, then this could be achieved by establishing a free medical care system (or a low price to all persons), as in the previous illustration, or through a system of subsidies that varied according to income levels. Equal financial access could be achieved under a subsidy system that reduced the price of medical care to low-income persons to zero; their consumption would thereby increase to Q_3. A subsidy to middle-income groups equal to $P_{mc} - P_{mc_2}$ would also increase their consumption to Q_3. At consumption level Q_3, the utilization of medical care for the three income groups would be equal. The aggregate increase in medical care use would go from Q_0 to Q_{5_0}. Equal financial access would require a more expensive subsidy ($Q_3 \times P_{mc}$ for the low-income group, plus $Q_3 \times P_{mc} - P_{mc_2}$ for the middle-income group) than would be required for achieving minimum provision, but it would

---

* For simplicity's sake it is assumed that the different proposals do not differ in their administrative costs nor in the response by suppliers to those proposals.

still be less costly than a medical care system that eliminated all financial barriers for everyone.

It is unlikely that the external demand for subsidization, based on the value that there should be equal financial access, would include the value judgment that the demands of higher-income persons should also be increased beyond levels that indicate what they currently would be willing to spend, and that this increase should be financed through higher taxes. If such persons are currently purchasing Q_3 amount of medical care, then the value to them of additional units of care is less than the price they would have to pay to consume it. It would be illogical for people to vote for an additional tax on themselves to purchase additional units of medical care when they were previously not willing to pay the equivalent amount of money to purchase those same units.

Equal treatment for equal needs expresses the third set of values that give rise to a demand for medical care subsidies. Since demands for medical care vary for more reasons than just financial ones, merely making the price of medical care free to all will not result in equal consumption. As shown in Figure 20-1, high-income groups would still consume more medical care at a zero price than the middle- and lower-income groups would. Thus, a free medical care system would not be able to achieve that set of values defined as equal treatment for equal needs. The value likely to be achieved through a free medical care system would be equal financial access, which, as we have shown, could be achieved at lower cost by a system of subsidies that varied by income level.

The only way in which equal treatment for equal needs could be achieved would be by differential subsidies, varying according to income level. For example, as shown in Figure 20-2, lowering the price of medical care to zero for both low- and middle-income groups would still not increase their utilization to where it equaled that of the high-income group. Only if the low- and middle-

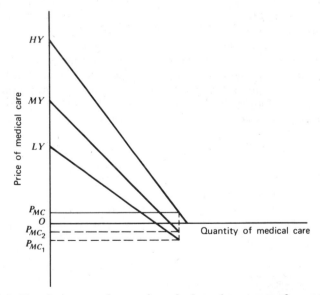

Figure 20-2. Equal treatment for equal needs through a system of negative prices.

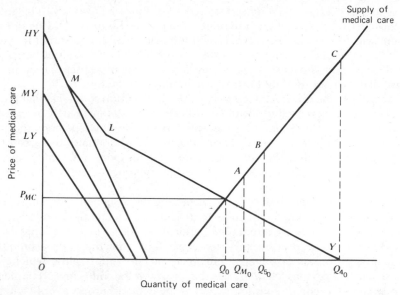

Figure 20-3. The cost of different demand subsidies when supply of medical care is relatively inelastic.

income groups were subsidized further, through a system of negative prices, could their utilization be equal. (Negative prices mean that such groups are paid to increase their use.) How large the negative prices would have to be would depend, in part, upon the consumption levels of the high-income groups. If high-income groups do not vote to increase their own consumption through subsidies which they will then have to repay in higher taxes, then the size of the subsidy required to increase the other groups' consumption to where it equals the higher income group's will be less.

It is unlikely that legislation could ever be passed that would actually pay people to increase their use of medical care. Instead, a negative price would be paid by means of a direct in-kind supply subsidy to low-income groups. For example, although the price of medical care to a low-income person would be zero, substantial travel and access costs might deter that person from using more medical services. Establishing clinics and neighborhood health centers in low-income areas and providing incentives for health personnel to practice there would increase access and decrease travel costs, thereby increasing use.

The cost in resources and the consequent increase in taxes required to achieve each of the three sets of values are even greater when the more realistic assumption is made that supply is not perfectly elastic but is, instead, relatively inelastic. Figure 20-3 is similar to Figure 20-1, except that the supply of medical care is less elastic. The consequence of a rising supply curve is that as demand is subsidized, the cost of a subsidy will be greater than if supply were more elastic. The cost of the subsidy necessary to achieve minimum provision is the utilization of the low-income group multiplied by the higher price of medical care (point A on the supply curve). This higher price will also be borne by those persons in society who favor subsidies that provide more medical care to low-income groups.* The taxes required to fund equal financial access will be greater than those required to achieve minimum provision. The price paid by the government will continue to increase, as will the price paid by those not receiving subsidies. As might be expected, as the price to those who are not being subsidized rises, and the cost of achieving a given set of values increases, the amount that they are willing to subsidize others will decline.

For national health insurance to have the redistributive effects that are desired by society, increased utilization must occur; it will most easily occur when the price elasticity of demand for medical services by those persons receiving subsidies is high. The greater the price elasticities of demand, the greater the increase in demand along an inelastic supply will be; therefore, rapidly increasing prices and total expenditures for the subsidy program will be the consequences.

It is precisely because of these expected higher costs that several proposals for national health insurance include approaches for changing the delivery system as well. In evaluating alternative national health insurance proposals, the demand proposals should be analyzed separately from the supply proposals. Presumably, proposals to enhance efficiency on the supply side, which were discussed in a previous chapter, can be incorporated into any NHI plan. A supply proposal becomes an integral part of the demand proposal only when its proponents are not willing to accept the criterion of economic efficiency in supply. Under one previous proposal for NHI, the Kennedy-Corman Health Security Act, which would have made medical care free to all, a great deal of emphasis is placed upon how the supply side will be financed and organized. Expenditure limits by regions and by type of provider would be established. As shown in Figure 20-3, total expenditures and prices would increase sharply under a free medical care system. Arbitrary establishment of dollar limits is an outgrowth of a political process and is unrelated to underlying supply and demand conditions. Expenditure limits would serve as a cost-control mechanism, but if cost control is the consequence of this approach, either intended or otherwise, the proponents of a free medical care system should be more explicit in defining the set of values that underlie this approach. They should also demonstrate how arbitrarily determined expenditure limits on the supply side would achieve these values.

The advocates of a free medical system might argue that it would still be possible to achieve the program's stated goals at a lower expenditure level than indicated by the supply curve in Figure 20-3, through greater efficiency. Since the advocates of a free medical system are opposed to competition as a way of determining the most efficient system and set of providers, reliance would have to be placed upon government to manage the medical system and to bring about greater efficiency in supply. Previous attempts by government to regulate or manage the supply of a good or service, both outside and within the medical care field, lend little credibility to the belief that the government will become an efficient and innovative manager in the near future. It is more likely that the

---

* Because the supply of medical care is not elastic, it is necessary to think in terms of the postsubsidy market price that an income group will face when the price of medical care is subsidized. National health insurance based on a tax credit is one way of achieving this.

current medical care system will be frozen in existing patterns. The government has not been able to close the Veterans Administration, Public Health Service, or any municipal hospitals, when it wanted to do so on grounds of efficiency (similar to its difficulty in closing military bases), because of political pressure from employee groups and the constituencies of these facilities. It is likely that each provider group within each region would attempt to protect its expenditure allocation each year; such actions would prevent changes in methods of delivery where dollar allocations to providers would be affected.

The ability of government to bring about greater efficiency is not borne out by the evidence, even in the health field. Lengths of stay in Veterans Administration hospitals are much longer than in nongovernment hospitals (for similar diagnoses), and there has been little substitution away from hospitals, when medically possible, to less expensive services, such as ambulatory care. It is unlikely that the quality of managers in a medical system controlled by government would be improved. It is more likely that the quality of management would decline because such an all-inclusive system would preclude a point of reference outside of itself, by which managers could be evaluated. There also would be no incentives for managers to seek to change the system, and the financial rewards to good management would be greater in nongovernment-controlled sectors. Evidence to support this contention may be found not only in VA hospitals, but also in AMTRAK and the postal service. In the medical system, too, unions would become more powerful in the decisionmaking process, and, as in the postal service, might inhibit the introduction of laborsaving innovations.

For each of the sets of values examined—minimum provision, equal financial access, and equal treatment for equal needs—it was shown that these values can be more efficiently achieved if the subsidy varies by income level rather than if changes are sought through a system that either results in an equal price reduction to all or makes medical care free to everyone, regardless of income level. Although this analysis was theoretical, empirical data support these conclusions.

SOME EMPIRICAL EVIDENCE
FROM THE MEDICARE PROGRAM

Medicare is an existing in-kind demand subsidy to the aged. (Part A of Medicare provides hospital coverage while Part B is a voluntary insurance program primarily for physician services.) The benefits available to all the aged under Medicare are similar, as is the reduced price they must pay for the use of medical care. To use physician services (Part B of Medicare), an aged person was initially required to pay $50 as a deductible and 20% copayment above and beyond that deductible.* It would appear that the pricing mechanism was designed to insure either equal financial access to medical care or equal treatment for equal medical needs for the aged.

As long as demand for medical care among the aged differs according to income and accessibility, then, as shown in Figure 20-1, a similar price to all

---

* The deductible was raised to $60 in 1973. The inflation-adjusted value of the deductible declined to $27 in 1982.

TABLE 20-1. Medicare Reimbursements for Covered Services Under the Supplementary Medical Insurance Program and Persons Served, by Income, 1968 and 1977

Income Group	Persons Receiving Reimbursable Services Per 1,000 Medicare Enrollees	Medicare Reimbursement Per Reimbursable Service	Medicare Reimbursement Per Person Enrolled
		1968	
Under $5,000	431.7	$ 7.02	$ 78.77
Over $15,000	552.3	10.40	160.30
Ratio, over $15,000 to under $5,000 incomes	1.28	1.48	2.04
		1977	
At or near poverty line	773.4	6.43	60.32
High-income	801.7	5.82	57.72
Ratio, high-income to at or near poverty line	1.04	.91	.96

Source: For 1968 data: Karen Davis, "Equal Treatment and Unequal Benefits: The Medicare Program." *Milbank Memorial Fund Quarterly/Health and Society* 53(4): 457. Copyright Milbank Memorial Fund. Table 1. For 1977 data: G. Wilensky, L. Rossiter, and L. Finney, "The Medicare Subsidy of Private Health Insurance," Rockville, Md.: National Center for Health Services Research, National Health Care Expenditure Survey, 1983.

persons, such as the aged under Medicare, would result in differences in utilization. Guaranteeing the same price to high-income aged would result in a greater utilization level for them in comparison with the low-income aged because it would represent a smaller financial burden to them and because their travel costs are lower, owing to their location in areas where they are closer to medical providers.

According to data shown in Table 20-1, the aged with higher incomes were more likely to pay the deductible and use the Part B supplementary coverage under Medicare: 552.3 persons per 1,000 Medicare enrollees with incomes in excess of $15,000, 431.7 persons per 1,000 among those aged with incomes less than $5,000. Services used by the higher-income aged also cost the government more: $10.40 compared with $7.02 per reimbursable service. (These higher prices represent higher prices for the same services as well as possibly higher-quality services, as when specialists are used.) The Medicare reimbursement per person enrolled was more than twice as high for the higher-income aged, $160.30 compared with $78.77. By 1977 the difference between the income groups lessened.

When Medicare utilization is examined for differences according to race, large disparities persist, as shown in Table 20-2. Whites are more likely to use physician services than nonwhites; one reason is that nonwhites receive more of their ambulatory services from hospital outpatient departments than do whites.

TABLE 20-2. Persons Served and Medicare Reimbursement Per Person Served, by Race, 1968 and 1977

	Persons Served Per 1,000 Enrollees		Reimbursement Per Person Served		Medicare Reimbursement per Person Enrolled
	Physician Services	Hospital Outpatient Services	Physician Services	Hospital Outpatient Services	
1968					
Whites	394.9	71.6	$199.44	$39.02	$82.70
Blacks and other races	279.4	89.9	173.37	50.43	54.20
Ratio, white to other	1.413	.796	1.150	.774	1.526
1977					
Whites	770.	227.	60.01	70.46	62.23
Blacks	652.	315.	42.99	47.57	43.04
Ratio, whites to blacks	1.18	.72	1.40	1.48	1.45

Source: Davis, Karen. 1975. Equal Treatment and Unequal Benefits: The Medicare Program. *Milbank Memorial Fund Quarterly/Health and Society* 53:468, 469. The 1977 data are from G. Wilensky, L. Rossiter, and L. Firney, "The Medicare Subsidy of Private Health Insurance," National Center for Health Services Research, National Health Care Expenditure Survey, 1983.

TABLE 20-3. Average Physician Visits for the Elderly, by Health Status and Family Income, Adjusted for Other Determinants, 1969 and 1977

	Health Status[a]		
	Good	Average	Poor
1969			
Family income:			
Under $5,000			
No aid[b]	2.78	5.64	10.47
Aid	3.86	7.52	13.42
$5,000–9,999	3.14	6.60	11.70
$10,000–14,999	3.75	7.27	12.98
$15,000 and over	5.35	9.53	16.98
1977[c]			
At or near poverty line			
No Medicaid	3.72	6.56	9.06
Medicaid	5.89	7.36	10.43
Middle-income	4.21	7.31	10.66
High-income	4.34	7.30	—[d]

Source: 1969 data are from Karen Davis, *National Health Insurance: Benefits , Costs and Consequences* (Washington, D.C.: Brookings Institution, 1975), p. 85. The 1977 data are from G. Wilensky, L. Rossiter, and L. Finney, "The Medicare Subsidy of Private Health Insurance," National Center for Health Services Research, National Health Care Expenditure Survey, 1983.

[a] Good health status is defined as absence of any chronic conditions, limitations of activity, or restricted activity days. Average and poor health are defined as at the mean and twice the mean level, respectively, of the three morbidity indicators used.

[b] Aid indicates public assistant recipients.

[c] For 1977 data, respondents were asked to characterize their own health status relative to people of the same age.

[d] Cell size too small to estimate.

The Medicare reimbursement is also on the average higher for whites than for nonwhites.

If Medicare were based upon the assumption that there should be equal treatment for equal needs, then one would expect to observe an equal number of physician visits according to level of medical need. This is unlikely to occur when all aged recipients face the same price but differ according to income, race, and accessibility, as shown in Table 20-3. Regardless of health status, aged persons with higher incomes had more physician visits than the aged with lesser incomes. Of those aged who are classified as being in poor health, in 1969 the low-income aged (less than $5,000 in income) had 10.47 physician visits per year compared with 16.98 visits per aged person with a high income (greater than $15,000 per year). When the 1977 data are examined, differences still exist according to income level, although they have lessened. Those aged on Medicaid generally show high visit rates, presumably because of their low out-of-pocket price. Visit rates for the high-income aged have declined since 1969.

The smaller difference in visit rates among aged in different income groups and the decrease in visit rates among the high income aged may be explained as follows. Between 1969 and 1977 the "real" price (adjusted for inflation) has gone down for the low-income aged, hence increasing their visit rates, while the "real" price faced by the high income aged has increased, thereby decreasing their visit rates. Physicians serving low-income aged are likely to accept Medicare assignment; that is, they are willing to accept the Medicare fee as the price for their services. Increases in Medicare fees have been limited by the Medicare Fee Index, which has increased much more slowly than the rate of inflation. Thus the "real" price of a physician visit to low-income aged has declined. The physician assignment rate, those physicians participating in Medicare, has declined over time. Physicians are also less likely to take assignment for those aged who have higher incomes. All aged are required to pay a deductible and a copayment. However, the high-income aged person going to a nonparticipating physician must also pay the full difference between what Medicare reimburses as the physician's fee and the physician's actual fee. Physicians not accepting assignment have also been able to raise their fees more rapidly than the increases permitted under the Medicare Fee Index. Thus high-income aged, using nonparticipating physicians, have experienced an increase in the "real" prices they pay for physician visits.

The 1969 data are therefore consistent with the expectation that visit rates will differ when different income groups face the *same* price. The 1977 data (and the change from 1969) are also consistent with what would be expected when different income groups pay *different* prices for physician visits.

Based on our experience with Medicare, it is obvious that a lower, but similar, price to all aged persons will achieve neither equal financial access nor equal treatment for equal needs. As could have been hypothesized, based on the earlier theoretical discussion, Medicare is an inefficient approach for achieving either of the above sets of values, because the higher-income persons use a greater number of services than lower-income persons and the services they use are more costly. If the Medicare subsidy varied according to income level (which would result in higher administrative costs), the same services could be provided to the low-income aged at a lower total cost. Not only would there be an overall smaller level of utilization under Medicare if the subsidy varied by income, but the rise in medical prices would also be less, since there would be a smaller overall increase in demand. The record of the Medicare program should be kept in mind when specific proposals for national health insurance are analyzed in the following section.

SPECIFIC CRITERIA FOR EVALUATING NATIONAL HEALTH INSURANCE PLANS

Before discussing specific proposals for national health insurance, it would be useful to have a common set of criteria by which these alternative plans may be evaluated.

THE BENEFICIARIES

Based on the previous discussion of the different sets of values held by society regarding redistribution of medical care, it may be said that the primary recipients of national health insurance should be those who are or might become medically indigent. The medically indigent are those persons who have low incomes and cannot buy as much medical care as society would prefer them to have; those persons whose medical expenses are large in relation to their incomes are potentially medically indigent. A person in the latter category may not necessarily have a low income, inasmuch as in the event of a serious illness, even persons with middle incomes might be hard pressed to pay their medical bills.

Subsidies under national health insurance, therefore, should vary according to income (they should be larger for low-income persons and decline as income increases), and subsidies should be available so that an upper limit on liability for medical expenses could be set to protect even higher-income persons from suffering an undue financial hardship. Since what constitutes a financial hardship depends upon one's income, the maximum medical liability for a person should also be related to one's income in the form of a fraction of that income. (An alternative approach to eliminating potential financial hardship would be to require everyone to have a major-medical or catastrophic insurance coverage. Because what is catastrophic for a low-income person may not be for a high-income person, a uniform definition may set the level too low for high-income persons, thereby encouraging greater use on their part once the limit is reached.)

The primary beneficiary groups included under national health insurance should be categorized according to both income and the size of the medical bill in relation to income. Categorizing population groups by age is a less direct approach for determining current medical need and potential financial hardship. Although many of the aged are low-income, not all of them require the same degree of financial subsidy; many younger persons may have greater medical and financial needs than some of the aged.

As discussed in Chapter 6 on health insurance, it would not be efficient for the government to provide subsidies to higher-income persons for a large fraction of their medical expenses. As long as there is moral hazard, the cost of subsidies to higher income families will be greater than the value of the additional care received by these persons. Subsidies for medical care under national health insurance should be decreased with increased incomes.

How large the subsidies for medical care should be for low income persons is basically a value judgment. Some persons would prefer that the poor receive all their medical care, including preventive care, without any charge; others would prefer a less generous subsidy. Any plan for national health insurance should be able to incorporate either of these conflicting values by varying the degree of subsidization in relation to income levels.

INCENTIVES FOR EFFICIENCY

A second criterion by which alternative health insurance plans should be judged is whether there are any incentives to encourage the efficient use of medical resources. The efficient use of resources may be accomplished in several ways. First, the combination of medical services that is least costly for providing a medical treatment should be used. If the benefit coverage is restricted to just hospital care, thereby excluding ambulatory and other nonhospital services, then more of the care will be provided in the hospital even though it would be less costly to substitute ambulatory, nursing home, and home care services. Second, consumers (particularly the nonpoor) should be provided with some incentives to seek out less costly providers and not to overutilize. An approach that has been suggested for providing consumers with both of these incentives is to include deductibles and copayments: deductibles, in addition to reducing the administrative cost of handling many small bills and thereby reduce the overall cost of national health insurance, would, together with copayments, provide the consumers with a monetary incentive to be aware of the provider's prices. In this way, cost savings could be achieved at the "front end," instead of having to exclude coverage for costly, but necessary, procedures and, as under Medicare, set an upper limit on the number of hospital days for which an aged person is covered.

The providers of medical services should also have incentives for efficiency under any national health insurance plan. Ideally, physicians should bear some fiscal responsibility for their use of medical resources. Suggestions for improving provider efficiency are varied and include allowing the providers to compete for patients once the patients have greater financial responsibility for their expenses, having providers and provider organizations compete on the prices established for delivering specified services, and increasing regulation and control by government for achieving a greater efficiency.

EQUITABLE FINANCING

A third criterion for evaluating alternative NHI plans is the equitability of their financing. If the basis of NHI is the desire on the part of those who are not poor to have those who have lower incomes and are less fortunate receive more medical services, then the most equitable method of financing should be that those who are not poor would bear a higher proportion of the costs of NHI.* An equitable method of financing would be one in which the contribution was greater for those with higher incomes. Greater reliance on the income tax would be more equitable than relying on a social security tax; income taxes generally rise with increased incomes, but social security taxes are a fixed percentage of income up to a specified level of income. Social security taxes are in fact regressive, because they constitute a larger fraction of income from a low-income person than from a high-income person.

Another problem with the social security tax approach to financing national health insurance is that it raises the cost of labor to industry. An increase in social security taxes represents a greater proportional increase in the cost of labor for lower-income workers than for high-income workers. The firm would therefore substitute some highly skilled labor for unskilled labor. The firm would also substitute capital for labor in its production of goods, owing to the general in-

---

*Compulsory catastrophic coverage is justified on different grounds. If someone does not have catastrophic coverage and suffers a large medical expense that has to be subsidized by the community, then that person, who may not have a low income, is shifting the risk, hence the cost, of catastrophic coverage to the rest of the community. If all persons have an equal chance of incurring a catastrophic illness of equal cost, then they should make an equal contribution.

crease in the cost of labor relative to the cost of capital. The composition of goods and services in society would also be affected by this increased tax on labor.

Although a social security tax is less equitable than an income tax and will cause an increase in unemployment among lower-skilled workers, it is favored by some as a method for financing national health insurance. The most likely explanation is that it is not obvious that this is a tax on workers or consumers. Since the social security tax is placed on the employer, many persons are unaware that the tax will be passed on to consumers in the form of higher prices for the goods and services they purchase, or that it causes an increase in the cost of employees, hence a decrease in their demand by industry.

In addition to these three criteria—the population group to be covered, incentives for efficiency, and the method of financing—two other supplementary goals are usually mentioned. First, the national health insurance plan should not be very costly to administer, so that as much of the money as possible goes to pay medical rather than administrative expenses. Second, it should be politically acceptable to the public, the providers, and the government. Political acceptability includes such issues as methods of reimbursing providers, whether there is a role for insurance companies and Blue Cross–Blue Shield, how large a tax increase would be necessitated by the program, and the impact on the federal budget. These aspects will subsequently be discussed in more detail.

ALTERNATIVE PROPOSALS
FOR NATIONAL HEALTH INSURANCE

Using the criteria that have been presented, a brief evaluation will be undertaken of the current system for financing care and of several types of proposals that either are popular or appear to have legislative support.

THE CURRENT SYSTEM
FOR FINANCING MEDICAL EXPENSES

Tax Subsidies for the Purchase of Health Insurance

In the past, the federal government financed the purchase of medical care and insurance for the nonpoor by allowing as a tax deduction one-half of health insurance premiums (up to $150), by permitting deductions on the income tax return of medical expenses in excess of 3 percent of income, and by excluding from taxable income insurance premiums paid by the employer on behalf of the employee.* It has been estimated that the cost, in terms of lost federal taxes, of these subsidies was approximately $23 billion in 1982. The beneficiaries of these subsidies are all persons who are employed and who file tax returns, but, as shown earlier, the major beneficiaries are those in higher-income groups. A deduction from income is worth more to a person in a higher-income bracket than to a person with a lower income. For example, employer-paid premiums for

---

* Starting in 1983, medical expenses, including health insurance premiums paid by the individual, must be in excess of 5 percent of income.

health insurance totaling $1,000 will cost the person in a 15 percent tax bracket $850, whereas they will cost a person in the 50 percent bracket only $500. If the true actuarial value of that premium is $800 (the remaining $200 going for administrative cost), then the person in the 50 percent bracket will demand more insurance because it costs him *less* than the actuarial value of that insurance.

The consequences of the current system for tax subsidies are that higher-income persons receive greater benefits than lower-income persons and it results in "too much" health insurance coverage for the higher-income person. It becomes worthwhile for higher-income persons to insure (through their employer) against small, routine medical expenses. This is because the cost of the insurance is less than the cost of those services if high-income persons were to pay for it themselves. The coverage that exists in the current system is generally shallow, covering many small and moderate bills, but not covering catastrophic illnesses. Coverage for hospital and surgical expense is much more complete (particularly the front-end expenses) than coverage for nonhospital expenses, thereby discouraging the use of less costly substitutes for hospital care. Efficiency in the use of resources is also not encouraged. Patients have little incentive to shop for lower-cost hospitals when they are covered by a service benefit policy. The method of hospital reimbursement has been cost-based, thereby decreasing the hospitals' incentives for efficiency.

Medicare

Medicare, a federal program to cover the medical expenses of the aged, was started in 1966. It was extended to all persons with chronic renal disease in 1974. Although the aged have obviously benefited from this program, a number of aspects could certainly be improved. All aged, regardless of their income levels, are presently included. The benefits and the prices the aged must pay, the deductibles and copayments for both hospital and physician services, are all the same for each aged person. The aged with higher incomes can afford to purchase more medical services and to buy supplementary coverage for those gaps not covered by Medicare. The catastrophic coverage under Medicare is not complete and the services covered are not comprehensive. There are limited benefits for posthospital care such as skilled nursing and home care. Before Medicare, in 1966, the average out-of-pocket expense for an aged person was $236.72; in 1980, the average out-of-pocket expense for an aged person was $768.24 (2). Because the prices the aged must pay under Medicare are not income-related, a number of the aged will find it difficult to pay the necessary out-of-pocket expenses. What occurs, in fact, is that because of the large out-of-pocket expenses and the gaps in benefit coverage, approximately 20 percent of the aged must rely on Medicaid.

Medicare is financed by a social security tax which, as discussed above, is regressive. Persons with a lower income contribute a higher fraction of their income.

Hospitals used to be reimbursed according to their costs, which did not provide any incentives for efficiency. Recently, however, the federal government has become less generous in its hospital reimbursement policies. (Medicare now reimburses hospitals according to a classification system, such as their case mix, and an inflation factor.) The method of reimbursement for physician services was the physicians' "usual, customary, and reasonable" fee, but as the costs of the Medicare program began to increase beyond the government's estimates, a fee index was developed and limits were placed on physician fee increases. The consequence of this action was to decrease physician participation.

Medicaid

Medicaid, which also began in 1966, is a federal-state matching program whose designated beneficiary group is the poor. The role of the federal government is primarily one of sharing the costs of the program with the states, who are themselves responsible for defining the eligibility requirements and determining the benefit coverage. As is the case with the Medicare program, although the beneficiaries of Medicaid have been helped, there are also a number of problems with the current program.

Because the program is administered by each state, there are wide variations in eligibility requirements and in services covered. In some states, people may lose all of their eligibility if their income rises so that it is slightly above the cut-off level; in other words, eligibility is not graduated according to income level. Although the beneficiary group is the poor, it has been estimated that approximately one-third to one-half of the population below the poverty level do not receive Medicaid benefits (3) because of differences in eligibility among states. Even within a state there are variations in access and use of services between white and nonwhite persons and between urban and rural dwellers.

Medicaid is financed through general tax revenues from the states and from federal income taxes. This is a more equitable method of financing than a social security tax. Because the increases in Medicaid costs have risen so rapidly—from $3.45 billion from federal and state governments in 1968 to $29.7 billion in 1981—states have found themselves under pressure to reduce their share of the rising Medicaid costs. The methods usually used have been to reduce eligibility, reduce benefits, and reduce the amount paid to medical providers. This latter approach has, in some places, resulted in two different systems of medical care: one for the Medicaid patient and the other for everyone else. Lower levels of reimbursement for Medicaid patients have limited the willingness of many providers to serve Medicaid patients. With the difficulties that some states have in meeting the increases in expenditures for Medicaid, the gaps in Medicaid are unlikely to be resolved without additional financing from sources other than the states.

PROPOSALS FOR FINANCING MEDICAL EXPENSES

The Committee for National Health Insurance

The most comprehensive of all the proposals for NHI is the plan developed by the Committee for National Health Insurance (CNHI); in legislative form it has been sponsored by Senator Kennedy. Under this proposal the entire population would be covered and the benefits would be uniform for all. An important characteristic of this plan is that there are no out-of-pocket expenses for basic medical services. Covered services under this plan are generally more inclusive than those currently provided in many high-option insurance packages: coverage is provided for home health care, dental care to age 25 (to be phased in), and limited vision care.

Greater comprehensiveness of benefit coverage is desirable in that it provides an incentive to the patient and the physician to prescribe less costly services. Increased benefit coverage is also advantageous in that it will increase the coverage of low-income persons. For persons with individual insurance coverage, where the premium represents a much smaller fraction of the actuarial value of the coverage, the administrative costs of insuring such persons should be lower.

There are, however, some difficulties with the broad coverage in this bill. Since the price of medical care is the same for all income groups (zero), differences will still exist in utilization of services, owing to the value of waiting time, the location of the provider, and the race of the patient. As previously discussed, to increase the use of services by the poor will require "negative" prices, although this has not been proposed. Equal financial access or equal treatment for equal needs could be more efficiently achieved with a system of differential subsidies. Another problem is encountered with regard to the high-income group: currently, many persons do not purchase coverage for drugs or dental services because of the relatively high transaction costs involved and the problem of moral hazard. Including such services among the benefits to be covered in effect requires these persons to purchase such services. They are clearly worse off, since they now have to purchase services they previously chose not to purchase when they had a choice.

Under a medical care system with no out-of-pocket expenses, patients will have an incentive to overutilize services and to demand the highest-quality care from specialists and hospitals. Hospitals, on their part, will try to oblige patients and their physicians. To prevent medical expenditures under such a system from rapidly escalating, cost control measures would have to be imposed on the providers. It is likely, therefore, that a medical system with no out-of-pocket expenses will be subject to arbitrary expenditure limits. It is unlikely that these limits will be related to changes in consumer demands or to input price increases that result from economywide price increases. If the resources provided are less than what is demanded by consumers, some form of rationing will have to occur. One such method is through increased waiting times. Allocation by time costs is inefficient, both because those who have lower time costs may not have greater medical needs and because the value of time spent in waiting is lost. An allocation process similar to waiting times would be allocating according to the patient's elasticity of demand for the particular services. Those services with more elastic demands are less likely to be provided than those services with less elastic demands. Emergency, acute, and catastrophic care are more likely to be provided than health education and preventive care for children and adults, although both the proponents and opponents of such a system would like to see more of the latter provided. The emphasis of the current system on the acutely sick patient is unlikely to be changed.

The proposed method of financing is a combination of social security taxes and income taxes; the inequitable nature of social security financing and its adverse impact on employment has been discussed previously.

The medical system proposed by the CNHI is to be administered by a single federal agency. Part of the increase in administrative costs under the new system will be offset by the decrease in administrative costs inherent in the current insurance system. The creation of a new agency to allocate resources and to control inflation throughout the entire medical system is likely to result in large administrative costs. The steady growth of bureaucratic agencies in government can rarely, if ever, be justified on grounds of achieving greater efficiency in production.

As to its political feasibility, the CNHI proposal has received a great deal of opposition from various provider interest groups. Physicians have opposed it because it would change their method of reimbursement and method of practice. Hospitals would receive predetermined allocations from a single source, which would limit their ability to grow and add services. Insurance companies and Blue Cross–Blue Shield would be eliminated. An additional aspect of the question of political feasibility is the fear on the part of the executive branch of the federal government that the federal budget would require either additional taxes or cutbacks in other programs (and fewer new programs) if medical costs continue to increase as they have in the recent past. As a result of this opposition, it is considered highly unlikely that such a comprehensive proposal would be enacted.

Mandating National Health Insurance Through Employers (4)

Requiring employers to provide health insurance benefits to their employees and families offers a number of political advantages to an administration. First, it offers the illusion that federal expenditures are unaffected. For those population groups that are not employed, additional federal expenditures would be required. However, for the vast majority of the population who are employed, and their families, additional federal revenues would not be needed. Congress would not have to pass a special tax to raise revenues for the program and other federal programs would be seemingly unaffected by a mandated NHI program. Second, a mandated program does not disturb the current system of delivery of medical services nor does it change the role of private insurance companies. A mandated program would have the effect of increasing the demand for insurance and, consequently, for medical services. Important interest groups, the health insurance companies and provider groups, should be expected to support it. Third, mandating a minimum set of insurance benefits permits unions and higher-income employees to retain their current negotiated benefits, which are generally higher than the mandated benefits.

Although an employer-mandated NHI program does not have the political drawbacks that other NHI programs (to be discussed) have, there are still problems with such an approach. To start with, federal revenues, hence expenditures, are affected by a mandated NHI program. Employer-purchased health insurance is not considered as taxable income to the employee; instead it is a business expense. Increased business expenses reduce the business's taxable revenues. Mandated employer premiums are an additional cost for each of the firm's employees. This cost is eventually borne by the worker in terms of lower wages. For those firms whose employees' insurance coverage is less than the mandated amount, it is equivalent to requiring the workers to trade some of their taxable income for nontaxable health insurance coverage. The federal government will lose revenue as taxable income is used to purchase health benefits. For those firms whose employees currently have insurance coverage in excess of the mandated amount, there should be no change in federal revenues. It is important for estimating the size of this federal revenue loss to determine the number of employees whose current insurance coverage is below the mandated amount, and by how much.

Firms with large numbers of employees generally have health insurance coverage greater than that which would be mandated. Firms with 100 or more employees constitute approximately 50 percent of all employees, while firms with fewer than 20 employees and firms with 20–99 employees account for 24 and 25 percent of employees, respectively (5). Thus the firms most likely to be affected by a mandated program would be the smaller firms. Phelps estimates that, as of 1980, an "intermediate" plan, one in which the employer contribution is $430 for an individual employee and $1,100 for an employee with a family, would result in an increase of $20 billion in new insurance premiums (6). As inflation pushes more people into higher marginal tax brackets, the loss of federal revenues from employer-paid premiums is constantly growing. However, the loss in federal revenues from a *mandated* program is decreasing. The additional loss in federal revenues as a result of an intermediate mandated NHI program was estimated to be approximately $7 billion in 1980.

There are also important indirect effects of a mandated employer program. A mandated program increases the cost of labor to the firm, thereby decreasing the firm's demand for labor. The decrease in demand for labor should be greater among unskilled workers whose wages may be close to the minimum wage. Skilled labor is less likely to be affected since they are likely to have benefits close to the mandated benefits, and the additional cost of the mandated program is likely to represent a small percentage of their wages. There should eventually be substitution toward skilled labor and capital away from unskilled labor. An increase in unemployment among unskilled labor should also occur. These effects, which are not obvious consequences of the legislation, are also costs which should be considered.

An additional difficulty with mandated employer insurance programs is that the problem of "overinsurance" still exists, i.e., employees have more comprehensive insurance than they otherwise would have because health insurance is a nontaxable fringe benefit. Increased health insurance coverage will only serve to exacerbate current concerns with utilization and rising medical prices.

Neither the benefits nor financing mechanisms of a mandated employer program are income related. The financing requirement is similar to a flat tax per worker, which more closely approximates a payroll tax, rather than an income tax, which would be more redistributive.

These concerns are addressed next.

Changes in the Tax Treatment of Employment-Based Health Insurance (7)

Currently, employer contributions to their employee's health insurance plans are not included as part of the employee's taxable income. This exclusion is equivalent to a discount on the purchase of insurance equal to the employee's

TABLE 20-4. Employer Contributions to Health Benefit Plans and Employee Tax Benefits, 1983

Annual Household Income	Households Receiving Contributions		
	Percentage Receiving Employer Contribution	Average Employer Contribution	Average Tax Benefit[a]
$ 0– 10,000	13	$ 636	$129
10,001– 15,000	31	972	269
15,001– 20,000	47	1,029	307
20,001– 30,000	59	1,375	460
30,001– 50,000	73	1,798	683
50,001–100,000	73	2,025	857
Over 100,000	62	1,761	886

Source: *Containing Medical Care Costs Through Market Forces* (Washington, D.C.: Congressional Budget Office, 1982), p. 27, Table 2, which is based on CBO estimates.

[a]Tax benefits include both federal tax reductions and the employer's and employee's share of federal payroll taxes. About three-quarters of the tax benefits are income tax reductions. State and local income tax reductions are excluded.

marginal tax rate. The consequence of this policy is a demand for more comprehensive insurance coverage.

To rectify the above situation it has been proposed that either employers' contributions toward their employees' insurance become completely taxable or that a dollar limit be established, such as $150 a month for a family, above which employer contributions become taxable. The proponents of such a change in the tax laws see a number of advantages, not least of which is that it will increase federal tax revenues. It has been estimated that by 1987 the loss in federal revenues from this tax exclusion will reach $45 billion (8). Eliminating the exclusion (or reducing it, which is politically more likely) results in taxing income that would be used to purchase more comprehensive insurance coverage.

Under the current tax system, those receiving the highest benefits from employer contributions also have the highest incomes. As shown in Table 20-4, both the percentage of households receiving employer contributions and the average employer contribution increase with higher household incomes. Thus placing a dollar limit on the size of the employer contribution that is nontaxable would be an improvement over the current system. A hoped for consequence of such a change in the tax law is that employees would purchase less health insurance, namely, policies with more deductibles and copayment features. Increased cost sharing should increase patient sensitivity to medical prices and result in a lessened demand for medical care. As a result, medical prices should not rise as rapidly.

There are political as well as technical difficulties in placing a limit on the employer's contribution. Unions that have bargained for and received health benefits that are greater than the dollar limit would be expected to oppose such a proposal. A dollar limit below their current negotiated benefit level would increase taxes on their member's wages and make them worse off. Another important interest group, the health insurance companies, would also be expected to oppose such a proposal. Placing a dollar limit on the employer's contribution that is tax free would decrease the demand for health insurance. There are also certain technical difficulties with such an approach; however, these are not insurmountable.

Since health care costs vary across the country, a dollar limit will enable employees in one part of the country to buy more health insurance than those located in areas with high medical prices. For example, the average tax benefit of those households receiving contributions is estimated to be $633 in the West and North Central regions and only $462 in the South (9). Although this problem can be resolved by indexing the dollar exclusion to an area's medical prices, it increases the administrative cost of the proposal. Further, employees belonging to large groups would still have a cost advantage in the purchase of insurance over the self-employed and those in small groups.

Placing a limit on the tax exclusion would decrease the demand for insurance by those with high incomes. Thus these proposals have a different objective than other NHI proposals; their purpose is to reduce the extent of overinsurance. Such a proposal would not, by itself, reform the current system of financing nor would it increase the demand for medical services by those receiving less than the taxable dollar limit. These tax limit proposals must be combined with proposals that increase the availability of insurance if lower-income populations are to have increased coverage. It is these latter proposals which are now examined.

Income-Related NHI Proposals

Tax Credit Proposals.   Legislative proposals favoring the use of a tax credit have been frequently introduced into Congress. Although such proposals differ in a number of respects, there appears to be some support in Congress for a tax credit approach.

A tax credit proposal would work in the following way. A taxpayer would be allowed to subtract from the amount of the tax he or she would otherwise be required to pay, a given dollar amount which would be used to purchase health insurance. Alternatively, the taxpayer could subtract from his or her taxes a specified fraction of his or her medical expenses. Individuals whose tax credit exceeded their tax liabilities would receive a refund for the difference. Currently, a taxpayer can only deduct those medical expenses from adjusted gross income. A total credit approach would channel greater benefits to lower-income taxpayers than the current medical expense deduction.

Tax credit proposals are varied. Some proposals are voluntary, others are compulsory. If a program is voluntary, then there is the problem of people not participating and possibly having to go on welfare if they are unable to meet a catastrophic expense. Some tax credit proposals would continue Medicare and Medicaid, others would incorporate them into a single tax credit system for everyone. If Medicare and Medicaid are to be retained, separate from the tax credit system, then these gaps and problems would have to be remedied. Some people have suggested that tax credits be used for the purchase of insurance; others have suggested that the credit be applied directly against medical expenses. Proposals which favor a credit against the purchase of a health insurance policy would reimburse a person a percentage of the premium based upon the person's income level. If the credit is against medical expenses, then the person could deduct a certain percentage of those expenses from his or her tax liability.

With regard to increasing the efficiency with which medical resources are used, the cost-sharing provisions of tax credit proposals provide an incentive for consumers to be concerned with the prices they pay, the amount of care they purchase, and the providers from whom they purchase services. Since tax credit proposals are generally comprehensive in benefit coverage (either with regard to the insurance package or in reimbursement of medical expenses), an incentive is provided to use less costly services when medically possible. A problem with all tax credit proposals is that they do not include a proposal for improving efficiency in the provision of care. It should be possible, however, to incorporate a number of supply proposals, such as those which stimulate the growth of prepaid delivery systems, into the tax credit proposal.

Tax credit proposals vary in terms of the benefits they provide to lower-income groups, how comprehensive their coverage is, how equitably they are financed, and the incentives they provide to consumers in their use of medical services. How close any tax credit proposal comes to meeting all the criteria discussed depends on the specific proposal that is offered.

Patient Cost Sharing and Catastrophic Proposals.   The idea behind patient cost sharing and catastrophic NHI proposals is to reduce the extent of overinsurance while assuring adequate coverage for those with lower incomes. Reducing over-insurance by introducing patient cost sharing should lower use of medical services and, consequently, reduce the rate of increase in medical prices. However, an important characteristic of such proposals is that the benefits should be income related.

The most recent evidence of the impact patient cost sharing has on medical service use are the preliminary results from the Rand Corporation Health Insurance Study (10). In this experiment, different insurance policies with varying levels of copayments were provided to families who were randomly selected. Copayments clearly had a large effect on use of services and expenditures. Families with cost sharing requirements of 25 percent (up to a maximum dollar limit per year) spent 19 percent less than families with complete coverage; their hospital admission rates were 21 percent lower and their expenditures on physician office visits were 20 percent less.

Proposals that emphasize catastrophic health insurance have been introduced in both the present and previous sessions of Congress. Different definitions are used, however, for defining catastrophic health expenditures. In some legislation, income-related definitions, such as expenditures exceeding 10 percent of a family's income, are used. In other proposals, absolute dollar amounts, such as $2,000 are used. Any definition based on an absolute dollar amount would not be as progressive in its distribution of benefits as would an income-related definition. What might be considered catastrophic to low-income families may be an average expenditure to high-income groups (11).

The advantage of federal catastrophic coverage is that federal dollars would be spent for a relatively small, although important, portion of total expenditures. Proponents of federal catastrophic coverage maintain that such insurance protection would be more equitable than the current medical expense deduction, which permits taxpayers who itemize to deduct from their income out-of-pocket medical expenses in excess of 5 percent of their adjusted gross income. Generally, low- and moderate-income persons do not itemize. Second, deductions are worth more to persons in higher tax brackets. Thus it is not surprising that the benefits of this tax provision go predominately to those with higher incomes. Another difficulty with the deduction is that the tax refunds would not be available until after the tax returns are filed.

Catastrophic insurance proposals are often combined with separate proposals for aiding low-income persons. An example of such a proposal is having the federal government become responsible for Medicaid, thereby providing for uniform eligibility and benefits to low-income persons. This would be an improvement over the current Medicaid program, which varies by state and excludes a large part of the population classified as poor. However, eligibility for public programs often has sharp cut-off points. Once a person's income exceeds the eligibility requirements, his or her medical benefits are completely eliminated. Thus, within a certain income limit, there may be a disincentive to earn more money because the loss in benefits would be greater than the increase in income. To rectify this situation, assistance for low-income persons should be gradually reduced as their income rises.

Persons who do not qualify for the low-income coverage, which includes the majority of the population, would have to rely on the current system. Since the demand for insurance is related to income and place of employment, low- and middle-income persons would continue to have less coverage and would be more likely to suffer financial hardship as a result of moderate medical expenses that do not qualify them for the catastrophic coverage. High-income persons would continue to have more insurance coverage, including coverage for those medical expenses that are considered small and routine. Thus, this proposal might also be combined with one which places a limit on the amount of employer paid contributions that are tax deductible.

One example of a catastrophic-type NHI proposal that has found favor with a number of economists is the following. Each family would be responsible for its own medical bills up to a certain percentage, e.g., 15 percent, of its income. Based upon the adjusted gross income on a family's tax return, the government would reimburse for medical expenses in excess of that percent. There are many variations on this basic approach. The maximum liability as a percent of income could be increased with higher family incomes. In place of what is basically a large deductible for anything below the maximum percentage, there would be a copayment feature up to the maximum percentage. For low-income families, there could be a small deductible and copayment that would not exceed a relatively small percentage of their income. The deductibles, copayments, and maximum liability could all increase with income (12). These different possible combinations are shown in Table 20-5.

Depending upon the extent to which society wishes to subsidize medical care, the deductible levels, copayments, and maximum limits can be set higher or lower than those shown in Table 20-5, which is merely illustrative. It is not necessary to require low-income groups to pay any deductibles or copayments. If a family incurred an expense in excess of its maximum limit, then government-guaranteed loans could be used to pay that expense until the family filed its tax return and was reimbursed by the government. An example of how this plan would work, using Table 20-5 as a source for discussion, is as follows. If a person with an income of $30,000 incurred medical expenses totaling $3,000 during a

TABLE 20-5. An Income-Related National Health Insurance Plan with Varying Deductibles, Copayments, and Maximum Liabilities

Adjusted Gross Income	Deductible	Copayment	Maximum Liability as a Percent of Income
Income level 1 (low)	$ 50	10%	5%
Income level 2	75	10	7
Income level 3	100	15	9
.	.	.	.
.	.	.	.
.	.	.	.
Income level N (high)	400	25	15

year, then the family would be liable for the first $400 and 25 percent of the remainder up to a limit of 15 percent of its income, which in this case would be $4,500. Thus, the family would pay $400 as a deductible and then 25 percent of the remaining $2,600, which is $650, for a total of $1,050. On its income tax return, the family would file for a refund of the difference between $3,000 and $1,050. The family in question may have a cash-flow problem until it is reimbursed from the government, making a government loan program necessary (13).

With this type of insurance program, there may be a demand for supplementary insurance to cover all or part of what the consumer would have to pay. Consumers should be able to purchase such supplementary insurance. Because there currently are tax subsidies for the purchase of health insurance and for payment of medical expenses (in excess of 5 percent of one's income), it would be a necessary part of this and other income-related insurance plans to take away such subsidies to prevent a situation wherein "too much" health insurance would be purchased.* (With the tax subsidies, the after-tax cost of the insurance to the higher-income consumer could be less than the actuarial value of the insurance. In this case, the consumer would demand too much insurance, because the actuarial value would be greater than the amount he or she had to pay for it.)

The advantages of an income-related insurance plan as just described would be as follows:

1. Those who would receive the largest subsidies would be those with the lowest incomes and those whose medical bills would represent a financial hardship. A means test would be necessary, but it would be no harder to administer and no more degrading than the current method of filing for deductions on one's income tax form.

---

*It has been argued that under NHI plans containing a deductible, the demand for supplementary insurance would be negligible if the favorable tax treatment of supplementary insurance were removed. It is unlikely that there would be any demand for supplementary insurance if the NHI plan covered only unreimbursed expenditures. See Emmett B. Keeler, Daniel T. Morrow, and Joseph P. Newhouse, "The Demand for Supplementary Health Insurance, or Do Deductibles Matter?" *Journal of Political Economy* 85 (4) (August 1977).

2. Because all medical services would be included under the expense limits, there should not be greater use of more costly services, as would be the case if certain services were covered while others were not. Instead, the services would be likely to be used with consideration given to both their price and effectiveness in treatment.

3. Since families with higher incomes would have to pay part of the cost of medical services, NHI would provide these families with an incentive to be concerned with the prices they paid.

4. By providing government protection against large medical expenses instead of insuring for small claims, not only would the administrative cost be reduced, but the NHI plan would also be providing coverage for those expenses that are generally more insurable. Consumers are more willing to pay an amount above the pure premium for large and unexpected expenses than they are for those that are small and routine.

To increase the use of medical care by low-income persons beyond what they would demand at a zero price, this type of income-related insurance plan would have to be supplemented with supply subsidies to low-income and rural areas in the form of neighborhood health centers and special incentives for health personnel to locate in certain areas.

There are several ways in which this system could be implemented. One is to use the current system of filing income tax returns. Another is to have the Internal Revenue Service issue each family a health care credit card that would have the appropriate cost-sharing and maximum liabilities information precoded. Using the patient's credit card, the provider would bill fees and charges to the IRS or to a fiscal intermediary. The IRS, in turn, would then bill the patient for the portion of the bill for which he or she would be responsible.

There are, however, several drawbacks to such an income-related insurance plan. There would be only a minimal role for health insurance carriers. This would lessen its chances for political acceptance. There is also no role for the government beyond the reimbursement of medical expenses by the Internal Revenue Service. It is politically unlikely that Congress and the government bureaucracy would go along with such a passive role for the government. A further problem is that once the maximum liability limit has been reached, the consumer and the provider have no incentives to limit the amount of care to just what is medically required. Similarly, if low-income persons were to have all, or a large part, of their medical expenses reimbursed, then there would need to be some means for outside limits to be placed on their total medical expenses. Otherwise, providers would be able to prescribe unlimited and unnecessary services at high prices just because they will be reimbursed by the government.

Lending support to the idea that cost constraints are still needed once a patient has reached a catastrophic level of medical expenses is the findings from a study by Zook et al.

> In any given year, about half of the resources in a typical hospital are consumed by only 13 percent of the patients. The most expensive one-fifth of patients accounts for nearly 70 percent of total resources. Since one person in ten is hospitalized each year, this implies that 1.3 percent of the nation's population may account for half of all charges in short-stay hospitals. This skewness is not

primarily a function of patient age. Though the aged account for nearly 40 percent of high-cost patients, there is a similar pattern of concentration within each age cohort. (In fact, some of the most expensive patients begin their "careers" at birth with non-lethal congenital abnormalities). (14)

The authors further state, "A reassessment of high-cost illness also makes it clear that catastrophic plans seldom give appropriate-incentives to hospitals and insurers to control costs. . . . By tempting hospitals to get the patient's bill up to $3,500 whenever possible (to reach a range in which there is full federal payment) it may exert a further inflationary impact on medical costs" (15).

Income Related Vouchers.   As a way of resolving some of these concerns while still retaining the basic features of an income-related insurance plan, a voucher system might be used. Under one such approach, Congress might specify a standard package of medical services that would become compulsory for everyone to purchase. Alternatively, there could be several standard packages, with the intermediate packages including deductibles and copayments, while the minimum package would be a catastrophic policy. The most generous standard package could be based on the medical needs of a low-income family. Everyone would receive a voucher, including the high-income family that may decide to purchase just the minimum standard catastrophic coverage. The percentage of the premium that would be paid for by the government would again be inversely related to income and paid for by a tax credit on the income tax return. The vouchers would be good only at a health plan approved by the government; the plans, which might take the form of health maintenance organizations (HMOs), prepaid health plans, or health care alliances, would have to offer each of the standard benefit packages. Everyone would have to register once a year with his or her voucher at one approved plan. Persons who had minimum standard benefit packages could purchase additional care from any provider; however, if they ever required care for what could be a catastrophic expense, then that would be provided by the approved health plan at which they had previously registered.

Approved health plans would compete for consumers and for their vouchers. If a voucher for a low-income family included a very generous set of benefits, then in order to attract consumers possessing such a voucher, a plan might choose to provide additional services. To prevent unscrupulous providers from taking advantage of a group of consumers, the government's responsibility for a plan's approval status might be exercised by placing limits on the number of consumers from any income or age group to be served by a given plan.*

Voucher proposals are also combined with other proposals, such as change in the tax treatment of employer paid health benefits. For example, a dollar limit may be placed on the employer contribution that is considered tax free to the employee. Employees choosing an insurance or health plan whose premium is

---

*Pauly also discusses use of a voucher system, but the voucher would have a flexible price. The advantage would be in avoiding having too many people who must make out-of-pocket payments, which would be the result if a voucher with a single price were set in the low range of potential costs. The disadvantage of a flexible-price voucher is that it would tend to discourage the seeking out of low-price plans. Mark V. Pauly, *Analysis of National Health Insurance Policies* (Washington, D.C.: American Enterprise Institute).

less than the amount of the tax exclusion would be entitled to receive a tax free rebate of the difference.

To stimulate reform of the delivery system, it has also been suggested that employers be required to offer their employees a choice between competing health plans, such as an HMO. Further, so as not to bias the employees' choice, the employer should contribute equally to whichever plan the employee chooses.

In some respects, a voucher system is more complicated than an income related proposal that simply works through the patient's tax return. Under a voucher system, the government would have to annually determine the value of its standard premiums for each actuarial category. Offsetting such higher administrative costs, however, are the incentives in a voucher plan that would exist for both consumers and providers. Because the voucher system is a form of prepayment, the consumer only has to choose which plan to join. They should find it easier to evaluate competing health plans than a set of individual providers. Under a voucher system, which would reimburse the health plan a predetermined amount, the provider would have no incentive to prescribe unnecessarily or to increase the cost of catastrophic medical care. A voucher system that is based on approved prepaid health plans would also encourage changes in the delivery of medical care (16).

Voucher proposals that offer a high- and low-option set of benefits have the potential problem of adverse selection. Those persons expecting to use medical services during the coming year would sign up for a high-option plan. As more people do this, the premium for the high-option plan increases more rapidly than it would otherwise. As the premium differences for the high- and low-option plans become larger, people from the high-option plan switch to the low-option plan. Eventually, the only people joining the high-option plan are those expecting to be high users in the coming year. The premiums reflect these different user groups and such a dual system no longer becomes viable. There are mechanisms, however, by which adverse selection can be lessened. Persons joining high-option plans can be charged an additional premium to reflect their higher potential risk. This additional premium would then be decreased the longer they belong to such plans (17).

Another potential problem with a voucher system that permits people to switch plans each year is that it results in high administrative costs, which are then reflected in the premiums. Currently, employees belonging to a group plan incur much smaller administrative costs.

These two problems, adverse selection and high administrative costs, are a concern in the design of NHI proposals that are based on individual vouchers.

The goals underlying NHI have changed over time. Earlier discussions of NHI assumed that there must be an increase in benefit coverage and in eligible population groups. NHI proposals are now viewed differently. Given its concern over the size of its budget, the federal government is more concerned with limiting its budgetary commitments under Medicare and Medicaid. Each president since Nixon has tried to shift the costs of proposed NHI programs off the federal budget onto employers and employees. Proponents of comprehensive NHI now seek support for their program as being a means for *controlling* health expenditures. Setting expenditure limits for each provider group is a means of limiting the annual increase in medical expenditures. Other proponents of NHI

favor it as a means by which the medical care system can be structurally re-
formed, such as by reducing the extent of overinsurance among employed
groups, increasing patient cost sharing, and/or creating competition among
qualified health plans.

The eventual outcome on NHI, if ever, will be a political compromise. Each
of the interest groups involved will seek to protect its members' interests. The
federal and state governments will seek to limit their budgetary commitments,
insurance companies and the Blues will attempt to retain as large a role as
possible, health care providers will attempt to protect their methods of reimbursement and their market shares, and business and labor will attempt to prevent the costs of any program from being shifted to them. Given the need for
political compromise if any NHI bill is to pass, it is difficult to predict whether
the goals of such legislation will be clearly specified or that economic efficiency
will be achieved.

This is not to imply that economic analysis is of no use in the political
process. Economic analysis can be a powerful tool in that it can sharpen the
debate and thereby influence the final outcome. Economics will have served this
purpose with regard to NHI if it can clarify the issues by separating those that
involve differences in the values underlying various goals of NHI from issues of
efficiency with regard to achieving a given set of NHI goals.

REFERENCES

1. The following is a selected list of such references: Karen Davis, *National Health
   Insurance: Benefits, Costs, and Consequences* (Washington, D.C.: The Brookings In-
   stitution, 1975). Robert D. Eilers and Sue S. Moyerman, eds., *National Health Insurance: Conference Proceedings* (Homewood, Ill.: Richard D. Irwin, Inc., 1971). Bridger
   M. Mitchell and William B. Schwartz, *The Financing of National Health Insurance*,
   Rand Publication R-1711 (Department of Health, Education and Welfare, 1976). Mark
   V. Pauly, ed., *National Health Insurance: What Now, What Later, What Never* (Washington, D.C.: American Enterprise Institute for Public Policy Research, 1980). *Catastrophic Health Insurance* (Washington, D.C.: Congressional Budget Office, Congress
   of the United States, 1977). *Tax Subsidies for Medical Care: Current Policies and
   Possible Alternatives* (Washington, D.C.: Congressional Budget Office, Congress of
   the United States, 1980). *Containing Medical Care Costs Through Market Forces*
   (Washington, D.C.: Congressional Budget Office, Congress of the United States, May
   1982).

2. *Containing Medical Care Costs Through Market Forces* (Washington, D.C.: Congressional Budget Office, Congress of the United States, 1982), p. 26.

3. Karen Davis, "Achievements and Problems of Medicaid," *Public Health Reports* 91(4)
   (1976): 316.

4. For a more complete discussion of this subject, upon which this section is based, see
   Charles E. Phelps, "National Health Insurance by Regulation: Mandated Employee
   Benefits," in Mark Pauly, ed., *National Health Insurance* (Washington, D.C.: Ameri-
   can Enterprise Institute for Public Policy Research, 1980).

5. *Ibid.*, p. 54.

6. Phelps provides tables that show the estimated increases in 1980 employer payments for different premium levels and employer share required; *ibid.*, pp. 69–70.

7. For a more complete discussion of this and related proposals, see *Tax Subsidies For Medical Care: Current Policies and Possible Alternatives* (Washington, D.C.: Congressional Budget Office, 1980). Also see *Containing Medical Care Costs Through Market Forces* (Washington, D.C.: Congressional Budget Office, 1982).

8. *Containing Medical Care Costs Through Market Forces, op. cit.*, p. 26.

9. *Ibid.*, p. 27.

10. Joseph P. Newhouse et al., "Some Interim Results From a Controlled Trial of Cost Sharing in Health Insurance," *New England Journal of Medicine*, December 17, 1981.

11. For a more complete discussion of catastrophic insurance, alternative proposals, and their estimated costs, see *Catastrophic Health Insurance* (Washington, D.C.: Congressional Budget Office, Congress of the United States, 1977).

12. Examples of income-related national health insurance plans similar to that described here have been proposed by the following: Jacob Meerman and Millard Long, "Aid for the Medically Indigent," *Vanderbilt Law Review*, December 1962, pp. 173–191; Mark V. Pauly, *Medical Care at Public Expense* (New York: Praeger Publishers, 1971); Charles Baird, "A Proposal for Financing the Purchase of Health Services," *Journal of Human Resources*, Winter 1970, pp. 89–105; Martin S. Feldstein, "A New Approach to National Health Insurance," *Public Interest*, Spring 1971, pp. 93–105; Alain C. Enthoven, *Health Plan* (Reading, Mass.: Addison-Wesley, 1980).

13. For a discussion of loans for medical services see Robert Eilers, "Postpayment Medical Expense Coverage: A Proposed Salvation for Insured and Insurer," *Medical Care*, May–June 1969.

14. Christopher Zook, Francis Moore, and Richard Zeckhauser, " 'Catastrophic' Health Insurance—A Misguided Prescription?," *The Public Interest* (Winter 1981): 68.

15. *Ibid.*, pp. 74–75.

16. Various people have proposed vouchers and competing health plans. One such proposal, which combines a voucher system and competition between qualified health plans, is Consumer Choice Health Plan. Alain Enthoven, *Health Plan* (Reading, Mass.: Addison-Wesley, 1980).

17. For a more complete discussion of adverse selection, see Paul B. Ginsburg, "Altering the Tax Treatment of Employment-Based Health Plans," *Milbank Memorial Fund Quarterly* (Spring 1981): 236–242.

CHAPTER 21

Concluding Comments on the Economics of Medical Care

The purpose of this book has been to demonstrate how the tools of economics can be applied to the study of medical care issues. Economic concepts define and clarify the different aspects of medical care, making them more susceptible to analysis. Differences in values among persons on particular issues can be separated from differences in the efficiency with which various approaches can achieve a specified set of values. In addition, economics offers criteria for determining whether particular policies increase or decrease *efficiency* and *equity* in medical care. Of course, economic analysis cannot resolve all of the concerns that health professionals and the public have with regard to medical care—different problems require different training and analytical expertise. Particularly suited to economic analysis are those problems that relate to issues of scarcity. Economics can illustrate the choices a society can make when its resources are insufficient to achieve everything it desires.

One decision that any society must make is how much of its limited resources to spend on medical care. It should be recognized that the choice in question is *not* how much to spend on health, but how much to spend on medical services. People do not desire increased health at any cost, as evidenced by their refusal to stop smoking, wear seat belts, and change their personal health habits. Medical services expenditures serve, to some extent, as a substitute for undertaking other activities to enhance health; part of the costs of neglecting these activities are borne by the population at large through taxes and higher medical care prices. Another decision any society must make is how much to spend on health, and although that is probably the more relevant choice, the emphasis of our current medical care system and the mechanisms for government financing of medical care is to provide more medical services. Increasing medical services is only one approach, and perhaps one of the most costly, to improving health.

554

Before it can be determined how much should be spent on medical care, it must be decided whether consumers or government will make the necessary decisions. It should again be recognized that this basic decision, which will determine the size and growth of the medical sector, depends upon resolving the issue of whose values are to dominate medical care. Are consumers to determine how much of their income is to be allocated to medical care, or is that decision to be made by a government agency? The answer will determine whether the consumer's or agency's preferences will dominate.

A market approach for allocating resources to different goods and services maximizes the consumer's preferences. Opponents of consumer decisionmaking in medical care argue that medical care is a special case in which a market approach may not be applicable, first of all because consumers may not be aware of their medical needs; second, because they may not spend as much as some persons believe they should on their medical needs; and third, because they do not have sufficient information to select among providers. Under such circumstances, opponents of a market approach propose substituting another mechanism for making the necessary allocation choices in medical care, but they do not explicitly state the criteria by which such a system of decisionmaking should be judged. The proponents of relying on consumer preferences recognize the limitations of the current medical system and how it affects consumer ability to make choices.

It seems clear that the amount, type, and quality of medical services being provided do not represent either consumer or third-party preferences. Consumers' demands for medical care are distorted both by their excess health coverage resulting from tax subsidies for the purchase of health insurance and by a lack of information on which to base their choices. The most knowledgeable purchaser in the medical market—the patient's physician—lacks the fiscal responsibility to be concerned with medical costs and also has a financial interest in the service he or she provides. These distortions in the medical care market result in the provision of either too many or too few of certain types of services. Instead of removing consumer decisionmaking, proponents of a market approach seek to improve the consumers' ability to make choices and satisfy their preferences. Before we can specify how much society should spend on medical care, we must identify who is to make that decision. Current proposals for financing medical care seek to reinstate consumer and provider incentives in the purchase of medical care.

The second basic decision to be made in any medical system is how medical services should be produced to ensure that output is provided at lowest cost. Rapidly increasing medical costs, duplication of expensive facilities and services, provision of unnecessary services, excessive testing, and unnecessary use of expensive settings all suggest that the efficiency with which medical care is provided could be improved. Again, society faces the choice of relying on greater regulation and controls implemented by government agencies, or relying on competitive market pressure to achieve greater efficiency. Not only do many persons in medical care have a basic distrust of a market system, but also they are concerned for the adequate protection of the consumer, should providers compete for profit. This concern for consumer protection has resulted in the development at a state level of a great many restrictions, which health professions and health institutions have actively participated in developing. However, restrictions on who can perform certain tasks, who may enter the health professions, and who may be reimbursed for providing medical services have not eliminated the public's concern that unnecessary services are being performed and that unethical health providers are present in the system. What they have accomplished is, in many instances, to effectively preclude workable competition in the provision of medical services. The concern with efficiency in supply and with containment of the rapidly escalating expenditures on medical services is at the forefront of public policy issues in medical care. New programs cannot be instituted and current medical benefits and beneficiaries may have to be reduced unless methods can be found to contain medical costs. It has been difficult to develop effective approaches to medical cost containment because those professions and organizations most likely to be adversely affected by any changes are also the most politically active.

The third basic decision that must be made in medical care involves questions of equity. How much medical care should be redistributed to different population groups and by what mechanisms? Issues of equity cannot be separated from issues of efficiency. The choice of how much medical care to provide to particular population groups will be affected by the costs of such programs. Proposals for national health insurance and for changes in the Medicare and Medicaid amendments are strongly influenced by expectations of the rapidity of medical cost increases and the enactment of cost-containment policies. Such proposals for financing medical care are currently being justified as much in terms of their ability to contain costs as for their success in redistributing medical services.

Currently, federal, state, and local governments are heavily involved in the financing of medical services. Demand financing programs include Medicare and Medicaid, as well as tax subsidies for the purchase of health insurance and the deductibility of medical expenses. Subsidy programs also increase demand by having the government become a direct provider of those services, such as through the Veterans Administration and U.S. Public Health Service hospitals and by federal, state, and local hospitals. Governments have also provided large subsidies to the providers of medical services by funding health professional education and making capital grants available to health institutions.

How well each of these subsidy programs redistributes medical services to those least able to afford them is questionable. Tax subsidy programs generally benefit those with higher incomes. Medicare beneficiaries with higher incomes use more medical services than those with lower incomes. Given a choice, many of those who receive care in government hospitals would prefer to receive their care in community hospitals. The large majority of the subsidies to education in the health professions are received by those who come from families with higher incomes and who subsequently enter those professions whose incomes are among the highest in the country. Recognizing that these huge subsidy programs provide redistributive benefits to different population groups is a first step in deciding whether the resulting redistributive effects are desirable. Second, it should be determined whether such subsidies could be provided more efficiently so that they are received by those most in need of care.

Requirements for additional funds and resources under any national health insurance program could be lessened if current government subsidies were more directly targeted to desired beneficiary groups. The political feasibility of achieving such a comprehensive strategy for redistribution is questionable. Each subsidy program has created a distinct constituency. Attempts to change the current distribution of subsidies will encounter strong political opposition from all those with an interest in continuing the current method. The potential beneficiaries of a more direct subsidy system are not organized enough to engage in the political process, as is indicated by the very fact of their need for such subsidies. Economic analysis of current, as well as of proposed, subsidy programs can indicate who is likely to receive such subsidies and whether such subsidies' stated objectives can be achieved more efficiently in another manner. Although such information may not determine the outcome of legislation, it is an input into the political process and raises the political costs to those who might otherwise benefit from less efficient subsidy schemes.

Of course the medical care industry is different from other industries. Economics can be of use to the study of medical care in several respects: it can help to clarify a number of policy issues, such as those involving redistribution and efficiency in the provision of medical services; it can be used to clarify legislation, both proposed and enacted, that affects the demand and supply sides of the medical markets; and it can be put to the more traditional tasks required in any industry, such as planning and forecasting. In addition to its tools—the prediction of changes in prices, quantities, and total expenditures, and the formulation of rules for cost minimization—economics provides a set of criteria for evaluating whether or not various policies achieve greater efficiency and equity in medical care. The application of these tools and criteria should result in an increased understanding of medical care issues, enable a person to separate differences in values from differences in approaches to achieving a given set of values, and indicate all of the costs and benefits of different choices in medical care.

Index